ACUTE EXACERBATIONS OF CHRONIC OBSTRUCTIVE PULMONARY DISEASE

LUNG BIOLOGY IN HEALTH AND DISEASE

Executive Editor

Claude Lenfant
Director, National Heart, Lung, and Blood Institute
National Institutes of Health
Bethesda, Maryland

ADDITIONAL VOLUMES IN PREPARATION

The opinions expressed in these volumes do not necessarily represent the views of the National Institutes of Health.

ACUTE EXACERBATIONS OF CHRONIC OBSTRUCTIVE PULMONARY DISEASE

Edited by

Nikos M. Siafakas
University Hospital of Heraklion
Heraklion, Crete, Greece

Nicholas R. Anthonisen
University of Manitoba
Winnipeg, Manitoba, Canada

Dimitris Georgopoulos
University Hospital of Heraklion
Heraklion, Crete, Greece

MARCEL DEKKER, INC.   NEW YORK · BASEL

Library of Congress Cataloging-in-Publication Data
A catalog record for this book is available from the Library of Congress.

ISBN: 0-8247-4128-5

This book is printed on acid-free paper.

Headquarters
Marcel Dekker, Inc.
270 Madison Avenue, New York, NY 10016
tel: 212-696-9000; fax: 212-685-4540

Eastern Hemisphere Distribution
Marcel Dekker AG
Hutgasse 4, Postfach 812, CH-4001 Basel, Switzerland
tel: 41-61-260-6300; fax: 41-61-260-6333

World Wide Web
http://www.dekker.com

The publisher offers discounts on this book when ordered in bulk quantities. For more information, write to Special Sales/Professional Marketing at the headquarters address above.

PRINTED IN THE UNITED STATES OF AMERICA

INTRODUCTION

Webster's dictionary defines the word chronic as follows: "Continuing for a long time; of a disease, of long duration: opposed to acute." Does this definition apply to chronic obstructive pulmonary disease (COPD)? It cartainly does, at least in the sense that if one has COPD, one has it forever! At best, we can hope to ease the symptoms and consequences of this disease, but as yet we cannot cure it. Ironically, though, COPD is very much characterized by acute episodes, which aggravate the symptoms in many cases. The progression and the severity of the disease are largely determined by the frequency of the exacerbations. Furthermore, these events may accelerate the course of COPD and increase its mortality, which is one of the highest in the United States—in fact, the fourth most common cause of death.

In light of these phenomena, it is abundantly clear that the acute exacerbations of COPD are, indeed, one of its most important aspects and a major concern for the physician caring for the COPD patient. Their effects reverberate within the health care system and throughout society at large, as well.

Thus, it should not be surprising to see this volume, titled *Acute Exacerbations of Chronic Obstructive Pulmonary Disease*, added to the series of monographs Lung Biology in Health and Disease. Since its inception this series has had two specific goals. One is to present new ideas and concepts to the readership in hope of stimulating research—most likely, fundamental research—at the cutting edge. The other goal is to provide physicians and other health care professionals with state-of-the-art clinical and therapeutic descriptions and discussions that will assist them in their search for better ways to care for their patients. These pursuits have resulted in some volumes on basic research and others on clinical issues; in some instances, both goals have been addressed. Many volumes on COPD have appeared, but this one is a prototype for what I have always hoped the series of monographs would achieve. It is truly a tribute to the editors.

Drs. Nikos M. Siafakas, Nicholas R. Anthonisen, and Dimitris Georgopoulos, as well as the remarkable cast of authors, are experts of great reputation in their field. Furthermore, they are truly international, just like COPD. The participation of contributors from so many countries adds a richness and scope that seems especially fitting for this volume about a disease that has no borders. Undoubtedly, the readership will benefit from the breadth of knowledge presented here and, hopefully, the patients will gain even more.

I am grateful to all contributors for the opportunity to introduce this valuable volume.

Claude Lenfant, M.D.
Bethesda, Maryland, U.S.A

PREFACE

Chronic obstructive pulmonary disease is a major health problem. It is the fourth leading cause of morbidity and mortality worldwide, and further increases in the prevalence and mortality of the disease can be predicted in the coming years. COPD is characterized by chronic inflammation throughout the airways, parenchyma, and pulmonary vasculature. These disturbances lead to airflow limitation that is not fully reversible and to a variety of symptoms such as productive cough and dyspnea. COPD is often associated with acute exacerbations of symptoms, an important hallmark of the disease. The economic and social burden of acute exacerbations of COPD is extremely high because management often requires hospital and, occasionally, intensive care unit admissions. This is particularly true in advanced stages of the disease as both the frequency and impact of acute exacerbations increase. The diagnosis and management of acute exacerbation of the disease are not always simple; they require a fair amount of medical knowledge and sophisticated approaches. Acute exacerbations of COPD have become a focal point for both researchers and clinicians, and a substantial amount of new information about exacerbations has been accumulated.

This book deals with all aspects of acute exacerbations of COPD, beginning with a chapter that defines it and ending with one that details future research. Each chapter focuses on the state of the art regarding a particular subject, summarizing and expanding the corpus of knowledge. Many internationally renowned experts have participated in this project and we are profoundly grateful to them for their efforts.

The book is divided into nine parts. Part One deals with the definition, epidemiology and economic burden of acute exacerbations of COPD. The effect of acute exacerbation on the natural history of the disease is also reviewed. Part Two includes topics related to pathophysiology, pathology, and biomarkers of acute exacerbations. Recent data indicate that acute exacerbations may reflect systemic disease and this issue is discussed as well. Parts Three and Four review the causes, which are not always obvious, the clinical spectrum, blood gas derangements, imaging, laboratory findings, and assessment of the severity of the acute exacerbations. The heart–lung interaction encountered during acute exacerbations and its influence on sleep, important but largely ignored issues, are also discussed, in addition to the decision-making process in patients with end-stage disease who present with acute exacerbations. Parts Five through Seven deal with the management of acute exacerbations either at home or in the hospital, including the management of patients in the intensive care unit. Reviews of new and old modes of therapy are also included. Special reference is made to the use of noninvasive mechanical ventilatory support as a means of avoiding intubation and its complications. Finally, Part Eight discusses the use of acute exacerbation as an outcome variable to test different therapeutic interventions, an issue that has important clinical and economic implications. The final chapter deals with future research, a hot topic in this era of limited resources for funding research.

This book will help readers understand many aspects of acute exacerbations of COPD. Furthermore, we hope this book will be provocative and stimulate additional research to expand our knowledge in this field.

Finally, we wish to thank Dr. Claude Lenfant for his guidance and support, as well as our wives, Penelope, Barbara, and Ioanna.

Nikos M. Siafakas
Nicholas R. Anthonisen
Dimitris Georgopoulos

CONTRIBUTORS

Alvar G. N. Agusti   Pulmonary Service, Son Dureta Hospital, Palma de Mallorca, Spain

Albert Alonso, M.D., Ph.D.   University of Barcelona-Corporació Sanitària Clínic (CSC), Barcelona, Spain

Nicolino Ambrosino   Pulmonary Division, Cardio-Thoracic Department, University Hospital, Cisanello-Pisa, Italy

Nicholas R. Anthonisen, M.D., Ph.D., F.R.C.P.(C)   Professor, Department of Medicine, University of Manitoba, Winnipeg, Manitoba, Canada

Peter J. Barnes, D.M., D.Sc., F.R.C.P.   Department of Thoracic Medicine, National Heart and Lung Institute, Imperial College London, London, England

Manel Borrell, M.D.   University of Barcelona-Corporació Sanitària Clínic (CSC), Barcelona, Spain

Roelinka Broekhuizen   Department of Respiratory Medicine, University Hospital Maastricht, Maastricht, The Netherlands

Zoheir Bshouty, M.D., Ph.D., F.R.C.P.C.   Associate Professor, Department of Internal Medicine, University of Manitoba, Winnipeg, Manitoba, Canada

Miguel Carrera   Pulmonary Service, Son Dureta Hospital, Palma de Mallorca, Spain

Bartolome R. Celli, M.D.   Tufts University School of Medicine, and Department of Pulmonary/Critical Care, St. Elizabeth's Medical Center, Boston, Massachusetts, U.S.A.

Enrico Clini, M.D.   Hospital Villa Pineta, Modena, Italy

Eva C. Creutzberg, Ph.D. Department of Pulmonary Diseases, University Hospital Maastricht, Maastricht, The Netherlands

Marc Decramer, P.T., Ph.D. Department of Pneumology and Rehabilitation Sciences, Katholieke Universiteit Leuven, Leuven, Belgium

M. Dentener, Ph.D. Department of Pulmonary Diseases, University Hospital Maastricht, Maastricht, The Netherlands

Paula de Toledo, Ph.D. Polytechnic University of Madrid, Madrid, Spain

Mark W. Elliot, M.D., F.R.C.P. St. James's University Hospital, Leeds, England

M. Engelen, Ph.D. Department of Pulmonary Diseases, University Hospital Maastricht, Maastricht, The Netherlands

Leonardo M. Fabbri, M.D. Department of Medical and Surgical Specialties, University of Modena and Reggio Emilia, Modena, Italy

Marios E. Froudarakis Department of Thoracic Medicine, University Hospital of Heraklion, Heraklion, Crete, Greece

Ghislaine Gayan-Ramirez, Ph.D. Department of Pneumology and Rehabilitation Sciences, Katholieke Universiteit Leuven, Leuven, Belgium

Dimitris Georgopoulos, M.D. Professor and Director, Department of Intensive Care Medicine, University Hospital of Heraklion, Heraklion, Crete, Greece

Federico P. Gómez, M.D. Department of Pulmonary Diseases, Hospital Clinic, University of Barcelona, Barcelona, Spain

Simon Gompertz Queen Elizabeth Hospital, Birmingham, England

Rik Gosselink, P.T., Ph.D. Department of Pneumology and Rehabilitation Sciences, Katholieke Universiteit Leuven, Leuven, Belgium

Carme Hernández Home Care Coordinator, Hospital Clinic, Barcelona, Spain

Peter K. Jeffery, M.Sc., Ph.D., D.Sc., F.R.C.Path. Professor of Lung Pathology, Department of Gene Therapy, National Heart and Lung Institute, Imperial College London, London, England

Amal Jubran, M.D. Division of Pulmonary and Critical Care Medicine, Edward Hines Jr., Veterans Affairs Hospital, and Loyola University of Chicago Stritch School of Medicine, Hines, Illinois, U.S.A.

Eumorfia Kondili, M.D. Department of Intensive Care Medicine, University Hospital of Heraklion, Heraklion, Crete, Greece

John Kottakis University General Hospital and Thrace Medical School, Alexandroupolis, Crete, Greece

William MacNee, M.B., Ch.B., M.D. (Hons), F.R.C.P.(G), F.R.C.P.(E) Professor of Respiratory and Environmental Medicine, University of Edinburgh, Edinburgh, Scotland

Katerina Malagari, M.D. Assistant Professor, 2nd Department of Radiology, University of Athens, Athens, Greece

Walter T. McNicholas, M.D., F.R.C.P.I., F.R.C.P.C. Department of Respiratory Medicine, St. Vincent's University Hospital and University College Dublin, Dublin, Ireland

Ioanna Mitrouska, M.D. Department of Thoracic Medicine, University Hospital of Heraklion, Heraklion, Crete, Greece

Maurizio Moretti University of Modena and Reggio Emilia, Modena, Italy

Dennis E. Niewoehner, M.D. Department of Pulmonary Medicine, Minneapolis Veterans Affairs Medical Center, Minneapolis, Minnesota, U.S.A.

Eva Papadopouli, M.D. University of Crete Medical School, Heraklion, Crete, Greece

Victor M. Pinto-Plata, M.D. Tufts University School of Medicine, and Department of Pulmonary/Critical Care, St. Elizabeth's Medical Center, Boston, Massachusetts, U.S.A.

Craig A. Piquette, M.D. Assistant Professor, Department of Pulmonary, Critical Care, and Sleep Medicine, University of Nebraska Medical Center, Omaha, Nebraska, U.S.A.

Roberto Porta Scientific Institute of Gussago, Gussago, Italy

E. Pouw, M.D., Ph.D. Department of Pulmonary Diseases, University Hospital Maastricht, Maastricht, The Netherlands

Yusheng Qiu, Ph.D., M.D. Research Associate, Department of Gene Therapy, National Heart and Lung Institute, Imperial College London, London, England

Clare D. Ramsey, M.D., F.R.C.P.C. Department of Medicine, University of Manitoba, Winnipeg, Manitoba, Canada

Scott D. Ramsey, M.D., Ph.D. Associate Member, Cancer Prevention Research Program/Tradition and Outcomes Research Group, Fred Hutchinson Cancer Research Center, Seattle, Washington, U.S.A.

Stephen I. Rennard, M.D. Profesor, Department of Pulmonary, Critical Care, and Sleep Medicine, University of Nebraska Medical Center, Omaha, Nebraska

Kathryn L. Rice, M.D. Department of Pulmonary Medicine, Minneapolis Veterans Affairs Medical Center, Minneapolis, Minnesota, U.S.A.

Josep Roca, M.D., Ph.D. University of Barcelona-Corporació Sanitària Clínic (CSC), Barcelona, Spain

Roberto Rodriguez-Roisin, M.D., F.R.C.P.(E) Department of Pulmonary Diseases, Hospital Clinic, University of Barcelona, Barcelona, Spain

Andrea Rossi Ospedali Riuniti di Bergamo, Bergamo, Italy

Marlna Saetta, M.D. Associate Professor, Department of Experimental and Clinical Medicine, University of Padua, Padua, Italy

Ernest Sala Pulmonary Service, Son Dureta Hospital, Palma de Mallorca, Spain

Sophia E. Schiza, M.D. University Hospital of Heraklion, Heraklion, Crete, Greece

Annemie M. W. J. Schols Department of Pulmonology, University Hospital Maastricht, Maastricht, The Netherlands

Sat Sharma, M.D., F.R.C.P.C. Department of Medicine, University of Manitoba, Winnipeg, Manitoba, Canada

Nikos M. Siafakas, M.D. Department of Thoracic Medicine, University Hospital of Heraklion, Heraklion, Crete, Greece

Martijn A. Spruit, P.T., Ph.D. Department of Pneumology and Rehabilitation Sciences, Katholieke Universiteit Leuven, Leuven, Belgium

Robert A. Stockley Department of Medicine, Queen Elizabeth Hospital, Birmingham, England

Sean D. Sullivan, Ph.D. Professor, Department of Pharmacy and Health Services, University of Washington, Seattle, Washington, U.S.A.

Thierry Troosters, P.T., Ph.D. Department of Pneumology and Rehabilitation Sciences, Katholieke Universiteit Leuven, Leuven, Belgium

Aiman Tulaimat, M.D. Loyola University of Chicago Stritch School of Medicine, Hines, Illinois

Nikos Tzanakis, M.D. Department of Thoracic Medicine, University of Crete Medical School, Heraklion, Crete, Greece

Graziella Turato, Ph.D. Assistant Professor, Department of Clinical and Experimental Medicine, University of Padua, Padua, Italy

J. Vernooy, M.Sc., Ph.D. Department of Pulmonary Diseases, University Hospital Maastricht, Maastricht, The Netherlands

Jørgen Vestbo, M.D., Ph.D. Consultant Physician, Department of Respiratory Medicine, Hvidovre University Hospital, Hvidovre, Denmark

Argyro Voloudaki, M.D. Department of Radiology, University Hospital of Heraklion, Heraklion, Crete, Greece

Jadwiga A. Wedzicha, M.A., M.D., F.R.C.P. Professor of Respiratory Medicine, St. Bartholomew's and Royal London School of Medicine and Dentistry, St. Bartholomew's Hospital, London, England

Emiel F. M. Wouters, M.D., Ph.D. Department of Pulmonary Diseases, University Hospital Maastricht, Maastricht, The Netherlands

Jie Zhu, Ph.D., M.D. Research Associate, Department of Gene Therapy, National Heart and Lung Institute, Imperial College London, London, England

CONTENTS

26. Invasive Mechanical Ventilation in Acute Exacerbation of Chronic Obstructive Pulmonary Disease   425

Dimitris Georgopoulos and Andrea Rossi

27. Weaning from the Ventilator   475

Amal Jubran and Aiman Tulaimat

28. Rehabilitation and Acute Exacerbations of Chronic Obstructive Pulmonary Disease   507

Nicolino Ambrosino and Roberto Porta

Part IX

ACUTE EXACERBATIONS OF CHRONIC OBSTRUCTIVE PULMONARY DISEASE

1

Definitions of Acute Exacerbations of Chronic Obstructive Pulmonary Disease

NIKOS M. SIAFAKAS

University Hospital of Heraklion
Heraklion, Crete, Greece

I. Definition of Chronic Obstructive Pulmonary Disease

In the 1990s, the two most commonly used definitions of chronic obstructive pulmonary disease (COPD) were those proposed by the European Respiratory Society (1) and American Thoracic Society (2). The ERS stated that "COPD is a disorder characterized by reduced maximum expiratory flow and slow forced emptying of the lungs—features which do not change markedly over several months. Most of the airflow limitation is slowly progressive and irreversible. The airflow limitation is due to varying combinations of airway disease and emphysema (1).

Similarly, the ATS defined COPD "as a disease state characterized by the presence of airflow obstruction due to chronic bronchitis or emphysema; the airflow obstruction is generally progressive, may be accompanied by airway hyperreactivity and may be partially reversible" (2). Both definitions separated asthma from COPD.

Recently, the NIH/WHO GOLD* definition seems more appropriate to describe the disease. It states that "COPD is a disease state characterized by airflow limitation that is not fully reversible. The airflow limitation is both progressive and

---

*NIH, National Institutes of Health; WHO, World Health Organization; GOLD, Global Initiative for Chronic Obstructive Lung Disease.

1

associated with an abnormal inflammatory response of the lungs to noxious particles of gases" (3).

In 2002, a joint ATS/ERS committee working on the diagnosis and management of COPD had agreed on the following definition: "COPD is a preventable and treatable disease state characterized by airflow limitation that is not fully reversible. The airflow limitation is usually progressive and is associated with an abnormal inflammatory response of the lungs to noxious particles or gases, primarily caused by cigarette smoking. Although COPD affects the lungs, it also produces significant systemic consequences." This definition must be approved by both scientific societies.

II. Definition of Acute Exacerbation of Chronic Obstructive Pulmonary Disease

Although it is well known that acute exacerbations of chronic obstructive pulmonary disease (AECOPD) are associated with an increase in health-care utilization, number of hospitalizations, and mortality, there is no widely accepted definition of this disorder (4).

In the late 1980s, Anthonisen et al. (5) defined AECOPD as the presence of any of one of the following conditions: (1) increased cough and sputum volume; (2) increased sputum purulence; (3) increased dyspnea—in other words, worsening of one of the common symptoms of COPD. In addition, the authors classified the severity of an acute exacerbation as type 1, when COPD patients report worsening of all three symptoms; type 2, when they had only two out of three symptoms; and type 3, when they had any one out of three symptoms. Furthermore, patients may have had fever, malaise, and chest congestion (5).

Since this classic paper (5), clinical symptoms were included in all subsequent definitions.

ATS in the last consensus document (2) states that "an acute exacerbation of COPD is difficult to define and its pathogenesis is poorly understood; impaired lung function can lead to respiratory failure requiring intubation and mechanical ventilation" which avoids giving a precise definition.

Similarly, the ERS consensus statement on the management of COPD bypasses a definition and goes straight to the management of this condition (1). Even the most recent, GOLD, although recognizing that exacerbations of respiratory symptoms requiring medical intervention are important clinical events in COPD, does not come with a precise definition of AECOPD (6).

Siafakas and Bouros reported a descriptive definition: "an acute, episode of deterioration, superimposed on stable COPD with increased dyspnea, reduced daily performance, with or without changes in sputum volume, color or purulence, coughing or body temperature, and/or alterations in mental status" (6). In this definition, the prime symptoms characterizing severity were worsening of dyspnea and alteration in mental status. Similarly, other authors placed emphasis primarily on symptoms (7–12).

Rodriguez-Roisin summarized the discussions of a workshop entitled "COPD: Working Toward a Greater Understanding." He reported that the participants proposed the following working definition of an exacerbation of COPD: "a sustained worsening of the patient's condition, from the stable state and beyond normal day-to-day variations, that is acute in onset and necessitates a change in regular medication in a patient with underlying COPD" (13).

This paper entitled "Toward a consensus definition for COPD exacerbations" proposed first to replace the term "acute exacerbation" with simple "exacerbation." However, in the above definition the authors use the phrase "that is acute in onset." The editors of this book believe that the term "acute exacerbation" describes the condition better than "exacerbation with acute onset." In addition "acute exacerbation of COPD" is the most commonly used term in medical literature.

In addition, the above definition introduces the health-care utilization factor (13). However, it is well known that health-care utilization is an extremely variable parameter depending on the health system of various countries, the economic status of the patient, and the patient's perception of symptom severity in order to seek medical attention.

More recently (Paris 2002), the ATS/ERS joint committee for the diagnosis and management of COPD agreed to propose the following definition: "An acute exacerbation of COPD (AECOPD) is an event in the natural course of the disease characterized by a change in the patient's baseline dyspnea, cough, and/or sputum beyond day-to-day variability." It also states that epidemiological studies should consider the need for additional pharmacological therapy or therapeutic interventions such as hospitalization, ventilatory support, etc. It remains to be seen whether this definition will be endorsed by both societies.

It is obvious that a very broad definition of AECOPD is required in order to cover the spectrum ranging from a mild episode that requires a few days in bed to a severe one that requires admission to ICU and life-saving ventilatory support. Thus, worsening of symptoms in a patient with COPD beyond the day-to-day variation is the common denominator of the condition defined as AECOPD.

References

1. Siafakas NM, Vermeire P, Pride NB, Paoletti P, Gibson J, Howard P, et al. Optimal assessment and management of chronic obstructive pulmonary disease (COPD). The European Respiratory Society Task Force. Eur Respir J 1995; 8:1398–1420.
2. American Thoracic Society. Standards for the diagnosis and care of patients with chronic obstructive pulmonary disease. Am J Respir Crit Care Med 1995; 152:S77–S121.
3. Pauwels RA, Buist SA, Calverley PMA, Jenkins CR, Hurd SS. On behalf of the GOLD Scientific Committee. Global strategy for the diagnosis management and prevention of chronic obstructive pulmonary disease. Am J Respir Crit Care Med 2001; 163: 1256–1276.
4. McCrory DC, Brown C, Gelfand SE, Bach PB. Management of acute exacerbations of COPD: a summary and appraisal of published evidence. Chest 2001; 119:1185–1189.

5. Anthonisen NR, Manfreda J, Warren CP, Hershfield ES, Harding GK, Nelson NA. Antibiotic therapy in exacerbations of chronic obstructive pulmonary disease. Ann Intern Med 1987; 106:196–204.
6. Siafakas NM, Bouros D. Management of acute exacerbation of chronic obstructive pulmonary disease. In: Postma DS, Siafakas NM, eds. Management of chronic obstructive pulmonary disease. Eur Respir Monogr 1998; 3(7):264–277.
7. Connors AF, Dawson NV, Thomas C, Harrell FE, Desbiens N Jr, Fulkerson WJ, Kussin P, Bellamy P, Goldman L, Knaus WA for the support investigators. Outcomes following acute exacerbation of severe chronic obstructive lung disease. Am J Respir Crit Care Med 1996; 154:959–967.
8. Seemungal TAR, Donaldson GC, Paul EA, Bestall JC, Jeffries DJ, Wedzicha JA. Effect of exacerbation on quality of life in patients with chronic obstructive pulmonary disease. Am J Respir Crit Care Med 1998; 157:1418–1422.
9. Plant PK, Owen JL, Elliott MW. Early use of non-invasive ventilation for acute exacerbations of chronic obstructive pulmonary disease on general respiratory wards: a multicentre randomised controlled trial. Lancet 2000; 355(9219):1931–1935.
10. Gravil JH, Al-Rawas OA, Cotton MM, Flanigan U, Irwin A, Stevenson RD. Home treatment of exacerbations of chronic obstructive pulmonary disease by an acute respiratory assessment service. Lancet 1998; 351(9119):1853–1855.
11. Niewoehner DE, Collins D, Erbland ML. Relation of FEV_1 to clinical outcomes during exacerbations of chronic obstructive pulmonary disease. Department of Veterans Affairs Cooperative Study Group. Am J Respir Crit Care Med 2000; 161:1201–1205.
12. Bach PB, Brown C, Gelfand SE, McCrory DC. American College of Physicians– American Society of Internal Medicine, American College of Chest Physicians. Management of acute exacerbations of chronic obstructive pulmonary disease: a summary and appraisal of published evidence. Ann Intern Med 2001; 134(7):600–620.
13. Rodriguez-Roisin R. Toward a consensus definition for COPD exacerbations. Chest 2000; 117:398S–401S.

2

Epidemiology of Exacerbations in Chronic Obstructive Pulmonary Disease

JØRGEN VESTBO

Hvidovre University Hospital
Hvidovre, Denmark

I. Introduction and Definition

The epidemiology of exacerbations in chronic obstructive pulmonary disease (COPD) does not differ from the epidemiology of other disorders. It attempts to describe the characteristics of this feature of COPD in the population and relies on usual epidemiological methodology. More than any other research area, however, epidemiology is set back by the lack of a simple definition of an exacerbation easily applied to larger population surveys. The recently proposed definition of an exacerbation as "a sustained worsening of the patient's condition, from the stable state and beyond normal day-to-day variations, that is acute in onset and necessitates a change in regular medication in a patient with underlying COPD" (1) needs to be made operational to be included in epidemiology. To be useful in epidemiology, information on exacerbations must be collected using questionnaires and/or diaries. In the initial testing of what later became the British Medical Research Council (MRC) questionnaire, Fletcher et al. included questions on "chest illness which has kept you in bed, off work, or indoors" and this phrasing presumably captures most moderate-to-severe exacerbations whereas its specificity is unknown. Before their systematic testing (2), it had been reported that "out-patients with chronic bronchitis tended to exaggerate the number and duration of past sickness absences," but

Fletcher et al. found no marked tendency to exaggerate or forget past illnesses. Also, variability in answers seemed acceptable (3). The concept of counting number of chest episodes was applied to several surveys in the 1950s but was then abandoned—paradoxically due to the findings by Fletcher et al. in their seminal study in East London (4). Questions on "chest illnesses" still remain in the latest version of the MRC questionnaire and they were included in the American Thoracic Society questionnaire from 1978 (5) but are not used—or at least not reported. No subsequent work has been done to try to define exacerbations for epidemiological purposes.

Alternative measures that can be applied in epidemiology are acute hospitalization that can serve as a proxy measure of severe exacerbations or exacerbations in severe COPD and episodes where acute treatment with corticosteroids, for example, is initiated. The latter information is increasingly available in large pharmacoepidemiological databases. Finally, the criteria based on worsening of symptoms used by Anthonisen et al. in their often-cited study on antibiotics in exacerbations in COPD (6) could be applied in epidemiology, but has not been.

II. Frequency of Exacerbations

Information on frequency can never be any better than the data on which it is based. For this reason, we have very little available population-based data on frequency of exacerbations.

In their paper on respiratory symptoms, Fletcher et al. (2) quote four studies assessing frequency of bronchitis chest illness using questionnaires. The populations studied are not well characterized in the paper but, apart from Fletcher's own cohort of London postmen, they are described as random samples of men and women aged 55 to 64, including approximately 350 men and 300 women. The percentage with one bronchitis chest illness within the last year varies from 4.8 to 11.6% among men, whereas 4.7 to 14.6 had experienced more than one. Percentages were similar in women.

Other data sources on exacerbations in the general population are sparse. Data on acute hospital admissions can be used to assess the number of severe exacerbations and therefore the most costly part of exacerbations. According to the Global Initiative for Chronic Obstructive Lung Disease (GOLD) (7), there were 448,000 hospitalizations or 1.7/1000 in 1997 in the United States, with COPD listed as primary diagnosis; the number of COPD admissions in the United Kingdom in 1999/2000 was 107,000 or 2.0/1000 (8). In Denmark, the number of admissions in 1997 was 21,000 or 4/1000 (9). Whereas uncertainty exists in classification and registration of admissions that can invalidate the tool for assessment of the exact size of the problem, these data can be used to monitor changes in the pattern of admissions over a period of time, given that the health service does not change markedly in the observation period. Figure 1 shows an example of such changes in hospitalizations for COPD for men and women in Denmark from 1979 to 1997. Risk factors for hospitalization for COPD and/or readmission include age (10–13), female

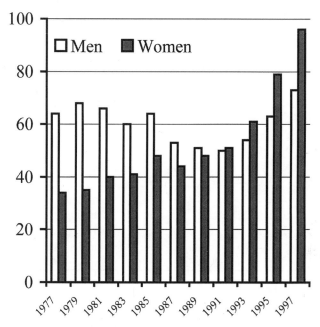

Figure 1 Annual number of bed days (per 1000) for COPD in Denmark.

gender (12), FEV_1 (10–13), previous admissions (14), smoking (11–14), chronic mucus hypersecretion (10,11), other respiratory symptoms (10), socioeconomic status (13), and underprescription of long-term oxygen treatment (14).

Among patients with established COPD, our information about frequency of exacerbations is also limited. Data usually come from more-or-less standardized collections of clinical data in departments with a specific interest in this particular area. However, with increasing use of large registers with information on hospitalizations, consultations with general practitioners, and prescriptions, it is possible to define larger cohorts for subsequent follow-up. An example of this comes from Sin and Tu in their register linkage study from Ontario (15), where a group of elderly COPD patients were defined on the basis of a recent hospital admission for COPD. In this group of elderly patients with presumably moderate-to-severe COPD, approximately 40% of patients not treated with inhaled corticosteroids experienced at least one readmission within 12 months.

Using hospital admissions in patients with established COPD as a crude measure of clinically significant exacerbations, we have learned a little about predictors. Age and severity of COPD still play a role, but, in addition, presence of chronic mucus hypersecretion (16), decreased health status (17), muscle weakness (18), comorbidities (16), and presumably withdrawal of inhaled corticosteroids (19,20) are also factors. Of more general importance is the rather consistent relationship between episodic outdoor particulate pollution and hospitalization for COPD (21,22).

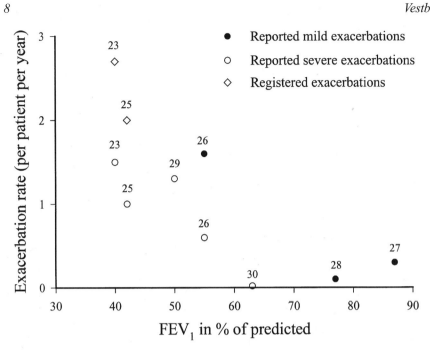

Figure 2   Exacerbation rates according to baseline lung function. Numbers are reference numbers.

Contrary to early belief (2), patients do not exaggerate the number of exacerbations. In fact, studies from East London have indicated that patients tend to underreport approximately half of their exacerbations when comparing recall with criteria modified from Anthonisen (6) registered on diary cards (23,24). Seemungal et al. (23) followed 70 well-characterized patients with COPD with a mean FEV of 1.05 L with MRC dyspnea scores ranging from 2 to 5. Patients completed daily diary cards and measured peak expiratory flow rate at home. They were seen by a doctor every 3 months. Exacerbations were defined based on symptoms and over a 12-month period 190 exacerbations were registered. Of these, 93 were reported at clinic visits and thus the reported exacerbation rate was 1.5 per patient per year and the registered rate was 2.7 per patient per year. Frequent past exacerbations, daily wheeze, and bronchitic symptoms were significant predictors of frequent exacerbations defined as 3+ exacerbations per year. In a subsequent study (25) in which the cohort had been expanded and where the observation period was 2.5 years, the same group found 504 exacerbations in 101 patients, which gives a registered exacerbation rate of 2 per patient per year; again, only 50% of registered exacerbations were reported (Fig. 2).

Self-reported number of exacerbations and/or diary cards are often used in various forms in clinical trials for monitoring adverse events, but previous studies were too small to provide information on frequency and distribution of COPD exacerbations. An important source of information on frequency and severity of COPD

Table 1 Study Characteristics and Exacerbation Rates in Placebo Arms of Recently Published Large Controlled Trials of Inhaled Corticosteroids in COPD

Ref.	Mean age (yrs)	n	Mean FEV$_1$ L/%pred	M/F ratio	Current smokers %	Exacerbation rate No. per year[a]
26	64	139	1.5/55	78/22	49	1.6/0.6[b]
27	59	145	2.4/87	60/40	76	0.3[c]
28[d]	52	643	2.5/77	72/28	100	0.1[e]
29	64	370	1.4/50	74/26	54	−/1.3[b]
30	56	557	2.2/63	62/38	90	−/0.02[f]

[a]Calculated using number of patients randomized to placebo.
[b]Moderate-to-severe exacerbations treated with antibiotics and/or corticosteroids.
[c]Episodic worsening of cough and phlegm.
[d]Information on exacerbations not in the paper but from oral presentations.
[e]Rate of patients experiencing at least one exacerbation (per year).
[f]Visit to a physician for respiratory reasons.

exacerbations, however, has been the knowledge obtained form the placebo arms of recent well-conducted, large, randomized controlled trials in COPD, mainly investigating the effect of inhaled corticosteroids in COPD (26–30). All of these studies included some measure of exacerbation, although exacerbation rate and frequency have not been the primary effect parameter in any of the studies. Table 1 shows the characteristics of these studies with the exacerbation rate calculated. None of these studies had exacerbation rate as a primary endpoint, but in most of them it was included among secondary endpoints. The placebo arms have been used for calculating exacerbation rates. For practical purposes, mostly moderate-to-severe exacerbations have been counted because they can be defined on the basis of contact with a doctor or prescription of systemic corticosteroids and/or antibiotics.

Subsequent large trials in COPD have all included exacerbations as primary or secondary endpoints and additional information can be obtained as these studies are published.

References

1. Rodriguez-Roisin R. Toward a consensus definition for COPD exacerbations. Chest 2000; 117:398–401S.
2. Fletcher CM, Elmes PC, Fairbarn AS, Wood CH. The significance of respiratory symptoms and the diagnosis of chronic bronchitis in a working population. Br Med J 1959; 3:257–266.
3. Fairbarn AS, Wood CH, Fletcher CM. Variability in answers to a questionnaire on respiratory symptoms. Br J Prev Soc Med 1959; 13:175–193.
4. Fletcher CM, Peto R, Tinker CM, Speizer FE. The Natural History of Chronic Bronchitis and Emphysema. Oxford: Oxford University Press, 1976.
5. World Health Organization. Methods for cohort studies of chronic airflow limitation. Copenhagen: WHO Regional Office for Europe, 1982.

6. Anthonisen NR, Manfreda J, Warren CPW, Hershfield ES, Harding GKM, Nelson NA. Antibiotic therapy in exacerbations of chronic obstructive pulmonary disease. Ann Intern Med 1987; 106:196–204.

7. Pauwels R, Buist A, Calverley P, Jenkins C, Hurd S. Global strategy for the diagnosis, management and prevention of chronic obstructive pulmonary disease. NHLBI/WHO global initiative for chronic obstructive lung disease (GOLD) workshop summary. Am J Respir Crit Care Med 2001; 163:1256–1276.

8. British Thoracic Society. The Burden of Lung Disease. London: British Thoracic Society, 2001.

9. The Danish National Board of Health, www.sst.dk. Accessed December 10, 2001.

10. Vestbo J, Rasmussen FV. Respiratory symptoms and FEV_1 as predictors of hospitalization and medication in the following 12 years due to respiratory disease. Eur Respir J 1989; 2:710–715.

11. Vestbo J, Prescott E, Lange P, The Copenhagen City Heart Study Group. Association of chronic mucus hypersecretion with FEV_1 decline and COPD morbidity. Am J Respir Crit Care Med 1996; 153:1530–1535.

12. Prescott E, Bjerg AM, Andersen PK, Lange P, Vestbo J. Gender differences in smoking effects on lung function and risk of hospitalization for COPD: results from a Danish longitudinal population study. Eur Respir J 1997; 10:822–827.

13. Prescott E, Lange P, Vestbo J, The Copenhagen City Heart Study Group. Socioeconomic status, lung function, and admission to hospital for COPD. Results from the Copenhagen City Heart Study. Eur Respir J 1999; 13:1109–1114.

14. Garcia-Aymerich J, Monsó E, Marrades RM, Escarrabill J, Félez MA, Sunyer J, Antó J, The EFRAM investigators. Risk factors for hospitalisation for a chronic obstructive pulmonary disease exacernation. Am J Respir Crit Care Med 2001; 164:1002–1007.

15. Sin DD, Tu JV. Inhaled corticosteroids and the risk of mortality and readmission in elderly patients with chronic obstructive pulmonary disease. Am J Respir Crit Care Med 2001; 164:580–584.

16. Miravitlles M, Guerrero T, Mayordomo C, Sánchez-Agudo L, Nicolau F, Segú JL. Factors associated with increased risk of exacerbation and hospital admission in a cohort of ambulatory COPD patients: a multiple logistic regression analysis. Respiration 2000; 67:495–501.

17. Osman LM, Godden DJ, Friend JAR, Legge JS, Douglas JG. Quality of life and hospital readmission in patients with chronic obstructive pulmonary disease. Thorax 1997; 52:67–71.

18. Decramer M, Gosselink R, Troosters T, Vershueren M, Evers G. Muscle weakness is related to utilization of health care resources in COPD. Eur Respir J 1997; 10:417–423.

19. Jarad NA, Wedzicha JA, Burge PS, Calverley PMA for the ISOLDE study group. An observational study of inhaled corticosteroid withdrawal in stable chronic obstructive pulmonary disease. Respir Med 1999; 93:161–166.

20. O'Brien A, Russo-Magno P, Karki A, Hiranniramd S, Hardin M, Kaszuba M, Sherman C, Rounds S. Effects of withdrawal of inhaled steroids in men with severe irreversible airflow obstruction. Am J Respir Crit Care Med 2001; 164:365–371.

21. Anto JM, Vermeire P, Vestbo J, Sunyer J. Epidemiology of chronic obstructive pulmonary disease. Eur Respir J 2001; 17:982–994.

22. Sunyer J. Urban air pollution and chronic obstructive pulmonary disease: a review. Eur Respir J 2001; 17:1024–1033.

23. Seemungal TAR, Donaldson G, Paul EA, Bestall JC, Jeffries DJ, Wedzicha JA. Effect of exacerbation on quality of life in patients with chronic obstructive pulmonary disease. Am J Respir Crit Care Med 1998; 157:1418–1422.
24. Wedzicha JA. Mechanisms of exacerbations. In: Chadwick D, Goode JA, eds. Chronic Obstructive Pulmonary Disease: Pathogenesis to Treatment. London: Novartis Foundation, 2001.
25. Seemungal T, Donaldson GC, Bhowmik A, Jeffries DJ, Wedzicha JA. Time course and recovery of exacerbations in patients with chronic obstructive pulmonary disease. Am J Respir Crit Care Med 2000; 161:1608–1613.
26. Paggiaro PL, Dahle R, Bakran I, Filth L, Hollingworth K, Efthimiou J, on behalf of the international COPD study group. Multicentre randomised placebo-controlled trial of inhaled fluticasone propionate in patients with chronic obstructive pulmonary disease. Lancet 1998; 351:773–780.
27. Vestbo J, Sørensen T, Lange P, Brix A, Torre P, Viskum K. Long-term effect of inhaled budesonide in mild and moderate chronic obstructive pulmonary disease—a randomised, controlled trial. Lancet 1999; 353:1819–1823.
28. Pauwels RA, Löfdahl C-G, Laitinen LA, Schouten JP, Postma DS, Pride NB, Ohlsson SV. Long-term treatment with inhaled budesonide in persons with mild chronic obstructive pulmonary disease who continue to smoke. N Engl J Med 1999; 340:1948–1953.
29. Burge PS, Calverley PMA, Jones PW, Spencer S, Anderson JA, Maslen TK. Randomised, double-blind, placebo controlled study of fluticasone propionate in patients with moderate to severe chronic obstructive pulmonary disease; the ISOLDE trial. Br Med J 2000; 320:1297–1303.
30. The Lung Health Study Group. Effect of inhaled triamcinolone on the decline in pulmonary function in chronic obstructive pulmonary disease. N Engl J Med 2000; 343:1902–1909.

3

Effects of Acute Exacerbations on the Natural History of Chronic Obstructive Pulmonary Disease

SOPHIA E. SCHIZA

University Hospital of Heraklion
Heraklion, Crete, Greece

NICHOLAS R. ANTHONISEN

University of Manitoba
Winnipeg, Manitoba, Canada

I. Introduction

The natural history of chronic obstructive pulmonary disease (COPD) is characterized by slowly progressive limitation of expiratory airflow. This can be well assessed by simple spirometry and only two parameters, the FEV_1 and the FVC, need to be measured to obtain almost all the useful information available. Variations in natural history are probably related to differences in the dose and influence of various risk factors.

II. COPD and Exacerbations

COPD is often associated with acute exacerbations of symptoms. In patients with mild-to-moderate COPD, an exacerbation is associated with increased breathlessness, often accompanied by increases in cough and sputum production, and may require medical attention outside the hospital. Exacerbations in severe COPD are associated with acute respiratory failure and require hospitalization. The most common causes of an exacerbation are infection of the tracheobronchial tree and air pollution, but the cause of about one-third of severe exacerbations cannot be identified. Acute exacerbations of COPD are usually attended by decreases in lung function (1–5).

COPD is a leading cause of death, a major medical problem, and an increasing economic burden. Despite the fact that COPD patients may experience as many as 1.7 exacerbations per year, the influence of exacerbations on the progression of COPD has not been established. The vast majority of hospitalizations for COPD are for the management of acute exacerbations in patients with severe baseline disease. If baseline lung function is very poor, or if the change in lung function with the exacerbation is large, the exacerbations are potentially fatal. Hospital mortality of patients admitted for an acute exacerbation of COPD is approximately 10%, and the long-term outcome is poor. Mortality reaches 40% in 1 year, and is even higher for up to 59% for patients older than 65 years (6–11). These figures vary from country to country depending on the health-care system and the availability of intensive-care-unit beds (10). The long-term prognosis of COPD patients hospitalized for exacerbations remains poor (Fig. 1). Predictors of subsequent mortality include the overall health status of the individual (comorbidities), the prior functional status, the severity of the exacerbation, and indices of poor nutrition such as low body mass index and serum albumin (6).

In the 1960s, British investigators framed the hypothesis that airway obstruction in chronic bronchitis was due to repetitive and perhaps chronic airways infection. The so-called British hypothesis was based on the evidence that COPD patients, especially in Britain, have periodic exacerbations of chronic cough and

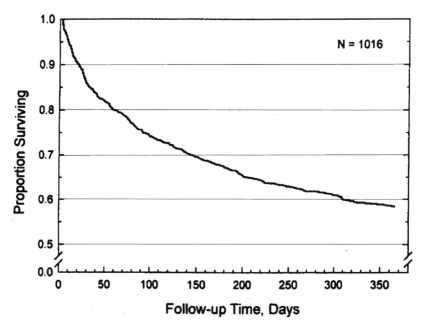

Figure 1 One-year survival in 1016 patients with COPD hospitalized for exacerbations. The in-hospital mortality was 11%. (From Ref. 6 with permission.)

sputum with clinical evidence of airways obstruction, and sputum cultures reveal the same organisms as those associated with exacerbations, mainly *H. influenza* and *S. pneumoniae* (12–15). Repetitive airways infection, perhaps triggered by viruses, caused permanent damage to the airways and lungs resulting in the airways obstruction (16). That hypothesis implied that antimicrobial therapy might avert the chronic airways obstruction.

Fletcher et al. designed a study in order to test the British hypothesis. They studied 792 London transit workers over 8 years, with assessment of smoking habits, sputum, chest infections, and FEV_1 (17). The results were published in 1976. They found that chronic cough and sputum were not necessarily associated with rapid decline of FEV_1. They concluded that there were two components of COPD (chronic cough and sputum), which were largely independent of each other but usually coexisted because smoking caused both and predisposed to repetitive "chest infections." Rapid decline in FEV_1 was also associated with smoking, but was less common and did not relate to either chronic cough and sputum or to chest colds.

The Fletcher results were corroborated by two other long-term studies. Howord et al. and Bates et al. found that acute respiratory illnesses did not influence the rate of decline of lung function (18,19). Although the British hypothesis was not entirely discarded by infectious disease specialists, it was discounted by COPD experts (20,21).

One study did indicate that infectious episodes were associated with rapid decline of FEV_1, but it examined a small group of heterogeneous patients (22).

The presence of chronic cough and sputum has been related to mortality and individuals with symptomatic chronic bronchitis, after correction for confounding

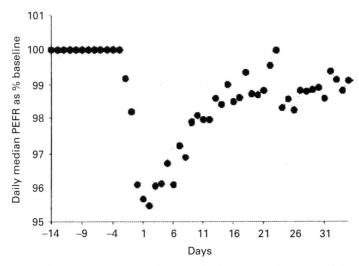

Figure 2 Median peak-flow data for 504 exacerbation in 91 patients over 14 days before the exacerbation to 35 days after its onset. Peak flows are expressed as a percentage of that observed at baseline. (From Ref. 27 with permission.)

variables, had higher mortality rates as showed in two large studies (23,24). Further studies of rate of decline of FEV_1 in smokers contradicted the Fletcher results in that decline was faster in people with chronic cough and sputum than in those without after statistical correction for baseline lung function and smoking habits (25,26).

While many studies have shown recovery of lung function during these events, pre-exacerbation function had been unknown, and so the extent of the recovery was also unknown. This gap in the literature has been at least partially filled by the studies of Seemungal et al., who prospectively followed COPD patients and measured lung function before, during, and after outpatient exacerbations (27). They found transient decrease in lung function with recovery; however, they noted that in 25% of patients recovery was not complete 35 days after onset and that in 7% of patients there was not complete recovery at 3 months (Fig. 2). A retrospective analysis of the Lung Health Study (LHS) was designed to test the influence of smoking cessation and inhaled bronchodilators (28). The frequency of acute respiratory illnesses was assesed by questionaire at annual visits, a common technique in such studies (29). Acute respiratory illnesses were about twice as common in participants with chronic cough and sputum as in those without these symptoms. These findings were in accord with the data of Fletcher et al. (17). Of great interest was the influence of respiratory illnesses on rate of decline of FEV_1 over the 5-year study duration. In people who quit smoking, respiratory illnesses had no influence on rate of decline, but in participants who continued to smoke there was an increased rate of decline that was proportional to exacerbation frequency (Fig. 3). The increase in rate of decline amounted to 7 mL/year for one respiratory infection, and approximately twice this number for two. The authors noted that in smokers

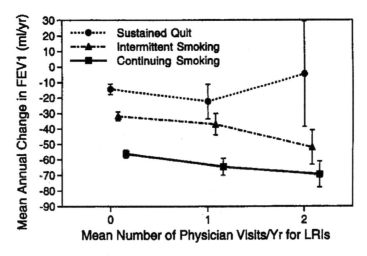

Figure 3   Effect of lower respiratory infections (LRI) on annual decline of FEV_1 in the Lung Health Study. There was no effect in people who stopped smoking at the onset of the study, but in those who continued to smoke, LRI were associated with an increased loss of lung function. (From Ref. 28 with permission.)

with repetitive acute respiratory illnesses, the effect may be important. Obviously, the association of acute respiratory illnesses with accelerated decline of lung function did not prove a cause-and-effect relationship, but such a relationship is inherently credible and in agreement with the incomplete recovery of function noted by Seemungal et al. (27). The LHS findings contradicted those of Fletcher and others, possibly because the LHS had more participants and better lung function measurements, and possibly because the LHS analyzed smokers and nonsmokers separately.

Therefore, it is possible that acute exacerbations of COPD do influence the long-term course of the disease by causing accelerated decline in lung function, and that this effect, more common in those with chronic bronchitis, may be an important one.

References

1. Felix-Davies D, Westlake EK. Corticotrophin in treatment of acute exacerbations of chronic bronchitis. Br Med J 1956; 1:780–782.
2. Albert RK, Martin TR, Lewis SW. Controlled clinical trial of methylprednisolone in patients with chronic bronchitis and acute respiratory insufficiency. Ann Intern Med 1980; 92:753–758.
3. Anthonisen NR, Manfreda J, Warren CPW, Hershfield ES, Harding GKM, Nelson NA. Antibiotic therapy in exacerbations of chronic obstructive pulmonary disease. Ann Intern Med 1987; 106:196–204.
4. Davies L, Angus RM, Calverly PMA. Oral corticosteroids in patients admitted to hospital with exacerbations of chronic obstructive pulmonary disease: a prospective randomized controlled trial. Lancet 1999; 354:456–460.
5. Niewoehner DE, Erblend ML, Deupree RH, Collins D, Gross NJ, Light RW, Anderson P, Morgan NA. Effect of systemic glucocorticoids on exacerbations of chronic obstructive pulmonary disease. N Engl J Med 1999; 340:1941–1947.
6. Connors AF, Dawson NV, Thomas C, Harrell FE Jr, Desbiens N, Fulkerson WJ, Kussin P, Bellamy P, Goldman L, Knaus WA, for the SUPPORT Investigators. Outcomes following acute exacerbation of severe chronic obstructive lung disease. Am J Respir Crit Care Med 1996; 154:959–967.
7. Bates DV, Klassen GA, Broadhurst CA, Peretz DI, Anthonisen NR, Smith HJ. Management of respiratory failure. Ann NY Acad Med 1965; 121:781–786.
8. Seneff MG, Wagner DP, Wagner RP, Zimmerman JE, Knaus WA. Hospital and 1-year survival of patients admitted to intensive care units with acute exacerbation of chronic obstructive pulmonary disease. JAMA 1995; 274:1852–1857.
9. Fuso L, Incalzi RA, Pistelli R, Muzzolon R, Valente S, Pagliari G. Predicting mortality of patients hospitalized for acutely exacerbated chronic obstructive pulmonary disease. Am J Med 1995; 98:272–277.
10. Ely EW, Baker AM, Evans GW, Haponik EF. The distribution of costs of care in mechanically ventilated patients with chronic obstructive pulmonary disease. Crit Care Med 2000; 28(2):408–413.
11. Burk RH, George RB. Acute respiratory failure in chronic obstructive lung disease. Arch Intern Med 1973; 85:865–868.
12. Fletcher CM. Chronic bronchitis. Am Rev Respir Dis 1959; 80:483–494.

13. Stuart-Harris CH. The pathogenesis of chronic bronchitis and emphysema. Scot Med J 1965; 10:93–107.
14. Laurenzi GA, Potter RT, Kass EH. Bacteriologic flora of the lower respiratory tract. N Engl J Med 1961; 265:1273–1278.
15. Fisher M, Akhtar AJ, Calder MA, Maffatt MAJ, Stewart SM, Zealley H, Crofton JW. Pilot study of factors associated with exacerbations in chronic bronchitis. Br Med J 1969; 4:187–192.
16. Cherry JD, Taylor-Robinson D, Willers H, Stehnouse AC. A search for mycoplasma infections in patients with chronic bronchitis. Thorax 1971; 26:62–67.
17. Fletcher C, Peto R, Tinker C, Speizer FE. The Natural History of Chronic Bronchitis and Emphysema. Oxford: Oxford University Press, 1976.
18. Howard P. A long-term follow-up of respiratory symptoms and ventilatory function in a group of working men. Br J Indust Med 1970; 27:326–333.
19. Bates DV. The fate of the chronic bronchitic: a report of the 10-year follow-up in the Canadian Department of Veterans Affairs coordinated study of chronic bronchitis. Am Rev Respir Dis 1973; 108:1043–1065.
20. Cole P. Host-microbe relationships in chronic respiratory infection. Respiration 1989; 55:5–8.
21. Murphy TF, Sethi S. Bacterial infection in chronic obstructive pulmonary disease. Am Rev Dis 1992; 146:1067–1083.
22. Kanner RE, Renzetti AD, Klauber MR, Smith CB, Golden CA. Variables associated with changes in spirometry in patients with obstructive lung diseases. Am J Med 1979; 67:44–50.
23. Annesi I, Kauffmann FE. Is respiratory mucus hypersecretion really an innocent disorder? Am Rev Respir Dis 1986; 134:688–693.
24. Speizer FE, Fay ME, Dockery DW, Ferris BG Jr. Chronic obstructive pulmonary disease mortality in six US cities. Am Rev Respir Dis 1989; 140:S49–S55.
25. Sherman CB, Xu X, Speizer FE, Ferris GB Jr, Weiss ST, Dockery DW. Longitudinal lung function decline in subjects with respiratory symptoms. Am Rev Respir Dis 1992; 146:855–859.
26. Vestbo J, Prescott E, Lange P, The Copenhagen City Heart Study Group. Association of chronic mucus hypersecretion with FEV_1 decline and chronic obstructive lung disease morbidity. Am J Resp Crit Care Med 1996; 153:1530–1535.
27. Seemungal TAR, Donaldson GC, Bhowmik A, Jeffries DJ, Wedzicha J. Time course and recovery of exacerbations in patients with chronic obstructive pulmonary disease. Am J Respir Crit Care Med 2000; 161:1608–1613.
28. Kanner RE, Anthonisen NR, Connett JE for the Lung Health Study Research Group. Lower respiratory illnesses promote FEV_1 decline in current smokers but not in ex-smokers with mild chronic obstructive pulmonary disease. Am J Respir Crit Care Med 2001; 164:358–364.
29. Antonisen NR, Connett JE, Kiley J, Altose M, Bailey W, Buist AS, Conway W, Enright P, Kanner RE, O'Hara P, et al. Effects of smoking intervention and the use of an inhaled anticholinergic bronchodilator on the rate of decline of FEV_1. J Am Med Assoc 1994; 272:1497–1505.

4

Economic Burden of Acute Exacerbations of Chronic Obstructive Pulmonary Disease

SCOTT D. RAMSEY

Fred Hutchinson Cancer
   Research Center
Seattle, Washington, U.S.A.

SEAN D. SULLIVAN

University of Washington
Seattle, Washington, U.S.A.

I. Introduction

The worldwide social burden of chronic obstructive pulmonary disease (COPD) in terms of days lost to disability is expected to increase from twelfth to fifth among all chronic diseases from 1990 to 2020 (1). In the United States, COPD affects approximately 1.9 million Americans and is one of the fastest growing causes of morbidity and mortality (2,3). Given COPD's prevalence and the duration of illness, its economic impact—in terms of medical treatment expenditures and work loss due to morbidity and premature mortality—is substantial for all societies. Studies have shown that the primary "cost-driver" for COPD in developed countries is hospital care for exacerbations, accounting for nearly 70% of all direct medical costs for this disease (1). Therefore, new treatments to reduce the severity or frequency of exacerbations could have a tremendous impact on the overall economic burden of the disease.

With constrained resources and ever-rising health-care expenditures, evaluating the economic impact of new therapies has become nearly as important as understanding their clinical impact. This chapter reviews the available evidence regarding the economic impact of acute exacerbations of chronic obstructive pulmonary disease (AECOPD). It will then review studies exploring the cost-effectiveness of treatments aimed at reducing the frequency and severity of AECOPD. Finally, it will outline a framework for evaluating the cost-effectiveness of new therapies designed to reduce this aspect of the COPD burden.

II. Issues for Evaluating the Economic Burden of AECOPD

Treatment of COPD contains many elements: prevention of slow progression of the disease (primarily smoking cessation), treatment of chronic day-to-day symptoms, and treatment of exacerbations related to COPD. The clinical definition of an exacerbation is protean and is reviewed in Chapter 1 of this book. From the economic perspective, we define a COPD exacerbation as an event that results in a rise in medical expenditures needed to treat a sudden, transient increase in severity of symptoms. The event can vary in duration, and ends with either death or a return to baseline or near-baseline health status. It is important to note that both the initial event and the "tail end" of an AECOPD can be difficult to define both from a clinical and economic perspective. This fact can complicate efforts to estimate costs attributable to AECOPD.

Defining the beginning and end of an AECOPD for economic evaluations is further complicated because researchers can take two general approaches: one based on using medical records (charts) to determine the beginning and end of the exacerbation; the second based on administrative claims records. These two methods may yield different durations of illness, and therefore different costs attributable to the exacerbation.

Although a health services definition of an AECOPD is defined as a rise in medical expenditures to treat a transient increase in severity of symptoms, the expenditures will be for a variety of services in several settings, such as drug or oxygen costs, clinic visits, emergency room visits, and hospital days. At one extreme might be a mild exacerbation that causes the patient to increase the use of his bronchodilator medication without ever visiting a physician; at the other would be one that requires an extensive stay in an intensive care unit. Depending on the database that is available for estimating costs, one may miss exacerbations of mild severity or portions of the event where care was used in a way that could not be captured.

Another issue that may limit comparability of economic studies of AECOPD relates to the type of costs that are included in the analysis. Costs can be divided into direct medical, direct nonmedical, and productivity costs.

Direct medical costs include all medical goods and services used to treat the illness. Usually, these costs are the easiest ones to identify and thus are part of most economic studies. Direct nonmedical costs include items related to an AECOPD event but not directly linked to the health-care system. Such costs can include hired caregiver expenses, costs to the family, lost wages of family caregivers, and transportation and parking costs for patients visiting their physicians. Because these costs usually are not reimbursed by health insurance and are difficult to track, they are often excluded from economic studies. As a result, almost no information exists on the value of direct nonmedical costs in COPD. This might be an important oversight, particularly for developing countries. For example, transportation costs may be one of the largest expenses for those who have to travel from remote areas to receive care. Productivity costs refer to the value of lost wages resulting from illness and from seeking treatment. They are particularly difficult to estimate and are usually excluded from economic evaluations. Nevertheless, productivity reduced by sporadic absences related to AECOPD is important, because it limits income and may inhibit the person's ability to maintain regular employment.

International comparisons of the cost of AECOPD are influenced by country-specific variations in patterns of care for this condition.

Important clinical issues limit the comparability of economic evaluations of AECOPD. First, the definition of COPD can vary. For example, in the Netherlands, COPD and asthma are often considered to be a spectrum of the same disease, and thus patients with both conditions are evaluated together. Second, the severity of illness of cohorts of patients followed vary from study to study. Those who are more severely affected are likely to have a greater number and more severe exacerbations (the latter translating into more use of medical resources). Patients also vary from study to study in the number and severity of comorbidities. Comorbidities also influence resource use when individuals suffer an AECOPD. Finally, duration of follow-up is critical. Longer follow-up times will influence the number of exacerbations captured in the database.

III. Economic Evaluations of AECOPD

To summarize the evidence regarding the economic impact of AECOPD, we searched the Medline (4), EconLit, and the United Kingdom's National Health Service Economic Evaluation Database (NHS-EED) (5). Articles were searched using the MESH headings "Pulmonary Disease, Chronic Obstructive" AND "Economics" AND the term "exacerbation(s)." To limit studies that reflected recent trends in therapy, only articles dating from 1985 were reviewed. A total of 20 articles were retrieved from Medline, 1 from EconLit, and 34 from the NHS-EED.

IV. Results: Economic Burden of AECOPD

Few studies have reported the cost of exacerbations in persons with COPD; the studies that have are summarized in Table 1. The comparability of these studies is limited due to variations in perspectives, data sources, and methods. In addition, practice patterns for AECOPD will vary by country of origin, further limiting comparability.

V. Cost-Effectiveness Studies of Treatments for AECOPD

Cost-effectiveness studies are now common in medicine and have been applied to therapies for AECOPD. Cost-effectiveness studies examine the value of expenditure for new treatments for AECOPD compared to existing therapies. Treatments for AECOPD can be broadly classified into two categories: (1) those aimed at reducing

Table 1   Studies Reporting Costs of Exacerbations of COPD

Study and origin (Ref.)	Method of identifying AECOPD	Average duration (SD)	Cost elements included	Average cost (SD) per exacerbation per person (year of costs)
USA (6)	Medical record	8.9 (3.3)	All	$942 (2173)[a] (1994)
UK (7)	Administrative data[b]	NA	All	£193[c] (1994)
Spain (8)	Medical record	NA	All	$159 (100) (1996)
USA (9)	Medical record	9 (5 to 15)[d]	Hospital	$7100 ($4100 to $16,000)[d] (1994)

[a]Costs for treatment using "first-line" antibiotic choices. Duration and costs for therapy using "second-line" or "third-line" therapies were lower. Charges were recorded rather than costs.
[b]Considered only costs for persons with at diagnosis of chronic bronchitis (ICD-9 code 491).
[c]Costs per year rather than per exacerbation.
[d]Interquartile range.

the frequency of AECOPD and (2) those aimed at reducing the severity when an exacerbation occurs. Ever-tightening health budgets will force payers to scrutinize the value for expenditures of new therapies more closely. In this context, it is an opportune time to review the important issues involved for conducting robust cost-effectiveness studies of treatments for AECOPD.

A.   Methodological Issues

Researchers have developed guidelines for conducting economic evaluations, or cost-effectiveness analyses (CEA) of health-care interventions (10,11). Items of particular interest to AECOPD evaluations are reviewed here.

Time Horizon

Chronic obstructive pulmonary disease is a lifelong illness, and AECOPD can be expected to occur during the course of illness. As noted above, the duration of follow-up will influence the number of exacerbations captured in the database. This issue is important for CEA because short durations of follow-up may not capture a representative sample of exacerbations (or none at all). Patients in one sample may have very high costs (or frequencies) while others have low costs due to statistical variation rather than true differences related to therapy. Ideally, costs and outcomes should be tracked for a minimum of 12 months' time to capture a sufficient number of exacerbations and to account for seasonal variation.

Credible Alternatives to the Intervention of Interest

New interventions for AECOPD must be compared with the standard of care for persons with similar age, gender, and comorbidity profiles. For this reason, economic evaluations based on placebo-controlled studies usually are inappropriate. Economic evaluations of new drugs should not be based on efficacy trials, unless the trials include the full complement of usual therapy in the absence of the new treatment, for example.

Selecting a Measure of Effectiveness

What is the best measure of effectiveness for treatments for AECOPD? The measure of effectiveness should capture the impact of the AECOPD on the individual *over time*. Frequency, severity, and duration of the events are important measures of success. Finally, quality of life and survival—the summary measures of the impact of any medical treatment—should ideally be evaluated. The episodic nature and varying severity of AECOPD make it particularly challenging for the researcher to capture all these issues in a single measure of effectiveness.

The most widely accepted measure combining quality of life and survival time is the quality-adjusted-life-year (QALY) (11). Because QALYs are well studied, stem from a solid theoretical foundation, and allow decision makers to compare health-care interventions both within and across diseases, we recommend this measure for studies in AECOPD whenever feasible. The difficulty for using QALYs as a measure of effectiveness in AECOPD stems from their potential lack of responsiveness to treatments, particularly those that impact severity rather than frequency. Other "clinical" measures of outcome, such as days without an exacerbation or days without oxygen, also are often meaningful to both patients and clinicians. One must use care with these measures, however, because some can influence both the numerator and denominator of a CEA (e.g., exacerbations). Such "double counting" can severely influence the interpretability of these measures.

We suggest including at least one measure that captures quality of life in any economic evaluation of AECOPD. The measure can be "generic" such as health-state utilities that are used to derive QALYs, or disease-specific, that is, has questions that are particularly relevant to persons with pulmonary disease. Providing multiple measures of effectiveness improves decision makers' understanding of the economic impact of the treatment and complements the measure of effectiveness that is chosen to derive the cost-effectiveness ratio.

B. Analysis Issues

Measuring Costs

Medical care costs are characterized by certain distributional properties that must be accounted for in an analysis. Failure to account for these issues will result in biased estimates of cost and, possibly, misguided conclusions for the study.

First, costs accrue unevenly over time, and months or years can go by with "zeros" in the database. Second, costs are skewed, with small numbers of patients having very high costs compared with other, larger numbers of patient groups across populations. Third, observations can be censored, that is, incomplete due to disenrollment or loss of follow-up. Fourth, retrospective studies are subject to uncontrolled factors that can confound the analysis.

Important recent advances in cost estimation can effectively address these issues. In rare cases where censoring is not an issue, two-part models with log transformation of dependent variables have traditionally been used to estimate costs in the setting of masses of observations with value equal to zero and skewed data (12,13). More recently, generalized linear models have addressed the issue of skewness with a more flexible and probably more robust modeling format (14,15). Although almost universally present in economic databases, censoring has only recently been recognized as an issue that can bias cost studies (16,17). Methods have been developed to estimate costs in the face of censoring, including multivariate methods that can address potential confounding in retrospective analyses (18).

Adjusting for Comorbidity

Individuals with AECOPD often have more comorbidity than age and gender-matched persons without COPD because of the impact of smoking on developing coronary artery disease, cancers, and other illnesses. In addition, persons with COPD may come from different socioeconomic groups than those without the disease because smoking is disproportionate among those with lower socioeconomic standing and in certain racial and ethnic groups (19,20). To estimate the impact of COPD on burden-of-illness or CEA studies, one must control for these factors. If persons in the two treatment groups differ in terms of their comorbidity status, this must be accounted for in the analysis.

Various methods used to control for comorbidity have been adapted to adjust for the impact of comorbid conditions on costs of care in multivariate analyses (21–24). It is important that the method accounts both for the *mix* of conditions and the *severity* of each condition as they impact cost. Some studies have focused on diagnoses for hospitalizations (25), but more recent studies show that comorbidities found largely in the ambulatory setting can also be important (12). Other studies have relied on pharmacy claims as measures of severity (13,26), although such data are frequently unavailable from administrative or clinical trial databases.

VI. Cost-Effectiveness Studies of Therapies for AECOPD

We searched for studies reporting the cost-effectiveness of treatments for exacerbations of COPD (Table 2). The databases used included the ones noted above for the burden of illness of AECOPDs. The search was limited to treatments for AECOPDs. Preventive therapies that may reduce the frequency exacerbations, but are difficult to separate for therapies aimed at treating chronic symptoms, are not included. In addition, studies of therapies for acute exacerbations of chronic bronchitis that are not clearly limited to patients with coexisting COPD, are excluded.

The few available studies vary widely in terms of treatments considered. All consider hospital costs only for individuals with severe exacerbations. Survival is a common outcome, but measures that incorporate quality of life were not uniform.

Table 2 Cost-Effectiveness Studies of Treatments for Persons with AECOPD

Study (Ref.)	Population	Treatment	Analysis method	Measure of effectiveness	Outcomes
27	Severe exacerbations requiring hospitalization, clinical criteria	Noninvasive positive pressure ventilation vs. standard therapy	Meta-analysis of trials	Survival, hospital days	Mortality OR: 0.22 [0.1–0.66] Savings per patient $3244 (1996, $CDN)
28	Exacerbations requiring mechanical ventilation	Pulmonary artery catheter vs. no catheter	Decision model	QALYs[a]	$77,407/QALY (1992, $US)
19	Severe exacerbations requiring hospitalization clinical criteria	Pulmonologist vs. generalist care	Analysis of observational data	Survival	OR 30-day mortality with pulmonologists: 1.6 [0.98–2.5] Costs $6400 in each arm (1994 $US), ($p = 0.99$)
20	Mild-to-moderate COPD exacerbation by clinical criteria	Home support vs. hospital admission	Piggyback CEA alongside RCT[b]	Spirometry, respiratory-specific QOL,[c] patient and physician satisfaction	No difference in QOL £877 for home care vs. £1753 (1997, £UK) for hospital care[d]

[a]Quality-adjusted life years.
[b]Randomized, controlled trial.
[c]QOL—quality of life measured by the Chronic Respiratory Disease Questionnaire.
[d]Confidence intervals or tests for statistical significance of cost difference not provided.

VII. Conclusions

Despite the incidence and economic and human burden of acute exacerbations for persons with COPD, very little economic information is available regarding this condition. Cost-effectiveness studies of treatments for AECOPDs are also important, particularly for decision makers that must make resource allocation decisions under budget constraints. Future studies of the burden of AECOPD and cost-effectiveness studies of new treatments for AECOPD should consider standardized criteria for case finding, identifying relevant costs, and specifying duration of follow-up.

References

1. Sullivan SD, Ramsey SD, Lee TA. The economic burden of COPD. Chest 2000; 117 (2 suppl):5S–9S.
2. American Lung Association, 1993.
3. Staton GW Jr, Ingram RH Jr. Chronic obstructive diseases of the lung. In: Rubenstein E, Federman DD, eds. Sci Am Med 1995; 3:1–25.
4. http://www.ncbi.nlm.nih.gov/entrez/query.fcgi?db = PubMed. Accessed February 4, 2003.
5. http://agatha.york.ac.uk/nhsdhp.htm. Accessed February 4, 2003.
6. Destache CJ, Dewan N, O'Donohue WJ, Campbell JC, Angelillo VA. Clinical and economic considerations in the treatment of acute exacerbations of chronic bronchitis. J Antimicrob Chemother 1999; 43(Suppl A):107–113.
7. McGuire A, Irwin DE, Fenn P, Gray A, Anderson P, Lovering A, MacGowan A. The excess cost of acute exacerbations of chronic bronchitis in patients aged 45 and older in England and Wales. Value Health 2001; 4(5):370–375.
8. Miravitlles M, Murio C, Guerrero T, Gisbert R. Pharmacoeconomic evaluation of acute exacerbations of chronic bronchitis and COPD. Chest 2002; 121(5):1449–1455.
9. Connors AF Jr, Dawson NV, Thomas C, Harrell FE Jr, Desbiens N, Fulkerson WJ, Kussin P, Bellamy P, Goldman L, Knaus WA. Outcomes following acute exacerbation of severe chronic obstructive lung disease. The SUPPORT investigators (Study to Understand Prognoses and Preferences for Outcomes and Risks of Treatments). Am J Respir Crit Care Med 1996; 154(4 Pt 1):959–967.
10. Drummond MF, Jefferson TO. Guidelines for authors and peer reviewers of economic submissions to the BMJ. The BMJ Economic Evaluation Working Party. Br Med J 1996; 313(7052):275–283.
11. Siegel JE, Torrance GW, Russell LB, Luce BR, Weinstein MC, Gold MR. Guidelines for pharmacoeconomic studies. Recommendations from the panel on cost effectiveness in health and medicine. Panel on Cost Effectiveness in Health and Medicine. Pharmacoeconomics 1997; 11(2):139–168.
12. Klabunde CN, Potosky AL, Legler JM, Warren J. Development of a comorbidity index using physician claims data. J Clin Epidemiol 2000; 53(12):1258–1267.
13. Von Korff M, Wagner EH, Saunders K. A chronic disease score from automated pharmacy data. J Clin Epidemiol 1992; 45(2):197–203.
14. Manning WG, Mullahy J. Estimating log models: to transform or not to transform? J Health Econ 2001; 20(4):461–494.

15. Blough DK, Ramsey SD. Using generalized linear models to assess medical care costs. Health Serv Outcomes Res Methodol 2000; 1:185–202.

16. Hallstrom AP, Sullivan SD. On estimating costs for economic evaluation in failure time studies. Med Care 1998; 36(3):433–436.

17. Lin DY, Feuer EJ, Etzioni R, Wax Y. Estimating medical costs from incomplete follow-up data. Biometrics 1997; 53(2):419–434.

18. Etzioni RD, Feuer EJ, Sullivan SD, Lin D, Hu C, Ramsey SD. On the use of survival analysis techniques to estimate medical care costs. J Health Econ 1999; 18(3):365–380.

19. Regueiro CR, Hamel MB, Davis RB, Desbiens N, Connors AF Jr, Phillips RS. A comparison of generalist and pulmonologist care for patients hospitalized with severe chronic obstructive pulmonary disease: resource intensity, hospital costs, and survival. SUPPORT Investigators. Study to Understand Prognoses and Preferences for Outcomes and Risks of Treatment. Am J Med 1998; 105(5):366–372.

20. Skwarska E, Cohen G, Skwarski KM, Lamb C, Bushell D, Parker S, MacNee W. Randomized controlled trial of supported discharge in patients with exacerbations of chronic obstructive pulmonary disease. Thorax 2000; 55(11):907–912.

21. Fishman PA, Shay DK. Development and estimation of a pediatric chronic disease score using automated pharmacy data. Med Care 1999; 37(9):874–883.

22. Deyo RA, Cherkin DC, Ciol MA. Adapting a clinical comorbidity index for use with ICD-9-CM administrative databases. J Clin Epidemiol 1992; 45(6):613–619.

23. Naessens JM, Leibson CL, Krishan I, Ballard DJ. Contribution of a measure of disease complexity (COMPLEX) to prediction of outcome and charges among hospitalized patients. Mayo Clin Proc 1992; 67(12):1140–1149.

24. McGuire TE. An evaluation of diagnosis-related group severity and complexity refinement. Health Care Financ Rev 1991; 12(4):49–60.

25. Charlson ME, Pompei F, Ales KL, MacKenzie CR. A new method of classifying prognostic comorbidity in longitudinal studies: development and validation. J Chronic Dis 1987; 40(5):373–383.

26. Lamers LM. Pharmacy costs groups: a risk-adjuster for capitation payments based on the use of prescribed drugs. Med Care 1999; 37(8):824–830.

27. Keenan SP, Gregor J, Sibbald WJ, Cook D, Gafhi A. Noninvasive positive pressure ventilation in the setting of severe, acute exacerbations of chronic obstructive pulmonary disease: more effective and less expensive. Crit Care Med 2000; 28(6):2094–2102.

28. Smith KJ, Pesce RR. Pulmonary artery catherization in exacerbations of COPD requiring mechanical ventilation: a cost-effectiveness analysis. Respir Care 1994; 39(10):961–967.

5

Pathophysiology of Acute Exacerbations of Chronic Obstructive Pulmonary Disease

WILLIAM MacNEE

University of Edinburgh
Edinburgh, Scotland

I. Introduction

Exacerbation of a disease implies worsening of the underlying pathophysiological process that characterizes the condition. Indeed the term exacerbate (derived from the Latin *exacerberi*, to irritate) has a dictionary definition (to make more violent, more severe) that suggests this. However, with respect to chronic obstructive pulmonary disease (COPD), it is not clear if we are justified in using the term "an exacerbation *of* COPD," which implies worsening of the underlying disease or "an exacerbation *in* COPD," which does not necessarily suggest worsening of the underlying disease process. However, since it has been shown that the cause of an acute exacerbation in COPD is not determined in around 30% of cases (1), this implies that in some cases exacerbations could be part of a cyclical worsening of the disease process itself, with or without known triggers. Indeed patients report that their condition is better or worse on some days than others, without obvious precipitating factors, although factors other than infection and air pollution, which are considered to be the major precipitants, seem to exacerbate symptoms and may lead to an exacerbation in a patient with COPD, (such as changes in weather and temperature and changes in physical activity). However, whether an exacerbation of COPD is an extension of the disease itself or is different from the disease process is still a matter of debate. Indeed, the term exacerbation—an endogenous or exogenous irritation—correctly describes the possible processes that create an exacerbation.

There is no generally accepted definition of an exacerbation of COPD. However, an operational definition has been produced recently (2): "a sustained worsening of the patient's condition, from the normal stable state and beyond normal day-to-day variations, that is acute in onset and necessitates a change in regular medication, in a patient with underlying COPD." Thus an acute exacerbation is a syndrome and its recognition is characterized by worsening of symptoms, particularly breathlessness, that exceeds day-to-day variations and does not respond to treatment with the patient's regular medication.

Considering the huge health-care burden in mortality and morbidity from COPD, and the fact that exacerbations account for a large proportion of this burden, it is perhaps surprising that there is a relative paucity of studies in COPD exacerbations. However, acute exacerbations in COPD (AECOPD) have been difficult to study because of the acute nature of the disease, compounded by the lack of a generally accepted definition of an AECOPD. A description of the pathophysiology of COPD is also complicated by the fact that AECOPD are heterogeneous, both in their etiology, known and unknown causes, and in their severity, which ranges from mild exacerbations, which can be managed by the patient at home with an increase in therapy, to severe exacerbations requiring hospital admission, on occasion leading to acute on chronic respiratory failure. Furthermore, the severity of the exacerbation clearly relates to the underlying disease severity. An exacerbation in patients with severe underlying COPD, with perhaps established chronic respiratory failure, is likely to result in more severe adverse effects than in a patient with mild COPD.

The severity of the underlying disease is also a risk factor for the frequency of AECOPD. This is clear from recent large studies of inhaled corticosteroids. The mean number of exacerbation rates in the patients in the ISOLDE study (3), where the FEV_1 was 50% predicted, was 1.90 exacerbations per year, compared to 0.37 exacerbations per year in the Copenhagen City Lung Study, where the FEV_1 was 87% predicted (4). Chronic hypermucus secretion is also a risk factor for AECOPD (5). Recent data from the Lung Health Study has shown a relationship between exacerbations of COPD requiring medical intervention and continued cigarette smoking associated with chronic hypermucus secretion (6). The presence of systemic features in patients with COPD is also a risk factor for AECOPD, as shown by the fact that low body mass index ($BMI < 20 \, kg/m^3$), limited exercise tolerance measured by 6-min walking distance ($\leq 367 \, m$), significant gas exchange impairment ($PO_2 \leq 65 \, mmHg$, $PaCO_2 > 44 \, mmHg$) are all predictive factors for hospitalization in AECOPD.

The cardinal symptom of the syndrome of an AECOPD is increased dyspnea, which may have multiple causes, including changes in pulmonary mechanics and gas exchange (7,8).

It has traditionally been considered that the clinical picture of an AECOPD depends on the degree of worsening of airflow limitation, together with the severity of the underlying COPD and the association of other comorbidities (9). The current view is that this increase in airflow limitation results from increased inflammation in the airways, precipitated by a known or unknown trigger factor for the exacerbation. Until recently, there was relatively little information to support or refute this view. In recent years, however, there have been several studies that have assessed both the symptomatic, physiological, and inflammatory changes in exacerbations of COPD. However, these studies have to be interpreted in light of the heterogeneity of both the underlying disease and of the exacerbation. Most studies have been cross-sectional, usually with assessments made at one time point in the exacerbation with a lack of longitudinal studies in AECOPD.

II. Inflammation in AECOPD

Around 60 to 70% of exacerbations of COPD appear to have a precipitating cause, or at least an associated factor, commonly either viral or bacterial infection. A small proportion, around 10%, are probably associated with inhalation of environmental pollution, especially increases in particulate air pollution, and in about 30% a cause is not apparent. However, it is assumed that an increase in the inflammatory response in the large and small airways (i.e., a bronchitis and/or a bronchiolitis to a known or unknown trigger) results in an AECOPD. There is, however, a relative lack of histological descriptions of the pathology of AECOPD (10). Limited postmortem studies in patients who died during AECOPD show increased airspace inflammation, with inflammatory cell infiltration with a variety of cells in both airway and alveolar walls, exudation of mucus, and mucus plugging (10). However, the findings in patients who have died of the disease cannot be extrapolated to all exacerbations of COPD. Furthermore, similar information is not available for mild or moderate AECOPD. Whether or not in enhanced inflammatory response in the airways is present in all AECOPD is unknown, but this is assumed to be the case. It is known, however, that exacerbations of COPD are associated with events that cause the initiation of an inflammatory response in the airspaces as shown by increased sequestration of neutrophils in the pulmonary microcirculation and presumably also in the bronchial circulation (11), and that these cells may be primed to release reactive oxygen species (12). Recent studies in AECOPD, largely in patients with mild disease, consisting of chronic bronchitis without much airflow limitation, have shown a significant increase in both eosinophils and neutrophils both in sputum and in bronchial biopsy specimens (13). But, in contrast to exacerbations of asthma, where increased eosinophils are noted in the airways, in AECOPD these eosinophils do not degranulate (14) and are not associated with increased expression of IL-5 (15). The cause of this eosinophilia in the airways is not known, but may be due to viral infections and may only occur in a subset of patients characterized with "asthma-like features" who may be more responsive to corticosteroids. In more severe AECOPD, predominantly in patients with exacerbations caused by bacterial infection, there are increased numbers of neutrophils, increased myeloperoxidase (a marker of neutrophil activation), and increased levels of interleukin-8, an important neutrophil chemoattractant in the airway lumen, all indicating increased neutrophilic inflammation (16). These studies emphasize the difficulties in extrapolating the results of studies in a disease that itself is heterogeneous, where there are differences between patients in severity of the underlying disease when the patients are clinically stable. Furthermore, the etiology of the exacerbations may be different between and even within studies of AECOPD and, finally, there are potential conflicting effects of preceding treatment on the inflammatory response produced during an exacerbation. Similar problems have arisen in interpreting the nature of the acute inflammatory response in studies where markers of inflammation in both sputum, serum urine, and exhaled breath samples have been assessed (16–22). In general, these studies all seem to show evidence of increased mediators of bronchial inflammation, as shown by increased myeloperoxidase activity and increased levels of interleukins-6 and -8, tumor necrosis factor, and leukotreine B_4 in sputum in AECOPD (16,17). There is also evidence that oxidative stress is increased in the airways in AECOPD, which may enhance the inflammatory response by increasing gene expression for proinflammatory mediators (23). This is evidenced by increased levels of hydrogen peroxide, nitric oxide, and 8-isoprostane, a lipid peroxidation product in exhaled breath in AECOPD (21,22,24). There is also evidence of a systemic inflammatory response as shown by increased levels of serum acute phase proteins, such as $\alpha 1$-antitrypsin and C-reactive protein (25) and also systemic oxidative stress as shown by increased plasma levels of lipid peroxidation products and a decrease in the antioxidant capacity in the blood of patients during AECOPD (26). However, all of these studies are in relatively small numbers of patients with COPD, without recognition of the different clinical phenotypes or causes of the exacerbation. Few studies have made more than one measurement in patients in and out of an exacerbation and the time course of the changes in inflammatory events before and during the AECOPD have not been studied in detail.

It is therefore possible that markers of inflammation may rise in response to the exacerbation rather than triggering the exacerbation. Furthermore, most of the studies which have assessed inflammatory markers and cells have largely used samples derived from the large airways and it is likely that more important events in the exacerbation may occur in the small airways. Indeed, historical autopsy studies of patients dying of AECOPD describe a "bronchiolitis exudativa" and such a bronchiolitis has been described in 26% of patients with AECOPD at autopsy (27).

The inflammatory response in AECOPD could increase airflow limitation in small airways as a result of a number of events, such as vascular congestion of the airway mucosa and plasma exudation (28,29) triggered by increased inflammation (30) in already inflamed airways. Furthermore, goblet cell hyperplasia can occur rapidly (31) resulting in increased mucus hypersecretion (32) stimulated, for example, by the release of neutrophil elastase (33,34), which would result in increased airflow limitation and mucus plugging in the small airway lumen. Mucus hypersecretion in COPD could also be caused by a number of mediators such as leukotrienes, proteinases, and neuropeptides released from inflammatory cells.

It is presumed that the deterioration in symptoms, particularly breathlessness in AECOPD, is due to increased airflow limitation (35). There are, however, few sequential measurements of airflow limitation in patients with AECOPD. In a randomized controlled trial of antibiotic therapy in 448 COPD exacerbations in 173 patients with moderate-to-severe COPD (mean ± SD FEV_1 % predicted 33.9 ± 13.7%), Anthonisen and colleagues showed an improvement in peak flow during treatment of the exacerbation (Fig. 1) (36). The time course showed that the peak expiratory flow (PEF) had returned to the baseline value by day 14. Similarly, in a cohort of 155 patients with COPD in general practice followed over 3 years, Sachs and coworkers (35) studied 71 exacerbations in 55 patients. However, these were a younger group of patients (mean age 51.7 years) than in most studies of AECOPD of whom 50% were asthmatics. Small changes in PEF were shown to occur again over the course of 14 days, but there was still a slight decrease in the PEF compared with the stable baseline values in both studies at what was considered to be the time of the resolution of the exacerbation. Davies and colleagues (37)

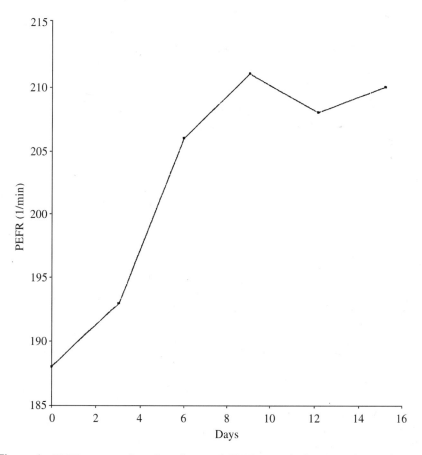

Figure 1 PEFR recovery from day of onset of COPD exacerbation. (Based on Ref. 36.)

measured FEV_1 repeatedly in a group of patients with AECOPD and showed an improvement in FEV_1 during treatment of the exacerbations, with a greater improvement in those treated with oral corticosteroid therapy compared with those given a placebo (Fig. 2). PEF readings may underestimate the degree of airflow limitation compared with FEV_1, which may be a more useful measurement, although there are no studies comparing these measurements in exacerbations (38).

Studies of the time course of recovery of AECOPD using spirometry or PEF are confounded by lack of a universal agreement on the day of onset of the exacerbation, which in some studies is taken as the day of presentation (36,38) and in others is defined in terms of the onset of a sustained increase in breathlessness (35). In a recent study of 101 patients with moderate-to-severe COPD (mean FEV_1 42% predicted) followed over a period of 2.5 years, there were 405 exacerbations. Over 60% of the exacerbations recorded were associated with increased dyspnea and around 20% with increased cough (39). However, exacerbations in this study were defined as the presence, for at least 2 consecutive days as recorded by the patient in a daily diary card, of an increase in any two major symptoms (dyspnea, sputum purulence, sputum amount) and one minor symptoms (wheeze, sore throat, cough, or symptoms of the common cold, which were nasal congestion/discharge), a definition modified from that used in the study by Anthonisen and colleagues (36). Based upon this definition, almost 50% of the exacerbations were not reported by the patients, confirming the findings of a previous study by the same group (40). This study also showed that adverse changes in symptoms (but not peak expiratory flow) occurred before the onset of the exacerbation (Fig. 3) and that there were very small decreases in peak flow at the onset of the exacerbation, such that the mean change in peak expiratory flow expressed as a percentage of baseline was 4.5%. Interestingly, there was no difference in the decrease in PEF, FEV_1, or FVC or increase in the symptom score at the onset of exacerbation between the reported and unreported exacerbations. Similarly, recovery times as measured by changes in PEF, FEV_1, or symptom score, which for PEF was around 7 days from the onset of the AECOPD, were not different between reported and unreported exacerbations. In this study only 75% of the patients were considered to have fully recovered their baseline PEFR at 5 weeks, but the changes from baseline were very small and, interestingly, antibiotic therapy had no effect on the time to or the completeness of the recovery from the exacerbation (40) (Fig. 4). The changes in FEV_1 during exacerbation in a smaller cohort of 34 patients who measured daily FEV_1 by hand-held spirometer, although highly significant, were very small, amounting to a mean fall in FEV_1 of 24 mL (range 16.1–84.3 mL). This study also showed significantly greater falls in peak expiratory flows in AECOPD, associated with increased dyspnea, increased wheeze, or symptoms of a cold, but not associated with other symptoms (40).

Thus there is limited information that increased airways obstruction, at least in terms of changes in FEV_1 and PEF, occur acutely in AECOPD and largely recover at the end of an exacerbation, although the changes in measurements of airflow obstruction are small. In the largest study of the time course of changes in pulmonary function in AECOPD there were no differences in the changes in measurements of airflow obstruction between those patients who reported an

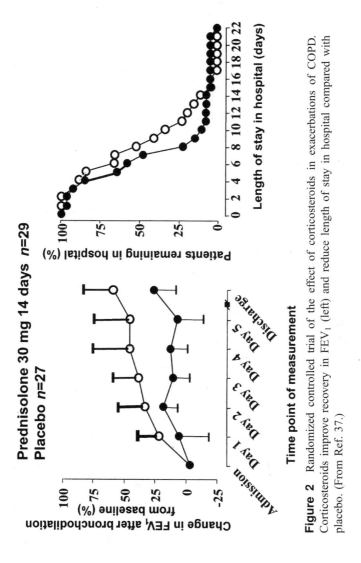

Figure 2 Randomized controlled trial of the effect of corticosteroids in exacerbations of COPD. Corticosteroids improve recovery in FEV$_1$ (left) and reduce length of stay in hospital compared with placebo. (From Ref. 37.)

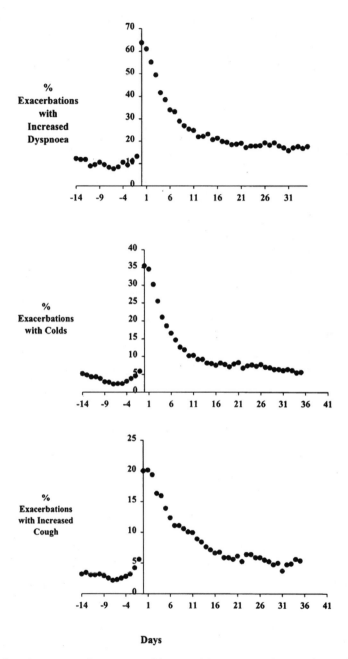

Figure 3 Time course of symptoms of increased dyspnea, nasal congestion, and cough for 504 exacerbations in 91 patients. Proportion of exacerbations with any one symptom over the 14 days before to 35 days after onset of exacerbation, expressed as a percentage of the total number of exacerbations. (From Ref. 40.)

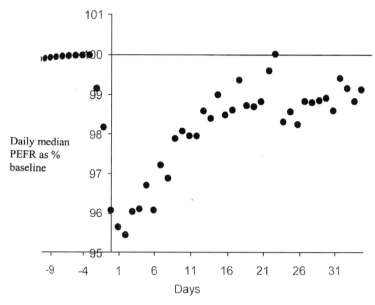

Figure 4 Median peak flow expressed as a percentage of baseline peak flow from 14 days prior to 35 days after onset of exacerbation for 504 exacerbations in 91 patients. (From Ref. 40.)

exacerbation and those in whom an exacerbation was obtained from a diary card of symptom scores, without the patient feeling the need to report it (40). Thus, during mild exacerbations of COPD, expiratory airflow is almost unchanged (13) and indeed is only slightly reduced during severe exacerbations (8,40).

Therefore, what are the mechanisms that underlie the increased symptoms in AECOPD? Expiratory airflow limitation, which is the hallmark of COPD, results from pathological changes that occur in large and small airways and in the lung parenchyma. Several factors, some of which are reversible and others irreversible, account for the airflow limitation (Table 1). These changes result in airway narrowing, with resulting increased resistance to airflow and loss of lung elastic

Table 1 Causes of Airflow Limitation in COPD

Irreversible	• Fibrosis and narrowing of airways
	• Loss of elastic recoil due to alveolar destruction
	• Destruction of alveolar support that maintains patency of small airways
Reversible	• Accumulation of inflammatory cells, mucus, and plasma exudates in bronchi
	• Smooth muscle contraction in peripheral and central airways
	• Dynamic hyperinflation during exercise

recoil, with a resultant decrease in driving pressure for expiratory flow. Airway narrowing results from several factors. Normally the lung parenchyma serves to keep the airways open. In emphysema, due to loss of the supporting alveolar walls, this effect is reduced. In addition, there is thickening and narrowing of bronchial and bronchiolar walls, constriction of bronchial smooth muscle, and intraluminal mucus and cell debris. In a normal subject, the expiratory limb of the maximum flow-volume loop reaches a peak flow at around 80% of the vital capacity (i.e., near total lung capacity). During tidal breathing, a very small proportion of the maximum flow-volume loop is used and inspiratory and expiratory flows remain far from the maximum. In this case, the pattern can be modified in any direction by increasing inspiratory and expiratory flow or increasing or decreasing lung volume. In a patient with severe COPD, the area of the expiratory flow-volume loop is markedly reduced compared to the normal subject and this reduction is proportional to the severity of the COPD (Fig. 5a,b). In this case, at any given lung volume, forced inspiratory and expiratory flows are reduced, as is forced vital capacity. The inspiratory limb of the flow-volume loop still remains far from the maximum possible value. By contrast, expiratory flows are very close to the values obtained at the same lung volume during forced expiration. Thus, tidal expiratory flow can be equal to forced expiratory flow and at times it can exceed it, resulting in expiratory flow limitation. This is a reflection of the collapsibility of the airways in severe COPD.

In order to compensate for airflow limitation, attempts can be made to increase inspiratory flow, allowing more time for exhalation, or overinflation can occur, which increases end-expiratory volume and functional residual capacity (FRC), but which takes advantage of higher expiratory flows at higher lung volumes due to both decreased airways resistance and increased elastic recoil. Eventually a new equilibrium is reached at some end-expiratory volume above FRC. This results in an inability to return to passive FRC before the next breath occurs, a process called dynamic hyperinflation. Both of these compensatory mechanisms result in an increased work of breathing and therefore place the inspiratory muscles, particularly the diaphragm, at a mechanical disadvantage due to length-tension effects. In addition, when the respiratory system rests above FRC at end-expiration, this creates a residual lung recoil pressure, producing a positive alveolar pressure (41). Thus, before air can enter the lung, alveolar pressure must be negative relative to atmospheric pressure. It follows that a proportion of the inspiratory muscle pressure generated with each breath will be wasted in overcoming the residual recoil pressure of the respiratory system. In addition, because breathing takes place at a higher lung volume, it occurs over the less compliant portion of the lung pressure–volume cycle and thus increases the work of breathing. This dynamic hyperinflation is probably a major contributor to the sensation of dyspnea in stable patients and probably also to the increased dyspnea in AECOPD (42). In patients with exacerbations of COPD, there is a further reduction in the forced expiratory flow-volume loop under these circumstances in severe exacerbations of COPD and the ability to compensate may be impossible.

Respiratory failure will occur against this background as a result of changes in the characteristics of the respiratory system, either an increase in the overall load

(A)

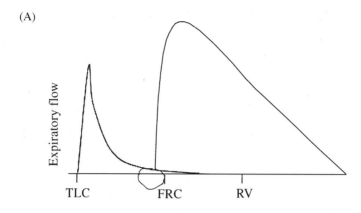

(B)

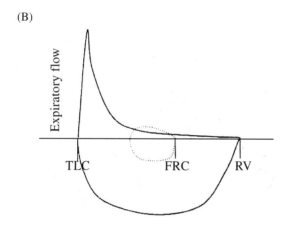

Figure 5 (A) Flow volume loop demonstrating the typical pattern seen in severe chronic obstructive pulmonary disease (solid line). Relative to the normal loop (dashed line), the total lung capacity (TLC) and residual volume (RV) are elevated, consistent with hyperinflation and gas trapping as is functional residual capacity (FRC). Expiratory flow limb is concave with a marked decrease in expiratory flows, particularly at lower lung volumes. (B) In severe airflow limitation, flows with tidal breathing (dashed line) often exceed maximal expiratory flow as determined by the maximal flow volume loop (solid line).

beyond the possible compensatory mechanisms or changes that impair the function or effectiveness of the respiratory muscles and central nervous system to compensate. In severe exacerbations, the primary physiological change is worsening of gas exchange, induced by increase in ventilation/perfusion ($V_{A/Q}$) inequality. As $V_{A/Q}$ relationships worsen, increased work of the respiratory muscles produces greater oxygen consumption, and hence decreased oxygen tensions, which further amplifies the gas exchange abnormalities (8). The pathological changes that result in abnormal $V_{A/Q}$ relationships in AECOPD are due to airway inflammation, edema, mucus hypersecretion, and bronchoconstriction, all of which may contribute to the changes in the distribution of ventilation. Hypoxic vasoconstriction of pulmonary arteries may modify the distribution of perfusion. Worsening gas exchange in AECOPD is also contributed to by abnormal patterns of breathing and fatigue of the respiratory muscles. All of these factors can lead to further deterioration in blood gases and worsening respiratory acidosis, which may lead to severe respiratory failure and death (8,43). Alveolar hypoventilation also contributes to hypoxemia, hypercapnia, and respiratory acidosis and also promotes pulmonary vasoconstriction, which increases pulmonary artery pressure and puts an added load on the right ventricle.

Other vascular events may play an adverse role in AECOPD. Although the most common cause of death in exacerbations of COPD is due to respiratory failure (44), other causes may contribute, including pulmonary thromboembolic disease. Postmortem studies have shown pulmonary arterial thrombi in a large proportion of patients with COPD who died in respiratory failure (45). Thrombi in small vessels occur in situ in patients with COPD, but it is not clear whether such events result in acute exacerbations.

The most common circumstance of death in patients with COPD is respiratory failure (44). In a cross-sectional study of 215 patients in whom detailed information was available at the time of death, Zielinski and colleagues found that the most common circumstances of death were respiratory failure (35%), cor pulmonale with edema (13%), pulmonary infections (12%), and pulmonary embolism (10%) (44). Although respiratory failure is a common cause of death, comorbidity also plays a role. Several studies have investigated which variables predict death after admission for an exacerbation of COPD and therefore identify at-risk subjects. In a cohort of 270 patients followed over 3 years from the index admission with an AECOPD, Incalzi and coworkers (46) found the predictors of mortality were age, signs of right ventricular hypertrophy, chronic renal failure, ischemic heart disease, and FEV_1.

Connors and colleagues (47) studied a prospective cohort of 1016 adult patients from five hospitals who were admitted with an exacerbation of COPD, with a $PaCO_2 > 5$ mmHg. In this population, survival was independently related to a number of factors, including the severity of the illness, body mass index, age, prior functional status, PaO_2, inspiratory oxygen fraction (FiO_2), congestive cardiac failure, serum albumin, and the presence of cor pulmonale (47). Poor treatment outcome, as assessed by a return visit with a respiratory problem requiring further treatment within 4 weeks following an exacerbation, was also related to the severity of the airways obstruction. Other factors associated with poor treatment outcome following an exacerbation are the use of home oxygen therapy, frequency of exacerbations, history of previous pneumonia, and the use of maintenance oral corticosteroids (48,49).

III. Respiratory Drive to Breathing

The pattern of breathing in acute exacerbations of COPD is clearly different from the chronic state. In stable COPD patients, the respiratory frequency increases and the tidal volume decreases as the disease progresses (50). In AECOPD, patients take shorter and smaller breaths with a respiratory frequency approximately twice as high as normal subjects.

The changes in blood gases in stable COPD patients have been attributed to several factors including decreased sensitivity of the respiratory centers, ventilation perfusion in homogeneity [increase in dead space $(V_D V_T)$], the Haldane effect, an increase in carbon dioxide production (VCO_2), mechanical limitation of active ventilation, changes in the central setting of respiratory timing, or a combination of all of these factors. The hypoxic drive to breathing is not the most important determinant of the activity of the respiratory center (51). In addition, administration of oxygen to patients with COPD in acute respiratory failure does not seem to induce a major change in breathing pattern (50,52,53). $P_{0.1}$ pressure, as a measure of respiratory drive, is usually high in stable COPD and increases further in acute respiratory failure.

IV. Gas Exchange

Ventilatory failure is defined conventionally by a higher than normal $PaCO_2$. $PaCO_2$ depends on both respiratory and nonrespiratory factors (54), metabolic regulation, as well as on respiratory variables. Under normal circumstances, in a steady state, CO_2 removal by the lungs equals the VCO_2. The relationship between ventilation of perfused alveoli ($V'A$) $PaCO_2$ is given by the equation

$$PaCO_2 = \frac{k \times V'CO_2}{V'A}$$

The normal response of the ventilatory system to any increase in VCO_2 or in $PaCO_2$ beyond the normocapnic level is by increasing minute ventilation ($V'E$). Only a fraction of the ventilation that remains available for gas exchange after the dead space ventilation is useful for CO_2 elimination:

$$PaCO_2 = \frac{k \times V'CO_2}{V'E \times (1 - VD/VT)}$$

One of the major determinants of $PaCO_2$ in hypercapnic respiratory failure is the VD/VT ratio, which is consistently increased in hypercapnic respiratory failure, while changes in VCO_2 are inconsistent (55–57).

Hypoxemia in respiratory failure is due to a combination of several factors (hyperventilation, ventilation perfusion mismatch, right-to-left shunt, diffusion alteration, and low mixed venous oxygen tension). As with the $PaCO_2$ the degree of heterogeneity of ventilatory and perfusion ratios seems the most important underlying determinant for PaO_2 (58). Hypoxemia itself produces pulmonary vasoconstriction, resulting in pulmonary hypertension (59), and may eventually lead to right ventricular dysfunction.

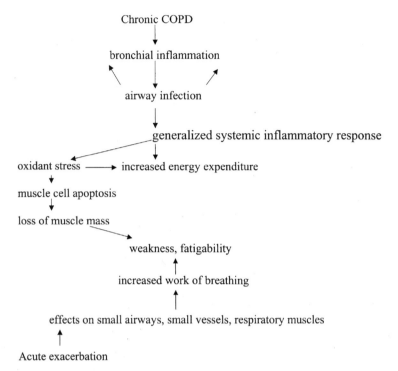

Figure 6 The pathophysiological and pathobiological factors and small lung vessels that occur during an acute exacerbation of chronic obstructive pulmonary disease. (Modified from Ref. 60.)

V.   Conclusion

It is clear that more information is required on the pathophysiology of AECOPD. Certainly more information is required to understand what an exacerbation of COPD really is before more specific treatments can be used both to prevent and to treat AECOPD. The simple view of the development of exacerbations needs to be extended by further research and, although inflammatory markers and biopsy studies help us to understand the events in the large airways, events in the smaller airways are clearly critical to both the pathology and the pathophysiology and hence the symptoms that develop in these patients. Understanding the mechanisms associated with changes in these airways could lead to benefits from new interventions in this condition (Fig. 6).

References

1. Chodosh S. Bronchitis and asthma. In: Gorbach SI, ed. Infectious Diseases. Philadelphia: WB Saunders, 1992:476–485.
2. Rodriguez-Roisin R. Toward a consensus definition for COPD exacerbations. Chest 2000; 117(5 suppl 2):398S–401S.

3. Burge PS, Calverley PM, Jones PW, Spencer S, Anderson JA, Maslen TK. Randomised, double blind, placebo controlled study of fluticasone propionate in patients with moderate to severe chronic obstructive pulmonary disease: the ISOLDE trial. Br Med J 2000; 320(7245):1297–1303.

4. Vestbo J, Prescott E, Lange P. Association of chronic mucus hypersecretion with FEV_1 decline and chronic obstructive pulmonary disease morbidity. Copenhagen City Heart Study Group. Am J Respir Crit Care Med 1996; 153(5):1530–1535.

5. Lange P, Nyboe J, Appleyard M, Jensen G, Schnohr P. Relation of ventilatory impairment and of chronic mucus hypersecretion to mortality from obstructive lung disease and from all causes. Thorax 1990; 45(8):579–585.

6. Kanner RE, Anthonisen NR, Connett JE. Lower respiratory illnesses promote FEV(1) decline in current smokers but not ex-smokers with mild chronic obstructive pulmonary disease: results from the lung health study. Am J Respir Crit Care Med 2001; 164(3):358–364.

7. Delafosse C, Similowski T, Derenne JP. Causes and pathophysiology of chronic obstructive pulmonary disease exacerbations. Monaldi Arch Chest Dis 1998; 53(3):305–311.

8. Barbera JA, Roca J, Ferrer A, Felez MA, Diaz O, Roger N, Rodriguez-Roisin R. Mechanisms of worsening gas exchange during acute exacerbations of chronic obstructive pulmonary disease. Eur Respir J 1997; 10(6):1285–1291.

9. Siafakas NM, Bouros D. Management of acute exacerbations of chronic obstructive pulmonary disease. In: Postma DS, Siafakas NM, eds. Management of Chronic Obstructive Pulmonary Disease. Eur Respir Monogr 1998; 3:264–277.

10. Pare PD, Hegele RG, Hogg JC. The lung pathology of acute exacerbations of chronic obstructive pulmonary disease. In: Derenne JP, Whitelaw WA, Similowski T, eds. Acute Respiratory Failure in COPD. New York: Marcel Dekker, 1996.

11. Selby C, MacNee W. Factors affecting neutrophil transit during acute pulmonary inflammation: minireview. Exp Lung Res 1993; 19(4):407–428.

12. Aaron SD, Angel JB, Lunau M, Wright K, Fex C, Le Saux N, Dales RE. Granulocyte inflammatory markers and airway infection during acute exacerbation of chronic obstructive pulmonary disease. Am J Respir Crit Care Med 2001, 163:349–355.

13. Saetta M, Di Stefano A, Maestrelli P, Turato G, Ruggieri MP, Roggeri A, Dalcagni P, Mapp CE, Ciaccia A, Fabbri LM. Airway eosinophilia in chronic bronchitis during exacerbations. Am J Respir Crit Care Med 1994; 150(6 Pt 1):1646–1652.

14. Lacoste JY, Bousquet J, Chanez P, Van Vyve T, Simony-Lafontaine J, Lequeu N, Fic P, Enander I, Godard P, Michel FB. Eosinophilic and neutrophilic inflammation in asthma, chronic bronchitis, and chronic obstructive pulmonary disease. J Allergy Clin Immunol 1993; 92(4):537–548.

15. Saetta M, Di Stefano A, Maestrelli P, Turato G, Mapp CE, Pieno M, Zanguochi G, Del Prete G, Fabbri LM. Airway eosinophilia and expression of interleukin-5 protein in asthma and in exacerbations of chronic bronchitis. Clin Exp Allergy 1996; 26(7): 766–774.

16. Crooks SW, Bayley DL, Hill SL, Stockley RA. Bronchial inflammation in acute bacterial exacerbations of chronic bronchitis: the role of leukotriene B4. Eur Respir J 2000; 15(2):274–280.

17. Bhowmik A, Seemungal TA, Sapsford RJ, Wedzicha JA. Relation of sputum inflammatory markers to symptoms and lung function changes in COPD exacerbations. Thorax 2000; 55(2):114–120.

18. Shindo K, Hirai Y, Fukumura M, Koide K. Plasma levels of leukotriene E4 during clinical course of chronic obstructive pulmonary disease. Prostaglandins Leukotr Essent Fatty Acids 1997; 56(3):213–217.

19. Drazen JM, O'Brien J, Sparrow D, Weiss ST, Martins MA, Israel E, Fanta CH. Recovery of leukotriene E4 from the urine of patients with airway obstruction. Am Rev Respir Dis 1992; 146(1):104–108.

20. Yamakami T, Taguchi O, Gabazza EC, Yoshida M, Kobayashi T, Kobayashi H, Yasui H, Ibata H, Adachi Y. Arterial endothelin-1 level in pulmonary emphysema and interstitial lung disease. Relation with pulmonary hypertension during exercise. Eur Respir J 1997; 10(9):2055–2060.

21. Agusti AG, Villaverde JM, Togores B, Bosch M. Serial measurements of exhaled nitric oxide during exacerbations of chronic obstructive pulmonary disease. Eur Respir J 1999; 14(3):523–528.

22. Dekhuijzen PN, Aben KK, Dekker I, Aarts LP, Wielders PL, van Herwaarden CL, Bast A. Increased exhalation of hydrogen peroxide in patients with stable and unstable chronic obstructive pulmonary disease. Am J Respir Crit Care Med 1996; 154(3 Pt 1):813–816.

23. Rahman I, MacNee W. Role of oxidants/antioxidants in smoking-induced lung diseases. Free Radic Biol Med 1996; 21(5):669–681.

24. Montuschi P, Collins JV, Ciabattoni G, Lazzeri N, Corradi M, Kharitonov SA, Barnes PJ. Exhaled 8-isoprostane as an in vivo biomarker of lung oxidative stress in patients with COPD and healthy smokers. Am J Respir Crit Care Med 2000; 162(3 Pt 1):1175–1177.

25. Dev D, Wallace E, Sankaran R, Cunniffe J, Govan JR, Wathen CG, Emmanuel FX. Value of C-reactive protein measurements in exacerbations of chronic obstructive pulmonary disease. Respir Med 1998; 92(4):664–667.

26. Rahman I, Skwarska E, MacNee W. Attenuation of oxidant/antioxidant imbalance during treatment of exacerbations of chronic obstructive pulmonary disease. Thorax 1997; 52(6):565–568.

27. Mitchell RS, Silvers GW, Dart GA, Petty TL, Vincent TN, Ryan SF, Filley GF. Clinical and morphologic correlations in chronic airway obstruction. Aspen Emphysema Conference, 1968, pp. 109–123.

28. Persson CG. Airway epithelium and microcirculation. Eur Respir Rev 1994; 4:353–362.

29. Persson CG, Erjefalt JS, Andersson M, Greiff L, Svensson C. Extravasation, lamina propria flooding and lumenal entry of bulk plasma exudate in mucosal defence, inflammation and repair. Pulm Pharmacol 1996; 9(3):129–139.

30. Lams BE, Sousa AR, Rees PJ, Lee TH. Immunopathology of the small-airway submucosa in smokers with and without chronic obstructive pulmonary disease. Am J Respir Crit Care Med 1998; 158(5 Pt 1):1518–1523.

31. Takeyama K, Dabbagh K, Lee H-M, Agusti C, Lausier JA, Veki IF, Grattan KM, Nadel JA. Epidermal growth factor system regulates mucin production in airways. Proc Natl Acad Sci USA 1999; 96:3081–3086.

32. Prescott E, Lange P, Vestbo J. Chronic mucus hypersecretion in COPD and death from pulmonary infection. Eur Respir J 1995; 8(8):1333–1338.

33. Takeyama K, Agusti C, Ueki I, Lausier J, Cardell LO, Nadel JA. Neutrophil-dependent goblet cell degranulation: role of membrane-bound elastase and adhesion molecules. Am J Physiol 1998; 275(2 Pt l):L294–L302.

34. Sommerhoff CP, Nadel JA, Basbaum CB, Caughey GH. Neutrophil elastase and cathepsin G stimulate secretion from cultured bovine airway gland serous cells. J Clin Invest 1990; 85(3):682–689.

35. Sachs AP, Koeter GH, Groenier KH, van der WD, Schiphuis J, Meyboom-de Jong B. Changes in symptoms, peak expiratory flow, and sputum flora during treatment with antibiotics of exacerbations in patients with chronic obstructive pulmonary disease in general practice. Thorax 1995; 50(7):758–763.

36. Anthonisen NR, Manfreda J, Warren CP, Hershfield ES, Harding GK, Nelson NA. Antibiotic therapy in exacerbations of chronic obstructive pulmonary disease. Ann Intern Med 1987; 106(2)196–204.

37. Davies L, Wilkinson M, Bonner S, Calverley PM, Angus RM. "Hospital at home" versus hospital care in patients with exacerbations of chronic obstructive pulmonary disease: prospective randomised controlled trial [In Process Citation]. Br Med J 2000; 321(7271):1265–1268.

38. Kelly CA, Gibson GJ. Relation between FEV1 and peak expiratory flow in patients with chronic airflow obstruction. Thorax 1988; 43(4):335–336.

39. Seemungal TA, Donaldson GC, Bhowmik A, Jeffries DJ, Wedzicha JA. Time course and recovery of exacerbations in patients with chronic obstructive pulmonary disease. Am J Respir Crit Care Med 2000; 161(5):1608–1613.

40. Seemungal TA, Donaldson GC, Paul EA, Bestall JC, Jeffries DJ, Wedzicha JA. Effect of exacerbation on quality of life in patients with chronic obstructive pulmonary disease. Am J Respir Crit Care Med 1998; 157(5 Pt 1):1418–1422.

41. Decramer M. Respiratory muscle interaction during acute and chronic hyperinflation. Monaldi Arch Chest Dis 1993; 48(5):483–488.

42. O'Donnell DE, Revill SM, Webb KA. Dynamic hyperinflation and exercise intolerance in chronic obstructive pulmonary disease. Am J Respir Crit Care Med 2001; 164(5):770–777.

43. Rodriguez-Roisin R. Pulmonary gas exchange in acute respiratory failure. Eur J Anaesthesiol 1994; 11(1):5–13.

44. Zielinski J, MacNee W, Wedzicha J, Ambrosino N, Braghiroli A, Dolensky J, Howard P, Gorselak K, Lahdensuo A, Strom K, Tobiasz M, Weitzenblum E. Causes of death in patients with COPD and chronic respiratory failure. Monaldi Arch Chest Dis 1997; 52(1):43–47.

45. Calverley PM, Howatson R, Flenley DC, Lamb D. Clinicopathological correlations in cor pulmonale. Thorax 1992; 47(7):494–498.

46. Incalzi RA, Fuso L, De Rosa M, Forastiere F, Rapiti E, Nardecchia B, Pistelli R. Co-morbidity contributes to predict mortality of patients with chronic obstructive pulmonary disease. Eur Respir J 1997; 10(12):2794–2800.

47. Connors AF Jr, Dawson NV, Thomas C, Harrell FE Jr, Desbiens N, Fulkerson WJ, Kussin P, Bellamy P, Goloman L, Knaus WA. Outcomes following acute exacerbation of severe chronic obstructive lung disease. The SUPPORT investigators (Study to Understand Prognoses and Preferences for Outcomes and Risks of Treatments) [published erratum appears in Am J Respir Crit Care Med 1997; 155(1):386]. Am J Respir Crit Care Med 1996; 154(4 Pt 1): 959–967.

48. Fuso L, Incalzi RA, Pistelli R, Muzzolon R, Valente S, Pagliari G, Gliozzi F, Ciappi G. Predicting mortality of patients hospitalized for acutely exacerbated chronic obstructive pulmonary disease. Am J Med 1995; 98(3):272–277.

49. Niewoehner DE, Collins D, Erbland ML. Relation of FEV(1) to clinical outcomes during exacerbations of chronic obstructive pulmonary disease. Department of Veterans Affairs Cooperative Study Group. Am J Respir Crit Care Med 2000; 161(4 Pt 1): 1201–1205.

50. Loveridge B, West P, Kryger MH, Anthonisen NR. Alteration in breathing pattern with progression of chronic obstructive pulmonary disease. Am Rev Respir Dis 1986; 134(5):930–934.

51. De Troyer A, Peche R, Yernault JC, Estenne M. Neck muscle activity in patients with severe chronic obstructive pulmonary disease. Am J Respir Crit Care Med 1994; 150(1): 41–47.

52. Aubier M, Murciano D, Milic-Emili J, Touaty E, Daghfous J, Pariente R, Derenne JP. Effects of the administration of O_2 on ventilation and blood gases in patients with chronic obstructive pulmonary disease during acute respiratory failure. Am Rev Respir Dis 1980; 122(5):747–754.

53. Sassoon CS, Hassell KT, Mahutte CK. Hyperoxic-induced hypercapnia in stable chronic obstructive pulmonary disease. Am Rev Respir Dis 1987; 135(4):907–911.

54. Ingram RH Jr, Miller RB, Tate LA. Acid-base response to acute carbon dioxide changes in chronic obstructive pulmonary disease. Am Rev Respir Dis 1973; 108(2):225–231.

55. Merton PA. Voluntary strength and fatigue. J Physiol 1954; 67:553–564.

56. Bellemare F, Bigland-Ritchie B. Assessment of human diaphragm strength and activation using phrenic nerve stimulation. Respir Physiol 1984; 58(3):263–277.

57. Merton PA, Hill DK, Morton HB. Indirect and direct stimulation of fatigued human muscles. CIBA Foundation Symposium 1981; 82:120–129.

58. Marthan R, Castaing Y, Manier G, Guenard H. Gas exchange alterations in patients with chronic obstructive lung disease. Chest 1985; 87(4):470–475.

59. Weitzenblum E, Sautegeau A, Ehrhart M, Mammosser M, Hirth C, Roegel E. Long-term course of pulmonary arterial pressure in chronic obstructive pulmonary disease. Am Rev Respir Dis 1984; 130(6):993–998.

60. Voelkel NF. Exacerbation of chronic obstructive pulmonary disease. In: Voekel NF, MacNee W, eds. Chronic Obstructive Lung Disease. London: BC Decker, Inc, 2002: 353–363.

6

Immunopathology of Chronic Obstructive Pulmonary Disease and Exacerbations of Bronchitis

PETER K. JEFFERY, JIE ZHU, and YUSHENG QIU

MARINA SAETTA and GRAZIELLA TURATO

National Heart and Lung Institute
Imperial College London
London, England

University of Padua
Padua, Italy

I. Introduction

By European consensus, COPD is defined as "a disorder characterized by reduced maximum expiratory flow and slow forced emptying of the lungs; features which do not change markedly over several months. Most of the airflow limitation is slowly progressive and irreversible" (1). The most recently published world guidelines on obstructive lung disease (GOLD) describe the airflow limitation as "associated with an abnormal inflammatory response of the lungs to noxious particles or gases" (2). Exacerbations of symptoms requiring medical intervention are important clinical events in COPD. Infection and air pollution are important triggers, but the cause of approximately one-third of severe exacerbations is unclear. Those in which infection is identified show increases of sputum volume and change in its color; fever may also be present.

At least three inflammatory conditions contribute to COPD: chronic bronchitis (mucus hypersecretion), chronic bronchiolitis (small airways disease), and emphysema. These conditions are interrelated but it is not clear whether they are part of a single spectrum of progression (with respect to anatomical location, severity, or time) or interrelated by their common association with smoking. While not all COPD is associated with smoking, the relationship between cigarette smoking and COPD is a strong one statistically. In genetically predisposed individuals, the inflammation initiated by cigarette smoke is probably responsible for most of the symptoms and pathological abnormalities associated with COPD and its progression. Even when relatively stable, there are influxes of inflammatory cells into the airways and lung parenchyma of patients with COPD. Severity of airflow limitation is associated with severity of airway inflammation even in stable disease (3–5). It is generally considered, but not proven, that at these tissue sites, such inflammatory cells release a myriad of inflammatory mediators that are ultimately toxic, damaging tissue and contributing to disease progression. Direct examination of airway and lung tissue support the presence of a marked inflammatory infiltrate even in stable phases of both chronic bronchitis and COPD. The pattern of inflammation is distinct to that found in asthma and to the balance of immune cells found in the airways of normal subjects (6,7). There is both enlargement and destruction of tissue structures and changes also occur in the pulmonary vasculature and, in advanced disease, the right heart (8).

The importance of exacerbations associated with the proinflammatory effects of acute infection requires clarification. With recurrent exacerbations, there is increased inflammation that changes in character. The increased infiltration of tissues by inflammatory cells is associated, in ways that are presently unclear, with increased symptoms, worsening of clinical status, and, it is hypothesized, with decline of lung function. Recent data have indicated that exacerbations may contribute to accelerated decline of lung function in those who continue to smoke (9). We have learned and continue to learn much about the immunopathology of the airway mucosa in patients with relatively stable disease. However, relatively little is known about that which occurs in association with an exacerbation no matter what its cause. This chapter reviews first what is known of the airway immunopathology of stable disease and then focuses on immunopathological observations of bronchial biopsies taken following an exacerbation (i.e., an acute clinical worsening in patients with chronic bronchitis or mild-to-moderate COPD). The focus is on changes in the bronchial wall as nothing is known concerning the immunopathological changes during exacerbations in the distal airways and lung parenchyma. Alterations identified in sputum and BAL are mentioned only in passing.

II. Stable Chronic Bronchitis and COPD in Smokers

Smoking tobacco per se induces an inflammatory response. Smoking shortens the transit time of neutrophils through the bone marrow, causes leukocytosis, and alters the immunoregulatory balance of T-cell subsets found in blood, bronchoalveolar lavage (BAL), and tissues of the conducting airways and lung (10–12). Smoking initiates a peripheral blood leukocytosis and a reversible decrease in the normally high CD4-to-CD8 cell ratio in blood of heavy smokers (i.e., >50 pack-years). There is also a significant reduction of the CD4-to-CD8+ cell ratio in BAL fluid but not in blood of a group of milder smokers (i.e., who have smoked on average

14 pack-years). The increase in the number of BAL and tissue CD8+ T-cells is positively associated with pack-years smoked (7,11,13).

A. Chronic Bronchitis

Histological examination of airway tissues (taken at resection for tumor) from smokers demonstrates that inflammatory cells are present in and around the area of mucus-secreting submucosal glands and that scores of inflammation show a better association with the subjects who have symptoms of mucus hypersecretion than does gland size per se (14). The safe use of the flexible fiberoptic bronchoscope as an investigative tool has allowed us the opportunity to investigate the changes that occur in the airway mucosa of proximal airways in relatively mild bronchitics and those that occur during the genesis of COPD. Of course, this assumes that what is sampled proximately reflects the inflammatory changes seen in smaller, more peripheral airways and lung parenchyma and there is emerging evidence to support this (5).

In bronchial biopsies of subjects with mild, stable chronic bronchitis and COPD, there is infiltration of the mucosa by inflammatory cells (6,7,15,16): this is associated with upregulation of cell-surface adhesion molecules of relevance to the inflammatory process (17). In the surface epithelium, where, in contrast to the subepithelium, CD8+ cells normally predominate, Fournier and colleagues origin-ally demonstrated by comparison with nonsmokers an increase in lymphocytes of all subsets in smokers with chronic bronchitis and mild COPD (18). In the subepithelial zone, in mild-to-moderate disease and in the absence of an exacerbation, bronchial lymphomononuclear cells appear to form the predominant cell type and neutrophils are scanty. The mononuclear component is composed of lymphocytes, plasma cells, and macrophages. Significant increases are reported in the numbers of CD45 (total leukocytes), CD3 (T-lymphocytes), CD25 (i.e., activated), and VLA-1 (late activa-tion) positive cells, presumed to be T-lymphocytes, and of macrophages (15). The endobronchial biopsy studies of O'Shaughnessy and coworkers have demonstrated that, by comparison with normal nonsmokers, T-lymphocytes and neutrophils increase in the surface epithelium while T-lymphocytes and macrophages increase in the subepithelium of smokers with COPD (6,19). In contrast to asthma, it is the CD8+ T-cell and not the CD4+ T-cell subset, which increases in number and proportion to become the predominant T-cell subset in COPD (Fig. 1). Furthermore, the increase of CD8+ cells shows a statistically significant negative association with forced expiratory volume in 1 s (FEV$_1$ expressed as a percentage of predicted). This novel distinction between the relative proportions of T-cell subsets of smokers with mild, stable COPD and nonsmoking mild asthmatics has received the support of subsequent studies of bronchial biopsies (13). The increase of the CD8/CD4 ratio seen in the mucosa also occurs deeper in the submucosa of the bronchial wall in association with submucosal mucus-secreting glands in bronchitic smokers (20). Mucous glands are also characterized by neutrophil infiltration (20) (Fig. 2a, b). Since neutrophil elastase is a remarkably potent secretagogue for cultured gland cells (21), the location of neutrophils within the bronchial glands may be crucial for the

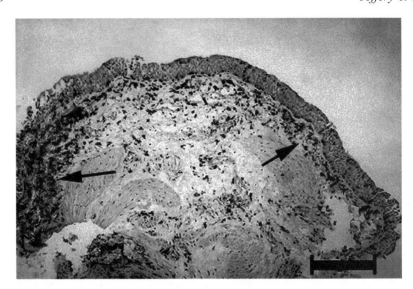

Figure 1 Histological section of an endobronchial biopsy of a large airway (i.e., second- or third-order bronchus) from a smoker with COPD. The mucosa, immunostained with anti-CD8 antibody, shows extensive inflammation composed predominantly of CD8+ T-cells both within and below the epithelium (arrows). Scale bar = 150 μm.

activation of the secretory function of gland cells and therefore for the induction of chronic sputum production in subjects with chronic bronchitis.

B. Chronic Bronchiolitis

Histologically, the earliest observed effect of cigarette smoke in small airways and surrounding alveoli is a marked increase in the number of macrophages and neutrophils, both in humans and experimentally in animal studies. The increase is seen within both the tissue and lumena and can be detected in BAL (22). Examination of small airways in lungs resected from smokers, stable at the time of surgery, shows that the same profile of CD8-predominant inflammation reported in bronchial biopsies of the larger airways occurs deeper in the lung in the small airways (23) (Fig. 3). As with the findings in the large conducting airways, there is a significant negative association of the numbers of CD8+ cells and FEV_1% of predicted in the small (peripheral) conducting airways also, suggesting an important role for these cells in the pathophysiology of COPD. However, the cytokine profile of these T-lymphocytes and their chemokine receptor expression has not been fully investigated. It has been recently shown that the T-cells infiltrating the peripheral airways in COPD express CXCR3, a chemokine receptor that is known to be preferentially expressed on type 1 cells (24). The fact that, in COPD, CXCR3-positive cells are CD8-positive and express IFN-γ suggests a Tc-1 immune response in this disease (25).

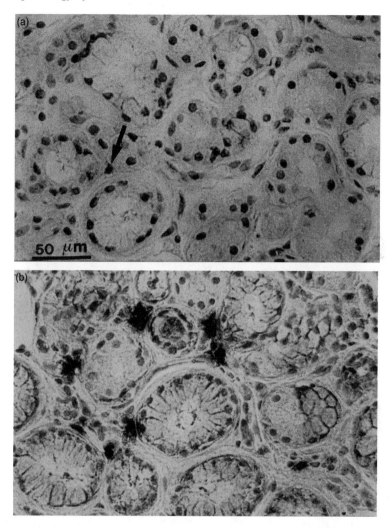

Figure 2 Neutrophil infiltration of the mucus-secreting bronchial submucosal glands in lung tissue resected from smokers: (a) the asymptomatic smokers show few cells (arrow) whereas (b) the smoker with symptoms of mucus hypersecretion (i.e., chronic bronchitis) has many neutrophils infiltrating between the secretory acini. Scale bar = 50 μm. Neutrophils detected by immunostaining sections with anti-human neutrophil elastase.

C. Emphysema

Normally, the macrophage is the resident phagocyte of the alveolus: neutrophils are rarely present (26). Neutrophils may be recruited to the lung parenchyma in smokers albeit the extent of tissue neutrophilia is variable. On exposure to cigarette smoke, there is recruitment of macrophages and phagocytosis of cigarette smoke components. A macrophage alveolitis and respiratory bronchiolitis are the early changes in

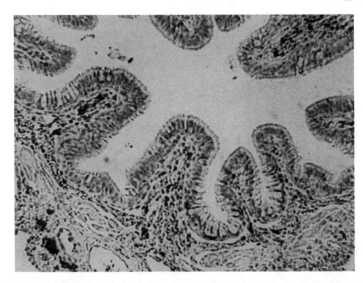

Figure 3 CD8 T-lymphocyte infiltration in a peripheral airway (bronchiole) in tissue resected from a smoker with COPD demonstrating the same CD8 T-cell predominance described in the mucosa of endobronchial biopsies of larger airways (bronchi). Immunostained with anti-CD8 antibody.

young cigarette smokers (27,28). As in the large and small conducting airways in COPD, CD8+ cells are also increased in the alveolar wall and their numbers show a similarly strong inverse correlation with $FEV_1\%$ of predicted as that seen in the small and large conducting airways (29,30). Thus the CD8+ cell increase is seen at both proximal and distal sites. This consistency of change indicates that sampling the large airways by biopsy does have the potential to provide information about the broad patterns of inflammation occurring more distally in the lung.

When COPD progresses, there is a further increase of CD8+ cells both in small airways and lung parenchyma, which is associated with an increase of other inflammatory cell types, as recently demonstrated in patients undergoing lung volume reduction surgery (LVRS) for severe emphysema (4,5). This enhanced inflammatory response is correlated with the degrees of airflow limitation, lung hyperinflation, CO diffusion impairment, and radiological emphysema, suggesting a role for this inflammatory response in the clinical progression of the disease.

D. Inflammation in Vessel Walls

Surprisingly, there are only a few studies that examine the inflammatory process in pulmonary arteries of subjects with COPD despite the fact that there is involvement of these vessels due to the close approximation of airways and pulmonary arteries and the spread of the inflammatory process from the bronchiolar wall to the adjacent vessel. An inflammatory process similar to that present in the conducting airways and in the lung parenchyma, consisting predominantly of increased numbers of

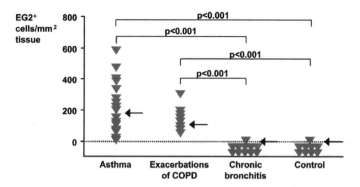

Figure 4 Counts of eosinophils in endobronchial biopsies of patients following an exacerbation of bronchitis (column 2) demonstrating their increased numbers as compared with chronic bronchitis in its stable phase and normal healthy controls (right). The increased numbers of eosinophils seen in exacerbations approaches that found in stable asthma (left). Immunostained with an antibody, EG2, against the cleaved or secreted form of eosinophil cationic protein.

CD8+ T-lymphocytes, has been reported in the adventitia of pulmonary arteries in smokers with COPD (30,31). The vascular infiltration of CD8+ cells correlates with the degree of airflow limitation in these subjects (30), supporting the role of vascular inflammation in the progression of the disease.

III. Mild Exacerbations of Bronchitis

COPD and asthma would seem to differ at the tissue level in a number of respects; for example, the marked tissue eosinophilia and thickening of the reticular basement membrane of asthma are not usually features of COPD (32). However, compared to normal healthy control tissue, there are a number of studies that report small, but significant, numbers of tissue eosinophils in subjects with chronic bronchitis or COPD (6,14,33), particularly during an exacerbation of the disease (32,33) (Fig. 4). Sputum eosinophilia is also reported in cases of "eosinophilic bronchitis" (i.e., patients without a history of asthma and without bronchial hyperresponsiveness but who respond to inhaled corticosteroids) (34–36). In a recent report, these patients with eosinophilic bronchitis have been shown to have a similar degree of eosinophilia, a similar thickening of the basement membrane but a lower number of mast cells in airway smooth muscle as compared to asthmatic patients (37).

In mild exacerbations of bronchitis, eosinophils are increased not only in bronchial tissue, but also in sputum and BAL indicating a similar inflammatory process in the airway wall and in the airway lumen. This eosinophilia is associated with a marked recruitment of tissue neutrophils (Fig. 5a) and with an increased expression of the cytokine TNF-α (Fig. 5b, c). TNF-α can induce an influx of inflammatory cells in the airway tissue either through a direct chemotactic effect or

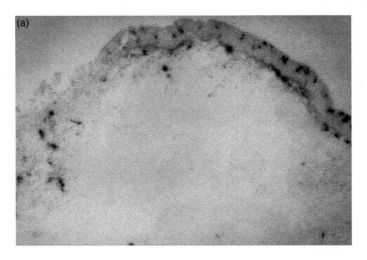

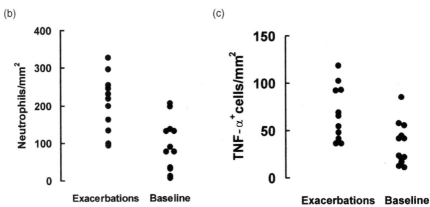

Figure 5   (a) Neutrophil infiltration of the bronchial epithelium of a smoker with mild COPD and an exacerbation of bronchitis. (b) Individual counts for neutrophils and (c) TNF-α in bronchial biopsies of subjects with chronic bronchitis examined during exacerbations and under baseline conditions. the results are expressed as number of cells per mm² of tissue examined. Immunostaining with anti-human neutrophil elastase.

through an increased expression of the adhesion molecules on endothelial cells. This latter mechanism is supported by the observation of an enhanced vascular expression of E-selectin in the bronchial mucosa of subjects with chronic bronchitis (17).

In asthma, the infiltration of tissue by eosinophils is an allergic reaction to allergen exposure. It is part of a response in which memory T-helper cells regulate specificity of the response. T-helper cells orchestrate the sequence of events via the production and secretion of interleukins (IL), notably IL-4 and IL-5, and eosinophil chemoattractants that include eotaxin, MCP-4 (monocyte chemoattractant protein), and regulated on activation, normal T-cell expressed and secreted (RANTES)

(38–40). These cytokines and chemokines are capable of multiple and interactive effects and IL-4 and IL-5 are required for tissue eosinophilia to occur. Importantly, the chemoattractant gradients that induce emigration and give direction to the movements of eosinophils within the tissues are provided by the secretion of chemokines produced by both inflammatory and structural cells, including airway surface epithelium and even bronchial smooth muscle (41,42). The molecular technique of ISH demonstrates that there is gene expression, for IL-4 and also for IL-5 in mild COPD. IL-4 has also recently been demonstrated in abundance in association with submucosal glands of patients with chronic bronchitis (43). However, study of endobronchial biopsies shows that the number of cells expressing these genes in stable bronchitis and in exacerbation are similar. The novel identification in chronic bronchitis of gene expression for the eosinophil chemoattractants, eotaxin, MCP-4, and RANTES, emphasizes the similarities that can exist in bronchial tissues between mild COPD when there is an exacerbation of bronchitis and exacerbations associated with asthma (44). As previously described in asthma, eotaxin mRNA is expressed by surface epithelium (40) and it appears to be strongly expressed by subepithelial mononuclear inflammatory cells. Gene expression and tissue distribution of MCP-4 in chronic bronchitis is similar to that of eotaxin. While eotaxin mRNA shows greater than normal expression in bronchitic smokers as compared to healthy nonsmokers, neither chemokine is upregulated significantly in association with an exacerbation nor does the number of cells expressing either of these chemokines show a significant association with the observed increase in the number of tissue eosinophils. The most striking finding associated with an exacerbation in mild disease is reported to be the upregulation of RANTES in both inflammatory and epithelial cells of the bronchial mucosa (Fig. 6a–c). It is suggested that the significant positive relationship between RANTES and tissue eosinophilia (Fig. 7) supports a role for this mechanism in the initiation of a tissue eosinophilia in the population of bronchitics with a recent exacerbation (44).

It is probable that the factors initiating the exacerbation are also responsible for the upregulation of RANTES. Although bacteria may also play a role (45–48), it is considered that viral infection is the most likely cause and inducer of epithelial RANTES during an exacerbation of bronchitis. Previous studies have shown that RSV upregulates RANTES experimentally following RSV inoculation of primary bronchial epithelial cells and the airway epithelial cell line BEAS 2 B. During the logarithmic phase of infectious virus production, only RANTES—and not MCP-1, MCP-3, or MIP-1α—is upregulated in an infection-dependent manner (49). To confirm these studies in vivo, RANTES has been measured in nasal lavage fluid obtained from children. RANTES is significantly increased in children with RSV infection as compared with the noninfected group in a stable phase of their disease. There is also evidence that both RANTES and IL-8 can be upregulated by inactive forms of RSV and can be detected along with MIP-1α in lower respiratory tract secretions in infants with RSV bronchiolitis (50). Additional evidence for the central role of RANTES production in response to viral infection comes from experimental studies of infection by influenza virus A (51). RANTES, IL-6, and IL-8 are released in significant amounts from the bronchial epithelial cell line, NCI-H292, and

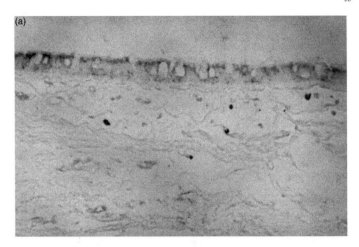

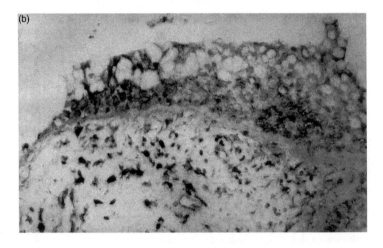

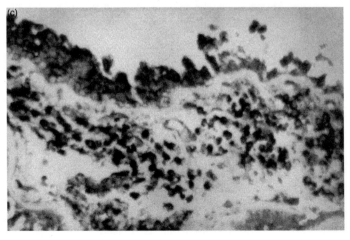

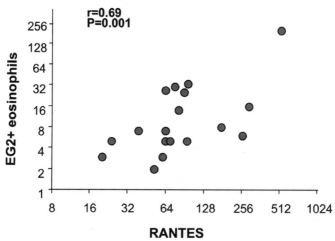

Figure 7 Graph showing the positive association between the increased numbers of tissue eosinophils (immunostained by EG2 antibody) and RANTES gene expression Data are $\log_2$-transformed). (From Ref. 44.)

RANTES mRNA and protein are detected in supernatants of cultured, primary bronchial and nasal polyp epithelial cells 24 to 72 h after influenza virus A infection. The supernatants of the virus-infected cells have potent chemotactic activity for eosinophils, which is attenuated after addition of anti-RANTES antibody (52). Sputum IL-6 has been shown to increase during exacerbations of patients with COPD and raised sputum levels of IL-8, measured during the stable phase of disease, are associated with relatively high exacerbation frequency (53). It would be instructive to measure RANTES in the sputa during such exacerbations.

The numbers of CD4+ cells are significantly lower in bronchitis as compared with normal healthy controls. In comparison with stable CB, exacerbations of CB are associated with an increased number of CD4+ cells and there is a relative fall in the CD8:CD4 ratio due primarily to the increase of the CD4 subset. The current working hypothesis proposed by Jeffery and colleagues (44) is that an exacerbation due to viral infection of airway surface epithelium in smokers with bronchitis induces a marked upregulation of epithelial RANTES. RANTES, acting through CCR3 receptors, is most responsible for the recruitment of tissue eosinophils in

---

Figure 6 Gene expression for RANTES (regulated on activation T-cell-expressed and secreted) in endobronchial biopsies. (a) There is very little gene expression for this eosinophil chemoattractant molecule in nonsmoking healthy controls. (b) There is increased expression in inflammatory cells beneath the epithelium and moderate expression in the epithelium of smokers with chronic bronchitis. (c) In exacerbations of bronchitis there is a marked increase of RANTES gene expression both in the epithelium and in subepithelial inflammatory cells. In situ hybridization demonstrating RANTES mRNA as black intracellular end-product. (From Ref. 44.)

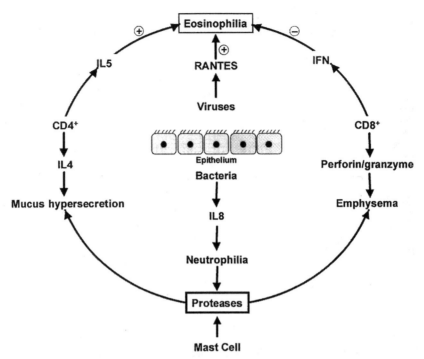

Figure 8 Proposed inflammatory mechanisms for exacerbations of COPD. The regulatory interleukins, IL-4 and IL-5 produced by CD4+ T-lymphocytes are associated with mucus hypersecretion and tissue eosinophilia. In contrast, the cytokines and effector molecules produced by CD8+ T-cells are associated with the cell lysis, development of emphysema and suppression of eosinaphilia. IFN = interferon gamma. IL = interleukin. (From Jeffery PK. The pathology of COPD and exacerbations. Eur Resp Rev 2002; 12:2–4.

virally induced exacerbations of bronchitis but also, via CCR3 and CCR4 receptors, recruits CD4+ memory cells (54) with consequent reduction of the normally high CD8:CD4 ratio present in stable disease. The prevailing balance between CD4+ and CD8+ cells at the time of an exacerbation may be critical (Fig. 8). There is evidence that RANTES acts synergistically with CD8+ cytolytic cells to enhance FAS-ligand-dependent apoptosis of virally infected cells (55,56). Thus when CD8+ cells predominate, exacerbations and increased RANTES may promote CD8-mediated tissue damage. Increased frequency of viral exacerbations may thus destroy airway and alveolar tissue directly, encouraging the development of microscopic emphysema (57). In this way, repeated exacerbations due to viral infection may accelerate decline in lung function in smokers whose CD8 T-cell numbers are already raised (6). This would be particularly important in a subset of individuals with an already high genetically determined CD8:CD4 ratio (58) and whose smoking habit has elevated the numbers of CD8+ cells even further (11). It would be reasonable to predict that CD8 cytolytic activity in response to viral exposure would be more vigorous than normal in such individuals and result in enhanced tissue destruction (41,42). This and other hypotheses require further investigation both in vitro and in vivo.

IV. Severe Exacerbations in COPD

The numbers of neutrophils are significantly increased in both sputum and bronchial biopsies in severe exacerbations of COPD compared to their stable phases (3,59–65). The recent results of examination of biopsies of patients hospitalized and intubated for their exacerbation demonstrate an approximately 100-fold increase of neutrophil numbers as compared with the stable phase of the disease (66). Neutrophil recruitment into airways is due, in part, to chemoattraction by neutrophil chemokines including IL-8, epithelial-derived neutrophil attractant-78 (ENA-78), growth-related protein-α, β, and γ (Groα, β, and γ), neutrophil-activating peptide-2 (NAP-2), and human granulocyte chemotactic protein 2 (GCP-2). IL-8 is well known as a potent chemoattractant and activating cytokine for neutrophils and, to a lesser extent, for eosinophils. Endothelial cells, fibroblasts, epithelial cells, alveolar macrophages, and neutrophils are able to release IL-8 in response to specific stimuli (TNF, IL-1, and endotoxin) (67). It is believed that these chemokines attract neutrophils via their interaction with specific receptors on the cell surface, namely, CXCR1 and CXCR2. IL-8 predominately binds to CXCR1 while Groα, β, and γ, NAP-2, GCP-2, ENA-78, as well as IL-8, bind mainly to CXCR2. Both receptors are highly expressed on neutrophils and macrophages and have been demonstrated to play functionally different roles on human neutrophils in vitro. The receptors are also found to be expressed on activated T-lymphocytes, mast cells, dentritic cells, basophils, and eosinophils; however, no functional significance for the presence of the receptors on these cells has been demonstrated in vivo.

It has been suggested that despite similar affinities for IL-8 and similar receptor numbers of CXCR1 and CXCR2, neutrophil chemotaxis is primarily mediated by the CXCR1 (68,69). Patel et al. (70) recently studied expression and function of such chemokine receptors in human peripheral blood leukocytes and reported that upregulation of the receptor expression and strong calcium responses were seen in neutrophils following stimulation with the CXCR1 and CXCR2 ligands, IL-8, GCP-2, and Gro-β. Using the molecular technique of ISH, CXCR1 and CXCR2 gene expression has been shown to be significantly increased in bronchial biopsies from subjects with severe exacerbations of COPD in comparison with both stable COPD and normal healthy nonsmoker controls (66). In comparison, the intensity of CXCR2 mRNA expression within the cells was stronger than that of CXCR1. There were significant positive correlations between the numbers of neutrophils and CXCR2 mRNA+ cells in severe exacerbations of COPD, which was not seen with CXCR1 mRNA+ cells. Considering CXCR1 and CXCR2 to be appropriate targets for treatment in severe exacerbations of COPD, such studies provide a basis for the development of potential and novel therapies to reduce exacerbation frequency and severity in the future.

Thus both eosinophil and neutrophil chemoattractants can be expressed also in chronic bronchitic smokers in association with a mild exacerbation of symptoms: in severe exacerbations requiring hospitalization, tissue neutrophilia appear to be the predominant alteration.

V. Summary and Conclusion

At least three inflammatory conditions contribute to COPD: chronic bronchitis (mucus hypersecretion), chronic bronchiolitis (small airways disease), and emphysema. In genetically predisposed individuals, the inflammation initiated by cigarette smoke is probably responsible for most of the symptoms and pathological abnormalities associated with COPD and its progression. Direct examination of airway and lung tissue support the presence of a marked inflammatory infiltrate even in stable COPD. The pattern of inflammation is distinct from that found in asthma. In stable COPD, significant increases are reported in the numbers of CD45 (total leukocytes), CD3 (T-lymphocytes), CD25 (i.e., activated), and VLA-1 (late activation) positive cells presumed to be T-lymphocytes, and of macrophages. By comparison with normal nonsmokers, T-lymphocytes and neutrophils increase in the surface epithelium while T-lymphocytes and macrophages increase in the subepithelium of smokers with COPD. In contrast to asthma, it is the CD8+ cells and not CD4+ T-cells that increase in number in COPD. Exacerbations of bronchitis in subjects with very mild COPD are associated with a marked recruitment of tissue neutrophils and also eosinophils. The novel identification in chronic bronchitis of gene expression for the eosinophil chemoattractants eotaxin, MCP-4, and RANTES, emphasizes the similarities that can exist in bronchial tissues between mild exacerbations in COPD and the inflammation of asthma. The most striking finding associated with an exacerbation in mild COPD is the upregulation of RANTES. The significant positive relationship between RANTES and tissue eosinophilia supports a role for this chemoattractant in exacerbations. Putative synergy between RANTES and CD8+ cells during repeated exacerbations due to viral infection may accelerate decline in lung function in smokers whose CD8 T-cell numbers are already raised. This would be particularly important in a subset of individuals with an already high genetically determined CD8:CD4 ratio and whose smoking habit has elevated the numbers of CD8+ cells even further.

Thus both eosinophil and neutrophil chemoattractants can be expressed also in chronic bronchitic smokers in association with an exacerbation of symptoms: in severe exacerbations requiring hospitalization, tissue neutrophilia appear to be the predominant alteration. The recent results of examination of biopsies of patients hospitalized and intubated for their exacerbation demonstrate an approximately 100-fold increase of neutrophil numbers as compared with the stable phase of the disease. Neutrophil recruitment into airways is due in part to chemoattraction by neutrophil chemokines including IL-8 and epithelial-derived neutrophil attractant-78 (ENA-78). There are significant positive correlations between the numbers of neutrophils and CXCR2 mRNA+ cells in severe exacerbations of COPD that are not seen with CXCR1 mRNA+ cells. Considering CXCR1 and CXCR2 to be appropriate therapeutic targets in severe exacerbations of COPD, these data provide a basis for the development of novel therapies aimed at the attenuation of exacerbation frequency and duration and, hopefully, a slowing of the relentless progression of COPD.

References

1. Siafakas NM, Vermeire P, Pride NB, Paoletti P, Gibson J, Howard P, Yernault, JC, Decramer M, Higenbottam T, Postma DS, Rees J. Optimal assessment and management of chronic obstructive pulmonary disease (COPD). Eur Respir J 1995; 8:1398–1420.
2. Pauwels R, Anthonisen N, Barnes PJ, Buist AS, Calverley P, Clark T, Fukuchi Y, Grouse L, Hogg JC, Jenkins C, Postma DS, Rabe KF, Ramsey SD, Rennard ST, Rodriguez-Roisin R, Siafakas N, Sullivan SD, Tan WC. Global initiative for chronic obstructive lung disease. National Heart, Lung, and Blood Institute, National Institutes of Health: 2001; 1–30.
3. Di Stefano A, Capelli A, Lusuardi M, Balbo P, Vecchio C, Maestrelli P, Mapp CE, Fabbri L, Donner CF, Saetta M. Severity of airflow limitation is associated with severity of airway inflammation in smokers. Am J Respir Crit Care Med 1998; 158:1277–1285.
4. Retamales I, Elliott WM, Meshi B, Coxson HO, Pare PD, Sciurba FC, Rogers RM, Hayashi S, Hogg JC. Amplification of inflammation in emphysema and its association with latent adenoviral infection. Am J Respir Crit Care Med 2001; 164:469–473.
5. Turato G, Zuin R, Miniati M, Baraldo S, Rea F, Beghe B, Monti S, Formichi B, Boschetto P, Harari S, Papi A, Maestrelli P, Fabbri LM, Saetta M. Airway inflammation in severe chronic obstructive pulmonary disease: relationship with lung function and radiologic emphysema. Am J Respir Crit Care Med 2002; 166:105–110.
6. O'Shaughnessy T, Ansari TW, Barnes NC, Jeffery PK. Inflammation in bronchial biopsies of subjects with chronic bronchitis: inverse relationship of CD8[+] T lymphocytes with FEV$_1$. Am J Resp Crit Care Med 1997; 155:852–857.
7. Lams BE, Sousa AR, Rees PJ, Lee TH. Subepithelial immunopathology of large airways in smokers with and without chronic obstructive pulmonary disease. Eur Respir J 2000; 15:512–516.
8. Jeffery PK. Remodeling in asthma and chronic obstructive lung disease. Am J Respir Crit Care Med 2001; 164:S28–S38.
9. Kanner RE, Anthonisen NR, Connett JE. Lower respiratory illnesses promote FEV(1) decline in current smokers but not ex-smokers with mild chronic obstructive pulmonary disease: results from the lung health study. Am J Respir Crit Care Med 2001; 164:358–364.
10. Miller LG, Goldstein G, Murphy M, Ginns LC. Reversible alterations in immunoregulatory T cells in smoking. Analysis by monoclonal antibodies and flow cytometry. Chest 1982; 82:526–529.
11. Costabel U, Bross KJ, Reuter C, Ruhle K-H, Matthys H. Alterations in immunoregulatory T-cell subsets in cigarette smokers. A phenotypic analysis of bronchoalveolar and blood lymphocytes. Chest 1986; 90:39–44.
12. van Eeden SF, Hogg JC. The response of human bone marrow to chronic cigarette smoking. Eur Respir J 2000; 15:915–921.
13. Lams BEA, Sousa AR, Rees PJ, Lee TH. Immunopathology of the small-airway submucosa in smokers with and without chronic obstructive pulmonary disease. Am J Respir Crit Care Med 1998; 158:1518–1523.

14. Mullen JBM, Wright JL, Wiggs BR, Pare PD, Hogg JC. Reassessment of inflammation of airways in chronic bronchitis. Br Med J 1985; 291:1235–1239.
15. Saetta M, Di Stefano A, Maestrelli P, Ferraresso A, Drigo R, Potena A, Ciaccia A, Fabbri LM. Activated T-lymphocytes and macrophages in bronchial mucosa of subjects with chronic bronchitis. Am Rev Respir Dis 1993; 147:301–306.
16. Di Stefano A, Turato G, Maestrelli P, Mapp CE, Paola Ruggieri M, Roggeri A, Boschetto P, Fabbri LM, Saetta M. Airflow limitation in chronic bronchitis is associated with T-lymphocyte and macrophage infiltration of the bronchial mucosa. Am J Respir Crit Care Med 1996; 153:629–632.
17. Di Stefano A, Maestrelli P, Roggeri A, Turato G, Calabro S, Potena A, Mapp CE, Ciaccia A, Covacev L, Fabbri LM, Saetta M. Upregulation of adhesion molecules in the bronchial mucosa of subjects with chronic obstructive bronchitis. Am J Respir Crit Care Med 1994; 149:803–810.
18. Fournier M, Lebargy F, Le Roy Ladurie F, Lenormand E, Pariente R. Intraepithelial T-lymphocyte subsets in the airways of normal subjects and of patients with chronic bronchitis. Am Rev Respir Dis 1989; 140:737–742.
19. O'Shaughnessy TC, Ansari TW, Barnes NC, Jeffery PK. Inflammatory cells in the airway surface epithelium of smokers with and without bronchitic airflow obstruction. Eur Respir J 1996; 9(suppl 23):14s.
20. Saetta M, Turato G, Facchini FM, Corbino L, Lucchini RE, Casoni G, Maestrelli P, Mapp CE, Ciaccia A, Fabbri LM. Inflammatory cells in the bronchial glands of smokers with chronic bronchitis. Am J Respir Crit Care Med 1997; 156:1633–1639.
21. Nadel JA. Role of mast cell and neutrophil proteases in airway secretion. Am Rev Respir Dis 1991; 144:S48–S51.
22. Reynolds HY. Bronchoalveolar lavage. Am Rev Respir Dis 1987; 135:250–263.
23. Saetta M. CD8+ T-lymphocytes in peripheral airways of smokers with chronic obstructive pulmonary disease. Am J Respir Crit Care Med 1998; 157:822–826.
24. Sallusto F, Lenig D, Mackay CR, Lanzavecchia A. Flexible programs of chemokine receptor expression on human polarized T helper 1 and 2 lymphocytes. J Exp Med 1998; 187:875–883.
25. Saetta M, Mariani M, Panina-Bordignon P, Turato G, Buonsanti C, Baraldo S, Bellettato CM, Papi A, Corbetta L, Zuin R, Sinigaglia F, Fabbri LM. Increased expression of the chemokine receptor CXCR3 and its ligand CXCL10 in peripheral airways of smokers with chronic obstructive pulmonary disease. Am J Respir Crit Care Med 2002; 165:1404–1409.
26. Saltini C, Hance AJ, Ferrans VJ, Basset F, Bitterman PB, Crystal RG. Accurate quantification of cells recovered by bronchoalveolar lavage. Am Rev Respir Dis 1984; 130:650–658.
27. Niewoehner DE, Klienerman J, Rice D. Pathologic changes in the peripheral airways of young cigarette smokers. N Engl J Med 1974; 291:755–758.
28. Cosio MG, Hale KA, Niewoehner DE. Morphologic and morphometric effects of prolonged cigarette smoking on the small airways. Am Rev Respir Dis 1980; 122:265–271.
29. Finkelstein R, Fraser RS, Ghezzo H, Cosio MG. Alveolar inflammation and its relation to emphysema in smokers. Am J Respir Crit Care Med 1995; 152:1666–1672.
30. Saetta M, Baraldo S, Corbino L, Turato G, Braccioni F, Rea F, Cavallesco G, Tropeano G, Mapp CE, Maestrelli P, Ciaccia A, Fabbri LM. CD8+ cells in the lungs of smokers with chronic obstructive pulmonary disease. Am J Respir Crit Care Med 1999; 160:711–717.

31. Peinado VI, Barbera JA, Abate P, Ramirez J, Roca J, Santos S, Rodriguez-Roisin R. Inflammatory reaction in pulmonary muscular arteries of patients with mild chronic obstructive pulmonary disease. Am J Respir Crit Care Med 1999; 159:1605–1611.

32. Jeffery PK. Differences and similarities between chronic obstructive pulmonary disease and asthma. Clin Exp Allergy 1999; 29(S2):14–26.

33. Lacoste J-Y, Bousquet J, Chanez P, Vyve TV, Simony-Lafontaine J, Lequeu N, Vic P, Enander I, Godard P, Michel F-B. Eosinophilic and neutrophilic inflammation in asthma, chronic bronchitis, and chronic obstructive pulmonary disease. J Allergy Clin Immunol 1993; 92:537–548.

34. Gibson PG, Hargreaves FE, Girgis-Gabardo A, Morris M, Denburg JA, Dolovich J. Chronic cough with eosinophilic bronchitis and examination for variable airflow obstruction and response to corticosteroid. Allergy 1995; 25:127–132.

35. Pizzichini E, Pizzichini MMM, Gibson P, Parameswaran K, Gleich GJ, Berman L, Dolovich J, Hargreave FE. Sputum eosinophilia predicts benefit from prednisone in smokers with chronic obstructive bronchitis. Am J Respir Crit Care Med 1998; 158:1511–1517.

36. Brightling CE, Monteiro W, Ward R, Parker D, Morgan MD, Wardlaw AJ, Pavord ID. Sputum eosinophilia and short-term response to prednisolone in chronic obstructive pulmonary disease: a randomised controlled trial. Lancet 2000; 356:1480–1485.

37. Brightling CE, Bradding P, Symon FA, Holgate ST, Wardlaw AJ, Pavord ID. Mast-cell infiltration of airway smooth muscle in asthma. N Engl J Med 2002; 346:1699–1705.

38. Ying S, Durham SR, Corrigan ChJ, Hamid Q, Kay AB. Phenotype of cells expressing mRNA for TH2-type (interleukin 4 and interleukin 5) and TH1-type (interleukin-2 and interferon-γ) cytokines in bronchoalveolar lavage and bronchial biopsies from atopic asthmatic and normal control subjects. Am J Respir Cell Mol Biol 1995; 12:477–487.

39. Humbert M, Ying S, Corrigan C, Menz G, Barkans J, Pfister R, Mend Q, Van Damme J, Opdenakker G, Durham SR, Kay AB. Bronchial mucosal expression of the genes encoding chemokines RANTES and MCP-3 in symptomatic atopic and nonatopic asthmatics: relationship to the eosinophil-active cytokines IL-5, GM-CSF, and IL-3. Am J Respir Cell Biol 1997; 16:1–8.

40. Sun Y, Robinson DS, Qiu M, Rottman J, Kennedy R, Ringler DJ, Mackay CR, Daugherty BL, Springer MS, Durham SR, Williams TJ, Kay AB. Enhanced expression of eotaxin and CCR3 mRNA and protein in atopic asthma. Association with airway hyperresponsiveness and predominant co-localization of eotaxin mRNA to bronchial epithelial and endothelial cells. Eur J Immunol 1997; 27:3507–3516.

41. Castleman WL. Bronchiolitis obliterans and pneumonia induced in young dogs by experimental adenovirus infection. Am J Pathol 1985; 119:495–504.

42. Cannon MJ, Openshaw PJM, Askonas BA. Cytotoxic T cells clear virus but augment lung pathology in mice infected with respiratory syncytial virus. J Exp Med 1988; 168:1163–1168.

43. Zhu J, Majumdar S, Qiu YS, Ansari T, Oliva A, Kips JC, Pauwels RA, De Rose V, Jeffery, PK. IL-4 and IL-5 gene expression and inflammation in the mucus-secreting glands and subepithelial tissue of smokers with chronic bronchitis: lack of relationship with CD8+ cells. Am J Resp Crit Care Med 2001; 164:2220–2228.

44. Zhu J, Qiu YS, Majumdar S, Gamble E, Matin D, Turato G, Fabbri LM, Barnes N, Saetta M, Jeffery PK. Bronchial eosinophilia and gene expression for IL-4, IL-5, and eosinophil chemoattractants in bronchitis. Am J Respir Crit Care Med 2001; 164:109–116.

45. Sadek MI, Sada E, Toossi Z, Schwander SK, Rich EA. Chemokines induced by infection of mononuclear phagocytes with mycobacteria and present in lung alveoli during active pulmonary tuberculosis. Am J Respir Cell Mol Biol 1998; 19:513–521.
46. Schrum S, Probst P, Fleischer B, Zipfel PF. Synthesis of the CC-chemokines MIP-1alpha, MIP-1beta, and RANTES is associated with a type 1 immune response. J Immunol 1996; 157:3598–3604.
47. Jedrzkiewicz S, Kataeva G, Hogaboam CM, Kunkel SL, Strieter RM, McKay DM. Superantigen immune stimulation evokes epithelial monocyte chemoattractant protein 1 and RANTES production. Infect Immun 1999; 67:6198–6202.
48. Sangari FJ, Petrofsky M, Bermudez LE. Mycobacterium avium infection of epithelial cells results in inhibition or delay in the release of interleukin-8 and RANTES. Infect Immun 1999; 67:5069–5075.
49. Becker S, Reed W, Henderson FW, Noah TL. RSV infection of human airway epithelial cells causes production of the beta-chemokine RANTES. Am J Physiol 1997; 272: L512–L520.
50. Harrison AM, Bonville CA, Rosenberg HF, Domachowske JB. Respiratory syncytical virus-induced chemokine expression in the lower airway: eosinophil recruitment and degranulation. Am J Respir Crit Care Med 2000; 159:1918–1924.
51. Adachi M, Matsukura A, Tokunaga H, Kokuba F. Expression of cytokines on human bronchial epithelial cells induced by influenza virus A. Int Arch Allergy Immunol 1997; 113:307–311.
52. Matsukura S, Kokubu F, Kubo H, Tomita T, Tokunaga H, Kadokura M, Yamamoto T, Kuroiwa Y, Ohno T, Suzaki H, Adachi M. Expression of RANTES by normal airway epithelial cells after influenza virus A infection. Am J Resp Cell Mol Biol 1998; 18:255–264.
53. Bhowmik A, Seemungal TA, Sapsford RJ, Wedzicha JA. Relation of sputum inflammatory markers to symptoms and lung function changes in COPD exacerbations [see comments]. Thorax 2000; 55:114–120.
54. Lloyd CM, Delaney T, Nguyen T, Tian J, Martinez AC, Coyle AJ, Gutierrez-Ramos JC. CC chemokine receptor (CCR)3/eotaxin is followed by CCR4/monocyte-derived chemokine in mediating pulmonary T helper lymphocyte type 2 recruitment after serial antigen challenge in vivo. J Exp Med 2000; 191:265–274.
55. Hadida F, Vieillard V, Mollet L, Clark-Lwis I, Baggiolini M, Debre P. Cutting edge: RANTES regulates Fas ligand expression and killing by HIV-specific CD8 cytotoxic T cells. J Immuno 1999; 161:1105–1109.
56. Kim JJ, Nottingham LK, Sin JI, Tsai A, Morrison L, Oh J, Dang K, Hu Y, Kazahaya K, Bennett M, Dentchev T, Wilson DM, Chalian AA, Boyer JD, Agadjanyan MG, Weiner DB. CD8 positive T cells influence antigen-specific immune responses through the expression of chemokines. J Clin Invest 1998; 15: 1112–1124.
57. Jeffery PK. Lymphocytes, chronic bronchitis and chronic obstructive pulmonary disease. In: Chadwick D, Goode JA, eds. Chronic Obstructive Pulmonary Disease: Pathogenesis to Treatment. Chichester: John Wiley & Sons Ltd, 2001:149–168.
58. Amadori A, Zamarchi R, De Silvestro G, Forza G, Cavatton G, Antonio Danieli G, Clementi M, Chieco-Bianchi, L. Genetic control of the CD4/CD8 T-cell ratio in humans. Nat Med 1995; 1:1279–1283.
59. Aaron SD, Angel JB, Lunau M, Wright K, Fex C, Le Saux N, Dales RE. Granulocyte inflammatory markers and airway infection during acute exacerbation of chronic obstructive pulmonary disease. Am J Respir Crit Care Med 2001; 163:349–355.

60. Saetta M, Di Stefano A, Maestrelli P, Turato G, Ruggieri P, Calcagni P, Mapp CE, Ciaccia A, Fabbri LM. Airway eosinophilia in chronic bronchitis during exacerbations. Am J Respir Crit Care Med 1994; 150:1646–1652.

61. Fahy JV, Kim KW, Liu J, Boushey HA. Prominent neutrophilic inflammation in sputum from subjects with asthma exacerbation. J Allergy Clin Immunol 1995; 95:843–852.

62. Wenzel SE, Szefler SJ, Leung DYM, Sloan SI, Rex MD, Martin RJ. Bronchoscopic evaluation of severe asthma. Persistent inflammation associated with high dose glucocorticoids. Am J Resp Crit Care Med 1997; 156:737–743.

63. Lamblin C, Gosset P, Tillie-Leblond I, Saulnier F, Marquette CH, Wallaert B, Tonnel AB. Bronchial neutrophilia in patients with noninfectious status asthmaticus. Am J Respir Crit Care Med 1998; 157:394–402.

64. Jatakanon A, Uasuf C, Maziak W, Lim S, Chung KF, Barnes PJ. Neutrophilic inflammation in severe persistent asthma. Am J Respir Crit Care Med 1999; 160:1532–1539.

65. Ordonez CL, Shaughnessy TE, Matthay MA, Fahy JV. Increased neutrophil numbers and IL-8 levels in airway secretions in acute severe asthma. Clinical and biologic significance. Am J Respir Crit Care Med 2000; 161:1185–1190.

66. Qiu YS, Zhu J, Bandi V, Fraire AE, Guntupalli KK, Jeffery PK. Neutrophil chemokine receptor (CXCR1&2) gene expression and biopsy neutrophilia in severe exacerbations of chronic obstructive pulmonary disease (COPD). Eur Resp J 2001; 18:501s.

67. Strieter RM, Lukacs NW, Standiford TJ, Kunkel SL. Cytokines. 2. Cytokines and lung inflammation: mechanisms of neutrophil recruitment to the lung. Thorax 1993; 48:765–769.

68. Chuntharapai A, Kim KJ. Regulation of the expression of IL-8 receptor A/B by IL-B: possible functions of each receptor. J Immunol 1995; 155:2587–2594.

69. Wuyts A, Proost P, Van Damme J. Interleukin-8 and other CXC chemokines. In: Thomson A, ed. The Cykotine Handbook, 3rd ed. San Diego: Academic Press, 2001:271–311.

70. Patel L, Charlton SJ, Chambers JK, Macphee CH. Expression and functional analysis of chemokine receptors in human peripheral blood leukocyte populations. Cytokine 2001; 14:27–36.

7

Biomarkers of Acute Exacerbations of Chronic Obstructive Pulmonary Disease

SIMON GOMPERTZ and ROBERT A. STOCKLEY

Queen Elizabeth Hospital
Birmingham, England

I. Introduction

It is now widely accepted that chronic obstructive pulmonary disease (COPD) is an inflammatory disease in which there is luminal, bronchial wall, and interstitial inflammatory cell activity (1–4) and resultant tissue damage (5). There is accumulating evidence that acute exacerbations of COPD (AECOPD) are associated with an increase in this inflammation and damage and that this is related predominantly to neutrophilic inflammation, although there may be subsets of patients with a bronchial eosinophilia (6–8). There is also evidence of increased oxidative stress during exacerbations (9,10). The problem in reviewing the literature is the general lack of information on the nature of the exacerbations described. The definitions of AECOPD have often been somewhat vague but have included an increase in symptoms for 2 or more days (11). The so-called "Anthonisen criteria" (12) of major symptoms (increased dyspnea, sputum volume, and sputum production) and minor symptoms (including sore throat, nasal discharge, fever, wheeze, and cough) have often been employed (5,11). It is clear, however, that corticosteroids (12,13), antibiotics (14,15) and antioxidants (16,17) may all have beneficial effects on some exacerbations. This suggests that inflammation, bacteria, and oxidative stress all play a role. An ideal biomarker would detect all such episodes or be specific to one subtype. At present, few authors have attempted to characterize the nature of their exacerbations in detail, which makes interpretation of the role of biomarkers often confusing rather than helpful. The aim of this chapter, therefore, is to discuss the various changes in inflammation and its markers that have been reported during AECOPD in order to describe the potential of these biomarkers for use as indicators of an impending or current exacerbation. These may have applications in the clinical management of patients with smoking-related chronic lung disease and the development of new treatments through future clinical research.

II. The Ideal Biomarker

The characteristics of an ideal biomarker include a molecule for which there is a relatively noninvasive test that may be performed even in patients with severe disease and one that can be undertaken repeatedly in the same individual (i.e., there should be good subject acceptability). The test should be specific for the process being assessed, have good reproducibility, and be sensitive to small and early changes in disease status, ideally in a linear fashion. Prospective studies of the levels of the parameter in the stable state and during the prodrome, onset, and resolution of different types of exacerbation should be available. The ideal biomarker would be easy and cheap to measure and sufficiently stable to allow measurement after a period of sample storage. The laboratory assays should have been well validated in appropriate specimens, including spiking experiments where appropriate (18). Ultimately a suitable biomarker could be used to identify impending exacerbations in prospective studies of COPD. It could also be used to facilitate early therapeutic intervention in the clinical setting and hence to avoid full-blown exacerbations and their economic impact (19) and personal consequences (20). It must be appreciated that many studies of AECOPD have involved incompletely characterized patients and/or different subsets of the COPD superfamily (19). Furthermore, different definitions of exacerbation have been employed (8,11,21,22) and it is therefore critical to define both the population of patients and the type of exacerbation to which a particular potential biomarker may be applicable. Changes in airway inflammatory cell numbers (in particular, neutrophils and eosinophils) occur during AECOPD and may provide useful markers of exacerbation in sputum and bronchoscopic specimens as well as influencing treatment. These changes have been described in detail elsewhere in this text and are not discussed further here.

III. Noninvasive Biomarkers

Biomarkers that are detected using noninvasive methods are more likely to be acceptable when repeated testing is required, for example, when patients are followed prospectively to identify the onset of an impending exacerbation or deterioration in inflammatory status. Samples can also be obtained noninvasively in patients with severe disease and from individuals who are acutely unwell at the time of exacerbation. Exhaled breath, airway secretions (spontaneous or induced sputum), blood, and urine provide noninvasive samples for the measurement of airway inflammation.

A. Exhaled Breath and Exhaled Breath Condensates

Measuring airway inflammation using exhaled breath and exhaled breath condensates is completely noninvasive. Furthermore, these samples can be measured repeatedly, even in patients with severe disease. At present, exhaled breath and condensate analyses are research tools but there is increasing evidence that they may have an important role in the diagnosis and management of lung disease in the future. This area forms the basis of a recent comprehensive review by Kharitonov et al. (23), which describes in detail the literature published so far. Much of the data are preliminary; however, the scanty evidence relating to changes during AECOPD is discussed below.

Exhaled Breath

Nitric Oxide

Nitric oxide (NO) is probably the most intensively studied exhaled marker of airway inflammation, but most of this effort has so far been directed at asthmatic patients. NO is derived from L-arginine by the enzyme NO synthetase that has 3 isoforms (NOS1–3) (23). Two of these enzymes are constitutively expressed (NOS1 and NOS3) and are activated by small rises in intracellular calcium concentration. The third member of the family, NOS2 or iNOS, is an inducible enzyme, which has much greater activity than the other two isoforms and is independent of calcium concentrations. The cellular source of NO in the airways is unclear, although epithelial cells throughout the bronchial tree would appear to be important. Inflammatory cells including alveolar macrophages, neutrophils, and eosinophils may also express NO synthetase (24); however, the vast majority of the NO is produced by the upper airways and sinuses rather than the lower respiratory tract (23).

Patients with stable COPD have relatively low levels of exhaled NO production (25,26). This could be related to current cigarette smoking (which downregulates NO production) (26,27), high previous cigarette consumption (28), and the conversion of NO to its product, peroxynitrite, during episodes of oxidative stress. In contrast, patients with unstable or severe disease may have higher mean (SEM) levels of nitric oxide than stable smokers or ex-smokers with COPD [12.1 ± 1.5, 4.3 ± 0.4, and 6.3 ± 0.6 parts per billion (ppb), respectively (Fig. 1) (29)]. However, these authors found that there was no difference in exhaled NO levels between patients with exacerbations ($n = 6$) and those with severe disease ($FEV_1 < 35\%$ predicted; $n = 6$). Much of the difference in NO between their subgroups of patients may have been related to differences in disease severity and a strong inverse correlation between FEV_1 and NO. Corradi et al. (28) reported significantly higher exhaled NO in patients with moderate-to-severe COPD than in healthy controls. They also described a relationship between exhaled NO and FEV_1; however, the correlation they found was a positive one, indicating that there may be many confounding influences on exhaled NO concentrations.

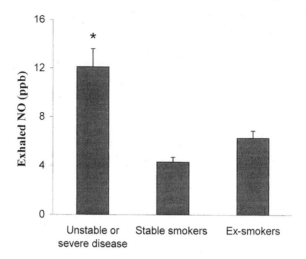

Figure 1   Nitric oxide concentrations in exhaled air from patients with unstable or severe COPD and stable COPD (current and ex-smokers). The asterisk indicates a significant difference compared to current smokers ($p < 0.0001$) and to ex-smokers ($p < 0.01$). ppb = parts per billion. (From Ref. 29.)

In a study employing sputum induction every 2 weeks for a 6-week period, a progressive worsening of airflow obstruction was observed associated with a significant increase in the fractional concentration of exhaled nitric oxide (FENO), (30). There was also a correlation between the changes in NO concentration and in the proportion of neutrophils in the sputum induction samples, suggesting that FENO may provide a useful marker of acutely worsening neutrophilic airway inflammation and obstruction. Agusti et al. (31) measured exhaled NO concentrations in 17 patients hospitalized with an exacerbation of COPD. NO was significantly elevated on admission (41.0 ± 5.1 ppb) and remained so at discharge 9 to 10 days later. When repeated at least 1 month after discharge, NO concentrations had fallen significantly ($p < 0.01$) to 15.8 ± 3.8 ppb and were no longer different from values for healthy nonsmoking controls.

Carbon Monoxide

Carbon monoxide (CO) is generated via activation of the inducible enzyme, hem oxygenase-1 (HO-1). A major limitation to the use of exhaled CO in COPD is the marked effect of continued smoking which masks any increase that would otherwise occur because of a worsening of the underlying disease process. Exhaled CO is understandably increased in cigarette smokers, but it is also increased in individuals with COPD who have given up smoking (32), suggesting that it is a marker of continued inflammation. Viral upper respiratory tract infections are thought to increase exhaled CO by inducing the expression of HO-1 (33). Five days of antibiotic treatment of purulent lower respiratory tract infections in otherwise healthy individuals is associated with a significant reduction ($p < 0.05$) in CO from 5.0 ± 2.8 to 3.4 ± 1.1 ppm (34). There are, however, no data describing the changes in exhaled carbon monoxide that occur during AECOPD.

Exhaled Breath Condensates

Exhaled breath condensates are obtained by cooling and freezing exhaled air. The samples obtained are derived from aerosolization of airway lining fluid during turbulent airflow in the mouth, oropharynx, tracheobronchial region, and alveoli; however, the proportional contribution of each compartment has yet to be deter- mined. Saliva may contain appreciable quantities of thromboxane B2, leukotriene B4 (LTB4), prostaglandin (PG)F2α, low levels of PGE2, and prostacyclin, and it is therefore important to minimize any salivary contamination (23). Furthermore, it is unclear whether the aerosolization rates of large and small molecules are the same. The collection procedure is, however, noninvasive, although low temperatures are required to collect labile mediators such as the lipid molecules and the samples should be stored at -70°C until analysis. A variety of molecules can be measured in exhaled breath condensates including hydrogen peroxide (H_2O_2), eicosanoids, products of lipid peroxidation, nitric oxide derivatives, proteins, and cytokines (23).

Hydrogen Peroxide (H_2O_2)

Inflammatory cell activation results in an increased production of O_2^-, which ultimately leads to the production of H_2O_2 (35). This molecule is less reactive than other oxygen species (23) and its solubility ensures that airway epithelial H_2O_2 equilibrates with air and thus expired H_2O_2 provides a potential marker of oxidative stress (36). Patients with stable COPD have increased exhaled hydrogen peroxide concentrations compared to normal subjects, suggesting continued airway inflammation (37,38) and these concentrations are increased further at exacerbation. Dekhuijzen et al. (37) reported H_2O_2 concentrations of $0.205 \pm 0.054\,\mu$M in patients with stable COPD compared with $0.600 \pm 0.075\,\mu$M in those with AECOPD ($p < 0.001$).

Eicosanoids and Products of Lipid Peroxidation

Arachidonic acid derivatives (eicosanoids) include the prostaglandins, isoprostanes, and leukotrienes. Prostaglandins are detectable in exhaled breath in COPD (39) but there is no published literature on the changes occurring during AECOPD. Leukotriene B4 (LTB4) is an important neutrophil chemoattractant that has been implicated in the increased luminal neutrophil infiltrate found at exacerbation (21,22,40). It has been detected in exhaled condensates from patients with COPD (23) as well as moderate and severe asthmatics (41), although there are no data relating to AECOPD. Nevertheless, it would be predicted to rise during such episodes in line with the increase seen in airway secretions during neutrophilic exacerbations (21,22,40).

Isoprostanes are formed by free radical–catalyzed lipid peroxidation of arachidonic acid. They are stable compounds that are detectable in all normal biological fluids and their concentrations are increased by systemic oxidative stress. The concentration of 8-isoprostane in exhaled breath condensates is increased in healthy cigarette smokers and is further increased in patients with COPD (39). Again, there are no data describing the changes occurring during AECOPD.

Products of lipid peroxidation and lipid peroxidation damage in tissues, cells, and body fluids may be quantified in a number of other ways. These include measurement of thiobarbituric acid reactive substances (TBARS), which are increased in exhaled condensate from asthmatics (42). However, there is little information from either stable or exacerbated individuals with COPD. More sophisticated assays include the measurement of primary (diene conjugates) and secondary (ketodiene) products of lipid peroxidation and these are elevated in exhaled condensate from patients with COPD and chronic bronchitis (23). However, there are no data relating products of lipid peroxidation to AECOPD.

NO-Related Products

Nitric oxide reacts with superoxide to produce peroxynitrite and can also be trapped by thiol-containing molecules to form S-nitrosothiols or oxidized to nitrate and nitrite. Nitrate and nitrite are reported (in unpublished observations) to be increased in COPD (23), and there may be a negative correlation between nitrogen intermediate formation and FEV_1 in stable disease (43); however, there is no published literature relating these products to AECOPD.

Proteins and Cytokines

The proinflammatory cytokines, interleukin-1β (IL-1β) and tumor necrosis factor-α (TNF-α) have been measured in exhaled breath condensates from a small number of patients with a variety of respiratory conditions including COPD (44). However, once again, there is little information on any changes that would be expected during AECOPD. Interleukin-8 (IL-8) has been implicated in the neutrophilic component of COPD (2,45,46) and cystic fibrosis (CF) (47), which is also a neutrophil-mediated bronchial disease. Further unpublished data (23) indicate that this important neutrophil chemoattractant is also slightly elevated in exhaled breath condensates from patients with stable CF and more markedly so in those with unstable disease. However, there is no information related to exhaled IL-8 levels in COPD in the stable state or at exacerbation.

B. Airway Secretions

Spontaneous Sputum

Sputum Color

Spontaneous sputum is derived from the airways and is composed of a pathological mixture of normal bronchial secretions, cells, cellular debris, and cleared microorganisms. It is a reflection of increased airway inflammation but is variably contaminated with saliva. However, there is good evidence that the degree of macroscopic purulence relates well to increasing neutrophilic inflammation (48,49) and increasing bacterial load (50) even in the stable state. A scientific color chart has been well validated for use with spontaneous sputum samples produced by patients with stable chronic bronchial disease (49) (Fig. 2). Exacer-

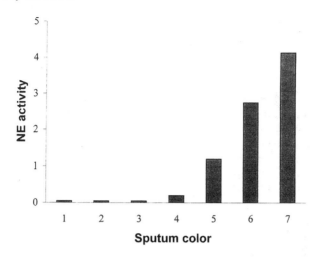

Figure 2 The relationship between neutrophil elastase (NE) activity (μM) and sputum color graded according to a 9-point color chart (Bronko Test, Heredilab Inc, Salt Lake City, Utah, USA). 0 = clear and colorless (no samples corresponded to this color number in this data set); numbers 1–8 indicate increasing purulence; 8 = the deepest green color observed in patients with cystic fibrosis (no samples corresponded to this color number in this data set). (From Ref. 49.)

bations characterized by worsening respiratory symptoms and purulent sputum (color numbers of 3–8) are associated with significant neutrophilic bronchial inflammation, positive sputum cultures, and significant systemic inflammation (22). With resolution of the exacerbation and declining airway inflammation there is a corresponding decrease in sputum color number. Exacerbations characterized by mucoid sputum (color numbers of 0–2) are not associated with significant neutrophilic bronchial inflammation, positive sputum cultures, or systemic inflammation (22). Furthermore, values on a 5-point color chart have been shown to correlate well with the symptoms of an exacerbation (51).

Sputum Microbiology

Although some 25 to 40% of patients with COPD have airways that are colonized in the stable state (50,52–54), exacerbations may be associated with bacterial (55) and viral (56,57) infection. Acquisition of airway micro-organisms (22,58) or an increase in their numbers (40,48) might therefore indicate an impending bacterial exacerbation. Colonization of airways in COPD is a dynamic process and acquisition and loss of bacteria may also occur without changes in symptoms; however, in patients with typical exacerbation symptoms, including, in particular, purulent sputum, a positive bacterial culture provides a useful confirmatory marker of AECOPD. Large changes in specific viral antibodies implicate acute viral infection as a cause of some exacerbations (58) and the combination of typical symptoms of AECOPD together with acute seroconversion would again support the diagnosis of exacerbation. Unfortunately, at present, this can only be determined in retrospect.

Biochemical Markers

A wide variety of derivatives of the inflammatory process have been measured in spontaneous sputum samples in stable state and during AECOPD, and some of these may provide useful markers of exacerbation. They can be divided into markers of cellular activation and degranulation, nonspecific markers of bronchial inflammation, antiproteinases, cytokines, and other chemoattractants (Table 1).

Purulent outpatient exacerbations of COPD are associated with increases in spontaneous sputum myeloperoxidase (MPO), neutrophil elastase (NE), protein leakage (as reflected in the sputum : serum albumin ratios) and, finally, LTB4 concentrations (22). It is worthy of comment that in this study there were no changes in IL-8 concentrations. However, more severe AECOPD requiring hospital admission has, also been shown to involve an increase in sputum IL-8 levels and sputum : serum α-1-antitrypsin ratios and the absolute level of bronchial inflammation is considerably greater (21). Time-course studies indicate that the bronchial concentration of these inflammatory parameters decreases rapidly as the acute exacerbation resolves; however, it is not known whether the increases precede the onset of clinical exacerbation or rise simultaneously with it. Nevertheless, these parameters are useful markers of purulent (bacterial) exacerbations and may therefore direct therapy. Indeed, Sethi et al. (59) have also reported that exacerbations

Table 1 Biochemical Markers of Airway Inflammation That Can Be Measured in Spontaneous Sputum

	Origin	Role
Myeloperoxidase (MPO)[a]	Neutrophil granules	Oxidative processes
Neutrophil elastase (NE)[a]	Neutrophil granules	Bacterial killing
Sputum : serum albumin ratio[b]	Serum	Nonspecific marker of bronchial leakiness
Sputum : serum A1AT ratio[b,c]	Serum	A1AT is an antiproteinase
SLPI[c]	Mucous glands and Clara cells	Antiproteinase
Interleukin-8 (IL-8)[d]	Macrophages, neutrophils, and airway epithelial cells	Potent neutrophil chemoattractant
Leukotriene B4 (LTB4)[d]	Macrophages, neutrophils	Potent neutrophil chemoattractant

A1AT = alpha-1-antitrypsin; SLPI = secretory leukoprotease inhibitor.
[a]Marker of cellular activation or degranulation.
[b]Nonspecifc marker of bronchial inflammation.
[c]Antiproteinase.
[d]Cytokine or other chemoattractant.

related to *Moraxella catarrhalis* or *Haemophilus influenzae* infection are associated with higher sputum concentrations of TNF-α (as well as NE and IL-8) than pathogen-negative exacerbations, suggesting a role in differentiating the different types of exacerbation and, hence, treatment.

Concentrations of the important bronchial antiprotease, secretory leukoprotease inhibitor (SLPI) are depressed at the onset of purulent exacerbations (60), probably secondary to the increase in elastase activity that results in a suppression of SLPI secretion (61,62). A decrease in stable state levels of SLPI might therefore be a useful indicator of increasing neutrophil influx and activation and impending neutrophilic exacerbation. Mucoid exacerbations, on the other hand, are associated with little change in any neutrophilic parameters except perhaps a slight increase in SLPI concentrations at presentation (60).

Induced Sputum

Induced sputum is a technique developed to obtain airway secretions from asthmatic patients (63,64) that has been adapted to the study of airway inflammation in smoking-related lung disease (2,11). Its use in COPD to date may have been confined largely to subjects who do not expectorate regularly and the results from these individuals may be different and, hence, not directly comparable to those who do expectorate spontaneously.

Microbiology in Induced Sputum

Outpatient exacerbations are associated with the acquisition of rhinovirus in induced sputum samples in nearly 25% of cases (10 out of 43) (57). In this study, the associated change in IL-6 concentrations in induced sputum was greatest in those with confirmed rhinovirus infection. Therefore, raised IL-6 may provide a more specific indication of viral AECOPD in this population.

Biochemical Markers in Induced Sputum

Endothelin-1 (ET-1) is a potent vaso- and bronchoconstrictor peptide that is produced by bronchial epithelium, pulmonary epithelium, and alveolar macrophages and is a cellular chemoattractant and upregulator of the inflammatory response (65). Increased spontaneous sputum concentrations and urinary excretion have been reported in patients with stable COPD (66,67). Furthermore, Roland et al. (65) found marked increases in sputum ET-1 concentrations during exacerbations of COPD ($n = 14$), from a median (IQR) of 5.37 (0.97–21.95) pg/mL in the stable state to 34.68 (13.77–51.95) pg/mL during the exacerbation ($p = 0.028$).

A nonpaired analysis of 81 samples (stable state, $n = 44$; AECOPD, $n = 37$) revealed raised IL-6 concentrations in induced sputum at exacerbation but no change in IL-8 levels (11). Other authors using sputum induction (68) have found raised concentrations of the matrix metalloprotein, MMP-9, at exacerbation, which persisted for up to 6 weeks. The implications are that it may take longer for some aspects of bronchial inflammation to resolve than for the exacerbation symptoms to subside and MMP, for example, could act as a marker of return to full biochemical stability.

Aaron et al. (69) followed patients prospectively for 15 months and reported exacerbations in 14 of 50 patients. Sputum induction was performed at baseline, at exacerbation, and 1 month later and demonstrated significant increases in both IL-8 and TNF-α from baseline to exacerbation, and these elevated values fell significantly 1 month after the AECOPD (Fig. 3). These two parameters might therefore prove to be suitable biomarkers of impending or active exacerbations in patients under long-

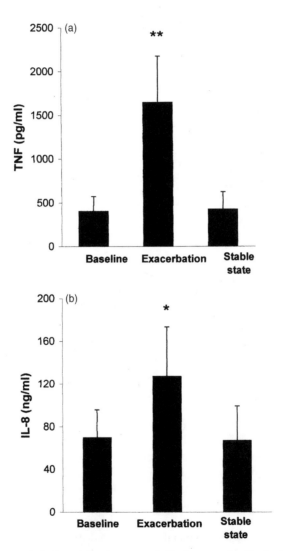

Figure 3   Changes in inflammation in sputum induction samples obtained prospectively at baseline, at exacerbation, and in the subsequent stable state for (a) TNF-α and (b) IL-8. The asterisks indicate significant differences; $*p = 0.05$ vs. baseline and $p < 0.05$ vs. stable state; $**p = 0.01$ vs. both baseline and stable state. (From Ref. 69.)

term follow-up. However, once again, further prospective studies with more frequent sampling would be required to determine whether these increases in inflammation preceded the clinical symptoms of exacerbation. Repetitive nebulization of hypertonic saline to obtain sputum induction samples may, however, cause increased neutrophilic inflammation in its own right (70) and thus limit the utility of this approach.

C. Blood

Raised plasma fibrinogen concentrations have been noted during exacerbations, particularly when there is purulent sputum or symptoms of a cold or cough (71). Bacterial exacerbations with purulent sputum requiring hospital admission are also associated with high serum C-reactive protein concentrations (CRP) (mean $\pm$ SE; 135 ± 36.2 mg/L) indicating a significant systemic acute-phase response (21). Even outpatient exacerbations characterized by purulent sputum are associated with elevated (median; IQR) concentrations of CRP albeit to a lesser degree (16.7; 6.2–40.3 mg/L) (22), whereas mucoid exacerbations are associated with low normal concentrations (4.6; 1.0–9.1 mg/L). This protein may therefore provide some guidance as to the nature of the episode and hence its treatment. Nevertheless, at present, it seems to add little to the observation of sputum color (22).

Absolute concentrations of endothelin-1 in plasma samples are an order of magnitude lower than those found in sputum from the same patients (0.54 ± 0.30 pg/mL) but rise significantly at AECOPD ($n = 28$; 0.67 ± 0.35 pg/mL; $p = 0.004$), again suggesting that this molecule may be a useful marker of exacerbation (65). The concentrations of the cytokine granulocyte-macrophage colony stimulating factor (GM-CSF) are also higher in serum from individuals with exacerbations of chronic bronchitis ($n = 5$; 13 ± 1 pg/mL) compared to stable subjects ($n = 8$, 1.4 ± 0.4 pg/mL; $p < 0.0001$) (6). Furthermore, patients with AECOPD have higher serum concentrations of MPO ($p < 0.01$) than those with stable disease (853 ± 168 µg/L vs. 469 ± 71 µg/L) and higher serum levels of ECP (22.2 ± 4.2 µg/L vs. 13.1 ± 2.7 µg/L; $p < 0.02$), suggesting increased activation of neutrophils and eosinophils, respectively (72).

Sahin et al. (73) demonstrated that erythrocyte glutathione peroxidase activity (a marker of antioxidant capacity) is deceased during exacerbations of COPD compared with the tenth day of treatment (45.54 ± 9.04 vs. 72.77 ± 9.68 units/g Hb). The same authors also found an increased concentration of the lipid peroxidation product, malondialdehyde, at the onset of the exacerbation (2.68 ± 1.28 nmol/mL) and this returned to the normal range by day 10 of treatment (1.08 ± 0.36 nmol/mL). Rahman et al. (9) measured the Trolox equivalent antioxidant capacity of plasma (TEAC) and the plasma levels of products of lipid peroxidation [thiobarbituric acid (TBA)–malondialdehyde (MDA) adducts] as markers of the overall plasma antioxidant–oxidant balance. They found that patients with exacerbations of COPD had lower plasma TEAC concentrations than those with stable disease (Fig. 4). Furthermore, in seven patients who were studied at exacerbation and in the stable state, TEAC levels increased from a mean (SEM)

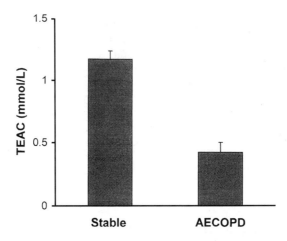

Figure 4 Plasma antioxidant capacity (TEAC) in patients with stable COPD ($n = 29$) and AECOPD ($n = 20$). The plasma TEAC levels are presented as mean and SEM and were lower for those individuals with an exacerbation. (From Ref. 9.)

value of 0.49 ± 0.09 mmol/L to 0.99 ± 0.19 mmol/L ($p < 0.001$). Plasma concentrations of TBA–MDA derivatives were also significantly higher in patients with unstable disease, confirming increased oxidant stress. Rahman et al. (10) subsequently followed 13 more patients prospectively throughout the course of an exacerbation and again reported low TEAC levels and high TBA–MDA levels on admission. By discharge, the TEAC concentrations had increased significantly and the TBA–MDA levels had fallen indicating an improvement in the antioxidant–oxidant balance.

D. Urine

Isoprostanes

The prostaglandin isomer, iPF$_{2\alpha}$-III, is a free-radical-dependent oxidation product of arachidonic acid for which there is a sensitive and specific assay. Pratico et al. (74) reported increased concentrations of iPF$_{2\alpha}$-III in urine from individuals with COPD when compared with matched control subjects and the concentration was related to disease severity. In five patients hospitalized for exacerbations of COPD (median; range) urinary isoprostane iPF$_{2\alpha}$ was increased at admission (125; 110–170 pmol/ mmol creatinine) and declined as clinical parameters improved (90; 70–110 pmol/mmol creatinine; $p < 0.001$).

Elastin Degradation Products

Degradation of extracellular matrix (including elastin) and hence tissue damage are features that are characteristic of COPD (75,76). Measurements of the specific elastin degradation products, desmosine and isodesmosine, in urine samples from patients with stable COPD are reproducible in the short term (5). These authors reported significantly higher ($p < 0.05$) urinary desmosine (mean $\pm$ SD; 17.15 ± 3.42 vs. $14.17 \pm 2.33 \, \mu g/g$ creatinine^{-1}) and isodesmosine (13.67 ± 2.87 vs. $10.59 \pm 2.17 \, \mu g/g$ creatinine^{-1}) concentrations in individuals with AECOPD compared to those with stable disease (5). However, the patients with exacerbations were significantly more obstructed than those with stable disease and some of the differences may be accounted for by a significant inverse relationship between urinary concentrations of the elastin degradation products and FEV_1.

E. Invasive Biomarkers

Bronchoscopy with bronchial lavage and bronchoalveolar lavage can be used to obtain samples from the smaller airways and alveoli, respectively, and can give an indication of luminal inflammation at these anatomical sites. However, broncho-scopy is an invasive technique that cannot readily be applied to patients with severe airflow obstruction, particularly during an exacerbation. Furthermore, repeated bronchoscopic examinations are unlikely to be acceptable in day-to-day clinical practice and may cause airway inflammation. Bronchial biopsies could provide some insight into the nature of bronchial wall inflammation but are even more invasive. Bronchoscopic sampling is therefore likely to remain a research tool and will not be used to provide useful biomarkers of AECOPD for day-to-day clinical practice. Nevertheless, the changes that have been detected in limited studies during exacerbations are described below.

The protected specimen brush (PSB) provides access to lower airway secre-tions through the bronchoscope without the risk of contamination of samples with upper respiratory tract commensals (55). PSB studies have demonstrated increased bacterial numbers and an increased proportion of patients with a positive bacterial isolate during exacerbations. Monso et al. (52) reported high bacterial loads [$> 10,000$ colony forming units/mL (cfu/mL)] in 24% of samples from patients with an AECOPD but in only 5% of those from stable patients ($p < 0.05$). Overall, a positive bacterial culture ($> 1000 \, cfu/mL$) was found in samples from 52% of the patients with an exacerbation but only 25% of those with stable disease ($p < 0.05$). In patients with symptoms suggestive of exacerbation quantitative culture of PSB specimens may be used as a marker of bacterial exacerbation. However, it must be emphasized that a significant proportion of patients will have positive cultures even while clinically stable.

Bronchoalveolar lavage (BAL) studies have revealed higher numbers of cells, including eosinophils and neutrophils, in samples from patients with nonpurulent exacerbations ($n = 8$) compared with patients in the stable state ($n = 5$) (6). The same study revealed greater concentrations of GM-CSF in BAL fluid from individuals with an exacerbation (54 ± 8 vs. $25 \pm 5 \, pgm/L$; $p = 0.009$).

Zhu et al. (77) reported increases in eosinophil numbers in bronchial biopsy specimens from chronic bronchitics during an exacerbation and this was associated with greater expression of the eosinophil chemoattractant, RANTES. However, over half of the patients studied (11/20) had no airflow obstruction and hence no COPD.

In a similar study (78), 16 of 21 patients with chronic bronchitis had airflow obstruction (76%). Eleven of these individuals were examined during an exacerbation and 10 in the stable clinical state. AECOPD was associated with a marked increase in the number of eosinophils in biopsy specimens ($p < 0.001$) and an increase in the proportion of patients with biopsies showing immunoreactivity for the eosinophil cytokine, interleukin-5 (1 out of 10 in the stable state and 5 out of 11 who had an exacerbation), although this difference failed to reach statistical significance ($p > 0.05$). The same group has also demonstrated increased numbers of cells staining for very late activation antigen-1 (VLA-1) and TNF-α during an exacerbation in a similar patient population (8), although the relationship to COPD remains uncertain.

V. Summary

The inflammatory processes underlying AECOPD have been described only relatively recently and our understanding of this area continues to expand. Suitable biomarkers of acute exacerbation will allow the onset of impending exacerbations to be detected and/or will provide laboratory confirmation of the clinical impression of a significant exacerbation. More importantly, the different patterns of markers may help determine the pathogenic nature and hence management of the episode. At present, although these tests may have clear applications in clinical research, their role in patient management is far from certain. The development of ideal biomarkers of AECOPD using noninvasive tests that can be performed repeatedly and in patients with severe disease remains a realistic aim. There are numerous potential candidates, including exhaled breath molecules (NO, H_2O_2), markers of oxidative stress (plasma TEAC and TBA–MDA; urinary isoprostane $PF_{2\alpha}$-III derivatives), and sputum parameters (neutrophilic inflammation and spontaneous sputum color). However, at present, none of these is able to predict an impending exacerbation, but they can confirm the clinical diagnosis of an AECOPD. As the nature of the subtypes of exacerbation becomes clearer (perhaps through the use of biomarkers), it may be possible to target management for each patient and episode more specifically.

References

1. Di Stefano A, Capelli A, Lusuardi M, Balbo P, Vecchio C, Maestrelli P, Mapp CE, Fabbri LM, Donner CF, Saetta M. Severity of airflow limitation is associated with severity of airway inflammation in smokers. Am J Respir Crit Care Med 1998; 158:1277–1285.
2. Keatings VM, Collins PD, Scott DM, Barnes PJ. Differences in interleukin-8 and tumor necrosis factor-α in induced sputum from patients with chronic obstructive pulmonary disease or asthma. Am J Respir Crit Care Med 1996; 153:530–534.
3. Lacoste J-Y, Bousquet J, Chanez P, Van Vyve T, Simony-Lafontaine J, Lequeu N, Vic P, Enander I, Godard P, Michel F-B. Eosinophilic and neutrophilic inflammation in asthma, chronic bronchitis and chronic obstructive pulmonary disease. J Allergy Clin Immunol 1993; 92:537–548.

4. Pesci A, Balbi B, Majori M, Cacciana G, Bertacco S, Alciato P, Donner CF. Inflammatory cells and mediators in bronchial lavage of patients with chronic obstructive pulmonary disease. Eur Respir J 1998; 12:380–386.

5. Viglio S, Iadarola P, Lupi A, Trisolini R, Tinelli C, Balbi B, Grassi V, Worlitzsch D, Doring G, Meloni F, Meyer KC, Dowson L, Hill SL, Stockley RA, Luisetti M. MEKC of desmosine and isodesmosine in urine of chronic destructive lung disease patients. Eur Respir J 2000; 15:1039–1045.

6. Balbi B, Bason C, Balleari F, Fiasella F, Pesci A, Ghio R, Fabiano F. Increased bronchoalveolar granulocytes and granulocyte/macrophage colony-stimulating factor during exacerbations of chronic bronchitis. Eur Respir J 1997; 10:846–850.

7. Maestrelli P, Saetta M, Di Stefano A, Calcagni PG, Turato G, Ruggieri MP, Roggeri A, Mapp CE, Fabbri LM. Comparison of leukocyte counts in sputum, bronchial biopsies and bronchoalveolar lavage. Am J Respir Crit Care Med 1995; 152:1926–1931.

8. Saetta M, Di Stefano A, Maestrelli P, Turato G, Ruggieri MP, Roggeri A, Calcagni P, Mapp CE, Ciaccia A, Fabbri LM. Airway eosinophilia in chronic bronchitis during exacerbations. Am J Respir Crit Care Med 1994; 150:1646–1652.

9. Rahman I, Morrison D, Donaldson K, MacNee W. Systemic oxidative stress in asthma, COPD, and smokers. Am J Respir Crit Care Med 1996; 154:1055–1060.

10. Rahman I, Skwarska B, MacNec W. Attenuation of oxidant/antioxidant imbalance during treatment of exacerbations of chronic obstructive pulmonary disease. Thorax 1997; 52:565–568.

11. Bhowmik A, Seemungal TAR, Sapsford RJ, Wedzicha JA. Relation of sputum inflammatory markers to symptoms and lung function changes in COPD exacerbations. Thorax 2000; 55:114–120.

12. Paggiaro PL, Dahle R, Bakrani I, Frith L, Hollingworth K, Efthmiou J. Multicentre randomised placebo-controlled trial of inhaled fluticasone propionate in patients with chronic obstructive pulmonary disease. Lancet 1998; 351:773–780.

13. Thompson WH, Nielson CP, Carvalho P, Charan NB, Crowley JJ. Controlled trial of oral prednisone in outpatients with acute COPD exacerbation. Am J Respir Crit Care Med 1996; 154:407–412.

14. Anthonisen NR, Manfreda J, Warren CPW, Hershfield ES, Harding GKM, Nelson NA. Antibiotic therapy in exacerbations of chronic obstructive pulmonary disease. Ann Intern Med 1987; 106:196–204.

15. Saint S, Bent S, Vittinghoff E, Grady D. Antibiotics in chronic obstructive pulmonary disease exacerbations. A meta-analysis. JAMA 1995; 273:957–960.

16. Decramer M, Dekhuijzen PN, Troosters T, van Herwaarden C, Rutten-van Molken M, van Schayck CP, Olivieri D, Lankhorst I, Ardia A. The Bronchitis Randomized On NAC Cost-Utility Study (BRONCUS): hypothesis and design. BRONCUS-trial Committee. Eur Respir J 2001; 17:329–336.

17. Pela R, Calcagni AM, Subiaco S, Isidori P, Tubaldi A, Sanguinetti CM. N-acetylcysteine reduces the exacerbation rate in patients with moderate to severe COPD. Respiration 1999; 66:495–500.

18. Stockley RA, Bayley D. Validation of assays for inflammatory markers in sputum. Eur Respir J 2000; 15:778–781.

19. Wilson R. The role of infection in COPD. Chest 1998; 113:242S–248S.

20. Seemungal TAR, Donaldson GC, Paul BA, Bestall JC, Jeffries DJ, Wedzicha JA. Effect of exacerbation on quality of life in patients with chronic obstructive pulmonary disease. Am J Respir Crit Care Med 1998; 157:1418–1422.

21. Crooks S, Bayley DL, Hill SL, Stockley RA. Bronchial inflammation in acute bacterial exacerbations of chronic bronchitis: the role of leukotriene B4. Eur Respir J 2000; 15:274–280.
22. Gompertz S, O'Brien C, Bayley DL, Hill SL, Stockley RA. Changes in bronchial inflammation during acute exacerbations of chronic bronchitis. Eur Respir J 2001; 17:1112–1119.
23. Kharitonov SA, Barnes PJ. Exhaled markers of pulmonary disease. Am J Respir Crit Care Med 2001; 163:1693–1722.
24. Saleh D, Ernst P, Lim S, Barnes PJ, Giaid A. Increased formation of the potent oxidant peroxynitrite in the airways of asthmatic patients is associated with induction of nitric oxide synthase: effect of inhaled glucocorticoid. FASEB J 1998; 12:929–937.
25. Rutgers SR, van der Mark TW, Coers W, Moshage H, Timens W, Kauffman HF, Koeter GH, Postma DS. Markers of nitric oxide metabolism in sputum and exhaled air are not increased in chronic obstructive pulmonary disease. Thorax 1999; 54:576–580.
26. Robbins RA, Floreani AA, Von Essen SG, Sisson JH, Hill GE, Rubinstein I, Townley RG. Measurement of exhaled nitric oxide by three different techniques. Am J Respir Crit Care Med 1996; 153:1631–1635.
27. Kharitonov SA, Robbins RA, Yates D, Keatings V, Barnes PJ. Acute and chronic effects of cigarette smoking on exhaled nitric oxide. Am J Respir Crit Care Med 1995; 152:609–612.
28. Corradi M, Majori M, Cacciani GC, Consigli GF, de'Munari E, Pesci A. Increased exhaled nitric oxide in patients with stable chronic obstructive pulmonary disease. Thorax 1999; 54:572–575.
29. Maziak W, Loukides S, Culpitt S, Sullivan P, Kharitonov SA, Barnes PJ. Exhaled nitric oxide in chronic obstructive pulmonary disease. Am J Respir Crit Care Med 1998; 157:998–1002.
30. Silkoff PE, Martin D, Pak J, Westcott JY, Martin RJ. Exhaled nitric oxide correlated with induced sputum findings in COPD. Chest 2001; 119:1049–1055.
31. Agusti AG, Villaverde JM, Togores B, Bosch M. Serial measurements of exhaled nitric oxide during exacerbations of chronic obstructive pulmonary disease. Eur Respir J 1999; 14:523–528.
32. Culpitt SV, Paredi P, Kharitonov SA, Barnes PJ. Exhaled carbon monoxide is increased in COPD patients regardless of their smoking habit. Am J Respir Crit Care Med 1998; 157:A787.
33. Yamaya M, Sekizawa K, Ishizuka S, Monma M, Mizuta K, Sasaki H. Increased carbon monoxide in exhaled air of subjects with upper respiratory tract infections. Am J Respir Crit Care Med 1998; 158:311–314.
34. Biernacki W, Kharitonov SA, Barnes PJ. Carbon monoxide in exhaled air in patients with lower respiratory tract infection. Eur Respir J 1998; 12(Suppl 27–28):345s–346s.
35. Gompertz S, Stockley RA. Inflammation—role of the neutrophil and the eosinophil. Semin Respir Infect 2000; 15:14–23.
36. Dohlman AW, Black HR, Royall JA. Expired breath hydrogen peroxide is a marker of acute airway inflammation in pediatric patients with asthma. Am Rev Respir Dis 1993; 148:955–960.
37. Dekhuijzen PN, Aben KK, Dekker I, Aarts LP, Wielders PL, van Herwaarden CL, Bast A. Increased exhalation of hydrogen peroxide in patients with stable and unstable chronic obstructive pulmonary disease. Am J Respir Crit Care Med 1996; 154:813–816.
38. Nowak D, Kasielski M, Pietras T, Bialasiewicz P, Antczak A. Cigarette smoking does not increase hydrogen peroxide levels in expired breath condensate of patients with stable COPD. Monaldi Arch Chest Dis 1998; 53:268–273.

39. Montuschi P, Collins JV, Ciabattoni G, Lazzeri N, Corradi M, Kharitonov SA, Barnes PJ. Exhaled 8-isoprostane as an in vivo biomarker of lung oxidative stress in patients with COPD and healthy smokers. Am J Respir Crit Care Med 2000; 162:1175–1177.

40. Hill AT, Campbell EJ, Bayley DL, Hill SL, Stockley RA. Evidence for excessive bronchial inflammation during an acute exacerbation of chronic obstructive pulmonary disease in patients with alpha(1)-antitrypsin deficiency (PiZ). Am J Respir Crit Care Med 1999; 160:1968–1975.

41. Hanazawa T, Kharitonov SA, Barnes PJ. Increased nitrotyrosine in exhaled breath condensate of patients with asthma. Am J Respir Crit Care Med 2000; 162:1273–1276.

42. Antczak A, Nowak D, Shariati B, Krol M, Piasecka G, Kurmanowska Z. Increased hydrogen peroxide and thiobarbituric acid-reactive products in expired breath condensate of asthmatic patients. Eur Respir J 1997; 10:1235–1241.

43. Ichinose M, Sugiura H, Yamagata S, Koarai A, Shirato K. Increase in reactive nitrogen species production in chronic obstructive pulmonary disease airways. Am J Respir Crit Care Med 2000; 162:701–706.

44. Scheideler L, Manke HG, Schwulera U, Inacker O, Hammerle H. Detection of nonvolatile macromolecules in breath. A possible diagnostic tool? Am Rev Respir Dis 1993; 148:778–784.

45. Chanez P, Enander I, Jones I, Godard P, Bousquet J. Interleukin 8 in bronchoalveolar lavage of asthmatic and chronic bronchitis patients. Int Arch Allergy Immunol 1996; 111:83–88.

46. Hill AT, Bayley DL, Campbell EJ, Hill SL, Stockley RA. Airways inflammation in chronic bronchitis: the effects of smoking and α-1-antitrypsin deficiency. Eur Respir J 2000; 15:886–890.

47. Richman-Eisehstat JBY, Jorens PG, Hebert CA, Ukei I, Nadel JA. Interleukin-8: an important chemoattractant in sputum of patients with chronic inflammatory airway diseases. Am J Physiol 1993; 264:L413–L418.

48. Stockley RA, O'Brien C, Pye A, Hill SL. Relationship of sputum colour to nature and outpatient management of acute exacerbations of COPD. Chest 2000; 117:1683–1645.

49. Stockley RA, Bayley D, Hill SL, Hill AT, Crooks S, Campbell EJ. Assessment of airway neutrophils by sputum colour: correlation with airways inflammation. Thorax 2001; 56:366–372.

50. Hill AT, Campbell EJ, Hill SL, Bayley DL, Stockley RA. Association between airway bacterial load and markers of airway inflammation in patients with stable chronic bronchitis. Am J Med 2000; 109:288–295.

51. Woolhouse I, Hill SL, Stockley RA. Symptom resolution assessed using a patient directed diary card during treatment of exacerbations of chronic bronchitis. Thorax 2001; 56: 947–953.

52. Monso E, Ruiz J, Rosell A, Manterola J, Fiz J, Morera J, Ausina V. Bacterial infection in chronic obstructive pulmonary disease. A study of stable and exacerbated outpatients using the protected specimen brush. Am J Respir Crit Care Med 1995; 152:1316–1320.

53. Soler N, Ewig S, Torres A, Filella X, Gonzalez J, Zaubert A. Airway inflammation and bronchial patterns in patients with stable chronic obstructive pulmonary disease. Eur Respir J 1999; 14:1015–1022.

54. Zalacain R, Sobradillo V, Amilibia J, Barron J, Achotegui V. Pijoan JI, Llorente JL. Predisposing factors to bacterial colonization in chronic obstructive pulmonary disease. Eur Respir J 1999; 13:343–348.

55. Wilson R. Bacterial infection and chronic obstructive pulmonary disease. Eur Respir J 1999; 13:233–235.

56. Gump DW, Phillips CA, Forsyth BR, McIntosh K, Lamborn KR, Stouch WH. Role of infection in chronic bronchitis. Am Rev Respir Dis 1976; 113:465–474.

57. Seemungal TA, Harper-Owen R, Bhowmik A, Jeffries DJ, Wedzicha JA. Detection of rhinovirus in induced sputum at exacerbation of chronic obstructive pulmonary disease. Eur Respir J 2000; 16:677–683.

58. Sethi S. Infectious etiology of acute exacerbations of chronic bronchitis. Chest 2000; 117:380S–385S.

59. Sethi S, Muscarella K, Evans N, Klingman KL, Grant BJ, Murphy TF. Airway inflammation and etiology of acute exacerbations of chronic bronchitis Chest 2000; 118:1557–1565.

60. Gompertz S, Unsall I, Bayley D, Hill SL, Stockley RA. Changes in sputum secretory leukoprotease inhibitor (SLPI) following non-bacterial and bacterial exacerbations of chronic bronchitis. Thorax 2000; 55(Suppl 3):A21.

61. Hill AT, Bayley D, Stockley RA. The interrelationship of sputum inflammatory markers in patients with chronic bronchitis. Am J Respir Crit Care Med 1999; 160:893–898.

62. Sallenave JM, Shulmann J, Crossley J, Jordana M, Gauldie J. Regulation of secretory leukocyte proteinase inhibitor (SLPI) and elastase-specific inhibitor (ESI/elafin) in human airway epithelial cells by cytokines and neutrophilic enzymes. Am J Respir Cell Mol Biol 1994; 11:733–741.

63. Fahy JV, Liu J, Wong H, Boushey HA. Cellular and biochemical analysis of ind-uced sputum from asthmatic and from healthy subjects. Am Rev Respir Dis 1993; 147: 1126–1131.

64. Pin I, Gibson PG, Kolendowicz R, Girgis-Gabardo A, Denburg JA, Hargreave FE, Dolovich J. Use of induced sputum cell counts to investigate airway inflammation in asthma. Thorax 1992; 47:25–29.

65. Roland M, Bhowmik A, Sapsford RJ, Seemungal TA, Jeffries DJ, Warner TD, Wedzicha JA. Sputum and plasma endothelin-1 levels in exacerbations of chronic obstructive pulmonary disease. Thorax 2001; 56:30–35.

66. Chalmers GW, Macleod KJ, Sriram S, Thomson LJ, McSharry C, Stack BH, Thomson NC. Sputum endothelin-1 is increased in cystic fibrosis and chronic obstructive pulmonary disease. Eur Respir J 1999; 13:1288–1292.

67. Sofia M, Mormile M, Faraone S, Carratu P, Alifano M, Di Benedetto G, Carratu L. Increased 24-hour endothelin-1 urinary excretion in patients with chronic obstructive pulmonary disease. Respiration 1994; 61:263–268.

68. Mercer PF, Shute JK, Bhowmik A, Wedzicha JA. Matrix metalloproteinases and TIMP-1 in sputum from patients before, during and after exacerbation. Am J Respir Crit Care Med 1999; 159:A189.

69. Aaron SD, Angel JB, Lunau M, Wright K, Fex C, Le Saux N, Dales RE. Granulocyte inflammatory markers and airway infection during acute exacerbation of chronic obstructive pulmonary disease. Am J Respir Crit Care Med 2001; 163: 349–355.

70. Pavord ID. Sputum induction to assess airway inflammation: is it an inflammatory stimulus? Thorax 1998; 53:79–80.

71. Seemungal TA, MacCallum P, Paul EA, Bhowmik A, Wedzicha JA. Elevated plasma fibrinogen increases cardiovascular risks in COPD patients. Am J Respir Crit Care Med 1999; 159:A403.

72. Fiorini G, Crespi S, Rinaldi M, Oberti E, Vigorelli R, Palmieri G. Serum ECP and MPO are increased during exacerbations of chronic bronchitis with airway obstruction. Biomed Pharmacother 2000; 54:274–278.
73. Sahin U, Unlu M, Ozguner F, Sutcu R, Akkaya A, Delibas N. Lipid peroxidation and glutathione peroxidase activity in chronic obstructive pulmonary disease exacerbation: prognostic value of malondialdehyde. J Basic Clin Physiol Pharmacol 2001; 12:59–68.
74. Pratico D, Basili S, Vieri M, Cordova C, Violi F, Fitzgerald GA. Chronic obstructive pulmonary disease is associated with an increase in urinary levels of isoprostane F2alpha-III, an index of oxidant stress. Am J Respir Crit Care Med 1998; 158:1709–1714.
75. Doring G. The role of neutrophil elastase in chronic inflammation. Am J Respir Crit Care Med 1994; 150:S114–S117.
76. Stockley RA, Hill SL, Burnett D. Proteinases in chronic lung infection. Ann NY Acad Sci 1991; 624:257–266.
77. Zhu J, Qiu YS, Majumdar S, Gamble E, Matin D, Turato G, Fabbri LM, Barnes N, Saetta M, Jeffery PK. Exacerbations of bronchitis: bronchial eosinophilia and gene expression for interleukin-4, interleukin-5, and eosinophil chemoattractants. Am J Respir Crit Care Med 2001; 164:109–116.
78. Saetta M, Di Stefano A, Maestrelli P, Turato G, Mapp CE, Pieno M, Zanguochi G, Del Prete G, Fabbri LM. Airway eosinophilia and expression of interleukin-5 protein in asthma and in exacerbations of chronic bronchitis. Clin Exp Allergy 1996; 26:766–774.

8

Acute Exacerbation of Chronic Obstructive Pulmonary Disease

A Systemic Disease?

EMIEL F.M. WOUTERS, M. DENTENER, J. VERNOOY, E. POUW, M. ENGELEN, and E. CREUTZBERG

University Hospital Maastricht
Maastricht, The Netherlands

I. Introduction

Chronic obstructive pulmonary disease (COPD) comprises a heterogeneous group of conditions, characterized by chronic airflow limitation and parenchymal destruction of lung parenchyma, with clinical manifestations of dyspnea, cough, sputum production, and impaired exercise tolerance. The clinical course of COPD is one of gradual progressive impairment, which may eventually lead to respiratory failure. Periods of relative clinical stability are interrupted by recurrent exacerbations. However, the definition of exacerbation is still imprecise and generally based on varying combinations of symptoms such as an increase in cough or sputum production, worsening of dyspnea, or changes in sputum purulence (1). An acute exacerbation has also been described as a sustained worsening of the patient's condition, from the stable state and beyond normal day-to-day variations, that is acute in onset and necessitates a change in regular medication in a patient with underlying COPD (2). This imprecise definition of COPD, largely based on experienced symptomatology by the patient without measurable parameters in order to define severity or outcome hampers at present every systematic approach of this disease condition. Based on the complexity of the sensation of breathlessness, generally considered as a key symptom during exacerbations, it can hypothesized that AECOPD is a heterogeneous condition in the clinical course of COPD. The imprecise pathogenesis related to infectious or noninfectious agents, as well as the wide variation in pathophysiological changes, make it very difficult to approach AECOPD as a unique disease condition, especially related to systemic effects. Systemic effects related to AECOPD can be considered as part of the pathogenesis or are related to complications of AECOPD, such as hypoxemia and hypercapnia. Systemic disease manifestations can also predispose the COPD patient to occurrence or recurrence of exacerbations or can contribute to the outcome of the treatment of AECOPD. Furthermore, considering an AECOPD as a sustained worsening of the patient's condition from the stable state and beyond normal day-to-day variations, systemic effects can be considered as part of this baseline or stable condition.

II. COPD: An Inflammatory Disease with Systemic Manifestations

Chronic obstructive pulmonary disease (COPD) is characterized by airway inflammation, which is considered to play a pathogenic role in this disorder. Polymorphonuclear leukocytes (PMN) are present at enhanced numbers in bronchoalveolar lavage fluid (BALF) and in sputum. In addition, an influx of macrophages and lymphocytes in bronchial mucosa, and enhanced levels of the proinflammatory cytokine tumor necrosis factor (TNF)α and the chemokine interleukin (IL)-8 in the sputum of patients with COPD, have been observed (3). Besides the local airway inflammation, indications for a systemic inflammatory process in COPD are also present. Similarly to the observation in the airways, increased amounts of PMN, which were activated as demonstrated by enhanced expression of the adhesion molecule CD11b/CD18, were detected in the circulation of COPD patients in a clinical stable condition (4). Furthermore, the expression of Gas, which is involved in many cell signaling pathways, was reduced, although the potential implications of that observation are unclear. In the latter study, a reduction of circulating levels of the soluble adhesion molecule ICAM-1 was detected, whereas Riise et al. detected enhanced levels of both sICAM-1 and sE-selectin (5). This discrepancy could be due to differences in severity of COPD in the two patient populations studied. In line with the observation of enhanced amounts of circulating PMN, cells that have a strong potential to produce oxygen radicals, proof for systemic oxidative stress in smokers and COPD patients was obtained by the observation of a reduction of the total antioxidative capacity, parallelled by enhanced levels of lipid peroxidation products, as indices of overall oxidative stress (6). Besides activation of PMN, activation status of circulating lymphocytes has also been demonstrated indicated by enhanced expression of cytochrome oxidase (7).

Changes in circulating levels of acute-phase proteins have been reported to accompany both acute and chronic inflammatory disorders (8). In line herewith, it has been demonstrated that in stable COPD patients, enhanced levels of both C-reactive protein (CRP) and the acute-phase protein LPS binding protein (LBP) are present (9,10). Furthermore, the acute-phase reactant and blood clotting factor fibrinogen has also been associated with COPD. A prospective epidemiological study in a cohort of 8955 subjects from a Danish general adult population study revealed that increased plasma levels of fibrinogen are associated with reduced lung function and increased risk of COPD, independent of smoking status (11).

The rise in the systemic levels of acute phase proteins suggest that the hepatocytes are activated to produce these reactants, although increasing evidence indicates that tissue-specific cells, like lung epithelial cells, are also able to produce acute-phase proteins (12). The formation of acute-phase proteins is strongly induced by cytokines such as IL-6 or TNF (8). Indeed, enhanced circulating levels of IL-6 (10) and TNF (10–13) have been reported in COPD. The detection of biological active TNF can be hampered by its short half-life (approximately 6 to 7 min), the formation of complexes with both soluble TNF-Rs and its renal clearance (14). Enhanced circulating levels of both sTNF-Rs (sTNF-R55 and sTNF-R75) have also been demonstrated in COPD (9,13,15). Since inflammatory stimuli, including TNF, will induce shedding of membrane-bound TNF-R, the enhanced levels of sTNF-R could reflect the enhanced inflammatory status of the patients (14,16).

Since in vitro studies have revealed that hypoxia will result into enhanced cytokine production by macrophages (17), Takabatake postulated that systemic hypoxemia observed in patients with COPD might contribute to the activation of the TNF system (13). Indeed, significant inverse correlations between PaO_2 and circulating TNF and sTNF-R levels in patients were detected. These results suggests that changes in circulation due to the deterioration of lung function will lead to enhanced levels of the systemic inflammatory markers, implying that they are not derived from leakage out of the local compartment. Further evidence for the hypothesis that the inflammatory processes in the airways and the systemic circulation are independent from each other comes from recent studies by Michel et al. (18). It was shown that healthy subjects exposed to the proinflammatory compound LPS via inhalation express differences in changes in body temperature, airway responsiveness (AR), and FEV_1. Subjects who had an increase in temperature showed an increase in indicators of inflammation in the blood (systemic response); those with an increase in AR showed an increase in indicators of airway inflammation (local response) but not in the blood; and those who had a decrease in FEV_1 did not shown an increase in inflammatory markers. The LPS-induced increase in body temperature and change in AR were not associated in a given subject, suggesting that the underlying mechanisms are dissociated. Further studies are urgently needed to assess whether these systemic changes are continuously present as part of the stable state of the COPD process or refelect day-to-day variations in the inflammatory state.

III. Systemic Inflammatory Responses During AECOPD

The events that increase the susceptibility of developing an exacerbation of COPD are poorly identified. Evidence indicates prominent changes in the local inflammatory profile during exacerbation, reflected by airway eosinophilia and increased levels of sputum proteins such as IL-8, myeloperoxidase (MPO), elastase, and endothelin-1 (19–22). In addition, changes in systemic inflammatory profile have been reported. Compared to patients in stable condition, the amounts of PMN in the circulation were further increased, although markers of activation could no longer be detected on the cells themselves (4). It could be hypothesized that this is due to sequestration of activated cells to the lungs, leaving the nonactivated cells behind. Activation of PMN during exacerbation has further been indicated by enhanced circulating levels of granulocyte/macrophage colony-stimulating factor, and of MPO (23,24). In the latter study, enhanced circulating levels of eosinophilic cationic protein were reported, suggesting that eosinophils are involved in the pathogenesis of exacerbation of COPD, in line with the observation of Saetta et al. (19). The oxidant–antioxidant imbalance, present in smokers and COPD patients, as reported above is even more pronounced during exacerbation of disease. Treatment of patients resulted in a return of this imbalance toward normal values (25).

Furthermore, also increased systemic levels of acute-phase proteins CRP, α_1-proteinase inhibitor, and α_1-antichymotrypsin were reported in patients with a clear bacterial infective exacerbation. Treatment of patients with antibiotics resulted in reduction of acute-phase proteins to levels present in stable conditions (20). Discrimination of exacerbations of chronic bronchitis patients on sputum color revealed that the enhancement of systemic CRP levels in purulent sputum exacerbations was significantly higher as compared to mucoid sputum exacerbation (21). Enhancement of systemic levels of fibrinogen and IL-6 was also detected during exacerbation of disease. In those patients with viral infection, a tendency toward higher levels of these mediators could be detected (26).

Besides activation of leukocytes and enhanced levels of acute-phase proteins a rise in circulating levels of the bronchoconstrictor peptide endothelin was also observed during exacerbation of disease (22). However, this enhancement was much more pronounced in sputum of the patients. Likewise, circulating levels of the leukotriene E4, which has bronchoconstrictive capacity, were elevated during exacerbation of COPD. Treatment with prednisolone resulted in reduction in the systemic levels of this leukotriene (27).

In general, the balance between pro- and anti-inflammatory mediators will determine the course of an inflammatory process. In a recent study, the hypothesis was made as to whether the chronic inflammatory process present in COPD is due to a defective anti-inflammatory mechanism (15). To this end, the systemic levels of the soluble forms of both TNF-Rs, and of IL-1RII, which could function as naturally occurring cytokine inhibitors (28), were analyzed in patients with stable COPD and compared with levels as present in control subjects. In addition, the time course of these inhibitors was studied in a group of patients hospitalized for an acute exacerbation of COPD during the first 7 days of hospitalization. Patients with stable COPD were characterized by a systemic inflammatory process indicated by an increased leukocyte count and enhanced levels of CRP and LBP. Both sTNF-Rs were only moderately enhanced and, therefore, were considered mainly as markers for a proinflammatory state (16). In contrast, sIL-1RII level was not different between patients and controls. These data suggest an imbalance in systemic levels of pro- and anti-inflammatory mediators in patients with stable COPD. During treatment of patients for exacerbation of disease, systemic levels of both CRP and LBP significantly declined, in line with other studies (20,21). The levels of both sTNF-Rs, however, showed only moderate changes. Furthermore, the levels of the anti-inflammatory mediator sIL-1RII strongly increased during treatment of exacerbation. This could be due to the effect of corticosteroids, which were part of the standard medications, known to induce shedding of membrane-bound IL-1RII (29). The authors speculated that the rise in sIL-1RII level could contribute to clinical improvement of patients.

Although the above-mentioned studies convincingly demonstrated the presence of a systemic inflammatory profile in COPD and a flare-up during exacerbation of disease, the source and the cause of this phenomenon still have to be elucidated. Since inflammatory processes are known to be affected by various factors like smoking status, bacterial colonization, treatment procedure, and other factors, in future studies of the role of inflammatory processes in the causes and progression of COPD, stratification of patient groups for these confounding factors is required.

IV. Muscle Wasting in COPD and During Acute Exacerbations

Systemic effects of a disease condition like COPD can be approached from structural or biochemical alterations in nonpulmonary structures or organs related to primary disease characteristics. Wasting of body cell mass (BCM) has to be considered as an important systemic manifestation, as a loss of more than 40% of actively metabolizing tissue is incompatible with life. The BCM represents the actively metabolizing and contracting tissue and can be clinically recognized by weight loss in general and loss of fat-free mass (FFM) in particular. Muscle mass is the single largest component of BCM and can be measured by assessment of FFM. In clinically stable patients with moderate-to-severe COPD, depletion of FFM has been reported in 20% of COPD outpatients and in 35% of those eligible for pulmonary rehabilitation (30,31). However, weight loss in COPD is not restricted to patients with moderate-to-severe COPD, but is also a frequent finding in mild COPD (32,33). During the last decade, it has been clearly shown that in addition to airflow limitation and loss of alveolar structure, respiratory and peripheral skeletal muscle weakness is an important determinant of dyspnea and exercise intolerance in COPD (34,35). Recent studies demonstrated that peripheral skeletal muscle dysfunction in COPD is characterized in part by reduced skeletal muscle mass (36). Moreover, FFM is a significant determinant of muscle strength (37), exercise capacity, and exercise response in patients with COPD (38–40). The functional consequences of being underweight and particularly of FFM depletion as quantified in exercise tests have also been reflected in a decreased health-related quality of life as measured by the St. George's Respiratory Questionnaire (SGRQ) (41). Patients with depleted FFM, regardless of body weight, also showed greater impairment in the activity and impact scores of the SGRQ and the domain invalidity of the Medical Psychological

Questionnaire for Lung Diseases, in comparison with depleted patients with relative preservation of FFM (42). The effects of FFM depletion on activity and impact of the SGRQ were mediated by a decreased exercise performance, but independent of exercise capacity a relationship was found between FFM depletion and the experienced invalidity of the patients.

Depletion of FFM can therefore been considered as an important determining factor of the "patient's condition," at least in a stable condition. In addition, several reports have provided evidence that weight loss negatively affects the prevalence and outcome of acute disease exacerbations. The risk of being hospitalized for an acute exacerbation is increased in patients with a low body mass index (BMI) (43). A low BMI and weight loss are also reported as an unfavorable index of outcome during an acute exacerbation of COPD (i.e., predicting the need for mechanical ventilation) (44). Furthermore, the survival time following disease exacerbation was independently related to the BMI (45). Early nonelective readmission in COPD patients for exacerbations is also found to be associated with weight loss during prior hospitalization and low body weight on prior admission for an acute exacerbation (46). Different metabolic alterations during acute exacerbations can contribute to weight loss and wasting of body cell mass: disturbances in energy metabolism, protein disturbances, or possible effects on muscle cell turnover.

A. Disturbances in Energy Balance

Depletion of FFM under chronic conditions like COPD can be approached by alterations in energy metabolism. Weight loss, in particular loss of fat mass (FM), occurs if energy, expenditure exceeds (EE) dietary intake. Total daily energy expenditure is usually divided into three components: (1) resting energy expenditure (REE), comprising sleeping metabolic rate and the energy cost of arousal; (2) diet-induced thermogenesis; and (3) physical activity-induced thermogenesis. Several studies have reported increases in REE in patients with COPD after adjustment for the metabolically active FFM. REE was found to be elevated in 25% of patients with COPD (47). Increasing evidence is present in the literature indicating that this increase in REE is related to the level of systemic inflammation (48,49). Ngyuen reported a significant relationship between REE and plasma levels of TNF-α. This polypeptide also triggers the release of other cytokines that mediate an increase in energy expenditure, as well as mobilization of amino acids and muscle protein catabolism. Otherwise, changes in total daily energy expenditure seem highly related to the energy spent for activities in patients suffering from COPD (50).

During acute exacerbations a temporary increase in metabolic rate has been reported (51). Especially during the initial days of onset of the exacerbation, an increase in REE can be measured. Remarkably, the improvement in energy balance during treatment of the acute exacerbation is accompanied by a significant improvement in symptoms such as dyspnea and fatigue (51).

In the same study, dietary intake was significantly lower than habitual intake and, especially during the initial phase, of the exacerbation, a negative energy balance could be demonstrated. These temporary disturbances in the energy balance during an acute exacerbation were related to increased leptin concentrations as well as to the systemic inflammatory response (52). Evidence was found that the elevated leptin concentrations during exacerbations were in turn under control of the systemic inflammatory response, and, presumably, the high-dose systemic glucocorticoid treatment. Leptin is a hormone produced by the adipose tissue and its circulating concentrations are proportional to the amount of fat mass. Leptin regulates the energy balance in a feedback mechanism in which the hypothalamus is involved (53). In animals, administration, of leptin results in a reduction in food intake (54) as well as in an increase in energy expenditure (55). The normal leptin feedback mechanism can be disturbed by several factors. In animals, administration of endotoxin, TNF-α or interleukin-1, inflammatory cytokines known for their anorectic effects, resulted dose-dependently in an upregulation of leptin mRNA in fat cells and in an increase in circulating leptin concentrations (56,57). Glucocorticosteroids stimulate leptin production directly or via the induction of insulin resistance, since glucose and insulin are also able to induce leptin expression (58–60). Besides function in weight homeostasis, leptin may also play a role in immunoregulation and ventilatory control (61,62). Whether these additional functions of leptin play a role during acute exacerbations of the disease deserves further attention.

B. Disturbances in Protein Metabolism

The ability to maintain homeostatic regulation of metabolic processes is an important key to survival of living organisms. While the regulation of energy balance in relation to weight loss has been extensively explored in COPD, investigation into intermediary metabolism is in its infancy. Protein turnover refers to a dynamic flux in protein metabolism whereby proteins are degraded and synthesized simultaneously. Protein turnover rates may differ considerably depending on function and specific need. Recently, substantial changes in whole-body protein metabolism after overnight fasting were reported in a group of clinically and weight-stable COPD patients. Significantly elevated levels of whole-body protein synthesis and breakdown were found (63), indicating a disease-related increase in whole-body protein turnover. Also in other chronic wasting diseases like cancer, human immunodeficiency virus infection, and advanced chronic renal failure, elevated levels for whole-body protein turnover were found (64–66). Several reports have provided evidence that weight loss negatively affects the prevalence and outcome of acute disease exacerbations of COPD (43–45). It can be hypothesized that these acute disease exacerbations induce a stepwise pattern of weight loss in COPD patients.

Weight loss and muscle wasting during an exacerbation has to be considered as a complex process, being a consequence of changes in the control of intermediary metabolism. Protein metabolism in disease states is regulated by various factors, which among others influence intermediary metabolism. The individual effects of several disease characteristics on intermediary metabolism have been investigated in healthy subjects and in other wasting conditions and are possibly also involved in COPD patients during acute phases of the disease process.

Factors Accelerating Protein Turnover in COPD

Increased Inflammatory Response

COPD is characterized by the presence of a chronic low-grade systemic inflammatory respons (15–68). Previous studies in other chronic wasting diseases showed that an acute inflammatory condition accelerates protein turnover (64,69). Evoked in inflammatory conditions, the acute-phase response includes hepatic synthesis of large quantities of proteins with a wide variety of functions. This is an energy-intensive process requiring large quantities of essential amino acids. The need for essential amino acids may drive the loss of skeletal muscle. In line with this, an inverse relationship between the acute-phase protein level and the total sum of plasma amino acid levels in stable patients with COPD is reported (70), suggesting that the elevated protein turnover in COPD may also be mediated by an activation of the cytokine network. It is likely that the increased inflammatory state associated with an exacerbation of COPD further accelerates protein turnover in these patients.

Intracellular Protein Degradation

The provision of the essential amino acids required for protein synthesis and energy metabolism requires the overall breakdown of cell proteins, especially in the muscles. Mammalian cells contain multiple proteolytic systems that serve distinct functions. However, most cellular proteins are degraded by a multienzymatic process, the ubiquitin-proteasome pathway (71). Degradation of proteins via this multistep pathway requires adenosine triphosphate (ATP) hydrolysis, the protein cofactor ubiquitin, and the 26S proteasome. The proteasome is a very large complex made up of at least 50 subunits, which may comprise as much as 1% of total cell proteins (72). Proteins are digested within the central core of the 26S proteasome, the 20S particle, which is a cylindrical complex containing three different proteolytic activities. In most cases, protein substrates are marked for degradation by covalent linkage of a chain of ubiquitin molecules. The ATP-ubiquitin-dependent proteolytic system can be activated by different factors: cytokines (71), glucocorticosteroids (73), acidosis (74), inactivity (75), or low insulin levels.

Proinflammatory cytokines such as TNF-α and IL-6 can activate the ubiquitin proteasome pathway. In stable COPD patients, muscle wasting was associated with increased serum levels of TNF-α as well as both TNF receptors, IL-6, and the soluble IL-6 receptor levels (76).

Acidosis

Respiratory acidosis often accompanies an exacerbation of COPD. Although no studies have been performed examining the effects of respiratory acidosis on intermediary metabolism, the protein metabolic effects of metabolic acidosis have extensively been studied in patients with chronic renal failure. Acidosis is known to increase degradation of proteins via stimulation of branched-chain amino acid (BCAA) dehydrogenase and to enhance the oxidation of the essential BCAAs (77,78). Moreover, acidosis stimulates cortisol secretion, which in itself results in proteolysis. In line with this, correction of acidosis for 4 weeks in hemodialysis patients decreased whole-body protein breakdown and synthesis (79). Glucocorti-costeroids are required, together with other signals, for the increase in mRNAs encoding ubiquitin and proteasome subunits and in ubiquitin-protein conjugates in muscles from rats in the fasting state (80,81). The chief factor opposing the catabolic effects of glucocorticosteroids is insulin (78). Activation of muscle proteolysis in the fasting state requires two signals: the presence of glucocorticosteroids and a decrease in insulin. In subjects who have an excess of glucocorticosteroids and are not in a fasting state, the high glucocorticoid level overcomes the inhibitory effect of insulin and causes muscle wasting (71). The catabolic response to acidification also requires glucocorticoids. These negative effects of systemic corticosteroid administration in the management of acute exacerbations are unexplored, yet based on the targeting of the primary organ failure (82).

Factors Reducing Protein Turnover in COPD

Hypoxia

An acute exacerbation in COPD is often accompanied by arterial hypoxemia. Hypoxia has been shown to depress muscle protein synthesis rate in animals and humans: 6 h of hypoxia (FiO_2: 11%) in rat decreased muscle protein synthesis rate by 14 to 17% (83). In line with this, ischemia and low flow conditions resulted in a reduced protein synthesis in perfused rat hindlimb muscle. Not only is PS an energy-consuming process (formation of peptide bindings, amino acid transport, RNA turnover) but also the ubiquitin proteosome pathway is ATP-requiring. Therefore, it is likely that in conditions of decreased ATP availability such as hypoxia, muscle protein turnover is depressed in COPD. However, it remains unclear whether and to what extent tissue hypoxia actually occurs during respiratory failure in COPD.

Insulin Resistance

Insulin has a central regulatory role in the regulation of intermediary metabolism. It inhibits glucose production by liver and kidney and stimulates peripheral glucose disposal. Previous longitudinal and cross-sectional studies found increased fasting insulin levels and a decreased fasting glucose/insulin ratio in stable COPD patients (37). Insulin resistance seems to be at the basis of this metabolic disturbance, although the few available data on COPD are not always consistent (84–86).

Insulin resistance also seems to be present during an exacerbation of COPD, based on the high insulin concentrations and the temporary increased glucose concentration (87). A significant correlation was found between glucose and sTNF-R55 in patients with COPD on day 7 of an acute exacerbation (68). Also TNF-α is known for its role in insulin resistance (78). In addition, the kinetics of glucose and insulin response during the exacerbation may (partly) be related to tapering off the systemic prednisolone treatment. Therefore, enhanced chronic and acute inflammatory state and glucocorticosteroid treatment will enhance peripheral insulin resistance in chronic wasting disease like COPD. In contrast, hypoxia is known to influence glucose metabolism by increasing glucose production and stimulating peripheral glucose transport, even in insulin-resistant human skeletal muscle. In healthy subjects, basal glucose production is almost twice as high at chronic altitude exposure as at sea level. This suggests that the balance between factors positively and negatively influencing insulin sensitivity in COPD will determine its effect on intermediary metabolism. It is not well understood whether insulin resistance regarding glucose metabolism also extends to the antiproteolytic effect of this hormone. Recently, an association was found between insulin levels and skeletal muscle amino acid status, and in particular that of the BCAAs in COPD (37). Also other studies examining the relationship between insulin and leucine metabolism indicate that hyperinsulinemia may negatively influence amino acid and thus protein metabolism. It is therefore very possible that insulin resistance, not only at the glucose level, but also at the protein level, may contribute to loss of muscle mass in COPD.

Corticosteroid Therapy

Glucocorticosteroids are often used in the treatment of an acute exacerbation of COPD (82). In Crohn's disease, corticosteroid use for 4 days resulted in decreased values for whole-body protein synthesis and breakdown (88). In contrast, in the same disease, corticosteroid use for 7 days resulted in an increase in whole-body PS and PB (89). In muscle of rheumatoid arthritis patients, negative effects have been shown on PS. Skeletal muscle protein synthesis was reduced when comparing a group of rheumatoid arthritis patients using 8 mg prednisolone/day for 9 years versus a group who were not using corticosteroids (90).

Physical Inactivity

The protracted decrease in muscle activity that accompanies bed rest is associated with muscle atrophy, weakness, and a loss of body nitrogen. Prolonged (14 days) bed rest showed a 50% decrease in skeletal muscle protein synthesis as measured by an arteriovenous flux model based on infusion of tracer as well as measured by fractional synthetic rate by tracer incorporation into muscle protein (91). These results indicate that the loss of body protein with physical inactivity is predominantly due to a decrease in protein synthesis and that this decrease was reflected in whole-body measures.

Depressed Dietary (Protein) Intake

An impaired energy balance in patients with COPD was reported during the first days of an acute exacerbation of their disease, predominantly due to severely depressed dietary intake (68). A depressed dietary (protein) intake is known to negatively influence protein balance. A study by Mortil showed that reduced or absent protein intake (short-term starvation) results in a sharp reduction in whole-body and muscle protein breakdown (92). Changes in protein synthesis are less reliable.

In conclusion, the pathogenesis of protein wasting during an acute exacerbation of COPD is multifactorally determined (Fig. 1). Whereas at the molecular level protein synthesis and degradation appear to be regulated by independent factors and mechanisms, in vivo the flux rates of free amino acids to protein synthesis and from protein degradation appear strictly related and changes in the opposite direction are

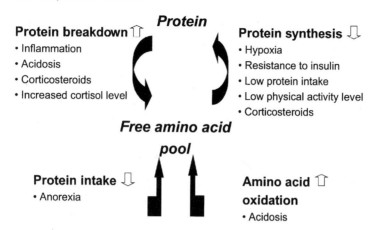

Protein breakdown ⇑
- Inflammation
- Acidosis
- Corticosteroids
- Increased cortisol level

Protein

Protein synthesis ⇓
- Hypoxia
- Resistance to insulin
- Low protein intake
- Low physical activity level
- Corticosteroids

Free amino acid

pool

Protein intake ⇓
- Anorexia

Amino acid ⇑
oxidation
- Acidosis

Figure 1 Factors contributing to disturbed protein turnover during AECOPD.

very rare. However, a small difference between rates of protein synthesis and breakdown determines protein accretion or loss. The inflammatory condition that evokes an acute-phase response is an important stressor increasing protein degradation in muscle during an acute exacerbation of COPD. It can be hypothesized that acute high-grade inflammation may negatively influence the balance between anabolic and catabolic responses at least partly through insulin resistance. Stressors like acidosis and increased cortisol secretion may further aggravate the acceleration in protein turnover.

A reduced protein-energy intake due to anorexia is likely the most common pathophysiological mechanism leading to decreased protein turnover. Other slow protein turnover conditions include low physical activity and insulin resistance. The presence of tissue hypoxia and insulin resistance and its modulating role in intermediary metabolism under conditions like an acute exacerbation of COPD remains elusive. Information on the exact contribution of each factor, and insight in the protein metabolic pathways and related mechanisms underlying muscle wasting during an acute exacerbation, is warranted in order to improve the efficacy of current treatment of muscle wasting.

V. Abnormalities in Gas Exchange During AECOPD: Effects on Muscle Energy Metabolism

Hypoxemia is a common finding during acute exacerbations of COPD. The consequences of hypoxemia and particularly impaired tissue oxygenation in the clinical course of acute exacerbations is poorly documented and at present impaired tissue oxygenation is mainly studied in relation to the energy-rich phosphate metabolism. Indeed, although over 100 enzymes require O_2 as a substrate, the most critical requirement for O_2 is to support mitochondrial ATP production.

In all cells, energy is needed for metabolic processes and maintenance of membrane potentials. In muscle cells, energy is further needed for cross-bridge cycling during contraction. Because muscle cell activity ranges from basal metabolic rate to vigorous contractile activity, muscle cells must be capable of large changes in metabolic activity. Therefore, energy metabolism is at present largely studied in muscle cells. Adenosine triphosphate (ATP) is the common energetic currency of the cell. Several strategies are available to muscle cells to ensure that enough ATP is generated under various circumstances. At the onset of contractile activity, energy is derived from a small pool of high-energy phosphates. To prevent a substantial decrease in ATP, phosphocreatine (PC) is available to provide phosphate for rephosphorylation of adenosine diphosphate (ADP) to ATP. Although in muscle cells relatively large quantities of PC are available, these stores can only supply energy for a short time. In the meantime, the rates of glycogenolysis and glycolysis accelerate to provide a more sustainable energy source (93,94). During glycolysis, glucose is metabolized to pyruvate in the cytosol. Pyruvate is either reduced to lactic acid, following an anaerobic pathway, or enters the mitochondrion to be metabolized aerobically. Within the mitochondrion, pyruvate is converted to acetyl CoA, which in turn enters the tricarboxylic acid cycle. In the inner mitochondrial membrane, reducing agents such as nicotinamide adenine dinucleotide, produced during glycolysis and in the tricarboxylic acid cycle, transfer electrons to O_2 to form H_2O. Energy derived from the passage of electrons along this so-called electron transport chain, is used to produce ATP in the oxidative phosphorylation process. In health, the processes of electron transport and oxidative phosphorylation are tightly coupled. Next to the formation of ATP via PC and the anaerobic glycolysis, the myokinase reaction $(2\ ADP \rightarrow AMP + ATP)$ is a third pathway for anaerobic formation of ATP (95).

Aerobic metabolism has several important advantages over anaerobic metabolism. First, it produces more energy: 38 ATP per mole of glucose versus 2 ATP per mole glucose in anaerobic glycolysis. Second, in aerobic metabolism, except for glucose lipid can be used as fuel via beta-oxidation (96).

Energy metabolism in resting muscle has been investigated in biopsy studies, evaluating muscle fiber-type distribution, muscle enzyme activities, and muscle high-energy phosphate content. By histochemical analysis using ATPase staining, a low proportion of type I fibers was positively related to the arterial PaO_2. In a recent study comparing COPD patients with age-matched healthy control subjects, the reduction in the proportion of type I fibers in quadriceps femoris muscle was confirmed and was found to be accompanied by an increase in the proportion of type IIb fibers (97). Furthermore, in COPD patients, the cross-sectional areas of type I, IIa, and IIab fibers were smaller as compared with the healthy controls (97). Further evaluation of energy metabolism in resting muscle of COPD patients comprised assessment of enzyme capacities in biopsies. Two studies investigated oxidative and glycolytic enzyme capacities in resting quadriceps femoris muscle of stable COPD patients. Jakobsson and coworkers (98) found decreased oxidative enzyme capacity as measured by a decreased citrate synthase (CS) capacity, and an increased glycolytic capacity, as measured by an increased phosphofructokinase (PFK) capacity. Maltais and coworkers (99) found a decreased CS and 3-hydroxyacyl-CoA dehydrogenase (HAD) capacity, but found PFK capacity to be unchanged.

Increased cytochrome oxidase capacity and upregulated mitochondrial gene expression of cytochrome oxidase have also been reported in resting quadriceps femoris muscle of stable COPD patients with chronic hypoxemia (100). Cytochrome oxidase is a key oxidative enzyme, being the terminal enzyme in the mitochondrial electron transport chain. It is as yet unclear how to interpret the variable results regarding parameters of oxidative metabolism. Further studies, investigating well-defined patient groups, and key enzymes of different metabolic pathways, are warranted.

Muscle high-energy phosphate content was analyzed in quadriceps femoris muscle comparing stable COPD patients to healthy control subjects (101). Muscle ATP and glycogen were lower and muscle creatine (C) and lactate were increased in COPD patients. In this study COPD patients were mildly hypoxemic (mean PaO_2 7.8 kPa). Comparing stable COPD patients with and without chronic respiratory failure (102) lower muscle ATP, PC, and glycogen levels, and higher C levels were found in patients with chronic respiratory failure. Furthermore, PaO_2 was positively and $PaCO_2$ was negatively related with muscle glycogen and PC. Present data stress the need to explore the role of hypoxemia and tissue oxygenation during these episodes of acute exacerbation of the disease process. Better insights in the alterations in energy metabolism can provide new therapeutic approaches in the management of the more severe acute exacerbations.

VI. Hypercapnia-Induced Changes in Energy Metabolism

The intracellular acidification that accompanies hypercapnia in skeletal muscle cells also affects the energy state of the muscle. It has been proposed that hypercapnia-induced acidosis results in glycolytic enzyme inhibition (103). Furthermore, it is well known that the creatine kinase reaction is near equilibrium in skeletal muscles (104) and that the equilibrium position of this reaction is pH-dependent (105).

Therefore, decreases in intracellular pH should result in a significant decrease in PCr levels in intact muscle (106). Meyer et al. (104) clearly demonstrated that the effects of intracellular acidification reflect both the creatine kinase equilibrium as well as the balance between all of the ATPase and ATPsynthetase reactions in the cell. They demonstrated that the effect of decreased pH in quiescent slow-twitch muscle is a relative stimulation of ATP synthesis or decrease in ATP hydrolysis rate, resulting in an increase in PCr levels.

Bioenergetics under hypercapnia-induced acidosis seems to be muscle fiber–type dependent: slow oxidative fibers, which have more mitochondria, are stimulated by acidosis (107) and fast fibers, which have fewer mitochondria, are depressed by acidosis (108–111). These findings again support a more systematic approach of energy metabolism in the assessment of AECOPD.

VII. Conclusion

Better insigths into the pathophysiology of COPD stress the complexity and heterogeneity of COPD. Growing evidence supports that AECOPD has to be considered as a complex inflammatory and metabolic derangement in the clinical course of the COPD patient. Gas exchange abnormalities complicating the acute exacerbation can have marked effects on energy and intermediary metabolism and on organ dysfunction. A more integrative approach of AECOPD can unravel new future therapeutic strategies in the management of AECOPD.

References

1. Anthonisen NR, Manfreda J, Warren CP, Hershfield ES, Harding GK, Nelson NA. Antibiotic therapy in exacerbations of chronic obstructive pulmonary disease. Ann Intern Med 1987; 106(2):196–204.
2. Rodriguez-Roisin R. Toward a consensus definition for COPD exacerbations. Chest 2000; 117(5 Suppl 2):398s–401s.
3. Barnes PJ. Medical progress: Chronic obstructive pulmonary disease. N Engl J Med 2000; 343:269–280.
4. Noguera A, Busquets X, Sauleda J, Villaverde JM, MacNee W, Agusti AGN. Expression of adhesion molecules and G proteins in circulating neutrophils in chronic obstructive pulmonary disease. Am J Respir Crit Care Med 1998; 158:1664–1668.
5. Riise FC, Larsson S, Löfdahl CG, Andersson BA. Circulating cell adhesion molecules in bronchial lavage and serum in COPD patients with chronic bronchitis. Eur Respir J 1994; 7:1673–1677.
6. Rahman I, Morrison D, Donaldson K, MacNee W. Systemic oxidative stress in asthma, COPD and smokers. Am J Respir Crit Care Med 1996; 154:1055–1060.
7. Sauleda J, Garcia Palmer JF, González G, Palou A, Agusti AGN. The activity of cytochrome oxidase is increased in circulating lymphocytes of patients with chronic obstructive pulmonary disease, asthma and chronic bronchitis. Am J Respir Crit Care Med 2000; 161;32:32–35.
8. Gabay C, Kushner I. Acute phase proteins and other systemic responses to inflammation. New Engl J Med 1999; 340:448–454.
9. Schols AM, Buurman WA, Staal van den Brekel AJ, Dentener MA, Wouters EFM. Evidence for a relation between metabolic derangements and increased levels of inflammatory mediators in a subgroup of patients with chronic obstructive pulmonary disease. Thorax 1996; 51:819–824.
10. Yasuda N, Gotoh K, Minatoguchi S, Asano K, Nishigaki K, Nomura M, Ohno, A, Watanabe, M, Sano, H, Kumada H, Sawa, T, Fujiwara H. An increase of soluble Fas, an inhibitor of apoptosis, associated with progression of COPD. Respir Med 1998; 92:993–999.
11. Dahl M, Tybjærg-hansen A, Vesto J, Lange P, Nordestgaard BG. Elevated plasma fibrinogeen associated with reduced pulmonary function and increased risk of chronic obstructive pulmonary disease. Am. J Respir Crit Care Med 2001; 164:1008–1111.
12. Dentener MA, Vreugdenhil ACE, Hoet PHM, Vernooy JHJ, Nieman FHM, Heumann D, Janssen YMW, Buurman WA, Wouters EFM. Evidence for production of the acute phase

protein LPS binding protein (LBP) by respiratory type II epithelial cells: implications for local defense to bacterial endotoxins. Am J Respir Cell Mol Biol 2000; 23:146–153.

13. Takabatake N, Nakamura H, Abe S, Inoue, S. Hino T, Saito H, Yuki H, Kato S, Tomoike H. The relationship between chronic hypoxemia and activation of the tumor necrosis factor-alpha system in patients with chronic obstructive pulmonary disease. Am J Respir Crit Care Med 2000; 161:1179–1184

14. Bemelmans MHA, Van Tits LJH, Buurman WA. Tumor necrosis factor: function, release and clearance. Crit Rev Immunol 1996; 16:1–11.

15. Dentener MA, Creutzberg EC, Schols AMWJ, Mantovani A, Van't Veer C, Buurman WA, Wouters EFM. Systemic anti-inflammatory mediators in COPD: increase in soluble interleukin-1 receptor II during treatment of exacerbations. Thorax 2001; 56:721–726.

16. Bigda J, Holtmann H. TNF receptors—how they function and interact. Arch Immunol Ther Exp Warsz 1997; 45:263–270.

17. Hempel SL, Monick MM, Hunninghake GW. Effect of hypoxia on release of IL-1 and TNF by human alveolar macrophages. Am J Respir Cell Mol Biol 1996; 14:170–176.

18. Michel O, Dentener M, Corazza F, Buurman W, Rylander R. Healthy subjects express differences in clinical responses to inhaled lipopolysaccharide that are related with inflammation and with atopy. J Allergy Clin Immunol 2001; 107:797–804.

19. Saetta M, Di Stefano A, Maestrelli P, Turato, G, Ruggieri MP, Roggeri A, Calcagni P, Mapp CE, Ciaccia A, Fabbri LMI. Airway eosinophilia in chronic bronchitis during exacerbations. Am J Respir Crit Care Med 1994; 150:1646–1652.

20. Crooks SW, Bayley DL, Hill SL, Stockley RA. Bronchial inflammation in acute bacterial exacerbations of chronic bronchitis: the role of leukotriene B4. Eur Respir J 2000; 15:274–280.

21. Gompertz S, O'Brien C, Bayley DL, Hill SL, Stockley RA. Changes in bronchial inflammation during acute exacerbations of chronic bronchitis. Eur Respir J 2001; 17:1112–1119.

22. Roland M, Bhowmik A, Sapsford RJ, Seemungal TA, Jeffries DJ, Warner TD, Wedzicha JA. Sputum and plasma endothelin-1 levels in exacerbations of chronic obstructive pulmonary disease. Thorax 2001; 56:30–35.

23. Balbi B, Bason C, Balleari E, Fiasella F, Pesci A, Ghio R, Fabiano F. Increased bronchoalveolar granulocytes and granulocyte/macrophage colony-stimulating factor during exacerbations of chronic bronchitis. Eur Respir J 1997; 10:846–850.

24. Fiorini G, Crespi S, Rinaldi M, Oberti E, Vigorelli R, Palmieri G. Serum ECP and MPO are increased during exacerbations of chronic bronchitis with airway obstruction. Biomed Pharmacother 2000; 54:274–278.

25. Rahman I, Skwarska E, MacNee W. Attenuation of oxidant/antioxidant imbalance during treatment of exacerbations of chronic obstructive pulmonary disease. Thorax 1997; 52:565–568.

26. Seemungal T, Harper-Owen R, Bhowmik A, Moris I, Sanderson G, Message SW, MacCallum P, Meade TW, Jeffries DJ, Johnston SL, Wedzicha JA. Respiratory viruses, symptoms, and inflammatory markers in acute exacerbations and stable chronic obstructive pulmonary disease. Am J Respir Crit Care Med 2001; 164:1618–1623.

27. Shindo K, Hirai Y, Fukumura M, Koide K. Plasma levels of leukotriene E4 during clinical course of chronic obstructive pulmonary disease. Prostaglandins Leuko Essent Fatty Acids 1997; 56:213–217.

28. Dinarello CA. Role of pro- and anti-inflammatory cytokines during inflammation: experimental and clinical findings. J Biol Regul Homeost Agents 1997; 11:91–103.

29. Orlando S, Sironi M, Bianchi G, Drummond AH, Boraschi D, Yabes D, Mantovani A. Role of metalloproteases in the release of the IL-1 type II decoy receptor. J Biol Chem 1997; 272:31764–31769.

30. Schols AM, Soeters PB, Dingemans AM, Mostert R, Frantzen PJ, Wouters EF. Prevalence and characteristics of nutritional depletion in patients with stable COPD cligiblc for pulmonary rchabilitation. Am Rcv Rcspir Dis 1993; 147(5):1151–1156.

31. Engelen MP, Schols AM, Baken WO, Wesseling GJ, Wouters EF. Nutritional depletion in relation to respiratory and peripheral skeletal muscle function in out-patients with COPD. Eur Respir J 1994; 7(10):1793–1797.

32. Wilson DO, Donahoe M, Rogers RM, Pennock BE. Metabolic rate and weight loss in chronic obstructive lung disease. J Parenter Enteral Nutr 1990; 14(1):7–11.

33. Landbo C, Prescott E, Lange P, Vestbo J, Almdal TP. Prognostic value of nutritional status in chronic obstructive pulmonary disease. Am J Respir Crit Care Med 1999; 160:1856–1861.

34. Gosselink R, Troosters T, Decramer M. Peripheral muscle weakness contributes to exercise limitation in COPD. Am J Respir Crit Care Med 1996; 153:976–980.

35. Hamilton AL, Killian KJ, Summers E, Jones NL. Muscle strength, symptom intensity, and exercise capacity in patients with cardiorespiratory disorders. Am J Respir Crit Care Med 1995; 152:2021–2031.

36. Bernard S, LeBlanc P, Whittom F, Carrier G, Jobin J, Belleau R, Maltais F. Peripheral muscle weakness in patients with chronic obstructive pulmonary disease. Am J Respir Crit Care Med 1998; 158(2):629–634.

37. Engelen MPKJ, Wouters EFM, Deutz NEP, Menheere PP, Schols AMWJ. Factors contributing to alterations in skeletal muscle and plasma amino acid profiles in patients with chronic obstructive pulmonary disease. Am J Clin Nutr 2000; 72(6): 1480–1487.

38. Baarends EM, Schols AMWJ, Mostert R, Wouters EFM. Peak exercise response in relation to tissue depletion in patients with chronic obstructive pulmonary disease. Eur Respir J 1997; 10(12):2807–2813.

39. Palange P, Forte S, Felli A, Galasseti P, Serra P, Carlone S. Nutritional state and exercise tolerance in patients with COPD. Chest 1995; 107:1206–1212.

40. Palange P, Forte S, Onorati P, Paravati V, Manfredi F, Serra P, Carlone S. Effect of reduced body weight on muscle aerobic capacity in patients with COPD. Chest 1998; 114(1):12–18.

41. Shoup R, Dalsky G, Warner S, Davies M, Connors M, Khan M, Khan F, ZuWallack R. Body composition and health-related quality of life in patients with obstructive airways disease. Eur Respir J 1997; 10(7):1576–1580.

42. Mostert R, Goris A, Weling-Scheepers C, Wouters E, Schols A. Tissue depletion and health related quality of life in patients with chronic obstructive pulmonary disease. Respir Med 2000; 94:859–867.

43. Kessler R, Faller M, Fourgaut G, Mennecier B, Weitzenblum E. Predictive factors of hospitalization for acute exacerbation in a series of 64 patients with chronic obstructive pulmonary disease. Am J Respir Crit Care Med 1999; 159(1):158–164.

44. Vitacca M, Clini E, Porta R, Foglio K, Ambrosino N. Acute exacerbations in patients with COPD: predictors of need for mechanical ventilation. Eur Respir J 1996; 9(7):1487–1493.

45. Connors AF Jr, Dawson NV, Thomas C, Harrell FE, Jr, Desbiens N, Fulkerson WJ, Kussin P, Bellamy P, Goldman L, Knaus WA. Outcomes following acute exacerbation of severe chronic obstructive lung disease. The SUPPORT investigators (Study to Under-

stand Prognoses and Preferences for Outcomes and Risks of Treatments). Am J Respir Crit Care Med 1996; 154(4 Pt 1): 959–967.

46. Pouw EM, Velde ten GPM, Croonen BHPM, Kester ADM, Schols AMWJ, Wouters EFM. Early nonelective readmission for chronic obstructive pulmonary disease is associated with weight loss. Clin Nutr 2000; 19(2):95–99.

47. Creutzberg EC, Schols AM, Bothmer-Quaedvlieg FC, Wouters EFM. Prevalence of an elevated resting energy expenditure in patients with chronic obstructive pulmonary disease in relation to body composition and lung function. Eur J Clin Nutr 1998; 52(6):396–401.

48. Schols AM, Mostert R, Soeters PB, Wouters EFM. Body composition and exercise performance in patients with chronic obstructive pulmonary disease. Thorax 1991; 46(10):695–699.

49. Nguyen LT, Bedu M, Caillaud D, Beaufrere B, Beaujon G, Vasson M, Coudert J, Ritz P. Increased resting energy expenditure is related to plasma TNF-alpha concentration in stable COPD patients. Clin Nutr 1999; 18(5):269–274.

50. Baarends EM, Schols AM, Pannemans DL, Westerterp KR, Wouters EFM. Total free living energy expenditure in patients with severe chronic obstructive pulmonary disease. Am J Respir Crit Care Med 1997; 155(2):549–554.

51. Vermeeren MA, Schols AM, Wouters EFM. Effects of an acute exacerbation on nutritional and metabolic profile of patients with COPD. Eur Respir J 1997; 10(10):2264–2269.

52. Creutzberg EC, Wouters EFM, Vanderhoven-Augustin IML, Dentener MA, Schols AMWJ. Disturbances in leptin metabolism are related to energy imbalance during acute exacerbations of COPD. Am J Respir Crit Care Med 2000; 162:1239–1245.

53. Campfield LA, Smith FJ, Burn P. The OB protein (leptin) pathway—a link between adipose tissue mass and central neural networks. Horm Metab Res 1996; 28:619–632.

54. Seeley RJ, Van Dijk G, Campfield LA, Smith FJ, Burn P, Nelligan JA, Bell SM, Baskin DG, Woods SC, Schwartz MW. Intraventricular leptin reduces food intake and body weight of lean rats but not obese Zucker rats. Horm Metab Res 1996; 28:664–668.

55. Hwa JJ, Ghibaudi L, Compton D, Fawzi FB, Strader CD. Intracerebroventricular injection of leptin increases thermogenesis and mobilizes fat metabolism in ob/ob mice. Horm Metab Res 1996; 28:659–663.

56. Grunfeld C, Zhao C, Fuller J, Pollack A, Moser A, Friedman J, Feingold KR. Endotoxin and cytokines induce expression of leptin, the ob gene product, in hamsters. J Clin Invest 1996; 97:2152–2157.

57. Sarraf P, Frederich RC, Turner EM, Ma G, Jaskowiak NT, Rivet DJ III, Flier JS, Lowell BB, Fraker DL, Alexander HR. Multiple cytokines and acute inflammation raise mouse leptin levels: potential role in inflammatory anorexia. J Exp Med 1997; 185:171–175.

58. Dagogo JS, Selke G, Melson AK, Newcomer JW. Robust leptin secretory responses to dexamethasone in obese subjects. J Clin Endocrinol Metab 1997; 82:3230–3233.

59. Mizuno T, Bergen H, Kleopoulos S, Bauman WA, Mobbs CV. Effects of nutritional status and aging on leptin gene expression in mice: importance of glucose. Horm Metab Res 1996; 28:679–684.

60. Bodkin NL, Nicolson M, Ortmeyer HK, Hansen BC. Hyperleptinemia: relationship to adiposity and insulin resistance in the spontaneously obese rhesus monkey. Horm Metab Res 1996; 28:674–678.

61. Lord GM, Matarese G, Howard LK, Baker RJ, Bloom SR, Lechler RI. Leptin modulates the T-cell immune response and reverses starvation-induced immunosuppression. Nature 1998; 394(6696):897–901.

62. O'Donnell CP, Schaub CD, Haines AS, Berkowitz DE, Tankersley CG, Schwartz AR, Smith PL. Leptin prevents respiratory depression in obesity. Am J Respir Crit Care Med 1999; 159:1477–1484.

63. Engelen MPKJ, Deutz NEP, Wouters EFM, Schols AMWJ. Enhanced levels of whole-body protein turnover in patients with chronic obstructive pulmonary disease. Am J Respir Crit Care Med 2000; 162(4 Pt 1):1488–1492.

64. Macallan DC, McNurlan MA, Milne E, Calder AG, Garlick PJ, Griffin GE. Whole-body protein turnover from leucine kinetics and the response to nutrition in human immunodeficiency virus infection. Am J Clin Nutr 1995; 61(4):818–826.

65. Jeevanandam M, Horowitz GD, Lowry SF, Brennan MF. Cancer cachexia and protein metabolism. Lancet 1984; 1(8392):1423–1426.

66. Melville S, McNurlan MA, Calder AG, Garlick PJ. Increased protein turnover despite normal energy metabolism and responses to feeding in patients with lung cancer. Cancer Res 1990; 50(4):1125–1131.

67. Dentener MA, Creutzberg EC, Schols AMWJ, Mantovani A, van't Veer C, Buurman WA, et al. Systemic anti-inflammatory mediators in COPD: increase in soluble interleukin 1 receptor II during treatment of exacerbations. Thorax 2001; 56(9): 721–726.

68. Creutzberg EC, Wouters EFM, Vanderhoven-Augustin IM, Dentener MA, Schols AMWJ. Disturbances in leptin metabolism are related to energy imbalance during acute exacerbations of chronic obstructive pulmonary disease. Am J Respir Crit Care Med 2000:162(4 Pt 1):1239–1245.

69. Morton RE, Hutchings J, Halliday D, Rennie MJ, Wolman SL. Protein metabolism during treatment of chest infection in patients with cystic fibrosis. Am J Clin Nutr 1988; 47(2):214–249.

70. Pouw EM, Schols AMWJ, Deutz NEP, Wouters EFM. Plasma and muscle amino-acid levels in relation to resting energy expenditure and inflammation in stable COPD. Am J Respir Crit Care Med 1998; 158:797–801.

71. Mitch WE, Goldberg AL. Mechanisms of disease: mechanisms of muscle wasting: the role of the ubiquitin–proteasome pathway. N Engl J Med 1996; 335:1897–1905.

72. Baumeister W, Walz J, Zuhl F, Seemuller E. The proteasome: paradigm of a self-compartmentalizing protease. Cell 1998; 92:367–380.

73. Wing SS, Goldberg AL. Glucocorticoids activate the ATP-ubiquitin-dependent proteolytic system in skeletal muscle during fasting. Am J Physiol 1993; 264:E668–E676.

74. Mitch WE, Medina R, Greiber S, May RC, England BK, Price SR, Bailey JL, Goldberg AL. Metabolic acidosis stimulates muscle protein degradation by activating the adenosine triphosphate-dependent pathway involving ubiquitin and proteasomes. J Clin Invest 1994; 93:2127–2133.

75. Wing SS, Haas AL, Goldberg AL. Increase in ubiquitin-protein conjugates concomitant with the increase in proteolysis in rat skeletal muscle during starvation and atrophy denervation. Biochem J 1996; 307:639–645.

76. Eid AA, Lonescu AA, Nixon LS, Lewis-Jenkins V, Matthews SB, Griffiths TI, Shale DJ. Inflammatory response and body composition in chronic obstructive pulmonary disease. Am J Respir Crit Care Med 2001; 164:1414–1418.

77. Garibotto G. Muscle amino acid metabolism and the control of muscle protein turnover in patients with chronic renal failure. Nutrition 1999; 15(2):145–155.

78. Mitch WE. Robert H Herman Memorial Award in Clinical Nutrition Lecture, 1997. Mechanisms causing loss of lean body mass in kidney disease. Am J Clin Nutr 1998; 67(3):359–366.

79. Graham KA, Reaich D, Channon SM, Downie S, Goodship TH. Correction of acidosis in hemodialysis decreases whole-body protein degradation. J Am Soc Nephrol 1997; 8(4):632–637.
80. Wing SS, Goldberg AL. Glucocorticoids activate the ATP-ubiquitin-dependent proteolytic system in skeletal muscle during fasting. Am J Physiol 1993; 264:E668–E676.
81. Price SR, England BK, Bailey JL, Van Vreede K, Mitch WE. Acidosis and glucocorticoids concomitantly increase ubiquitin and proteasome subunit mRNAs in rat muscle. Am J Physiol 1994; 267:C955–C960.
82. Niewoehner DE, Erbland ML, Deupree RH, Collins D, Gross NJ, Light RW, Anderson P, Morgan NA. Effect of systemic glucocorticoids on exacerbations of chronic obstructive pulmonary disease. Department of Veterans Affairs Cooperative Study Group. N Engl J Med 1999; 340:1941–1947.
83. Preedy VR, Smith DM, Sugden PH. The effects of 6 hours of hypoxia on protein synthesis in rat tissues in vivo and in vitro. Biochem J 1985; 228(1):179–185.
84. Hjalmarsen A, Aasebo U, Birkeland K, Sager G, Jorde R. Impaired glucose tolerance in patients with chronic hypoxic pulmonary disease. Diabetes Metab 1996; 22(1): 37–42.
85. Jakobsson P, Jorfeldt L, von Schenck H. Insulin resistance is not exhibited by advanced chronic obstructive pulmonary disease patients. Clin Physiol 1995; 15(6):547–555.
86. Jakobsson P, Jorfeldt L, von Schenck H. Fat metabolism and its response to infusion of insulin and glucose in patients with advanced chronic obstructive pulmonary disease. Clin Physiol 1995; 15(4):319–329.
87. Hotamisligil GS, Arner P, Caro JF, Atkinson RL, Spiegelman BM. Increased adipose tissue expression of tumor necrosis factor-alpha in human obesity and insulin resistance. J Clin Invest 1995; 95(5):2409–2415.
88. Thomas AG, Miller V, Taylor F, Maycock P, Scrimgeour CM, Rennie MJ. Whole body protein turnover in childhood Crohn's disease. Gut 1992; 33(5):675–677.
89. O'Keefe SJ, Ogden J, Rund J, Potter P. Steroids and bowel rest versus elemental diet in the treatment of patients with Crohn's disease: the effects on protein metabolism and immune functions. J Parenter Enteral Nutr 1989; 13(5):455–460.
90. Gibson JN, Poyser NL, Morrison WL, Scrimgeour CM, Rennie MJ. Muscle protein synthesis in patients with rheumatoid arthritis: effect of chronic corticosteroid therapy on prostaglandin F2 alpha availability. Eur J Clin Invest 1991; 21(4):406–412.
91. Ferrando AA, Lane HW, Stuart CA, Davis-Street J, Wolfe RR. Prolonged bed rest decreases skeletal muscle and whole body protein synthesis. Am J Physiol 1996; 270(4 Pt 1): E627–E633.
92. Motil KJ, Matthews DE, Bier DM, Burke JF, Munro HN, Young VR. Whole-body leucine and lysine metabolism: response to dietary protein intake in young men. Am J Physiol 1981; 240(6):E712–E721.
93. Spriet L, Soderlund L, Bergstrom M, Hultman E. Anaerobic energy release in skeletal muscle during electrical stimulation in man. J Appl Physiol 1987; 62:611–615.
94. Frits RH, Cellular mechanisms of muscle fatigue. Physiol Rev 1994; 74:49–94.
95. Sahlin K, Broberg S, Ren JM. Formation of inosine monophosphate (IMP) in human skeletal muscle during incremental dynamic exercise. Acta Physiol Scand 1989; 136:193–198.
96. Westerblad H, Lee JA, Lannergren J, Allen DG. Cellular mechanisms of fatigue in skeletal muscle. Am J Physiol 1991; 261:C195–C209.
97. Whittom F, Jobin J, Simard PM, Leblanc P, Simard C, Bernard S, Belleau R, Maltais F. Histochemical and morphological characteristics of the vastus lateralis muscle in COPD

patients. Comparison with normal subjects and effects of exercise training. Med Sci Sports Exerc 1998; 30:1467–1474.

98. Jakobsson P, Jordfelt L, Hendriksson J. Metabolic enzyme activity in the quadriceps femoris muscle in patients with severe chronic obstructive pulmonary disease. Am J Respir Crit Care Med 1995; 151:374–377.

99. Maltais F, Simard A, Simard C, Jobin J, Desgagnes P, LeBlanc P. Oxidative capacity of the skeletal muscle and lactic acid kinetics during exercise in normal subjects and in patient with COPD. Am J Respir Crit Care Med 1996; 153:288–293.

100. Sauleda J, Garcia-Palmer F, Wiesner RJ, Tarraga S, Harting I, Tomas P, Gomez C, Saus C, Palou A, Agusti AGN. Cytochrome oxidase activity and mitochondrial gene expression in skeletal muscle of patients with chronic obstructive pulmonary disease. Am J Respir Crit Care Med 1998; 157:1413–1417.

101. Jakobsson P, Jordfelt L. Long-term oxygen therapy may improve skeletal muscle metabolism in advanced chronic obstructive pulmonary disease patients with chronic hypoxaemia. Respir Med 1995; 89:471–476.

102. Jakobsson P, Jordfelt L, Brundin A. Skeletal muscle metabolites and fibre types in patients with advanced chronic obstructive pulmonary disease (COPD), with and without chronic respiratory failure. Eur Respir J 1990; 3:192–196.

103. Braunwald E. Control of myocardial oxygen consumption. Am J Cardiol 1971; 27: 416–432.

104. Meyer RA, Sweeney HL, Kushmerick MJ. A simple analysis of the "phosphocreatine shuttle." Am J Physiol 1984; 246:C365–C377.

105. Lawson JWR, Veech RL. Effects of pH and free Mg^{2+} on the K_{eq} of the creatine kinase reaction and other phosphate hydrolyses and phosphate transferases. J Biol Chem 1979; 254:6528–6537.

106. Sahlin K, Edstrom L, Sjoholm H. Fatigue and phosphocreatine depletion during carbon dioxide-induced acidosis in rat muscle. Am J Physiol 1983; 245:C15–C20.

107. Pannier JL, Weyne J, Leusen I. Effects of PCO_2, bicarbonate and lactate on the isometric concentrations of isolated soleus muscle of the rat. Pfluegers Arch 1970; 320:120–132.

108. Nioka S, Argov Z, Dobson GP, Forster RE, Subramanian HV, Veech RL, Chance B. Substrate regulation of mitochondrial oxidative phosphorylation in hypercapnic rabbit muscle. J Appl Physiol 1992 Feb; 72(2): 521–528.

109. Dawson MJ, Gadian DG, Wilkie DR. Muscular fatigue investigated by phosphorus nuclear magnetic resonance. Nature 1978; 274:861–866.

110. Hill DK. Preferred sites of adenine nucleotide in frog's striated muscle. J Physiol Lond 1960; 153:433–446.

111. Mukherjee A, Wong TM, Templeton G, Buja LM, Willerson JT. Influence of volume dilution, lactate, phosphate, and calcium on mitochondrial functions. Am J Physiol 1979; 237:H224–H238.

9

Causes of Acute Exacerbations of Chronic Obstructive Pulmonary Disease

JADWIGA A. WEDZICHA

St. Bartholomew's and Royal London School of Medicine and Dentistry
St. Bartholomew's Hospital
London, England

I. Introduction

Exacerbations of chronic obstructive pulmonary disease (COPD) are an important cause of the considerable morbidity and mortality found in COPD (1). Some patients are prone to frequent exacerbations that are an important cause of hospital admission and readmission, and these frequent exacerbations may have considerable impact on quality of life and activities of daily living (2). Strategies to reduce exacerbation frequency are urgently required and depend on an understanding of the etiological factors associated with exacerbations. COPD exacerbations are caused by a variety of factors such as viruses, bacteria, and possibly common pollutants (Fig. 1).

II. Viral Infections

COPD exacerbations are frequently triggered by upper respiratory tract infections and these are more common in the cold winter months (3) when there are more respiratory viral infections prevalent in the community. Patients may also be more prone to exacerbations during the winter because lung function in COPD patients shows small, but significant, decreases with reduction in outdoor temperature (3).

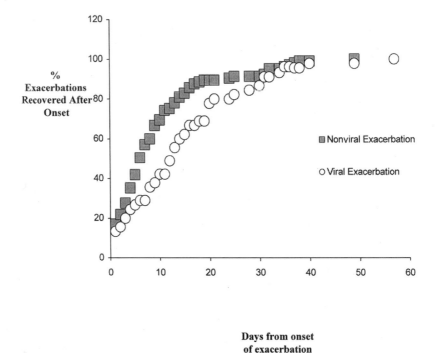

Figure 1   Graph showing the cumulative percentage of viral and nonviral exacerbations recovering symptomatically with respect to time after onset during 150 COPD exacerbations ($p = 0.006$). (Reproduced with permission from Ref. 5.)

Further evidence that respiratory viral infections are important triggers of exacerbations comes from the association of colds with exacerbations. In a prospective analysis of 504 exacerbations, where daily monitoring was performed, larger falls in peak flow were associated with symptoms of dyspnea and presence of colds, and were related to longer recovery time from exacerbations (4). We have recently reported that up to 64% of exacerbations were associated with symptomatic colds as assessed using daily diary card monitoring and thus it is likely that these exacerbations were precipitated by viruses (5). Viruses that may lead to respiratory tract infections are listed in Table 1.

A.   Detection of Respiratory Viruses

Rhinovirus is responsible for the common cold and is currently the most important cause of COPD exacerbation. Since the introduction of influenza immunization for patients with chronic lung disease, influenza has become a less prominent cause of exacerbation, although this is still likely to be an important factor at times of influenza epidemics. Together with enteroviruses, rhinoviruses belong to the picornavirus group of RNA viruses. Rhinoviruses are spread directly from one

Table 1 Etiology of COPD Exacerbations

Viruses
Rhinovirus (common cold)
Coronavirus
Influenza A and B
Parainfluenza
Adenovirus
RSV
Atypical organisms
Chlamydia pneumoniae
Mycoplasma pneumoniae
Bacteria
Haemophilus influenzae
Streptococcus penumoniae
Branhamella cattarhalis
Staphylococcus aureus
Pseudomonas aeruginosa
Common pollutants
Nitrogen dioxide
Particulates
Sulfur dioxide
Ozone

person to another by infected respiratory secretions. Although rhinovirus has been recognized as an important cause of asthma exacerbations (6,7), until recently rhinovirus had not been considered significant during exacerbations of COPD because techniques for detection used only isolation by cell culture and serology. This virus has fastidious growth requirements and over 100 serotypes, which make detection by culture or serological methods very difficult.

Early studies using serological and cell culture diagnostic methods reported relatively small effects of rhinovirus at COPD exacerbations. In a study of 44 chronic bronchitics over 2 years, Stott and colleagues found rhinovirus in 13 (14.9%) of 87 exacerbations of chronic bronchitis (8). In a more detailed study of 25 chronic bronchitics with 116 exacerbations over 4 years, Gump et al. found that only 3.4% of exacerbations could be attributed to rhinoviruses (9). In a study of 35 episodes of COPD exacerbation that used serological methods and nasal samples for viral culture, little evidence was found for a rhinovirus etiology of COPD exacerbation (10). Greenberg and colleagues recently also studied viral etiologies of COPD exacerbations and, using viral culture and serology, found that 27% of COPD exacerbations were associated with respiratory viruses, while 44% of acute respiratory illnesses in control subjects were associated with viruses (11). In COPD patients, rhinoviruses accounted for 43% of the virus infections and thus were responsible for about 12% of exacerbations.

B.   Virus Detection with PCR Techniques

The advent of polymerase chain reaction (PCR) techniques for viral detection enabled a more detailed evaluation of the role of viruses in asthma and COPD exacerbations. Studies in childhood asthma have shown that rhinovirus can be detected by polymerase chain reaction from a large number of these exacerbations (7). We have recently reported a study to evaluate the nature of respiratory viruses at COPD exacerbation using PCR techniques for the major respiratory viruses (5). Samples consisted of nasopharyngeal aspirates or throat swabs at exacerbation and also when patients were stable. Up to 40% of COPD exacerbations were associated with viral infections, although this may be an underestimate due to difficulties in sampling at the very onset of an exacerbation. Rhinovirus was the most common respiratory virus detected and found in 58% of viral exacerbations. The other viruses detected included coronavirus (11%), influenza A and B (16%), and parainfluenza, adenovirus, and *Chlamydia pneumoniae* were each detected in one exacerbation. The relatively low levels of influenza were related to the fact that 74% of the patients had received influenza immunization.

Viruses are less likely to be associated with exacerbations with increased sputum volume or purulence. This observation may explain the finding in the study reported by Anthonisen and colleagues that the effects of antibiotics were not significantly different from placebo in the treatment of exacerbations without the presence of purulent sputum (12). In our study, respiratory viruses were associated with a longer median symptom recovery time at exacerbation of 13 days compared to 6 days for nonviral exacerbations. Viruses were also found to be associated with a slower rate of symptom score resolution (Fig. 1). Thus viruses are associated with more severe exacerbations and therefore with greater morbidity. Measures to prevent viral infection may lead to a reduction in exacerbation frequency, exacerbation severity, and reduction in hospital admission, and thus may have important economic consequences.

Using the median number of exacerbations as a cut-off point, we have previously classified COPD patients as frequent and infrequent exacerbators (2). Quality of life was significantly worse in the frequent, compared to the infrequent, exacerbators. Factors predictive of frequent exacerbations included the exacerbation frequency in the previous year. This suggests that exacerbation frequency is an important determinant of health status in COPD and is thus an important outcome measure. In the study by Seemungal and colleagues of respiratory virus detection by PCR (5), at least one virus was detected in 64% of patients and these patients had a higher exacerbation frequency than patients where viruses were not detected. Thus patients with a history of frequent exacerbations may be more susceptible to respiratory viral infections and further work is required to study the nature of this susceptibility.

We also found that 19 exacerbations were associated with respiratory syncytial virus (RSV), although more patients had RSV detected in the stable state than at exacerbation. In none of these samples was RSV detected by culture or serology and detection disappeared when the sensitivity of the PCR was reduced, suggesting that the colonization with virus was low grade. However, we found that patients in whom RSV was detected were more likely to have elevated systemic inflammatory markers. This implies that RSV may be a cause of chronic infection in COPD and further evaluation of the role of RSV at COPD exacerbation is required. Viruses apart from RSV were detected in 16.2% of patients with stable COPD by PCR. Rhinoviruses were most commonly detected in the stable state as well as at exacerbation, and were found in 7.3% of stable COPD patients; coronaviruses were found in 5.9% of stable patients. There was a tendency for patients in whom these viruses were detected in stable COPD to give a history of more frequent exacerbations in the year prior to recruitment. Recent work by Retmales and colleagues shows that latent expression of adenoviral E1A protein in alveolar epithelial cells may amplify the effects of cigarette smoke–induced lung inflammation (13). Thus chronic viral infection may be linked to disease severity in COPD.

C. Detection of Rhinovirus in the Lower Airway

There is now increasing evidence from experimental rhinovirus infections that respiratory viruses can infect the lower airway (14,15). Seemungal and colleagues showed that rhinovirus can be recovered from induced sputum more frequently using PCR techniques than from nasal aspirates at exacerbation, suggesting that wild-type rhinovirus can infect the lower airway and contribute to inflammatory changes at exacerbation (16). They also found that exacerbations associated with the presence of rhinovirus in induced sputum had larger increases in airway IL-6 levels compared to exacerbations where rhinovirus was not detected. This suggests that viruses increase the severity of airway inflammation at exacerbation. This finding is in agreement with the data that respiratory viruses produce longer and more severe exacerbations and have a major impact on health care utilization (4,5).

D. Mechanisms of Virus-Induced Exacerbations

There are a number of mechanisms that may be involved in the association between viruses and exacerbations. The major group of rhinoviruses (accounting for 90% of total rhinovirus types) attach to airway epithelium through ICAM-1, inducing ICAM-1 expression, which promotes inflammatory cell recruitment and activation as seen in exacerbations (17). The minor rhinovirus group use members of the LDL-receptor family as cell surface receptors, although ICAM-1 surface expression may also be upregulated (17). There is some evidence for upregulation of ICAM-1 in the bronchial mucosa of patients with chronic bronchitis (18), and thus ICAM-1 is an important therapeutic target in COPD exacerbation associated with rhinoviruses.

In a prospectively followed cohort of patients from the East London COPD Study, inflammatory markers in induced sputum were related to symptoms and physiological changes at COPD exacerbation (19). At exacerbation, increases were found in induced sputum IL-6 levels and the levels of IL-6 were higher when exacerbations were associated with symptoms of the common cold (Fig. 2).

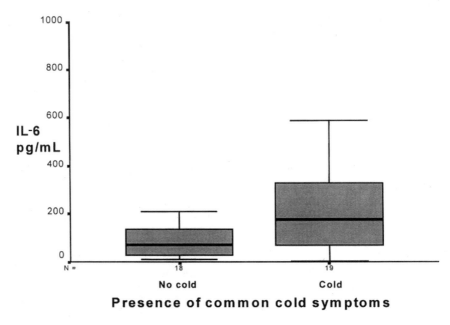

Figure 2   Induced sputum IL-6 levels in the absence and presence of a natural cold. Data are expressed as medians (IQR). (Reproduced with permission from Ref. 19.)

Experimental rhinovirus infection has been shown to increase sputum IL-6 in normal subjects and asthmatics (20–22). However, rises in cell counts and IL-8 were more variable with exacerbation and did not reach statistical significance, suggesting marked heterogeneity in the degree of the inflammatory response at exacerbation. The exacerbation IL-8 levels were related to sputum neutrophil and total cell counts, indicating that neutrophil recruitment is the major source of airway IL-8 at exacerbation. Lower airway IL-8 has been shown to increase with experimental rhinovirus infection in normal and asthmatic patients in some studies (21) but not in others (22). However, COPD patients have already upregulated airway IL-8 levels when stable due to their high sputum neutrophil load (23) and further increases in IL-8 would be unlikely. COPD exacerbations are associated with a less pronounced airway inflammatory response than asthmatic exacerbations (24), and this may explain the relatively reduced response to steroids seen at exacerbation in COPD patients relative to asthma (25–31).

Viral infections have been associated with increased oxidant stress that is increased at COPD exacerbation (32). Rhinovirus infection of human respiratory epithelial cells increases production of reactive oxygen species and stimulates the activation of nuclear factor kappa B (NF-κB), which is important in the regulation of the IL-8 gene (33). In patients with experimental rhinovirus infections, nasal IL-8 levels have been related to common cold symptoms (34). Viral infections can also induce the expression of stress-response genes (e.g., heme-oxygenase-1) and genes encoding antioxidant enzymes (e.g., glutathione peroxidase, MnSOD) (35) and these responses may be important in potentiating the effects of the virally mediated inflammation at COPD exacerbation. We have also shown that exacerbations are associated with increased airway and systemic endothelin-1 levels (36). Endothelin-1 is an important bronchoconstrictor peptide that has been found to be proinflammatory and mucogenic and has been also implicated in the pathogenesis of virally mediated inflammation (37). Sputum ET-1 levels increase at COPD exacerbation and these increases are related to sputum IL-6 levels. Further work with specific ET receptor antagonists may provide a new therapeutic option for virus-induced inflammation associated with COPD exacerbations.

E. Relation of Viruses to Systemic Inflammation in COPD

Recently, associations have been described between chronic bronchitis and death from cardiovascular disease (38). Plasma fibrinogen is an independent risk factor for cardiovascular disease (39) and we have shown that plasma fibrinogen is increased in COPD thus making COPD patients with moderate-to-severe disease more susceptible to ischemic events (40). At exacerbation we found further increased levels of plasma fibrinogen and Il-6, which is produced by blood monocytes and stimulates the production of fibrinogen in the liver. We found that plasma fibrinogen levels were higher in the presence of colds and respiratory viral infections at COPD exacerbation (5,40). This suggests that viral infections are associated with increased systemic inflammatory markers and also may predispose to an increased risk from vascular disease. Epidemiological studies have suggested that infections, especially those of the respiratory tract, may be involved in the onset of myocardial infarction and stroke (41) and thus patients who are frequent exacerbators with their recurrent infections may be particularly susceptible to cardiovascular disease.

III. Role of Bacterial Infection in COPD Exacerbation

The precise role of bacteria in COPD exacerbation has been difficult to evaluate because airway bacterial colonization in the stable state has been found in approximately 30% of COPD patients. The most common organism isolated is *Haemophilus influenzae*, but others isolated include *Streptococcus pneumoniae*, *Branhamella cattarhalis*, *Staphylococcus aureus*, and *Pseudomonas aeruginosa*. Bacterial colonization has been shown to be related to the degree of airflow obstruction and current cigarette smoking status, as well as associated with an increased exacerbation frequency (42–45). Soler and colleagues showed that the presence of potentially pathogenic organisms in bronchoalveolar lavage from COPD patients at bronchoscopy was associated with a greater degree of neutrophilia and higher TNF-α levels (43). In a large study, Hill and colleagues showed that the airway bacterial load was related to inflammatory markers (46). They also found that the bacterial species was related to the degree of inflammation, with *P. aeruginosa* colonization showing greater myeloperoxidase activity (an indirect measure of neutrophil activation).

Although bacteria such as *H. influenzae* and *Strep. pneumoniae* have been associated with COPD exacerbation, early studies have produced conflicting results on bacterial isolation during exacerbation (47). Evidence for the involvement of bacteria at COPD exacerbation has come from studies of antibiotic therapy. Acute exacerbations of COPD often present with increased sputum purulence and volume and antibiotics have traditionally been used as first-line therapy in such exacerbations. A study investigating the benefit of antibiotics in over 300 acute exacerbations demonstrated a greater treatment success rate in patients treated with antibiotics, especially if their initial presentation was with the symptoms of increased dyspnea, sputum volume, and purulence (12). Patients with mild COPD obtained less benefit from antibiotic therapy. However, a randomized placebo-controlled study investigating the value of antibiotics in patients with mild obstructive lung disease in the community concluded that antibiotic therapy neither accelerated recovery nor reduced the number of relapses (48). A meta-analysis of trials of antibiotic therapy in COPD identified only nine studies of significant duration and concluded that antibiotic therapy offered a small, but significant, benefit in outcome in acute exacerbations (49).

Recent studies have reexamined the effects of bacteria at acute exacerbation with more detailed evaluation of the nature of the COPD exacerbation and bacterial culture. Stockley and colleagues showed that COPD exacerbations associated with purulent sputum are more likely to produce positive bacterial cultures than exacerbations where the sputum production was mucoid (50). Sethi and colleagues have shown that exacerbations associated with *H. influenzae* and *B. catarrhalis* are associated with significantly higher levels of airway inflammatory markers and neutrophil elastase, compared to pathogen-negative exacerbations (51). Miravitlles and colleagues also showed that patients with the highest degree of functional impairment were more likely to have *P. aeruginosa* and *H. influenzae* isolated, although this group of patients are also more likely to have airway bacterial colonization (52). However, the degree of airway bacterial load may be a more important determinant of airway infection at exacerbation rather than the type of bacteria isolated, as different types of bacteria and different strains may be present in individual patients at exacerbation, especially those with more severe COPD. Bandi and colleagues have recently reported that different strains of *H. influenzae* were recovered from the upper and lower airway in patients with chronic bronchitis (53). At exacerbation, there was a low recovery of *H. influenzae* in the lower airway due to early administration of antibiotics but, in 87% of biopsies taken from acute exacerbations in intubated patients, *H. influenzae* could be detected intracellularly. Thus, during an exacerbation, there is intracellular invasion of *H. influenzae* and this will contribute to the increased airway inflammation associated with exacerbation. However, in view of the presence of airway bacterial colonization, detection of bacteria at exacerbation does not prove the bacterial etiology of the exacerbation and important viral–bacterial interactions may exist and require further study.

IV. Other Infective Agents

A. *Chlamydia pneumoniae*

Chlamydia pneumoniae has also been related to exacerbations in COPD patients. Using IgM and IgG antibody titers, *C. pneumoniae* has been identified as the etiological factor in 5% of outpatient COPD exacerbations (54). This is similar to the results obtained by Blasi and coworkers who identified *C. pneumoniae* in 4% of COPD exacerbations (55). A recent study by Mogulkoc and colleagues in a relatively small sample of patients with exacerbations detected high IgG titers to *C. pneumoniae* in 7 of 49 exacerbations, suggesting that *C. pneumoniae* was associated with about 16% of COPD exacerbations (56). Karnak and colleagues detected serological evidence of recent *C. pneumoniae* infection in 34% of COPD patients having acute exacerbations, although microbiological examination of the sputum found potentially pathogenic microorganisms in 60% of the COPD patients, suggesting that *C. pneumoniae* was not the sole agent responsible for the exacerbation (57).

However, one of the problems with relating *C. pneumoniae* infection to exacerbation is that many COPD patients have had exposure to previous *C. pneumoniae* infection and thus chlamydial serology is not the best technique for evaluating the cause of COPD exacerbation. In addition, chronic infection with *C. pneumoniae* may be a feature of COPD. One study using tissue samples from lung resections found increased immunohistochemical staining for *C. pneumoniae* in patients with COPD as compared to that in patients with normal lung function (58). However, a recent study has suggested that the presence of antibodies to *C. pneumoniae* has no effect on the natural history of COPD (59) and thus the significance of persistent antibodies against *C. pneumoniae* is not known. Evaluation of the role of *C. pneumoniae* at COPD exacerbation is required using sensitive PCR techniques both when the patients are stable and at exacerbation.

B. *Mycoplasma pneumoniae*

Mycoplasma pneumoniae is an uncommon cause of COPD exacerbation with less than 1% of exacerbations diagnosed by complement fixation or culture methods (9,60). Another, more recent, study that also uses serological techniques found that *M. pneumoniae* was associated with only 6% of COPD exacerbations (56). However, the results of sample analysis for *M. pneumoniae* using PCR has not been reported.

C. Pollution

There has been considerable interest in the effects of air pollution on COPD exacerbation, especially with respect to the effects of common pollutants on hospital admissions. COPD patients have been found to have increased hospital admissions, suggesting increased exacerbation when increasing environmental pollution occurs. During the December 1991 pollution episode in the United Kingdom, COPD mortality as well as hospital admissions were increased in elderly COPD patients (61). Data from a study of air pollution in six European cities (APHEA project) showed that the relative risks for COPD admissions for a 50 $\mu g/m^3$ increase in daily mean level of pollutant, with lags for the effects seen from 1 to 3 days, were 1.02 for SO_2, NO_2, and total suspendable particles, and 1.04 for ozone (62). Analysis of data form Birmingham, Alabama, also showed that inhalation of particles was a 1.27 relative risk for admissions for COPD (63). A study from Australia suggested an increase of 4.6% in COPD admissions with NO_2 exposure (64). Generally, the most convincing relationship between COPD admission has been with particulate pollution.

Although there are considerable epidemiological data that increased pollutants are associated with COPD admission, the mechanisms involved are largely unknown. As COPD exacerbations are closely linked to respiratory infections, the hypothesis that pollutants can increase susceptibility to viral infections has been proposed. Another possibility is that pollutants may directly increase the infectivity of the virus, although it is more likely that the effects are mediated through increased airway inflammation, as both viruses and NO_2 can lead to increases in expression of inflammatory markers in airway epithelial cells (65,66). One study investigated the effect of NO_2 exposure in a controlled chamber on the susceptibility to infection with influenza and found some small increases in effect with the combination of virus and pollutant (67). Another recent study investigated the effect of personal exposure of NO_2 and the risk of airflow obstruction in asthmatic children with respiratory infections (68). This study suggested that with higher personal pollutant exposure there was a greater risk of an asthmatic exacerbation following a respiratory infection. Thus similar mechanisms may be operating in patients with COPD and further studies are required on the association of pollution and infection. It is likely that the adverse effects of pollutants in COPD are more likely to be associated with exacerbations either directly or through interactions with infective factors rather than affecting patients when in a stable clinical condition.

V. Conclusions

The etiology of COPD exacerbation is complex and a number of factors have been shown to be associated with exacerbations. However, the available evidence suggests that respiratory viruses, especially infections with rhinovirus, the cause of the common cold are the most important triggers of exacerbations. Respiratory viruses are also associated with more severe exacerbations and may have important interactions with cold temperature and common pollutants. Although bacteria have been implicated in COPD exacerbations for many years and antibiotics are used for therapy, there is much less information available about their actual role at exacerbation. Further research is required on the nature of interactions between viruses and bacteria. Respiratory viral infections are an important target for therapy in COPD and prevention of viral infection will reduce exacerbation frequency. Reduction of COPD exacerbation will have an important impact on the considerable morbidity and mortality associated with COPD.

References

1. Fletcher CM, Peto R, Tinker CM, Speizer FE. Natural History of Chronic Bronchitis and Emphysema. Oxford: Oxford University Press, 1976.
2. Seemungal TAR, Donaldson GC, Paul EA, Bestall JC, Jeffries DJ, Wedzicha JA. Effect of exacerbation on quality of life in patients with chronic obstructive pulmonary disease. Am J Respir Crit Care Med 1998; 151:1418–1422.
3. Donaldson GC, Seemungal T, Jeffries DJ, Wedzicha JA. Effect of environmental temperature on symptoms, lung function and mortality in COPD patients. Eur Resp J 1999; 13:844–849.
4. Seemungal TAR, Donaldson GC, Bhowmik A, Jeffries DJ, Wedzicha JA. Time course and recovery of exacerbations in patients with chronic obstructive pulmonary disease. Am J Respir Crit Care Med 2000; 161:1608–1613.
5. Seemungal TAR, Harper-Owen R, Bhowmik A, et al. Respiratory viruses, symptoms and inflammatory markers in acute exacerbations and stable chronic obstructive pulmonary disease. Am J Respir Crit Care Med 2001; 164:1618–1623.
6. Nicholson KG, Kent J, Ireland DC. Respiratory viruses and exacerbations of asthma in adults. Br Med J 1993; 307:982–986.
7. Johnston SL, Pattemore PK, Sanderson G et al. Community study of the role of viral infections in exacerbations of asthma in 9–11 year old children. Br Med J 1995; 310:1225–1229.
8. Stott EJ, Grist NR, Eadie MB. Rhinovirus infections in chronic bronchitis: isolation of eight possible new rhinovirus serotypes. J Med Microbiol 1968; 109:117.
9. Gump DW, Phillips CA, Forsyth BR. Role of infection in chronic bronchitis. Am Rev Respir Dis 1976; 113:465–473.
10. Philit F, Etienne J, Calvet A, et al. Infectious agents associated with exacerbations of chronic obstructive pulmonary disease and attacks of asthma. Rev Mal Respir 1992; 9:191–196.
11. Greenberg SB, Allen M, Wilson J, Atmar RL. Respiratory viral infections in adults with and without chronic obstructive pulmonary disease. Am J Respir Crit Care Med 2000; 162:167–173.
12. Anthonisen NR, Manfreda J, Warren CPW, Hershfield ES, Harding GKM, Nelson NA. Antibiotic therapy in exacerbations of chronic obstructive pulmonary disease. Ann Intern Med 1987; 106:196–220.
13. Retmales I, Elliott MW, Meshi B, et al. Amplification of inflammation in emphysema and its association with latent adenoviral infection. J Respir Crit Care Med 2001; 164:469–473.
14. Gern JE, Galagan DM, Jarjour NN, Dick EC, Busse W. Detection of rhinovirus RNA in lower airway cells during experimentally induced infection. Am J Respir Crit Care Med 1997; 155:1159–1161.
15. Papadopoulos NG, Bates PJ, Bardin PG, et al. Rhinoviruses infect the lower airways. J Infect Dis 2000; 181:1875–1884.
16. Seemungal TAR, Harper-Owen R, Bhowmik A, Jeffries DJ, Wedzicha JA. Detection of rhinovirus in induced sputum at exacerbation of chronic obstructive pulmonary disease. Eur Resp J 2000; 16:677–683.
17. Papi A, Johnston SL. Rhinovirus infection induces expression of its own receptor ICAM-1 via increased NF-κB mediated transcription. J Biol Chem 1999; 274:9707–9720.

18. Di Stefano A, Maestrelli P, Roggeri A, et al. Upregulation of adhesion molecules in the bronchial mucosa of subjects with chronic obstructive bronchitis. Am J Respir Crit Care Med 1994; 149:803–810.

19. Bhowmik A, Seemungal TAR, Sapsford RJ, Wedzicha JA. Relation of sputum inflammatory markers to symptoms and physiological changes at COPD exacerbations. Thorax 2000; 55:114 200.

20. Fraenkel DJ, Bardin PG, Sanderson G, Dorward M, Lau C, Johnston SL, Holgate ST. Lower airways inflammation during rhinovirus colds in normal and in asthmatic subjects. Am J Respir Crit Care Med 1995; 151:879–886.

21. Grunberg K, Smits HH, Timmers MC, et al. Experimental rhinovirus 16 infection: effects on cell differentials and soluble markers in sputum of asthmatic subjects. Am J Respir Crit Care Med 1997; 156:609–616.

22. Fleming HE, Little EF, Schnurr D, et al. Rhinovirus-16 colds in healthy and asthmatic subjects. Am J Respir Crit Care Med 1999; 160:100–108.

23. Keatings VM, Collins PD, Scott DM, et al. Differences in interleukin-8 and tumour necrosis factor in induced sputum from patients with chronic obstructive pulmonary disease and asthma. Am J Respir Crit Care Med 1996; 153:530–534.

24. Pizzicini MMM, Pizzichini E, Clelland, et al. Sputum in severe exacerbations of asthma: kinetics of inflammatory indices after prednisone treatment. Am J Respir Crit Care Med 1997; 155:1501–1508.

25. Albert RK, Martin TR, Lewis SW. Controlled clinical trial of methylprednisolone in patients with chronic bronchitis and acute respiratory insufficiency. Ann Intern Med 1980; 92:753–758.

26. Emerman CL, Connors AF, Lukens TW, May ME, Effron D. A randomised controlled trial of methylprednisolone in the emergency treatment of acute exacerbations of chronic obstructive pulmonary disease. Chest 1989; 95:563–567.

27. Bullard MJ, Liaw SJ, Tsai YH, Min HP. Early corticosteroid use in acute exacerbations of chronic airflow limitation. Am J Emerg Med 1996; 14:139–143.

28. Murata GH, Gorby MS, Chick TW, Halperin AK. Intravenous and oral corticosteroids for the prevention of relapse after treatment of decompensated COPD. Chest 1990; 98:845–849.

29. Thompson WH, Nielson CP, Carvalho P, et al. Controlled trial of oral prednisolone in outpatients with acute COPD exacerbation. Am J Respir Crit Care Med 1996; 154:407–412.

30. Davies L, Angus RM, Calverley PMA. Oral corticosteroids in patients admitted to hospital with exacerbations of chronic obstructive pulmonary disease: a prospective randomised controlled trial. Lancet 1999; 354:456–460.

31. Niewoehner DE, Erbland ML, Deupree RH, et al. Effect of systemic glucocorticoids on exacerbations of chronic obstuctive pulmonary disease. N Engl J Med 1999; 340:1941–1947.

32. Rahman I, Skwarska E, MacNee W. Attenuation of oxidant/antioxidant imbalance during treatment of exacerbations of chronic obstructive pulmonary disease. Thorax 1997; 52:565–568.

33. Biagioli MC, Kaul P, Singh I, Turner RB. The role of oxidative stress in rhinovirus induced elaboration of IL-8 by respiratory epithelial cells. Free Radical Biol Med 1999; 26:454–462.

34. Turner RB, et al. Association between nasal secretion interleukin-8 concentration and symptom severity experimental rhinovirus colds. Clin Infect Dis 1998; 26:840–846.

35. Choi AMK, Knobil K, Otterbein SL, Eastman DA, Jacoby DB. Oxidant stress responses in influenza virus pneumonia: gene expression and transcription factor activation. Am J Physiol 1996; 271:L383–L391.
36. Roland MA, Bhowmik A, Sapsford RJ, Seemungal TAR, Jeffries DJ, Warner T, Wedzicha JA. Sputum and plasma endothelin-1 in exacerbations of chronic obstructive pulmonary disease. Thorax 2001; 56:30–35.
37. Carr MJ, Spalding LJ, Goldie RG, et al. Distribution of immunoreactive endothelin ion the lungs of mice during respiratory viral infection. Eur Resp J 1998; 11:79–85.
38. Jousilahti P, Vartiainen E, Tuomilehto J, Puska P. Symptoms of chronic bronchitis and the risk of coronary disease. Lancet 1996; 348:567–572.
39. Meade TW, Ruddock V, Stirling Y, Chakrabarti R, Miller GJ. Fibrinolytic activity, clotting factors and long term incidence of ischaemic heart disease in the Northwick Park Heart Study. Lancet 1993; 324:1076–1079.
40. Wedzicha JA, Seemungal TAR, MacCallum PK, et al. Acute exacerbations of chronic obstructive pulmonary disease are accompanied by elevations of plasma fibrinogen and serum IL-6 levels. Thromb Haemostasis 2000; 84:210–215.
41. Meier CR, Jick SS, Derby LE, Vasilakis C, Jick H. Acute respiratory tract infections and risk of first-time acute myocardial infarction. Lancet 1998; 351:1467–1471.
42. Zalacain R, Sobradillo V, Amilibia J, et al. Predisposing factors to bacterial colonization in chronic obstructive pulmonary disease. Eur Resp J 1999; 13:343–348.
43. Soler N, Ewig S, Torres A, Filella X, Gonzalez J, Zaubet A. Airway inflammation and bronchial microbial patterns in patients with stable chronic obstructive pulmonary disease. Eur Resp J 1999; 14:1015–1022.
44. Monso E, Rosell A, Bonet G, et al. Risk factors for lower airway bacterial colonization in chronic bronchitis. Eur Resp J 1999; 13:338–342.
45. Patel IS, Seemungal TAR, Wilks M, Lloyd Owen S, Donaldson GC, Wedzicha JA. Relationship between bacterial colonisation and the frequency, character and severity of COPD exacerbations. Thorax 2002; 57:759–764.
46. Hill AT, Campbell EJ, Hill SL, Bayley DL, Stockley RA. Association between airway bacterial load and markers of airway inflammation in patients with chronic bronchitis. Am J Med 2000; 109:288–295.
47. Wilson R. Bacterial infection and chronic obstructive pulmonary disease. Eur Respir J 1999; 13:233–235.
48. Sachs APE, Koeter GH, Groenier KH, Van der Waaij D, Schiphuis J, Meyboom-de Jong B. Changes in symptoms, peak expiratory flow and sputum flora during treatment with antibiotics of exacerbations in patients with chronic obstructive pulmonary disease in general practice. Thorax 1995; 50:758–763.
49. Saint S, Bent S, Vittinghoff E, Grady D. Antibiotics in chronic obstructive pulmonary disease exacerbations. A meta-analysis. JAMA 1995; 273:957–960.
50. Stockley RA, O'Brien S, Pye A, Hill SL. Relationship of sputum colour to nature and outpatient management of acute exacerbations of COPD. Chest 2000; 117:1638–1645.
51. Sethi S, Muscarella K, Evans N, et al. Airway inflammation and aetiology of acute exacerbations of chronic bronchitis. Chest 2000; 118:1557–1565.
52. Miravitlles M, Espinosa C, Fernandez-Laso E, Martos JA, Maldonado JA, Gallego M. Relationship between bacterial flora in sputum and functional impairment in patients with acute exacerbations of COPD. Chest 1999; 116:40–46.
53. Bandi V, Apicella MA, Mason E, et al. Nontypeable *H. influenzae* in the lower respiratory tract of patients with chronic bronchitis. Am J Respir Crit Care Med 2001; 164:2114–2119.

54. Beaty CD, Grayston JT, Wang SP, Kuo CC, Reto CS, Martin TR. Chlamydia pneumoniae, strain Twar, infection in patients with chronic obstructive pulmonary disease. Am Rev Respir Dis 1991; 144:1408–1410.

55. Blasi F, Legnani D, Lombardo VM, Negretto GG, Magliano B, Pozzoli R, Chiodo F, Fasoli A, Allegra L. Chlamydia pneumoniae infection in acute exacerbations of COPD. Eur Respir J 1993; 6:19–22.

56. Mogulkoc N, Karakurt S, Isalska B, et al. Acute purulent exacerbation of chronic obstructive pulmonary disease and Chlamydia pneumoniae infection. Am J Respir Crit Care Med 1999; 160:349–353.

57. Karnak D, Beng-sun S, Beder S, Kayacan O. Chlamydia pneumoniae infection and acute exacerbation of chronic obstructive pulmonary disease. Resp Med 2001; 95:811–816.

58. Wu L, Skinner SJ, Lambie N, Vuletic JC, Blasi F, Black PN. Immunohistochemical staining for Chlamydia pneumoniae is increased in lung tissue from subjects with chronic obstructive pulmonary disease. Am J Respir Crit Care Med 2000; 162:1148–1151.

59. Strachan DP, Carrington D, Mendall M, Butland BK, Yarnell JW, Elwood P. Chlamydia pneumoniae serology, lung function decline and treatment for respiratory disease. Am J Respir Crit Care Med 2000; 161:493–497.

60. Smith CB, Golden CA, Kanner RE, Renzetti AD. Association of viral and Mycoplasma pneumoniae infections with acute respiratory illness in patients with chronic obstructive pulmonary diseases. Am Rev Respir Dis 1980; 121:225–232.

61. Anderson HR, Limb ES, Bland JM, Ponce de Leon A, Strachan DP, Bower JS. Health effects of an air pollution episode in London, December 1991. Thorax 1995; 50:1188–1193.

62. Anderson HR, Spix C, Medicna S, et al. Air pollution and daily admissions for chronic obstructive pulmonary disease in 6 European cities: results from the APHEA project. Eur Respir J 1998; 11:992–993.

63. Schwartz J. Air pollution and hospital admissions for the elderly in Birmingham, Alabama. Am J Epidemiol 1994; 139:589–598.

64. Morgan G, Corbett S, Wlodarczyk J. Air pollution and hospital admissions in Sydney, Australia 1990 to 1994. Am J Pub Health 1998; 88:1761–1766.

65. Subauste MC, Jacoby DB, Richards SM, Proud D. Infection of a human respiratory epithelial cell line with rhinovirus. J Clin Invest 1995; 96:549–557.

66. Johnston SL, Papi A, Bates PJ, Mastronarde JG, Monick MM, Hunninghake GW. Low grade rhinovirus infection induces a prolonged release of IL-8 in pulmonary epithelium. J Immunol 1998; 160:6172–6181.

67. Goings SA, Kulle TJ, Bascom R, et al. Effect of nitrogen dioxide exposure on the susceptibility to influenza A virus infection in healthy adults. Am Rev Respir Crit Care Med 1989; 1349:1075–1081.

68. Linaker CH, Coggon D, Holgate ST, et al. Personal exposure to nitrogen dioxide and risk of airflow obstruction in asthmatic children with upper respiratory infection. Thorax 2000; 55:930–933.

10

Symptoms and Signs of Acute Exacerbation of Chronic Obstructive Pulmonary Disease

EUMORFIA KONDILI and
DIMITRIS GEORGOPOULOS

NICHOLAS R. ANTHONISEN

University Hospital of Heraklion
Heraklion, Crete, Greece

University of Manitoba
Winnipeg, Manitoba, Canada

I. Introduction

The diagnosis of chronic obstructive pulmonary disease (COPD) is usually made on the basis of history and physical examination with laboratory studies being used to validate the initial clinical impression (1–3). Acute exacerbation of symptoms is an important characteristic of the disease and has a great impact on the quality of life as well as on the economic burden of the disease (1–3). Since exacerbations are usually defined in terms of symptoms, they are essential to making the diagnosis. Acute exacerbations of symptoms are usually associated with worsening of lung function, which may or may not be reflected in various signs. The symptoms and, to a much lesser degree, the signs of acute exacerbations are used to assess both their severity and the response to therapy.

It has been stated that the most common causes of acute exacerbations of COPD are air pollution and infections of the tracheobronchial tree (4–10). However, in the majority of patients, the cause of acute exacerbations cannot be determined, and the role of infection and air pollution in their etiology is controversial (3). Nevertheless, during acute exacerbation the patient may present with the common symptoms and signs of infection of the upper respiratory tract, such as fever, sore throat, and nasal congestion or discharge (11,12).

As a general statement, the symptoms and signs of acute exacerbation depend on the cause of exacerbation (if apparent), the degree of additional airflow limitation and blood gas derangement, the severity of the underlying COPD, comorbidities, and body build. Although specific severity criteria are not well defined, severity of exacerbations varies widely, from being mere nuisances to being life threatening, largely depending on the degree of airways obstruction and associated blood gas abnormalities. The most commonly used system to assess the severity of an acute exacerbation was developed by Anthonisen et al. (11) and was based only on symptom description. Acute exacerbation was defined as the presence of any one of the following three symptoms: (1) increased sputum volume; (2) increased sputum purulence; and (3) increased dyspnea. Patients with type 1 (severe) exacerbations have all three of the above symptoms; those with type 2 (moderate) have two of three of the symptoms; patients with type 3 (mild) exacerbations have one of these symptoms, as well as one of the following clinical criteria: an upper respiratory tract infection in the past 5 days, fever without another apparent cause, increased wheezing, increased cough, or increase in respiratory or heart rate by 20% above baseline (11). Classifying the severity of an acute exacerbation is useful for epidemiological purposes and may have therapeutic implications and prognostic value. Indeed, it has been shown that patients with severe exacerbations are at highest risk of treatment failure and more likely to experience benefit from antibiotic therapy than those with mild exacerbations (11,13).

Finally, it should be noted that other conditions may mimic the symptoms of an acute exacerbation, such as pneumonia, congestive heart failure, pneumothorax, pleural effusion, pulmonary embolism, and arrhythmia (3). For this reason, it is essential during the assessment of the acute exacerbation to search for symptoms and signs of the above conditions and treat the patient accordingly.

II. Characteristics of Exacerbations

Worsening of dyspnea and increases in cough and sputum volume and sputum purulence are the most common symptoms characterizing an acute exacerbation (11,12). Anthonisen et al. (11) followed 362 exacerbations of COPD and observed that at the onset of the exacerbation the most common symptoms were worsening of dyspnea, increased sputum production, increased cough, wheezing, and sputum purulence (Table 1). Seemungal et al. (12) studied 101 patients with moderate-to-severe COPD over a period of 2.5 years and followed them regularly when stable and during 504 exacerbations. On the day of onset of exacerbation, reports of symptoms increased sharply (Fig. 1), with 64% of exacerbations associated with increased dyspnea, 26% with increased sputum volume, 42% with sputum purulence, 35% with symptoms of common colds, 35% with wheeze, 12% with sore throat, and 20% with cough (12).

III. Symptoms

Dyspnea, cough with or without sputum production, and wheezing are the most common symptoms in stable COPD patients. Although stable patients have good

Table 1 Symptoms at the Onset of Acute Exacerbation ($n = 362$) of COPD[a]

Symptoms	Proportion of appearance
Increased dyspnea	90%
Increased sputum production	70%
Sputum purulence	60%
Increased wheeze	70%
Increased cough	82%
Fever	30%

[a]*Source*: Based on Ref. 11.

days and bad days, there is never any time when they are entirely asymptomatic. Thus, it is very important in assessing acute exacerbations to obtain a detailed history of how long worsening or new symptoms have been present (12). This includes the frequency and severity of breathlessness and coughing attacks, sputum volume and color, limitation of daily activities, any previous episodes of exacerbation, and whether the patient may require hospitalization. Finally, current therapy should be carefully reviewed. Knowledge of the severity of symptoms of an individual patient when stable greatly contributes to evaluating whether new or worse symptoms are present. Quantitative assessment of symptoms, although it is not an easy task, is therefore of great value.

Increased dyspnea or breathlessness is the most significant symptom in acute exacerbations of COPD. Dyspnea can be defined as an awareness of increased or inappropriate inspiratory effort. It is a symptom perceived by the patient and is believed to relate to an awareness of the motor command to breathe (14). It correlates with mouth occlusion pressure, swings in pleural pressure, and magnitude of dynamic hyperinflation in healthy subjects during loaded breathing at rest (15–17). Changes in the arterial blood gases, especially increases in arterial carbon dioxide tension ($PaCO_2$) increase the intensity of perceived effort for a given level of ventilation (18). The terms used to describe dyspnea may vary with the stimulus used to provoke it (19). However, patients with COPD commonly describe the sensation of dyspnea as being one of inspiratory difficulty (20).

O'Donnell et al. have shown that the intensity of breathlessness in moderate to advanced COPD is best related to increases in end-expiratory lung volumes during exercise, something that does not occur in normals (20). Furthermore, they have shown that the changes in dyspnea are mirrored by a mechanical ratio reflecting both the pressure developed by the respiratory muscles and the resulting change in tidal volume with each breath (20). These observations indicate that measurements such as inspiratory capacity may correlate better with the sensation of breathlessness than with FEV_1 or peak flow (17,21–23).

The quantification of dyspnea is an important goal in the overall assessment of the patient with COPD. Quantitative measurements of dyspnea provide baseline data to assess the efficacy of various therapeutic regimens and the stability of the patient

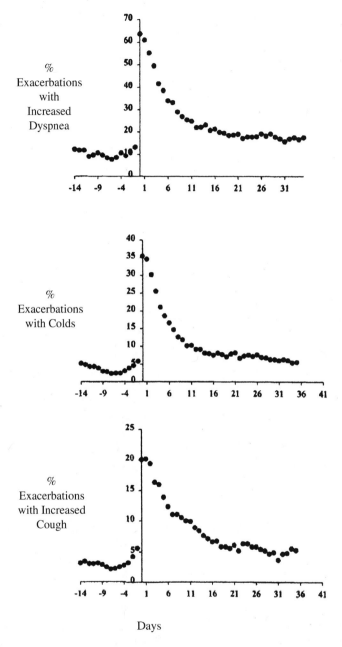

Figure 1 Time course of symptoms of increased dyspnea, nasal congestion, and cough for 504 exacerbations in 91 patients. Proportion of exacerbations with any one symptom over the 14 days before to 35 days after onset of exacerbation, expressed as a percentage of the total number of exacerbations.

over time. The MRC dyspnea scale may be used for dyspnea grading because it is simple and allows the patients to indicate the extent to which their breathlessness affects their mobility (24). The MRC dyspnea scale is a questionnaire consisting of five statements about perceived breathlessness: grade 1, "I only get breathless with strenuous exercise;" grade 2, "I get short of breath when hurrying on the level or up a slight hill;" grade 3, "I walk slower than people of the same age on the level because of breathlessness or have to stop for breath when walking at my own pace on the level;" grade 4, "I stop for breath after walking 100 yards or after a few minutes on the level;" grade 5, "I am too breathless to leave the house" (24). A relationship between MRC dyspnea grade and walking test performance has been established (25). The visual analog scale (VAS) (26), the oxygen cost diagram (27), the baseline dyspnea index (BEI) (28), and the Borg category scale (29) are some of the other techniques used for dyspnea quantification. The VAS consists of a vertical line 100 mm long connecting two points that represent "no breathlessness" and "greatest breathlessness" (26). The patient marks a point in the line that corresponds to his or her breathlessness and the distance above the "no breathlessness" point is an index of the severity of the dyspnea. The oxygen cost diagram is a type of VAS in which everyday activities are placed proportionally to their oxygen cost along the 100-mm vertical line (27). The baseline dyspnea index quantifies the intensity of dyspnea based on grades for components, including task magnitude, effort, and functional impairment (28). The Borg category scale is used for rating breathlessness during exercise testing (29). The clinical measurements of dyspnea by these methods are reproducible and can be completed in a few minutes. The results generally correlate with lung function and respiratory muscle strength (28).

The severity of dyspnea may be used as a guide to estimate lung function, although the latter should be evaluated with the appropriate tests. Dyspnea at rest or on minimal exertion indicates severe respiratory impairment. In stable COPD this sign indicates that the FEV_1 has fallen to less than 30% of predicted normal and the oxygen uptake is less than 15 mL/kg/min (23). In acute exacerbations of COPD there are a paucity of data because even simple lung function tests can be difficult for a sick patient to perform properly. Furthermore, individuals with similar lung function can be surprisingly variable in their symptom intensity. The situation is further complicated if it is taken into account that the intensity of dyspnea depends on the patient's body weight (30). Sahebjami et al. (30) quantitated dyspnea (using the MRC dyspnea scale) in 33 underweight and 56 normal-weight COPD patients and demonstrated that, despite the similar lung function, underweight patients were more dyspneic. Notwithstanding that the severity of dyspnea is multi-factorial, these results indicate that body weight may affect the process of patient evaluation.

Cough is an important respiratory defense mechanism that protects the airways from unwanted inhaled particulates and is the major method of clearing excess mucus production (31). In stable COPD patients, the cough is chronic, usually productive, occasionally episodic, and worse in the morning upon rising. The patient is seldom awakened from sleep by coughing (31). All these features should be considered when the patient reports an increased cough. Whether cough in COPD is a normal nonspecific physiological response to increased mucus production or is itself due to specific pathological changes in the airways is unknown (32,33).

Sputum production is a frequent complaint especially in the early stages of COPD but accurate measurements of volume are difficult as much is swallowed. The physicochemical and clinical significance of mucus production has been reviewed in detail (34). Typically, a normal person produces about 10 mL of colorless sputum, an amount that is unnoticed and swallowed. Therefore, as a general rule, any sputum production reported by the patient is abnormal. Patients with stable COPD usually produce white mucoid sputum usually in the morning and often throughout the day. Increases in sputum volume and change in color to yellow or green (purulent) are probably the most reliable symptoms of acute exacerbation due to endobronchial infection treatable with antibiotics (5,8,10–12,31). It should be noted that changes in sputum color do not always denote purulence, since eosinophil accumulation may cause yellow sputum and a yellow–green color may be imparted by myeloperoxidase (35). Foul-tasting or foul-smelling sputum is extremely rare in acute exacerbations of COPD and, if present, strongly suggests superinfection with anaerobic organisms.

As the severity of airflow limitation increases, sputum production may become more variable and many patients produce only small volumes daily (31). Whether this relates to impaction of mucus in the small airways, reduced goblet cell function, or smoking cessation is unclear. Some patients during exacerbations feel unable to raise sputum that they believe is present, and it is possible that due to increased airway resistance dynamic airway collapse during coughing prevents sputum expectoration. This may explain the observation that in some patients sputum production may increase during the recovery phase of exacerbations.

A history of wheezing is not unusual in patients with COPD and may indicate a reversible component of the disease (36). Between 35 to 70% of exacerbations are associated with wheeze and this symptom may correlate positively with the response to inhaled bronchodilators (36). However, bronchospasm is not the sole cause of wheezing. Some patients can produce convincing wheeze from their larynx as infactitious asthma (37). Whether these changes represent a way of increasing airway stability during expiration or are a psychological response has not been addressed. Many patients also experience wheeze with exertion, presumably because of increased gas flow through airways narrowed by inflammation or scarring (38). Finally, abdominal muscle contraction, common in severe exacerbation, may cause wheezing (39). Studies in asthmatic patients during induced bronchoconstriction indicate that wheeze does not occur at the onset of flow limitation but probably requires additional abdominal contraction (39). Nocturnal wheeze is uncommon in COPD and suggests asthma or heart failure.

Approximately 30% of patients with acute exacerbation have fever (11). However, fever should probably not be considered as a cardinal symptom of an exacerbation and other causes should be thoroughly investigated. Specifically, in the presence of fever, a chest x-ray should be performed to exclude pneumonia, since pneumonia is associated with high morbidity and mortality in COPD (13).

Occasionally patients with COPD complain of chest pain or hemoptysis. Chest pain usually is not due to the disease. Ischemic heart disease is frequent in any population of heavy smokers and may be difficult to distinguish from symptoms of esophageal reflux. Acid reflux occurs in up to 40% of COPD patients possibly reflecting mechanical inefficiency of the diaphragm and the use of xanthines and cigarette smoking (40–42). A sudden onset of chest pain, pleuritic and sharp in character, associated with worsening of dyspnea and diaphoresis, is against the diagnosis of acute exacerbation and strongly suggests pulmonary embolism or pneumothorax (43–46). Pneumothorax, although not very common in patients with COPD, may have serious consequences because of limited respiratory reserve (46). Pulmonary embolism may complicate COPD, particularly when right heart failure and pulmonary hypertension are present.

Hemoptysis may occur during acute exacerbations of COPD. The blood presumably originates in inflamed airways and the typical episode of hemoptysis consists of blood-streaked purulent sputum (47,48). Grossly bloody sputum is uncommon during exacerbations and should be investigated. Other causes of hemoptysis, such as pneumonia, tumor, bronchiectasis, or heart failure should always be considered (49).

Finally, mental status should be carefully evaluated. Psychiatric morbidity is high in stable COPD, reflecting both the social isolation the disease produces, its chronic nature, and the neurological effects of hypoxemia (50–53). In addition, sleep quality is impaired in advanced disease and this may also contribute to abnormal neuropsychiatric performance (54). Acute or subacute changes in mental status may indicate a severe exacerbation and impending acute respiratory failure (1–3). These patients usually need to be admitted to the intensive care unit (1–3).

IV. Physical Signs

Physical examination, although an integral part in the assessment of acute exacerbation of COPD, is not used either for definition or for classifying acute exacerbations. Usually physical signs are specific and sensitive only for severe obstruction to airflow. Indeed, in less severe cases, physical examination is often normal.

Respiratory distress elicited by minimal exertion such as undressing or entering the examining room is a sign of severely impaired lung function with an FEV_1 of less than 50% of predicted (55). The respiratory distress manifested by tachypnea and speaking in an interrupted fashion reflects expiratory flow limitation during tidal expiration, also indicative of severe disease (55). In order to meet the higher ventilatory demands encountered even during minimal exertion, these patients must increase end-expiratory lung volume (dynamic hyperinflation), a highly inefficient strategy from an energetic point of view (56). They frequently sit leaning forward with their arms resting on a stationary object, allowing the muscles connecting the limb girdle and the rib cage such as the latissimus dorsi to perform an inspiratory function (31). Some patients also develop pursed-lip breathing (pursing the lips during expiration) with exertion. Although the reason for adopting this strategy remains uncertain, flow limitation during tidal expiration with deformation of the airways downstream from the choke point may be responsible (57).

Indeed, it has been shown that the collapse of airways downstream of the choke point increases the sense of dyspnea (57). Pursed-lip breathing, by increasing the intraluminal pressure in large airways, may reduce the unpleasant sensation related to airways deformation during tidal expiration (58). Also pursed-lip breathing tends to decrease respiratory frequency and this may reduce dynamic hyperinflation and improve gas exchange.

The pattern of breathing should be assessed carefully. Patients with stable COPD invariably demonstrate resting breathing frequency above 16 breaths/min (59). Breathing frequency is roughly proportional to the disease severity, with hypercapnia being associated with rates of 20 to 25 breaths/min (60,61). However, breathing frequency is an unreliable sign of evolving hypercapnia or hypoxemia and should not be used during exacerbations as a substitute for arterial blood gas analysis (62). Accessory muscle use indicates severe disease, excessive work of breathing, and diaphragmatic dysfunction or fatigue. In these patients, FEV_1 is less than 1 L (63). Contrary to widespread belief, the sternocleidomastoid muscles are usually inactive during resting breathing in stable COPD (64). Contraction of these muscles during resting breathing indicates an acute exacerbation of the disease and is an ominous sign of impending acute respiratory failure (64).

Expiratory muscle activity may be detected during acute exacerbation (65,66). The functional significance of this activity is uncertain. Expiratory muscle contraction cannot increase expiratory flow when it is limited during tidal breathing, but it may cause greater deformation of the airways downstream of the flow-limiting segments (65,67). It has been proposed that contraction of expiratory muscles may place the diaphragm in a better position for pressure generation by altering its shape and length. However, this advantage is likely to be lost as soon as inspiration begins when expiratory muscles relax (68).

During acute exacerbations, several breathing patterns have been associated with fatigue of the inspiratory muscles due to excessive work of breathing combined with reduced muscle efficiency. Nevertheless, inspiratory muscle fatigue is extremely difficult to characterize accurately and these associations have not been verified. It is clear, however, that both paradoxical breathing and respiratory alternans occur in patients with very severe ventilatory limitation, usually with acute respiratory failure (69,70).

Paradoxical breathing consists of an inward motion of the upper abdominal wall with inspiration (71). This sign in stable COPD is mainly due to pulmonary hyperinflation, which causes the diaphragm to be flatter and lower than that in normal subjects and thus the apposition zone between diaphragm and ribcage is reduced in size (72). On the other hand, paradoxical breathing in a patient with acute exacerbation of COPD may be due to diaphragmatic fatigue (73,74). With severe hyperinflation, the patient may breath close to total lung capacity where the normal curvature of the diaphragm is reversed and the apposition zone disappears. As a result contraction of the diaphragm pulls the lower ribs inward and the abdominal pressure becomes negative as pleural pressure falls due to vigorous activity of the ribcage inspiratory muscles. Thus, during inspiration, the dimensions of the abdominal wall may be reduced rather than increased. In this situation, the ribcage inspiratory muscles are the only functional muscles of respiration (73,74). These patients are not able to sustain adequate ventilation indefinitely and, if not treated, inspiratory muscle fatigue and overt respiratory failure will ensue.

Respiratory alternans is a cyclic alteration in breathing movements so that the diaphragm dominates a series of breaths with outward movement of the abdominal wall during inspiration, and then a series of breaths are taken largely using ribcage muscles with expansion of the ribcage and reduced or even paradoxical abdominal motion (75,76). This sign is not observed in stable COPD but may be observed during acute exacerbation and respiratory failure. The Hoover sign is an inward motion of the lower lateral ribcage with inspiration and is seen in severe COPD (77). It is probably similar in significance to paradoxical breathing, although other potential causes have been cited (71,78). Increased thoracic anteroposterior diameter, reduced anterioposterior motion of the ribcage, tracheal tug or pulsus paradoxus, and continuous chest wall incursion (inward movement) that persists up until the moment the next inspiration occurs are other signs that may indicate dynamic hyperinflation in patients with acute exacerbation of COPD (79). However, these signs are not very sensitive and may not be present in patients with substantial dynamic hyperinflation.

Peripheral edema, jugular venous distention, and hepatomegaly have been considered as signs of pulmonary hypertension and right ventricular failure (cor pulmonale) (80). None of these signs, however, are specific for cor pulmonale (80). Peripheral edema can be due to other causes such as hypoalbuminemia, renal dysfunction, or venous obstruction, which may occur in patients with severe COPD. Furthermore, the jugular venous pressure is usually difficult to assess in COPD patients with severe acute exacerbation because of accessory muscle activity and large swings in intrathoracic pressure due to dynamic hyperinflation. Finally, hepatomegaly may be elusive due to downward displacement of the liver by the diaphragm.

Percussion of the chest is not very helpful in patients with acute exacerbation of COPD. The tympanic percussion may reflect a sign of pulmonary hyperinflation, but this is neither a sensitive nor a specific sign. Note that pneumothorax, as a cause of tympanic percussion, must be ruled out when this sign is present. Some physicians use percussion to estimate diaphragmatic motion during inspiration (81). However, there is considerable disagreement as to whether diaphragmatic motion can be determined accurately by percussion.

Unlike percussion, auscultation of the chest may give valuable information during exacerbations, especially if findings had been noted when the patient was stable. Abnormal sounds on auscultation such as wheezing, crackles, rales, and decreased breath sounds are commonly heard during an acute exacerbation (49).

Diminished breath sounds is a common auscultatory finding in pulmonary emphysema (82–86). This finding is independent of parenchyma destruction and well correlated with the degree of flow limitation. Schreur et al. (86) compared lung sound intensity in normal and emphysematous subjects at standardized airflows and demonstrated that there was no significant difference in lung sound intensity at any flow rate between normal and emphysematous subjects, suggesting that the reduction in lung sound intensity in patients with emphysema is predominantly due to airflow limitation.

Wheezing—a high-pitched continuous sound best heard over the trachea or the neck area—is an important sign of severe flow limitation (39,87–89). Wheezing heard during unforced tidal breathing has been shown to be a specific sign of flow limitation, and its intensity correlated with the severity of the limitation as well as with the bronchodilator response (89). Wheezing, however, is not a sensitive sign and obstruction can be present in the absence of wheezing.

Discontinuous adventitious sounds (crackles or rales) are commonly found in chest auscultation of COPD patients during an acute exacerbation, but are not uncommon in stable patients either (49). These sounds (well heard at the lung bases), begin at the onset of the inspiration, last for less than 20 ms, and represent the explosion of gas bubbles in pulmonary secretions (88,90–92). The timing of their occurrence differentiates them from the end-inspiratory crackles, usually heard in congestive heart failure and restrictive lung diseases (91,92).

Dynamic hyperinflation may be suspected by listening for the persistence of breath sounds during exhalation up until the moment the next breath occurs (93). Kress et al. (93) have shown that this sign combined with the persistence of chest wall incursion at the end of expiration has a good specificity (0.91) but relatively poor sensitivity (0.72) for the presence of dynamic hyperinflation and intrinsic positive end-expiratory pressure. Although these results were obtained in mechanically ventilated patients, they underscore the value of clinical examination in detecting the presence of dynamic hyperinflation (93).

Cardiac auscultation is an essential part of the examination in patients with acute exacerbations of COPD. It should be noted that heart sounds are often difficult to hear due to hyperinflation and the presence of adventitious sounds. Usually, in these patients heart sounds are best heard in the subxiphoid area (94). Tachycardia and arrhythmias are common and should be treated (11,13,95,96). In a recent study, an increase in heart rate above 100 beats/min was found in 18% of exacerbations (13). Signs of cor pulmonale, such as right ventricular gallop or an increase in the second sound, may be detected indicating pulmonary hypertension, while murmurs of pulmonary or tricuspid insufficiency may represent acute or chronic right ventricular failure (79,80). A systolic left parasternal heave indicates right ventricular hypertrophy (80). These signs, however, are often not present in COPD patients with acute exacerbations and are relatively insensitive for detecting pulmonary hypertension or right ventricular dysfunction (79,80).

References

1. Siafakas NM, Vermeire P, Pride NB, et al., on behalf of the Task Force. ERS Consensus Statement. Optimal assessment and management of chronic obstructive pulmonary disease (COPD). Eur Respir J 1995; 8:1398–1420.
2. Celli B, Snider GL, Heffner J, et al., for the American Thoracic Society. Standards for the diagnosis and care of patients with chronic obstructive pulmonary disease. Am J Respir Crit Care Med 1995; 152:S77–S120.

3. National Heart, Lung, and Blood Institute Workshop Report. Global strategy for diagnosis, management, and prevention of Chronic Obstructive Pulmonary Disease.
4. Voelkel NF, Tuder R. COPD exacerbations. Chest 2000; 117:376S–379S.
5. Stockley RA, O'Brien C, Pye A, Hill SL. Relationship of sputum color to nature and outpatient management of acute exacerbations of COPD. Chest 2000; 117:1638–1654.
6. Sethi S. Infection etiology of acute exacerbations of chronic bronchitis. Chest 2000; 117:380S–385S.
7. Miravitlles M, Espinosa C, Fernandez-Laso E, Martos JA, Maldonado JA, Gallego M, and study group of bacterial infections in COPD. Relationship between bacterial flora in sputum and functional impairment in patients with acute exacerbations of COPD. Chest 1999; 116:40–46.
8. MacFarlane JT, Colville A, Guion A, MacFarlane RM, Rose DH. Prospective study of etiology and outcome of adult lower-respiratory-tract infections in the community. Lancet 1993; 341:511–514.
9. Anderson HR, Spix C, Medina S, Schouten JP, Castellsague J, Rossi G, et al. Air pollution and daily admissions for chronic obstructive pulmonary disease in 6 European cities: results from the APHEA project. Eur Respir J 1997; 10:1064–1071.
10. Eller J, Ede A, Schaberg T, Niederman MS, Mauch H, Lode H. Infective exacerbations of chronic bronchitis. Relation between bacteriologic etiology and lung function. Chest 1998; 113:1542–1548.
11. Antonisen NR, Manfreda J, Warren CPW, Hershfield ES, Harding GK, Nelson NA. Antibiotic therapy in exacerbation of chronic obstructive pulmonary disease. Ann Intern Med 1987; 106:196–204.
12. Seemungal TAR, Donaldson GC, Bhowmik A, Jeffries DJ, Wedzicha JA. Time course and recovery of exacerbations in patients with chronic obstructive pulmonary disease. Am J Respir Crit Care 2000; 1615:1608–1613.
13. Dewan N, Rafique S, Kanwar B, Satpathy H, Ryschon K, Tillotson GS, Niederman MS. Acute exacerbation of COPD. Factors associated with poor treatment outcome. Chest 2000; 117:662–671.
14. Killian KJ, Gandevia SC. Sense of effort and dyspnea. In: Adams L, Guz A, eds. Respiratory Sensation. New York; Marcel Dekker, 1996: 181–200.
15. Clague JE, Carter J, Pearson MG, Calverley PMA. Relationship between inspiratory drive and perceived inspiratory drive and perceived inspiratory effort in normal man. Clin Sci 1990; 78:493–496.
16. Bradley TD, Chartrand DA, Fitting JW, et al. The relationship of inspiratory effort sensation to fatiguing patterns of the diaphragm. Am Rev Respir Dis 1986; 134:1119–1124.
17. Tantucci C, Ellaffi M, Duguet A, Zelter M, Similowski T, Derenne JP, Milic Emili J. Dynamic hyperinflation and flow limitation during metacholine-induced bronchoconstriction in asthma. Eur Respir J 1999; 14(2):295–301.
18. Clague JE, Carter J, Pearson MG, Calverley PMA. Physiological determinants of inspiratory effort sensation during CO_2 rebreathing in normal subjects. Clin Sci 1993; 85:637–642.
19. Elliott MW, Adams L, Cockroft A, MacRae KA, Murphy K, Guz A. The language of breathlessness: use by patients of verbal descriptors. Am Rev Respir Dis 1991; 144: 826–852.
20. O'Donnell DE, Bertley JC, Chan LKL, Webb KA. Qualitative aspects of exertional breathlessness in chronic airflow limitation. Am J Respir Crit Care Med 1997; 155:109–115.

21. Lougheed MD, Lam M, Forket L, Webb KA, O'Donnell DE. Breathlessness during acute bronchoconstriction in asthma. Pathophysiologic mechanisms. Am Rev Respir Dis 1993; 148:1452–1459.
22. Sulk J, Volta CA, Ploysongsang Y, Eltayara L, Olivenstein R, Milic-Emili J. Flow limitation and dyspnea in healthy supine subjects during metacholine challenge. Eur Respir J 1999; 14:1326–1331.
23. American Medical Association. The respiratory system. In: Guides to the Evaluation of Permanent Impairment, 2nd ed. Chicago: publisher, 1984; 85–101.
24. MRC, Committee on the aetiology of chronic bronchitis. Standardized questionnaire on respiratory symptoms. Br Med J 1960; 2:1665.
25. Bestall JC, Paul EA, Garrod R, Garnham R, Jones PW, Wedzicha JA. Usefulness of the Medical Research Council (MRC) dyspnea scale as a measure of disability in patients with chronic obstructive pulmonary disease. Thorax 1999; 54:581–586.
26. Mahler DA. Dyspnea: diagnosis and management. Clin Chest Med 1987; 8:215–230.
27. McGavin CR, Artvinli M, Vaoe H, McHardy GJR. Dyspnoea, disability and distance walked: comparison of estimates of exercise performance in respiratory disease. Br Med J 1978; 2:241–243.
28. Mahler DA, Weinberg DH, Well CK, Freistein AR. The measurement of dyspnea: contents, interobserver agreement, and physiologic correlates of two new clinical indexes. Chest 1984; 85:751–758.
29. Borg G. Psychophysical bases of perceived exertion. Med SCl Sports Exerc 1982; 14:377–381.
30. Sahebjami H, Sathianpitayakul E. Influence of body weight on the severity of dyspnea in chronic obstructive pulmonary disease. Am J Respir Crit Care Med 2000; 161:886–890.
31. Calverley PMA, Georgopoulos D. Chronic obstructive pulmonary disease: symptoms and signs. In: Postma DS, Siafakas NM, eds. Management of Chronic Obstructive Pulmonary Disease. Eur Respir Monogr 1998; 3:6–24.
32. Choudry NB, Fuller RW, Pride NB. Sensitivity of the human cough reflex: effect of inflammatory mediators prostaglandin E_2, bradykinnin and histamine. Am Rev Respir Dis 1989; 140:137–141.
33. Choudry NB, Fuller RW. Sensitivity of the cough reflex in patients with chronic cough. Eur Respir J 1992; 5:296–300.
34. Wanner A, Salathe M, O'Riordan TG. Mucociliary clearance in the airways. Am J Respir Crit Care Med 1996; 154:1868–1902.
35. Robertson AJ. Green sputum. Lancet 1952; i:12–15.
36. Marini JJ, Pierson DJ, Hudson LD, Lakshminaranyan S. The significance of wheezing in chronic airflow obstruction. Am Rev Respir Dis 1979; 120:1069–1072.
37. Rodenstein DO, Francis D, Stanescu DC. Emotional laryngeal wheezing: a new syndrome. Am Rev Respir Dis 1983; 127:354–357.
38. Earis JE. Lung sounds. Thorax 1992; 47:671–672.
39. Spence DPS, Graham DR, Jamieson G, et al. The relationship between wheezing and lung mechanics during methacholine-induced bronchoconstriction in asthmatic subjects. Am J Respir Crit Care Med 1996; 154:290–294.
40. Mokhlesi B, et al. Increased prevalence of gastroesophageal reflux symptoms in patients with COPD. Chest 2001; 119(4):1043–1048.
41. David P, Denis P, Nouvet G, et al. Lung junction and gastro-oesophageal reflux during chronic bronchitis. Bull Eur Physiopathol Respir 1982; 18:81–86.
42. Berquist NE, Rachelefsky GS, Kadden M, et al. Effect of theophylline on gastro-oesophageal reflux in normal adults. J Allergy Clin Immunol 1981; 67:407–411.

43. Fraser RG, Pare PJA. Diagnosis of Diseases of the Chest, Vol. III, 2nd ed. Philadelphia: WB Saunders, 1979:1770–1776.
44. Goodwin JF. The Clinical diagnosis of pulmonary thromboembolism. In: Sasahara AA, Stein M, eds. Pulmonary Embolic Disease. New York: Grune and Stratton, 1965: 239–255.
45. Leading article. Prevention of pulmonary embolism. Br Med J 1973; 2:1–2.
46. Dines DE, Clagett OT, Payne WS. Spontaneous pneumothorax in emphysema. Proc Mayo Clin 1970; 45:481–487.
47. Johnston RN, Lockhart W, Ritchie RT, Smith DH. Haemoptysis. Br Med J 1960; 1:592–595.
48. Pode G, Stradling P. Routine radiography for haemoptysis. Br Med J 1964; 1:341–342.
49. Murray JF. History and physical examination. In: Murray JF, Nadel JA, eds. Textbook of Respiratory Medicine, Vol. 1, 2nd ed. Philadelphia: WB Saunders, 1994: 536–584.
50. Hjalmarsen A, Waterloo K, Dahl A, Jorde R, Viitanen M. Effect of long-term oxygen therapy on cognitive and neurological dysfunction in chronic obstructive pulmonary disease. Eur Neurol 1999; 42(1):27–35.
51. Stuss DT, Peterkin I, Guzman DA, Guzman C, Troyer AKJ. Chronic obstructive pulmonary disease: effects of hypoxia on neurological and neuropsychological measures. Clin Exp Neuropsychol 1997; 19(4):515–524.
52. Incalza R, Gemma A, Marra C, et al. Chronic obstructive pulmonary disease: an original model of cognitive decline. Am Rev Respir Dis 1993; 148:418–424.
53. Grandt I, Heaton RK, Mac Sweeny JA. Neuropsychologic findings in hypoxemic chronic obstructive pulmonary disease. Arch Intern Med 1982; 142:1470–1476.
54. Calverley PMA, Brezinova V, Douglas NJ, et al. The effect of oxygenation on sleep quality in chronic bronchitis and emphysema. Am Rev Respir Dis 1982; 126:206–210.
55. Hubmayr RD, Rodarte JR. Cellular effects and physiologic responses: lung mechanics. In: Cherniack NS, ed. Chronic Obstructive Pulmonary Disease. Philadelphia: W.B. Saunders, 1991: 79–95.
56. Younes M. Mechanisms of ventilatory failure. Curr Pulmonol 1993; 14:243–292.
57. O'Donnell DE, Sanii R, Anthonisen NR, Younes M. Effect of dynamic compression on breathing pattern and respiratory sensation in severe chronic obstructive pulmonary disease. Am Rev Respir Dis 1987; 135:912–918.
58. Spahija JA, Grassino A. Effects of pursed-lips breathing and expiratory resistive loading in healthy subjects. J Appl Physiol 1996; 80(5):1772–1784.
59. Loveridge B, Wets P, Kryger MH, Anthonisen NR. Alteration in breathing pattern with progression of chronic obstructive pulmonary disease. Am Rev Respir Dis 1986; 134:930–934.
60. Oliven A, Cherniack NS, Deal EC, Kelsen SG. The effects of acute bronchoconstriction on respiratory activity in patients with chronic obstructive pulmonary disease. Am Rev Respir Dis 1985; 131:236–241.
61. Gorini M, Misuri G, Corrado A, Duranti R, Iandelli I, De Paola E, Scano G. Breathing pattern and carbon dioxide retention in severe chronic obstructive pulmonary disease. Thorax 1996; 7:677–683.
62. Hey EN, Lloyd BB, Cunningham DJC, Juke MOM, Bolton DPG. Effects of various respiratory stimuli on the depth and frequency of breathing in man. Respir Physiol 1966; 1:193–205.
63. McFaden ER, Kiser R, Degroot WJ. Acute bronchial asthma: clinical and physiologic relations. N Eng J Med 1973; 288:221–224.

64. De Troyer A, Peche R, Yernault JC, Estenne M. Neck muscle activity in patients with severe obstructive pulmonary disease. Am J Respir Crit Care Med 1994; 150:41–65.
65. Inane V, Ripens F, Yernault JC, De Troyer A. Abdominal muscle use during breathing in patients with chronic airflow obstruction. Am Rev Respir Dis 1992; 146:16–21.
66. Inane V, Yernault JC, De Troyer A. Intrinsic PEEP in patients with chronic obstructive pulmonary disease. Am Rev Respir Dis 1993; 148:1037–1042.
67. Decramer M, Gosselink R, Derom E. Respiratory muscle mechanics in chronic obstructive pulmonary disease and acute respiratory failure. In: Derenne JP, Whitelaw WA, Similowski T, eds. Acute Respiratory Failure in Chronic Obstructive Pulmonary Disease. New York: Marcel Dekker, Inc., 1966: 47–64.
68. Yan S, Sinderby C, Bielen P, Beck J, Comtois N, Sliwinski P. Expiratory muscle pressure and breathing mechanics in chronic obstructive pulmonary disease. Eur Respir J 2000; 16:684–690.
69. Ashutosh K, Gilbert R, Auchincloss JH, Peppi D. Asynchronous breathing movement in patients with chronic obstructive pulmonary disease. Chest 1975; 67:553–557.
70. Cohen AC, Zagelbaum G, Gross D, et al. Clinical manifestations of inspiratory muscle fatigue. Am J Med 1982; 73:308–31668.
71. Roussos C. Function and fatigue of respiratory muscles. Chest 1985; 88 (suppl): 124S–132S.
72. De Troyer A. Effect of hyperinflation on the diaphragm. Eur Respir J 1997; 10: 708–713.
73. De Troyer A, Leeper JB, McKenzie DK, Gandevia S. Neural drive to the diaphragm in patients with severe COPD. Am J Respir Crit Care Med 1997; 155:1335–1340.
74. Decramer M. Hyperinflation and respiratory muscle interaction. Eur Respir J 1997; 10:934–941.
75. Cohen AC, Zagelbaum G, Gross D, et al. Clinical manifestations of inspiratory muscle fatigue. Am J Med 1982; 73:308–316.
76. Ashutosh K, Gilbert R, Auchincloss JH, Peppi D. Asynchronous breathing movement in patients with chronic obstructive pulmonary disease. Chest 1975; 67:553–557.
77. Hoover CF. Diagnostic significance of inspiratory movements of costal margins. Am J Med Sci 1920; 159:633.
78. Mead J. Functional significance of the area of apposition of diaphragm to ribcage. Am Rev Respir Dis 1979; 119:31–39.
79. Georgopoulos D, Anthonisen NR. Symptoms and signs of COPD. In: Cherniack NS, ed. Chronic Obstructive Pulmonary Disease: Diagnosis of Chronic Obstructive Pulmonary Disease. Philadelphia: WB Saunders, 1991: 357–363.
80. MacNee W. Pathophysiology of cor pulmonale in chronic obstructive pulmonary disease. Part 1. State of art. Am J Respir Crit Care Med 1994; 150:833–852.
81. Williams TJ, Ahmad D, Morgan WKC. A clinical and roentgenographic correlation of diaphragmatic movement. Arch Intern Med 1981; 141:878–880.
82. Schneider IC, Anderson AE. Correlation of clinical signs with ventilatory function in obstructive lung disease. Ann Intern Med 1965; 62:477–485.
83. Bohadana AB, Peslin R, Uffholtz H. Breath sounds in the clinical assessment of airflow obstruction. Thorax 1978; 33:345–351.
84. Nari JR, Turner-Warwick M. Breath sounds in emphysemas. Br J Dis Chest 1969; 63:29–37.
85. Schnedier IC, Anderson AE. Correlation of clinical signs with ventilatory function in obstructive lung disease. Ann Intern Med 1965; 62:477–485.

86. Schreur HJ, Sterk PJ, Vanderschoot J, van Klink HC, van Vollenhoven E, Dijkman JH. Lung sound intensity in patients with emphysema and in normal subjects standardized airflows. Thorax 1992; 47:674–679.
87. Meslier N, Charbonneau G, Racineux JL. Wheezes. Eur Respir J 1995; 11:1942–1948.
88. Loudon R, Murphy RLH, Jr. State of the art. Lung sounds. Am Rev Respir Dis 1984; 130:663–673.
89. Marini JJ, Pierson DJ, Hudson LD, Lakshminaranyan S. The significance of wheezing in chronic airflow obstruction. Am Rev Respir Dis 1979; 120:1069–1072.
90. Jones AY, Jones RD, Kwong K, Burns Y. The effects on sound generation of varying both gas flow rate and the viscosity of sputum-like gel in simple tubular mode. Lung 2000; 178:31–40.
91. Nath AR, Capel LH. Inspiratory crackles. Early and late. Thorax 1974; 29:223–227.
92. Nath AR, Capel LB. Inspiratory crackles and mechanical events of breathing. Thorax 1974; 29:695–698.
93. Kress JP, O'Conor MF, Schmidt GA. Clinical examination reliably detects intrinsic positive end-expiratory pressure in critically ill mechanically ventilated patients. Am J Respir Crit Care Med 1999; 159:290–294.
94. Hill NS. The cardiac exam in lung disease. Clin Chest Med 1987; 8:273–285.
95. Hudson LD, Kurt TL, Petty TL, Geuton E. Arrhythmias associated with acute respiratory failure in patients with chronic airway obstruction. Chest 1973; 63:661–665.
96. Kleiger RE, Senior RM. Long-term electrocardiographic monitoring of ambulatory patients with chronic airway obstruction. Chest 1974; 65:483–487.

11

Pulmonary Gas Exchange in Exacerbations of Chronic Obstructive Pulmonary Disease

FEDERICO P. GÓMEZ and ROBERTO RODRIGUEZ-ROISIN

Hospital Clínic
University of Barcelona
Barcelona, Spain

I. Introduction

The chief function of the lung is pulmonary gas exchange, which requires adequate levels of ventilation and perfusion of the alveoli. The lung must match pulmonary O_2 uptake ($\dot{V}O_2$) and elimination of CO_2 ($\dot{V}CO_2$) to the whole-body metabolic O_2 consumption and CO_2 production, whatever the O_2 and CO_2 partial pressures in the arterial blood. In normal conditions, the cardiovascular and the pulmonary systems interact to reach this adequate matching, both at rest and during stress conditions such as physical exercise.

In patients with chronic obstructive pulmonary disease (COPD), in particular during episodes of exacerbation, the interplay between the cardiovascular and pulmonary systems plays a critical pathophysiological role leading to either adaptive and compensatory effects or, conversely, accentuating the disease state requiring advanced medical support.

The diagnosis of exacerbation is mainly defined by the impairment of respiratory symptoms, such as progressive dyspnea and increased sputum production and cough requiring therapeutic intervention. Nevertheless, symptoms of impaired cardiovascular function are commonly present in patients with moderate-to-severe exacerbations and, in some instances, could account for the precipitating cause of the symptoms. Coexistence of left ventricular failure with pulmonary edema, or "cardiogenic" bronchial hyperresponsiveness, may mimic the classic respiratory behavior of COPD exacerbation, including gas exchange abnormalities. Similarly, development or impairment of preexisting pulmonary hypertension and right ventricular failure in hypoxemic patients is commonly seen as a complicating event during exacerbations while these conditions could themselves be precipitating conditions in some patients. Management of episodes of exacerbations of COPD should take into account cardiac and pulmonary interactions, especially in more severely affected patients in whom clinical and functional outcomes and survival could be critically affected.

This review outlines the interactions between the cardiovascular and pulmonary systems during episodes of exacerbation in patients with COPD in different clinical conditions, paying special attention to those factors that affect pulmonary gas exchange.

II. Pulmonary and Systemic Determinants of Oxygen and Carbon Dioxide Exchange

Adequate management of patients with respiratory failure in the clinical setting requires proper assessment of pulmonary gas exchange. Partial pressures of arterial respiratory blood gases (PaO_2 and $PaCO_2$) and pH are the directly measurable variables used by most clinicians for this purpose. Although respiratory blood gases have become increasingly easy to obtain in the intensive or emergency care setting, often the interpretation of the pathophysiological determinants of abnormal PaO_2 and/or $PaCO_2$ in the clinical arena is not straightforward. This is because arterial respiratory blood gases reflect not only the functional conditions of the lung as a gas exchanger, thereby their intrapulmonary determinants (i.e., ventilation–perfusion heterogeneities, increased intrapulmonary shunt, and/or alveolar to end-capillary diffusion limitation to oxygen), but also the conditions under which the lung operates, namely, the composition of inspired gas and mixed venous blood (i.e., minute ventilation, cardiac output, inspired PO_2 and oxygen uptake) (1–6). We will focus essentially on the determinants of arterial PO_2 and PCO_2 in the light of the evidences shown by means of the multiple inert gas elimination technique (MIGET) (3,7).

A. Intrapulmonary Factors

The highest efficiency of the lung as O_2 and CO_2 exchanger should be achieved when ventilation and blood flow to each individual alveolar unit are adequately balanced ($\dot{V}_A/\dot{Q} = 1.0$) and, consequently, homogeneity of $\dot{V}_A/\dot{Q}$ ratios among alveolar units is present. This so-called "perfect lung" is not seen in normal subjects because mild heterogeneities of pulmonary $\dot{V}_A/\dot{Q}$ ratios are always present due to the gravity and a slight amount of physiological post-pulmonary shunt (approximately 1%) due to both the Thebesian veins draining blood flow from the coronary veins directly to the left atrium and the bronchial venous blood going to pulmonary (arterialized) veins. The characteristic $\dot{V}_A/\dot{Q}$ distribution in normals obtained with the MIGET consists of narrow perfusion and ventilation distributions (second moment) centered around a $\dot{V}_A/\dot{Q}$ ratio of 1.0 (first moment). Mean values for the second moment of both blood flow and ventilation distributions range from 0.35 to 0.43 (8,9). The upper 95% confidence limit for the dispersion of perfusion distribution (log SD $\dot{Q}$) is 0.60 and for that of ventilation distribution (log SD $\dot{V}$) is 0.65 (10–13), but, at age 70 years, these are 0.70 and 0.75, respectively (14). No (or virtually no) perfusion to $\dot{V}_A/\dot{Q}$ ratios <0.005 (by convention, accepted as intrapulmonary shunt) is present (9). Likewise, the amount of ventilation to $\dot{V}_A/\dot{Q}$ ratios >100 (dead space) (including instrumental, anatomical, and physiological dead space) is approximately 30%. No perfusion to lung units with $\dot{V}_A/\dot{Q}$ ratios <0.1 (low $\dot{V}_A/\dot{Q}$) is observed; similarly, ventilation to lung units with $\dot{V}_A/\dot{Q}$ ratios >10 (high $\dot{V}_A/\dot{Q}$) is not present. In most instances, $\dot{V}_A/\dot{Q}$ mismatch is the predominant factor disturbing both pulmonary O_2 uptake and CO_2 output and, consequently, inducing hypoxemia and hypercapnia (15,16). It should be noted, however, that patients with $\dot{V}_A/\dot{Q}$ inequality exhibit hypoxemia but not hypercapnia regardless of their causal disease state. This is because increased activity of central chemoreceptors provokes a rise in total ventilation (extrapulmonary factor) that returns $PaCO_2$ back to normal values, but it is not as effective on PaO_2 because of the different shape of the oxygen and carbon dioxide dissociation curves (2,8). Particular features of uneven $\dot{V}_A/\dot{Q}$ relationships in different clinical conditions related to exacerbation of COPD are described below. The amount of $\dot{V}_A/\dot{Q}$ inequality observed in a given patient is essentially the combined end result of three distinct factors: (1) functional consequences of pulmonary impairment caused by the underlying disease; (2) efficiency of the ventilatory pattern (for a given minute ventilation, the combination of deep tidal volume and slow respiratory rate improves $\dot{V}_A/\dot{Q}$ balance); and (3) magnitude of hypoxic pulmonary vasoconstriction (increased arteriolar tone in low $\dot{V}_A/\dot{Q}$ areas constitutes a well-known compensatory phenomenon that reduces $\dot{V}_A/\dot{Q}$ inequality). Increased intrapulmonary shunt is the foremost factor causing hypoxemia in acute respiratory distress syndrome (ARDS). Since it refers to perfusion to unventilated alveolar units ($\dot{V}_A/\dot{Q}$ <0.005), it should be considered as a particular condition of $\dot{V}_A/\dot{Q}$ inequality. However, because its pathophysiological and therapeutic implications (hypoxemia refractory to high inspired oxygen therapy), it is considered a separate entity rarely involved as a cause of hypoxemia in patients with COPD, even in the most life-threatening conditions. Similarly, alveolar-end capillary diffusion limitation to oxygen is a rather uncommon cause of arterial hypoxemia in patients with COPD. It has been only demonstrated in idiopathic pulmonary fibrosis (17), both at rest and during exercise, and in the hepatopulmonary syndrome under resting conditions (18).

B. Extrapulmonary Factors

Extrapulmonary factors of primary importance are: (1) inspired O_2 fraction (F_IO_2); (2) total ventilation ($\dot{V}_E$); (3) cardiac output ($\dot{Q}_T$); and (4) metabolic rate ($\dot{V}O_2$). The importance of F_IO_2 as a key determinant of alveolar PO_2 (P_AO_2), and in turn of PaO_2, is indicated by the components of the ideal alveolar gas equation (2,8):

$$P_AO_2 = (Pb - PH_2O) \cdot F_IO_2 - PaCO_2/R + [PaCO_2 \cdot F_IO_2 \cdot (1 - R)/R],$$

where, Pb is the barometric pressure, PH_2O corresponds to the partial pressure of water vapor at $37°C$, and R is the respiratory exchange ratio ($\dot{V}CO_2/\dot{V}O_2$, $\dot{V}CO_2$ being carbon dioxide production). However, the relationships between F_IO_2 and PaO_2 are also modulated by the degree of pulmonary $\dot{V}_A/\dot{Q}$ inequality, as described in Refs. 1,2,4. Total ventilation is considered an extrapulmonary factor because it is essentially set by the respiratory centers (central drive). The impact of $\dot{V}_E$ on respiratory blood gases (PaO_2 and $PaCO_2$) also varies with the degree of $\dot{V}_A/\dot{Q}$ mismatch. However, as mentioned above, the increase in $\dot{V}_E$ is always more efficient to remove CO_2 from the blood (decrease $PaCO_2$) than to increase PaO_2. Because the CO_2 dissociation curve is almost linear in its working range, an increase in $\dot{V}_E$ to a lung with substantial $\dot{V}_A/\dot{Q}$ inequality continues to be effective in eliminating more CO_2. This is why arterial PCO_2 is so sensitive to changes in $\dot{V}_E$ (15,16). It should be noted that the equation:

$$P_ACO_2 = K \cdot \dot{V}CO_2/\dot{V}_A,$$

where P_ACO_2 is alveolar PO_2, K is a constant term, $\dot{V}CO_2$ is carbon dioxide production, and $\dot{V}_A$ is alveolar ventilation [$\dot{V}_A = \dot{V}_E(1 - V_D/V_T)$], can be meaningfully applied only to a single alveolar unit or to a homogeneous lung. But the above equation does not hold to describe the relationships between $PaCO_2$ and $\dot{V}_E$ in diseased lungs because effective alveolar ventilation cannot be assessed (15). By contrast, the nonlinear O_2 dissociation curve determines that an increase in $\dot{V}_E$ typically results in a modest gain in PaO_2. This is because the high $\dot{V}_A/\dot{Q}$ units that are operating in the "plateau" of the oxyhemoglobin dissociation curve are unable to compensate for the depressive effect on PaO_2 of the low $\dot{V}_A/\dot{Q}$ units.

It is important here to emphasize the role of mixed venous PO_2 ($P\bar{v}O_2$) and how extrapulmonary factors (other than inspired PO_2 and total ventilation) may contribute to reduce PaO_2 through the effects on $P\bar{v}O_2$. In this regard, a diminished $P\bar{v}O_2$ may result from: (1) a low cardiac output; (2) an increased oxygen uptake; and/or (3) a decreased blood oxygen content due to several alterations in the principal factors modulating the oxyhemoglobin dissociation curve. It should be noted that the impact of $P\bar{v}O_2$ on arterial PO_2 also varies with the pattern of $\dot{V}_A/\dot{Q}$ mismatch. The more affected $\dot{V}_A/\dot{Q}$ relationships, the greater deleterious impact of reduced $P\bar{v}O_2$ on arterial PO_2, hence amplifying its detrimental effects.

In addition to the four primary extrapulmonary factors, secondary variables such as hemoglobin concentration, hemoglobin P_{50}, body temperature, and blood acid–base status play an additional role in the clinical setting (19). Metabolic alkalosis deteriorates in critically sick patients with more severe respiratory failure needing mechanical support, both increased intrapulmonary shunt and $\dot{V}_A/\dot{Q}$ imbalance, whereas its correction by hydrochloric acid (HCl) improves overall pulmonary gas exchange (20). The most likely mechanism is that acidosis ameliorates the intrapulmonary determinants of hypoxemia, possibly causing an enhancement of hypoxic pulmonary areas of the lung; in contrast, shifts of the oxyhemoglobin dissociation curve related to the Bohr effect accounts for a marginal improvement in arterial oxygenation (20). In a canine model of permeability pulmonary edema (21), metabolic acidosis improved arterial oxygenation, and, to the contrary, metabolic alkalosis deteriorated it. Because cardiac output and minute ventilation remained unchanged, changes in intrapulmonary shunt and $\dot{V}_A/\dot{Q}$ mismatch, either enhancing or releasing hypoxic pulmonary vasoconstriction, respectively, mostly influenced pulmonary gas exchange.

As described by West et al. (4), it is possible to predict the arterial PO_2 expected from the measured $\dot{V}_A/\dot{Q}$ inequality and the particular combination of extrapulmonary factors that existed at the time of measurement. The MIGET algorithm, however, allows the observer to change any or all of the extrapulmonary factors (primary and/or secondary), and then to compute the expected value of arterial PO_2. Such flexibility is useful to understand not only potential expected effects of therapeutic interventions, but also to separately determine the quantitative role of each extrapulmonary factor when they change between two conditions of MIGET measurement. This can be particularly useful to analyze the underlying physiological effects of different ventilatory settings on arterial PO_2.

In clinical research, to analyze separately the influence of the increase in cardiac output, it is a simple matter to execute the MIGET algorithm using: (1) the data during mechanical ventilation; (2) the spontaneous breathing variables with the cardiac output measured during mechanical ventilation; and (3) all spontaneous breathing parameters to assess the individual influences on arterial PO_2 of each factor. By the same token, it is possible to use the $\dot{V}_A/\dot{Q}$ algorithm to differentiate separately, for example, the effect of increased intrapulmonary shunt versus that of $\dot{V}_A/\dot{Q}$ inequality on arterial PO_2.

III. Ventilation–Perfusion Inequality: Natural History

Regardless of the precipitating factor, episodes of exacerbation of COPD are characterized by worsening of pulmonary gas exchange that results in severe hypoxemia with or without hypercapnia (22). The characteristics of the $\dot{V}_A/\dot{Q}$ distributions and their interrelations with extrapulmonary factors are critical conditions that ultimately influence arterial blood gases. The mechanisms of gas exchange worsening during exacerbations have been well characterized using the MIGET technique. In this regard, Barberà et al. (23) have precisely addressed several aspects of the natural history of that dismal condition. Thus, a group of patients with COPD suffering from an episode of exacerbation were sequentially studied at the beginning of the exacerbation and more than 1 month later when they were clinically stable (23).

In stable conditions (23), these patients showed severe airflow limitation (mean $\pm$ SD) (FEV_1, 0.91 ± 0.19 L, $29 \pm 6\%$ predicted) that worsens during exacerbations $(0.74 \pm 0.17\,L)$. In all cases, the exacerbation was attributed to nonspecific bronchial infection without evidences of heart failure or requirement of mechanical ventilation. Gas exchange abnormalities in patients with severe exacerbations of COPD who still breathe spontaneously were characterized, as expected, by the decrease in PaO_2 $(PaO_2$ $53 \pm 12\,mmHg$, at $F_IO_2 = 0.21$; $PaO_2/F_IO_2 = 245 \pm 58\,mmHg)$ and the increase of $PaCO_2$ $(51 \pm 12\,mmHg)$ accompanied by a further worsening of $\dot{V}_A/\dot{Q}$ relationships compared with stable conditions (Fig. 1). The pattern of $\dot{V}_A/\dot{Q}$ abnormalities included a low (L) bimodal perfusion pattern, characterized by a low $\dot{V}_A/\dot{Q}$ mode or a broad unimodal blood flow and ventilation pattern mainly due to the increased perfusion in poorly ventilated areas with low $\dot{V}_A/\dot{Q}$ ratios, as shown by the increase in log SD $\dot{Q}$ $(1.10 \pm 0.29$ during exacerbations, 0.96 ± 0.27 under stable conditions) and in areas of low $\dot{V}_A/\dot{Q}$ $(9.2 \pm 12.9\%$ of $\dot{Q}_T$ during exacerbations, $4.1 \pm 8.6\%$ of $\dot{Q}_T$ in stable conditions), the latter also reflected in the former. This $\dot{V}_A/\dot{Q}$ pattern of abnormalities is consistent with the presence of airway narrowing induced by inflammation, bronchospasm, bronchoconstriction, mucus secretion, increased intrinsic positive end-expiratory pressure (PEEP), and/or gas trapping and dynamic hyperinflation during exacerbations. By contrast, intrapulmonary shunt, which was relatively trivial under stable conditions, increased marginally during exacerbations (to less than 5% of cardiac output). This gives further support to the finding that increased intrapulmonary shunt is not a crucial mechanism contributing to hypoxemia in COPD, probably because these patients never have completely occluded airways, possess efficient collateral ventilation, and/or preserve an active hypoxic pulmonary vaso-

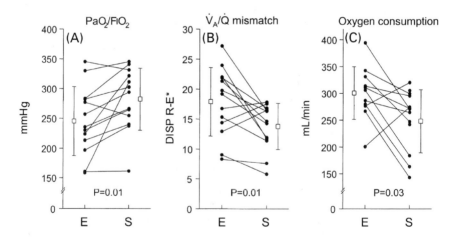

Figure 1 Change in (A) ratio of arterial oxygen tension to inspired oxygen fraction (PaO_2/F_IO_2); (B) ventilation–perfusion $(\dot{V}_A/\dot{Q})$ inequality (expressed as the dispersion of the retention minus excretion of inert gases corrected by dead space (DISP R-E*)); and (C) oxygen consumption $(\dot{V}O_2)$, from acute exacerbations (E) to stable conditions (S). Open symbols and vertical bars denote mean $\pm$ SD. (From Ref. 23.)

constriction. Likewise, dead space was substantially increased with values above the normal 30% of overall ventilation ($41 \pm 7\%$ of $\dot{V}_E$).

On the side of extrapulmonary factors, both cardiac output and $\dot{V}O_2$ were significantly increased during exacerbations (6.1 ± 2.4 L/min and 300 ± 49 mL/min, respectively) compared with the results observed during stable conditions (respectively, 5.1 ± 1.7 L/min and 248 ± 59 mL/min). By contrast, minute ventilation was moderately increased during exacerbations, essentially due to a high respiratory frequency (21 ± 7 breath/min) with a sustained tidal volume (526 ± 154 mL). In spite of this slight increase in $\dot{V}_E$, the ventilatory pattern during exacerbations was essentially unchanged in comparison with the values observed under stable conditions ($\dot{V}_E$, 10.5 ± 2.2 L/min vs. 9.2 ± 1.8 L/min, respectively). Dead space, increased during exacerbations, did not differ at all with the values observed during stable conditions ($43 \pm 9\%$ of $\dot{V}_E$). These findings reinforce the concept that the increased $\dot{V}_A/\dot{Q}$ inequality is a very important determinant for the development of hypercapnia during COPD exacerbations, regardless of the development of both muscle fatigue and alveolar hypoventilation (23).

Of particular interest in the analysis of these results is that the moderate increase in $\dot{V}_A/\dot{Q}$ imbalance did not completely explain the worsening of arterial oxygenation, implying that other factors contributed to reduce PaO_2 (23) (Fig. 2). Among them, the principal factor involved was the increased $\dot{V}O_2$ which, according to the Fick principle, produce a reduction in $P\bar{v}O_2$. Indeed, $P\bar{v}O_2$ calculated by mass balance in COPD patients was actually reduced during exacerbation (32 ± 7 mmHg) in comparison with stable condition (37 ± 5 mmHg; $p < 0.01$) (23). Such a decreased $P\bar{v}O_2$ may further reduce PaO_2 by a direct effect but also, and more importantly, by amplifying the impact of increase $\dot{V}_A/\dot{Q}$ inequality on end-capillary PO_2 (2). The increase in $\dot{V}O_2$ was attributed to an increased oxygen demand of the respiratory muscles as a result of the increase in airway resistance and the efforts to overcome dynamic hyperinflation, let alone the effects of a high dose of short-acting β_2-agonists (24) and/or an increased metabolic activity. It is important to emphasize that, other things being equal, the negative effect of increased $\dot{V}O_2$ on $P\bar{v}O_2$ was partially counterbalanced by an increase in cardiac output that tends to increase oxygen concentrations of mixed venous blood without altering the degree of $\dot{V}_A/\dot{Q}$ inequality. Accordingly, it was estimated that 46% of the decrease in arterial oxygenation during exacerbations was caused by increased $\dot{V}_A/\dot{Q}$ inequality, 28% to the combined changes in oxygen consumption and in cardiac output, and the remaining 26% to the amplifying effects that a decreased $P\bar{v}O_2$ has on $\dot{V}_A/\dot{Q}$ mismatch in further decreasing end-capillary PO_2 (23).

Additional studies of COPD patients during exacerbations have shown comparable results (25–27). This is the case of the study performed by Díaz et al. (25) in patients with exacerbations of COPD with hypercapnic respiratory failure, while breathing spontaneously before the application of noninvasive positive pressure ventilation (NIPPV). This subset of patients, studied within 36 h of admission to the emergency room, was more severely affected than those alluded to above (23) showing a worse, rapid, and shallow breathing (f, 26 ± 5 breath/min; V_T, 311 ± 42 mL), a more pronounced hypercapnia ($PaCO_2$, 66 ± 10 mmHg), and

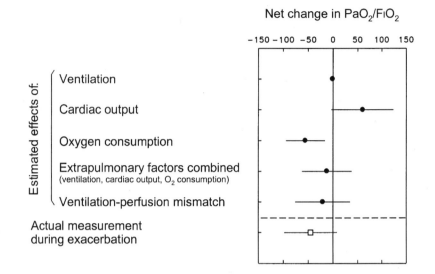

Figure 2 Theoretical analysis of the relative contributions of the factors that determined the change in the ratio of arterial oxygen tension to inspired oxygen fraction (PaO_2/F_1O_2) during an exacerbation of chronic obstructive pulmonary disease (COPD). Values are the mean difference in PaO_2/F_1O_2 measured under stable clinical conditions minus that predicted to results from a specific change, at the level corresponding to exacerbation, in: minute ventilation ($\dot{V}_E$), cardiac output ($\dot{Q}$), oxygen consumption ($\dot{V}O_2$), and ventilation–perfusion ($\dot{V}_A/\dot{Q}$) inequality (closed symbols). The open symbol shows the actual change in PaO_2/F_1O_2 during exacerbation. Lines indicate the 95% confidence intervals.

a greater dead space ($60 \pm 7\%$ of $\dot{V}_E$). However, the general pattern of $\dot{V}_A/\dot{Q}$ abnormalities was qualitatively similar to that observed during less severe exacerbations, showing a moderate-to-severe increase in $\dot{V}_A/\dot{Q}$ inequality (log SD $\dot{Q}$, 1.08 ± 0.23), increased perfusion to areas with low $\dot{V}_A/\dot{Q}$ ratios (low $\dot{V}_A/\dot{Q}$, $13 \pm 11\%$ of $\dot{Q}_T$), and a marginal contribution of increased intrapulmonary shunt ($5 \pm 5\%$ of $\dot{Q}_T$) (25). Inert gas data from two additional studies have confirmed the depicted general traits of $\dot{V}_A/\dot{Q}$ abnormalities, although in both studies patients were included some time later during the sequence of the time course of the exacerbation (26,27).

These gas exchange findings shown during exacerbations of COPD contrast with the larger degree of $\dot{V}_A/\dot{Q}$ inequality developed during acute severe asthma. In acute exacerbated asthmatics needing hospitalization but not requiring ventilatory support (28), the changes in the $\dot{V}_A/\dot{Q}$ relationships were much more dramatic, including a greater impairment during the exacerbation and a near normalization after recovery. Accordingly, the log SD $\dot{Q}$ changed from 1.41 ± 0.12 in the acute phase to 0.53 ± 0.07 during stable conditions (28). This greater degree of $\dot{V}_A/\dot{Q}$ imbalance may imply that airway narrowing during asthma attacks is much more pronounced than during COPD exacerbations, leading to the development of a greater proportion of alveolar units with low $\dot{V}_A/\dot{Q}$ ratios. This is consistent with a very active smooth muscle contraction in peripheral airways acting together with airway wall thickening induced by submucosal edema, which further enhances airway narrowing. The possible influences of the different extrapulmonary factors in the patients with asthma are less clear. By contrast, dead space remained relatively stable with mild increases.

In the study by Barberà et al. (23), 10 of the patients admitted to the hospital for an exacerbation of COPD were reevaluated sequentially during their hospital stay. Accordingly, measurements of $\dot{V}_A/\dot{Q}$ distributions were performed within the first week (day 6 ± 1) of hospitalization and at discharge (day 15 ± 13), along with the measurements performed at admission and some time later during stable conditions. This time sequence allowed a more detailed description of the outcomes studied and gave additional insights into the interrelation between pulmonary and extrapulmonary factors governing pulmonary gas exchange in COPD. The time course of spirometric and gas exchange measurements developed during the follow-up study is illustrated in Figure 3. FEV_1 increased progressively during hospitaliza-

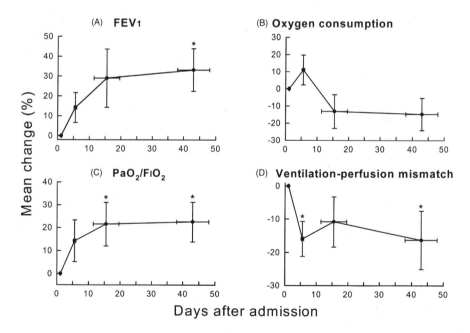

Figure 3 Sequential evolution of spirometric and gas exchange measurements during hospitalization and after discharge (day 15 ± 4). Values are the mean ($\pm$SEM) percentage change from the value obtained at the initial study of (A) forced expiratory volume in one second (FEV_1); (B) oxygen consumption ($\dot{V}O_2$); (C) ratio of arterial oxygen tension to inspired oxygen fraction (PaO_2/F_IO_2); and (D) ventilation–perfusion ($\dot{V}_A/\dot{Q}$) inequality (expressed as DISP R-E*). The asterisks indicate significant differences ($p < 0.05$) compared with the values at the initial assessment.

tion, reaching at discharge the levels seen under stable conditions. A similar favorable time course was observed by and large for gas exchange variables, although with specifics depending on the parameter analyzed. Thus, $\dot{V}_A/\dot{Q}$ distributions expressed as an overall index of heterogeneity (DISP R-E*) reached the maximal improvement at day 6 of hospitalization and did not change significantly thereafter, whereas the PaO_2/F_IO_2 ratio improved some later, at the end of the hospital stay. The further increase in $\dot{V}O_2$ observed at day 6, most likely related to the increment in metabolic rate possibly due to the effects of the massive use of β_2-agonists as alluded to, could account for this lack of increase in PaO_2/F_IO_2 in spite of a simultaneous improvement of $\dot{V}_A/\dot{Q}$ distributions at this point in time. These findings emphasize the possible influence of pharmacological interventions on extrapulmonary factors that could affect pulmonary gas exchange during exacerbation. Treatments that may reduce cardiac performance (diuretics, negative inotropic agents) should be employed with caution as they could be inappropriate in part for the purposes of an optimal gas exchange (23).

A. Mechanical Ventilation

Invasive Mechanical Ventilation

Mechanical ventilation is often a necessary intervention for life support in patients with COPD during severe exacerbations and acute respiratory failure. Studies of COPD patients needing mechanical ventilation have shown essentially similar qualitative $\dot{V}_A/\dot{Q}$ patterns, although quantitatively more severe than those observed in patients breathing spontaneously. During mechanical ventilation in patients with exacerbations of COPD, Torres et al. (29) reported a bimodal perfusion pattern or broad unimodal pattern in six out of eight patients, whereas only one patient showed a pure high $\dot{V}_A/\dot{Q}$ distribution pattern. The increased severity of the abnormal $\dot{V}_A/\dot{Q}$ distributions in patients mechanically ventilated during COPD exacerbations is reflected by the greater dispersion of $\dot{V}_A/\dot{Q}$ distributions, as shown by the elevated values of log SD $\dot{Q}$ (1.37 ± 0.30) reported by Castaing et al. (30), Rossi et al. (1.33 ± 0.16) (31), and Torres et al. (29) (1.40 ± 0.1). The main difference with the findings observed in patients breathing spontaneously is that in mechanically ventilated patients there is an additional greater amount of increased intrapulmonary shunt, although never greater than 10% of cardiac output (29) (Fig. 4). This suggests that some airways could be completely occluded, possibly by inspissated bronchial secretions. However, in patients with COPD, a substantial increase in intrapulmonary shunt, excluding atelectasis, pleural effusions, pneumonia, or pulmonary edema, should also alert the clinician about the possibility of a reopening of the foramen ovale due to the increase in right atrial pressure promoted by the inception of mechanical ventilation. In the presence of a true shunt, 100% oxygen breathing fails to increase PaO_2 substantially ($>300–350$ mmHg).

As expected, the improved efficiency of the ventilatory pattern during mechanical ventilation is reflected by the larger tidal volume, the less affected dispersion of ventilation (log SD $\dot{V}$), and a near-normal dead space. The importance of this ventilatory profile becomes evident when patients are weaned from the

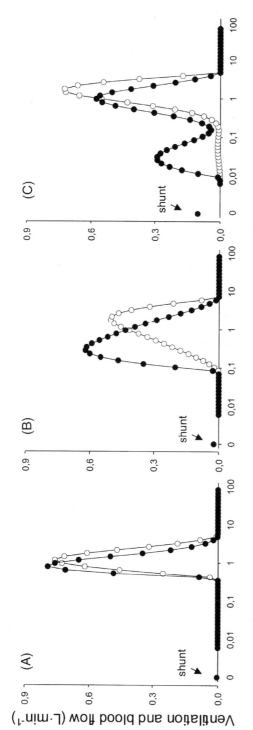

Ventilation/perfusion ratio

Figure 4 Representative distributions of alveolar ventilation (open symbols) and pulmonary blood flow (closed symbols) (Y-axis) plotted against $\dot{V}_A/\dot{Q}$ ratio on a log scale (X-axis) from (A) a healthy, young individual at rest, breathing room air showing a normal $\dot{V}_A/\dot{Q}$ pattern; (B) a patient with chronic obstructive pulmonary disease (COPD) breathing spontaneously during an exacerbation, with a broad unimodal blood flow and ventilation pattern mainly due to the increased perfusion in poorly ventilated areas with low $\dot{V}_A/\dot{Q}$ ratios; and (C) an exacerbated patient with COPD during mechanical ventilation, showing a type low (L) bimodal perfusion pattern.

ventilator (see below). By contrast, mechanical ventilation impacts negatively on the hemodynamic profile by reducing cardiac output, oxygen delivery, and, consequently, $P\bar{v}O_2$ (29). Arterial PO_2 will reflect the integrated effects of all these changes.

At the time of weaning from mechanical ventilation in patients with COPD, both cardiac output and ventilatory pattern play a crucial influencing role for the purposes of gas exchange. The change from mechanical ventilation to spontaneous breathing in a COPD patient may increase considerably cardiac output (29,32) due to the abrupt increment of the preload of the right ventricle secondary to the marked elevation of venous return (following the reduction in intrathoracic pressure due to the less positive pressure). The consequent increase in pulmonary blood flow may be preferentially redistributed to poorly ventilated areas with low $\dot{V}_A/\dot{Q}$ ratios, leading to a further worsening of $\dot{V}_A/\dot{Q}$ mismatch. In fact, the perfusion to areas with low $\dot{V}_A/\dot{Q}$ ratios increased significantly from $9.4 \pm 4.4\%$ of cardiac output (during mechanical ventilation) to $19.6 \pm 5.3\%$ (during spontaneous ventilation) during weaning in a group of COPD patients (29). It is of note that only a small increase of the shunt fraction has been observed despite the marked increase in cardiac output. On the other hand, the removal of the patient from the ventilator may lead to the development of a less efficient ventilatory pattern due to a fall in tidal volume together with an increase in the respiratory rate (rapid and shallow breathing) without changes in total minute ventilation ($\dot{V}_E$). As a result, both the dispersion of the alveolar ventilation (log SD $\dot{V}$) and the overall $\dot{V}_A/\dot{Q}$ heterogeneity (DISP R-E*) increase leading to further $\dot{V}_A/\dot{Q}$ mismatch. In addition to the changes in hemodynamics and ventilatory pattern, an eventual rise in $\dot{V}O_2$ due to the increase in the metabolic requirements of respiratory muscles during weaning may potentially decrease mixed venous PO_2 which, in turn, may have a deleterious effect on PaO_2. On the other hand, the increase of cardiac output also increases the $P\bar{v}O_2$ which, as previously stated, has a direct beneficial effect on pulmonary gas exchange.

Combining inert gas data and isotopic scans, Beydon et al. (33) complemented and extended these data in a group of patients with COPD after more than 5 days of attempted weaning from the ventilator. It was suggested that the abnormal ventilatory pattern during spontaneous breathing was the major determinant of $\dot{V}_A/\dot{Q}$ mismatch by showing that the critical alteration of the ventilation during weaning led to the development of basal regions of very low $\dot{V}_A/\dot{Q}$ ratios.

Noninvasive Mechanical Ventilation

Noninvasive positive pressure ventilation (NIPPV) is an increasing demanding therapeutic approach for management of respiratory failure that can reduce both hypercapnia and respiratory acidosis, thus preventing tracheal intubation in several clinical situations, such as COPD exacerbation. The effects of NIPPV on $\dot{V}_A/\dot{Q}$ distributions of exacerbated patients with COPD and hypercapnic respiratory failure have been investigated in detail (25). Ten patients admitted to the hospital with hypercapnic respiratory failure (PaO_2, 44 ± 8 mmHg; $PaCO_2$, 71 ± 13 mmHg; F_IO_2,

0.22 ± 0.01, at admission in the emergency room) were studied at baseline, and after 15 and 30 min of NIPPV, implemented by pressure support (10 to 16 cmH$_2$O) and PEEP (up to 5 cmH$_2$O) combination. Compared to baseline (Fig. 5), NIPPV clearly showed a beneficial effect on pulmonary gas exchange demonstrated by the reduction of PaCO$_2$ and the increase in both PaO$_2$ and pH. This improvement was essentially due to a more optimal ventilatory pattern induced by an increased tidal volume, minute ventilation, and alveolar ventilation associated with a reduction in breathing frequency. By contrast, dead space remained constant. It is of note that, contrary to the hypothesis that noninvasive ventilation could result in recruitment of nonventilated or poorly ventilated alveolar units, the implementation of NIPPV to this group of patients did not produce any beneficial influence on their underlying $\dot{V}_A/\dot{Q}$ inequalities (DISP R-E*, 17 ± 5 at baseline; 17 ± 6, and 16 ± 5 after 15 and 30 min of NIPPV, respectively). Similar to what has been observed during the use of invasive ventilatory support, a significant reduction in both cardiac output and oxygen delivery were seen during NIPPV, although in this case the changes were of

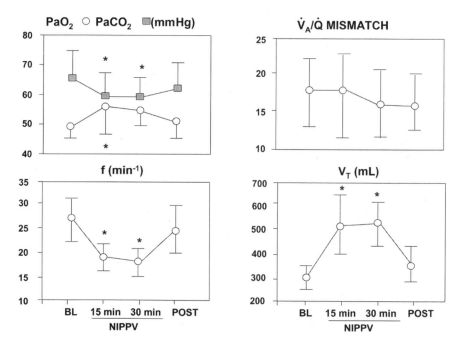

Figure 5 Sequential time course (mean ± SD) of ventilatory and gas exchange measurements at baseline (BL), during 15 and 30 min of noninvasive positive pressure ventilation (NIPPV) and after withdrawal (POST), in patients with COPD and hypercapnic respiratory failure. Whereas arterial oxygen tension (PaO$_2$) and arterial carbon dioxide tension (PaCO$_2$) improves, no changes were observed in $\dot{V}_A/\dot{Q}$ inequality (expressed as DISP R-E*). The improvement in respiratory blood gases was due to a more optimal ventilatory pattern, induced by an increased tidal volume ($\dot{V}_T$) associated with a reduction in breathing frequency (f). (Reproduced from Ref. 25.)

little magnitude and did not result in any detrimental effect on either arterial PO_2 or $P\bar{v}O_2$. However, it should be underscored that delivery of high-pressure ventilatory support to these patients may enhance the deleterious effect of NIPPV on cardiac output (by depressing it) or pulmonary gas exchange as well as increasing the patient's discomfort. One intriguing finding of this study was that $AaPO_2$ increased, thus apparently reflecting gas exchange impairment during NIPPV in spite of the moderate improvement in PaO_2 and the decrease of $PaCO_2$ by a similar amount. As $AaPO_2$ was calculated using the actual R (i.e., $\dot{V}CO_2/\dot{V}O_2$), which was increased during NIPPV as a result of an enhanced pulmonary clearance of the body stores of CO_2 and a mild reduction in O_2 consumption, the paradoxical increase in $AaPO_2$ could be explained by the observed increase in R, but not as an indicator that the lung was less efficient as a gas exchanger during NIPPV.

In summary, taken together all these findings point to the view that respiratory gas disturbances (arterial hypoxemia and hypercapnia) are the integrative endpoint of $\dot{V}_A/\dot{Q}$ abnormalities plus the interaction of overall indices of gas exchange, namely, total alveolar ventilation, cardiac output, and the metabolic demands including O_2 consumption and CO_2 production.

IV. Gas Exchange Response to High Oxygen Breathing

Controlled oxygen therapy is the cornerstone for hospital treatment of COPD exacerbations. Adequate levels of oxygenation (PaO_2 >60 mmHg or SaO_2 >90–92%) are easy to achieve in uncomplicated exacerbations, but CO_2 retention can occur insidiously with little change in symptoms. In clinical practice, however, physicians administer low inspired O_2 concentrations (either 0.24 or 0.28) delivered through high-flow masks to patients with COPD and acute respiratory failure. This provides modest but effective increases in PaO_2 (of the order of 10–15 mmHg) without inducing detrimental CO_2 retention, to optimize O_2 delivery to peripheral tissues by facilitating reasonable levels of oxygen saturation.

The response to high oxygen concentrations in patients with COPD is similar regardless of the clinical severity of the disease. With little $\dot{V}_A/\dot{Q}$ mismatch, PaO_2 rises almost linearly as the inspired O_2 is increased. As the severity of $\dot{V}_A/\dot{Q}$ inequality worsens, the rate of rise of PaO_2 is reduced and becomes more curvilinear. We have shown in patients with COPD and acute respiratory failure needing mechanical ventilation that full nitrogen washout of alveolar units, even in patients with poorly ventilated alveolar units with low or very low $\dot{V}_A/\dot{Q}$ ratios, is rapid and that steady-state conditions are easily reached even before 30 min (34). The coexistence of a modest increased intrapulmonary shunt, however, should decrease the elevation of PaO_2, other things being equal.

Although $\dot{V}_A/\dot{Q}$ inequality is no longer a barrier to O_2 exchange when 100% O_2 is breathed, 100% O_2 always worsens $\dot{V}_A/\dot{Q}$ mismatch, as assessed by a significant increase in the dispersion of blood flow (log SD $\dot{Q}$), without changes in intrapulmonary shunt or the dispersion of alveolar ventilation; in contrast, pulmonary arterial pressure and pulmonary vascular resistance remain essentially unchanged. The impairment in $\dot{V}_A/\dot{Q}$ relationships indicates release or abolition of hypoxic pulmonary vasoconstriction. The total absence of further increases in intrapulmonary shunt suggests that reabsorption atelectasis does not take place, suggesting that either collateral ventilation is very efficient or regional airway obstruction is never complete, or both. By contrast, in patients with ARDS a mild-to-moderate increase in shunt (of the order of 25%) without release of hypoxic pulmonary vasoconstriction results (34). This response suggests the presence of critical alveolar units (with low inspired $\dot{V}_A/\dot{Q}$ ratios) unstable and vulnerable to high O_2 concentrations over time. These units tend to collapse easily, hence leading to the development of reabsorption atelectasis (35). When there is no release of hypoxic vasoconstriction, the amount of shunt is always greater, regardless of the F_IO_2. The contention is that alveolar units with poorly ventilated $\dot{V}_A/\dot{Q}$ ratios are not able to redistribute blood flow if their vascular resistance remains unaltered. Alternatively, in patients with COPD, it has been shown that breathing high inspired O_2 concentrations reduces the degree of airways resistance (36). This should tend to improve the distribution of ventilation, other factors being equal, thus reducing the amount of areas with low $\dot{V}_A/\dot{Q}$ ratios and, consequently, the dispersion of pulmonary blood flow.

Using traditional gas exchange measurements, such as Bohr's dead space, Aubier et al. (37) concluded that, in patients with COPD and acute respiratory insufficiency breathing spontaneously, the administration of 100% O_2 resulted in a remarkable increase in $PaCO_2$. Since the respiratory muscles maintained ventilation at nearly the same level as when breathing room air, they suggested that the increase in $PaCO_2$ was mainly attributed to an increased dead space; additional mechanisms included a small reduction in both tidal volume and the Haldane effect, namely, the changes in the CO_2 dissociation curve facilitating the release of CO_2 from bicarbonate and also from that directly bound as carbamate during 100% O_2. This conclusion has been disputed by Stradling (38), who advocated that the increase in $PaCO_2$ could be explained entirely by the latter two mechanisms together with that from flattening the slope of the CO_2 pressure/content relationship with a rise in $PaCO_2$. Our group has also shown an increase in $PaCO_2$ during 100% O_2 breathing in COPD patients needing mechanical support (34). Conceivably, the increased dead space and the experimental evidence that increased $\dot{V}_A/\dot{Q}$ disturbances can worsen not only the O_2 transfer but also CO_2 exchange are behind this increase. We estimated that the hyperoxia-induced increments of $PaCO_2$ in this subset of patients could be attributed almost entirely to the simultaneous increased dead space, thereby indicating a marginal role of the Haldane effect. This was further supported by the persistence of hypercapnia when maintenance F_IO_2 was restarted. The increased dead space suggests redistribution of pulmonary blood flow from high $\dot{V}_A/\dot{Q}$ ratios to poorly but still ventilated units (low $\dot{V}_A/\dot{Q}$ ratios). An alternative or complementary mechanism could be bronchodilation secondary to the hypercapnia, as postulated by Sydney et al. (27) in patients with COPD breathing spontaneously during exacerbations. A similar conclusion was reached when data derived from a computer model of the pulmonary circulation were compared with data from a case series of patients with COPD (39). In this study, changes in physiological dead space were sufficient to account for the hypercarbia developed by patients with exacerbations of COPD when treated with supplemental oxygen.

Robinson et al. (27) have shown recently, in hyperoxia-induced CO_2-retaining patients with COPD that during exacerbations ventilation fell by an average of 20% and that the dispersion of alveolar ventilation (log SD $\dot{V}$), as a reflection of an inert gas measurement of alveolar dead space, increased by about 25% while breathing 100% O_2. Likewise, patients who were CO_2 retainers showed a significant increase in alveolar dead space, indicating a higher CO_2 retention, perhaps related to bronchodilation. Moreover, there was an increase in the dispersion of pulmonary blood flow (i.e., areas with low $\dot{V}_A/\dot{Q}$ ratios) from release of hypoxic vasoconstriction, regardless of the presence or absence of CO_2 retention.

V. Effects of Pharmacological Interventions

A. Bronchodilators

High doses of inhaled bronchodilators are commonly employed for the treatment of severe exacerbations of COPD, both at home and during hospital management (40–44). Short-acting inhaled β_2-agonists and/or anticholinergics are usually recommended, principally based on their spirometric effects. Nevertheless, the effects of these bronchodilating agents on the cardiopulmonary function and the major factors that may affect pulmonary gas exchange during episodes of COPD exacerbations have not been assessed in full.

In patients with severe COPD suffering from an exacerbation, Karpel et al. (45) compared the effects of the short-acting inhaled β_2-agonist, metaproterenol, with those of the anticholinergic ipratropium, in a double-blind, randomized trial using conventional arterial blood gas measurements in the emergency room setting. At 30 min after administration, patients receiving ipratropium showed a small, but significant, rise in PaO_2 (from 68.5 ± 4.0 to 74.5 ± 4.3 mmHg), while those treated with metaproterenol had a significant fall in PaO_2 (from 64.8 ± 4.3 to 58.6 ± 5.1 mmHg). These differences were noted when neither of the two drugs had reached their maximal bronchodilatory effect and disappeared at 90 min when both drugs had reached a similar improvement in FEV_1. The investigators attributed these changes to pulmonary vasodilatation induced by the β_2-agonist, whereas it was speculated that ipratropium has less effect on pulmonary circulation or that anticholinergics are not as well absorbed. In addition, they speculated that the changes in arterial PO_2 could be more pronounced in patients with more severe hypoxemia on initial presentation, an issue that still remains unsolved when the case is an exacerbation. Interestingly enough, this is the only investigation of the acute effects of short-acting bronchodilators in the setting of COPD exacerbations, a lack of information that is available in acute severe asthma. Yet, the assessment of these agents has been done under stable conditions, a fact that will be reviewed in detail for the sake of comparison.

Thus, in patients with advanced COPD in stable condition Ringsted et al. (46) studied the effects of a continuous intravenous infusion of terbutaline (β_2-agonist bronchodilator). They explored the role of the pulmonary vascular tone in modulating gas exchange in these patients. Following terbutaline, cardiac output increased and systemic blood pressure and pulmonary vascular resistance decreased. In addition, while PaO_2 decreased and $P\bar{v}O_2$ and O_2 delivery increased, $PaCO_2$ remained unchanged. There was further $\dot{V}_A/\dot{Q}$ worsening, as assessed by increases both in the perfusion to low $\dot{V}_A/\dot{Q}$ ratios and in the dispersion of blood flow. Although FEV_1 and minute ventilation increased, these increments were not significant. Thus, the $\dot{V}_A/\dot{Q}$ worsening could have resulted from an increased dispersion of pulmonary blood flow and/or a decrease in the overall $\dot{V}_A/\dot{Q}$ ratio due to the increased cardiac output, not efficiently counterbalanced by the simultaneous increased minute ventilation. The concomitant significant increase in $P\bar{v}O_2$ may have also contributed to further worsen $\dot{V}_A/\dot{Q}$ mismatch by releasing hypoxic pulmonary vasoconstriction. However, from these data it was not possible to differentiate between increased cardiac output, inducing an increase in the amount of dispersion of pulmonary blood flow, or an active reduction in pulmonary vascular tone. In the same study, it was shown in another small group of patients with COPD with more airflow obstruction, more hypoxemia, more hypercapnia, and more pulmonary hypertension, that cardiac output increased in response to terbutaline without changes in concomitant pulmonary hemodynamics (i.e., pulmonary artery pressure, pulmonary vascular resistance). Minute ventilation increased modestly, but without improvement in the indices of airflow obstruction. Yet respiratory arterial blood gases did not change, nor did the underlying $\dot{V}_A/\dot{Q}$ abnormalities. In summary, despite the fact that terbutaline caused an increased cardiac output and, consequently, mixed venous PO_2 similar to the former group of patients, this subset of patients with more severe airways obstruction, higher pulmonary hypertension, and worse pulmonary gas exchange, did not modify their gas exchange profile following terbutaline. Conceivably, hypoxic vascular response could have played a pivotal role in modulating pulmonary gas exchange before and after the administration of the drug. Thus, these patients with more severe COPD could have weaker or even absent hypoxic vascular response. This lack of hypoxic vascular response in advanced severe COPD could be related to either severe chronically established alveolar hypoxia or to structural changes in the pulmonary circulation coupled with areas of parenchymal destruction due to emphysema, or both. This is in keeping with the concept that the progressive increase of pulmonary vascular resistance seen in advanced COPD is not only due to irreversible structural vascular lesions but also includes a reversible vascular component. This interpretation would be consistent with the work of Barberà et al. (47) investigating the influence of the structure of pulmonary arteries and the contribution of the hypoxic vascular response in preserving an adequate matching of ventilation and blood flow in patients with mild COPD.

The acute effects of salmeterol, a long-acting β_2-adrenergic agonist in stable patients with COPD, have been compared with those of salbutamol and ipratropium, given in recommended doses, using conventional arterial blood gas measurements (48). Arterial blood gases were measured at baseline and at intervals to 120 min on separate days in a double-blind, crossover design. The decline in PaO_2 following salmeterol was of lesser magnitude but more prolonged, of about $-2.8\,mmHg$ at 30 min, than that after salbutamol, of about $-3.5\,mmHg$ at 20 min; after ipratropium, the corresponding change was about $-1.3\,mmHg$ at 20 min. These marginal decrements of PaO_2, almost entirely explained by increases in the $AaPO_2$, hence suggesting further $\dot{V}_A/\dot{Q}$ worsening, were more evident in those patients with higher baseline PaO_2 values. The study, which did not show differences among the three agents, concluded that despite small negative changes in PaO_2 after each of the three bronchodilators, the decreases were marginal, transient, and above all, of doubtful clinical relevance.

We have also compared the short-term effect on gas exchange of fenoterol, another short-acting β_2-agonist, against that of ipratropium bromide, both given by nebulization, in a double-blind, placebo-controlled study in a series of patients with severe COPD and mild-to-moderate hypoxemia (49). It was shown that while fenoterol slightly decreased mean PaO_2 (about 6 mmHg) due to further worsening in the dispersion of pulmonary blood flow, gas exchange remained unaltered after ipratropium. Although pulmonary hemodynamics were not measured, it was suggested that the pulmonary vascular tone was probably decreased, hence inducing further $\dot{V}_A/\dot{Q}$ mismatch. This varies from the effects of intravenous salbutamol given to patients with acute severe asthma (50), in whom PaO_2 remains unchanged despite marked increases in cardiac output and further $\dot{V}_A/\dot{Q}$ worsening. This suggests that fenoterol may have a greater direct effect on the pulmonary vasculature, which decreases the vascular tone. At doses used in clinical practice, it has been shown that fenoterol causes more adverse effects (namely, cardiac, metabolic, and systemic) than salbutamol or terbutaline in patients with mild asthma (51). The most likely explanation is that fenoterol has been marketed at a higher dose than the other two β_2-agonists, despite having in vitro the same potency than isoproterenol; furthermore, it is suggested that fenoterol may be less selective for β_2 receptors.

The effects on $\dot{V}_A/\dot{Q}$ distributions on the intravenous administration of aminophylline have been also investigated in a group of patients recovering from an exacerbation of COPD (26). Although aminophylline, at therapeutic plasma levels, did not exhibit any significant effect on $\dot{V}_A/\dot{Q}$ distributions for the whole group, individual patients, particularly those with substantial low $\dot{V}_A/\dot{Q}$ areas at baseline, showed deteriorations in their $\dot{V}_A/\dot{Q}$ distributions in response to the drug in spite of a slight, but significant, improvement of the FEV_1. In addition, the same patients who worsen gas exchange during aminophylline infusion showed a further increase in blood flow to low $\dot{V}_A/\dot{Q}$ areas when breathing 100% oxygen, suggesting that the partial release of hypoxic pulmonary vasoconstriction could be the most likely mechanism implicated in the deleterious effect of aminophylline on gas exchange in some patients.

B. Other Agents

Inhalation of nitric oxide (NO) can improve arterial oxygenation due to the reduction of increased intrapulmonary shunt in patients with acute respiratory distress syndrome (ARDS). By contrast, in patients with stable COPD in whom hypoxemia is caused essentially by $\dot{V}_A/\dot{Q}$ imbalance rather than by shunt, inhaled NO can worsen gas exchange by inhibiting hypoxic pulmonary vasoconstriction; hence the hypoxic regulation of the matching between ventilation and perfusion. Blanch et al. (52) investigated the effects of inhaled NO in patients with severe COPD (FEV_1, 0.91 ± 0.11 L) mechanically ventilated due to acute respiratory failure, most of them with a superimposed pneumonia, which is expected to increase the intrapulmonary shunt. Compared with a parallel group of patients with ARDS, patients with COPD showed a similar degree of decrease in pulmonary artery pressure and pulmonary vascular resistance (PVR), but demonstrate an unpredictable effect on arterial PO_2 in response to inhaled NO. Whereas patients with ARDS had improved PaO_2, mean values of PaO_2 where not affected by NO inhalation in patients with COPD, although four out of nine patients experienced a decrease in PaO_2. These findings reinforce the notion that the net results of inhaled NO on gas exchange depends on the balance between the different effects on the normal and abnormal areas that receive the gas (53). This could be the case of a COPD patient with pneumonia, in which areas with different degrees of $\dot{V}_A/\dot{Q}$ inequality coexist with increased intrapulmonary shunt. Improvements of gas exchange with inhaled NO may be due to shift of blood flow from nonventilated to ventilated lung units accessible to NO by increasing blood flow to normal areas. Nevertheless, inhaled NO oxide can reach poorly ventilated lung units with low $\dot{V}_A/\dot{Q}$ ratios and then dilate pulmonary arteries already constricted by hypoxia, thus impairing $\dot{V}_A/\dot{Q}$ balance and reducing PaO_2. Similar detrimental effects on gas exchange have been shown following the use of vasoactive agents, such as dopamine and dobutamine, in patients with COPD and acute respiratory failure needing artificial ventilation (54), prostaglandin E1 (55), atrial natriuretic factor (56), and acetylcholine (57).

There have been three other studies (30,58,59) in patients with COPD and different degrees of ventilatory respiratory failure in which, by investigating the effects of oral almitrine bismesylate, a peripheral chemoreceptor, the influence of pulmonary vascular tone played a key role in improving pulmonary gas exchange. In the first report (59), it was observed in a few patients, some with hypercapnic respiratory failure, that respiratory arterial blood gases improved significantly due to $\dot{V}_A/\dot{Q}$ amelioration. The only associated hemodynamic change was a modest increase in pulmonary vascular resistance without increases in pulmonary artery pressure. In another study (30), in patients requiring mechanical ventilation because of severe respiratory failure, conventional and inert gas exchange indices improved significantly together with a small, but significant, decrease in cardiac output and a mild increase in pulmonary vascular resistance. In all three studies, there was essentially a redistribution of pulmonary blood flow from regions of low $\dot{V}_A/\dot{Q}$ units to areas with normal $\dot{V}_A/\dot{Q}$ ratios. An even more dramatic improvement in pulmonary gas exchange, by markedly reducing the amount of shunt [of an order of magnitude much greater than that induced by NO (60)], has been shown in patients with ARDS following intravenous almitrine (61). In both disorders, COPD and ARDS, it was suggested that enhancement of hypoxic pulmonary vasoconstriction was possible at the origin of the overall improvement in pulmonary gas exchange. However, this beneficial effect on gas exchange in patients with COPD needs to be balanced against some of the unwanted side effects of almitrine, such as peripheral neuropathy and body weight loss, particularly if long-term administration of the drug is decided upon.

Acknowledgments

Supported by the Fondo de Investigación Sanitaria (FIS 00/0617) and the Departament de Recerca, Universitatsi Societat de l'Informació (DURSI) (2001 SGR00386) de la Generalitat de Catalunya.

References

1. West JB. Ventilation-perfusion inequality and overall gas exchange in computer models of the lung. Respir Physiol 1969; 7:88–110.
2. West JB. State of the art: ventilation-perfusion relationships. Am Rev Respir Dis 1977; 116:919–943.
3. Roca J, Wagner PD. Contribution of multiple inert gas elimination technique to pulmonary medicine. 1. Principles and information content of the multiple inert gas elimination technique. Thorax 1994; 49:815–824.
4. West JB, Wagner PD. In: West, JB, ed. Pulmonary gas exchange. Bioengineering Aspects of the Lung. New York: Marcel Dekker, Inc., 1977:361–457.
5. Dantzker DR. The influence of cardiovascular function on gas exchange. Clin Chest Med 1983; 4:149–159.
6. Wagner PD. Ventilation-perfusion inequality in catastrophic lung disease. In: Prakash O, ed. Applied Physiology in Clinical Respiratory Care. The Hague: Martinus Nijhoff, 1982: 363–379.
7. Light RB. Intrapulmonary oxygen consumption in experimental pneumococcal pneumonia. J Appl Physiol 1988; 64:2490–2495.
8. West JB. Ventilation/Blood Flow and Gas Exchange, 4th ed. Oxford: Blackwell Scientific Publications, 1985.
9. Wagner PD, Laravuso RB, Uhl RR, West JB. Continuous distributions of ventilation-perfusion ratios in normal subjects breathing air and 100% O_2. J Clin Invest 1974; 54:54–68.
10. Hammond MD, Gale GE, Kapitan KS, Ries A, Wagner PD. Pulmonary gas exchange in humans during normobaric hypoxic exercise. J Appl Physiol 1986; 61:1749–1757.
11. Hammond MD, Gale GE, Kapitan KS, Ries A, Wagner PD. Pulmonary gas exchange in humans during exercise at sea level. J Appl Physiol 1986; 60:1590–1598.
12. Wagner PD, Gale GE, Moon RE, Torre-Bueno JR, Stolp BW, Saltzman HA. Pulmonary gas exchange in humans exercising at sea level and simulated altitude. J Appl Physiol 1986; 61:260–270.
13. Gale GE, Torre-Bueno JR, Moon RE, Saltzman HA, Wagner PD. Ventilation-perfusion inequality in normal humans during exercise at sea level and simulated altitude. J Appl Physiol 1985; 58:978–988.
14. Cardus J, Burgos F, Díaz O, Roca J, Barberà JA, Marrades RM, Rodriguez-Roisin R, Wagner PD. Increase in pulmonary ventilation-perfusion inequality with age in healthy individuals. Am J Respir Crit Care Med 1997; 156:648–653.

15. West JB. Causes of carbon dioxide retention in lung disease. N Engl J Med 1971; 284:1232–1236.
16. Weinberger SE, Schwartzstein RM, Weiss JW. Hypercapnia. N Engl J Med 1989; 321:1223–1231.
17. Agusti AG, Roca J, Gea J, Wagner PD, Xaubet A, Rodriguez-Roisin R. Mechanisms of gas-exchange impairment in idiopathic pulmonary fibrosis. Am Rev Respir Dis 1991; 143:219–225.
18. Martínez GP, Barberà JA, Visa J, Rimola A, Pare JC, Roca J, Navasa M, Rodes J, Rodriguez-Roisin R. Hepatopulmonary syndrome in candidates for liver transplantation. J Hepatol 2001; 34:651–657.
19. Hansen JE, Clausen JL, Levy SE, Mohler JG, Van Kessel AL. Proficiency testing materials for pH and blood gases. The California Thoracic Society experience. Chest 1986; 89:214–217.
20. Brimioulle S, Kahn RJ. Effects of metabolic alkalosis on pulmonary gas exchange. Am Rev Respir Dis 1990; 141:1185–1189.
21. Brimioulle S, Vachiery JL, Lejeune P, Leeman M, Melot C, Naeije R. Acid-base status affects gas exchange in canine oleic acid pulmonary edema. Am J Physiol 1991; 260:H1080–H1086.
22. Curtis JR, Hudson LD. Emergent assessment and management of acute respiratory failure in COPD. Clin Chest Med 1994; 15:481–500.
23. Barberà JA, Roca J, Ferrer A, Felez MA, Diaz O, Roger N, Rodriguez-Roisin R. Mechanisms of worsening gas exchange during acute exacerbations of chronic obstructive pulmonary disease. Eur Respir J 1997; 10:1285–1291.
24. Amoroso P, Wilson SR, Moxham J, Ponte J. Acute effects of inhaled salbutamol on the metabolic rate of normal subjects. Thorax 1993; 48:882–885.
25. Díaz O, Iglesia R, Ferrer M, Zavala E, Santos C, Wagner PD, Roca J, Rodriguez-Roisin R. Effects of noninvasive ventilation on pulmonary gas exchange and hemodynamics during acute hypercapnic exacerbations of chronic obstructive pulmonary disease. Am J Respir Crit Care Med 1997; 156:1840–1845.
26. Barberà JA, Reyes A, Roca J, Montserrat JM, Wagner PD, Rodriguez-Roisin R. Effect of intravenously administered aminophylline on ventilation/perfusion inequality during recovery from exacerbations of chronic obstructive pulmonary disease. Am Rev Respir Dis 1992; 145:1328–1333.
27. Robinson TD, Freiberg DB, Regnis JA, Young IH. The role of hypoventilation and ventilation-perfusion redistribution in oxygen-induced hypercapnia during acute exacerbations of chronic obstructive pulmonary disease. Am J Respir Crit Care Med 2000; 161:1524–1529.
28. Roca J, Ramis L, Rodriguez-Roisin R, Ballester E, Montserrat JM, Wagner PD. Serial relationships between ventilation-perfusion inequality and spirometry in acute severe asthma requiring hospitalization. Am Rev Respir Dis 1988; 137:1055–1061.
29. Torres A, Reyes A, Roca J, Wagner PD, Rodriguez-Roisin R. Ventilation-perfusion mismatching in chronic obstructive pulmonary disease during ventilator weaning. Am Rev Respir Dis 1989; 140:1246–1250.
30. Castaing Y, Manier G, Guenard H. Improvement in ventilation–perfusion relationships by almitrine in patients with chronic obstructive pulmonary disease during mechanical ventilation. Am Rev Respir Dis 1986; 134:910–916.
31. Rossi A, Santos C, Roca J, Torres A, Félez MA, Rodriguez-Roisin R. Effects of PEEP on VA/Q mismatching in ventilated patients with chronic airflow obstruction. Am J Respir Crit Care Med 1994; 149:1077–1084.

32. Lemaire F, Teboul JL, Cinotti L, Giotto G, Abrouk F, Steg G, Macquin-Mavier I, Zapol WM. Acute left ventricular dysfunction during unsuccessful weaning from mechanical ventilation. Anesthesiology 1988; 69:171–179.
33. Beydon L, Cinotti L, Rekik N, Radermacher P, Adnot S, Meignan M, Harf A, Lemaire F. Changes in the distribution of ventilation and perfusion associated with separation from mechanical ventilation in patients with obstructive pulmonary disease. Anesthesiology 1991; 75:730–738.
34. Santos C, Ferrer M, Roca J, Torres A, Hernandez C, Rodriguez-Roisin R. Pulmonary gas exchange response to oxygen breathing in acute lung injury. Am J Respir Crit Care Med 2000; 161:26–31.
35. Dantzker DR, Wagner PD, West JB. Proceedings: instability of poorly ventilated lung units during oxygen breathing. J Physiol 1974; 242:72P.
36. Astin TW. The relationships between arterial blood oxygen saturation, carbon dioxide tension, and pH and airway resistance during 30% oxygen breathing in patients with chronic bronchitis with airway obstruction. Am Rev Respir Dis 1970; 102:382–387.
37. Aubier M, Murciano D, Milic-Emili J, Touaty E, Daghfous J, Pariente R, Derenne JP. Effects of the administration of O_2 on ventilation and blood gases in patients with chronic obstructive pulmonary disease during acute respiratory failure. Am Rev Respir Dis 1980; 122:747–754.
38. Stradling J. Effects of the administration of O_2 on ventilation and blood gases in patients with chronic obstructive pulmonary disease during acute respiratory failure. Am Rev Respir Dis 1987; 135:274.
39. Hanson CW, III, Marshall BE, Frasch HF, Marshall C. Causes of hypercarbia with oxygen therapy in patients with chronic obstructive pulmonary disease. Crit Care Med 1996; 24:23–28.
40. Standards for the diagnosis and care of patients with chronic obstructive pulmonary disease. American Thoracic Society. Am J Respir Crit Care Med 1995; 152:S77–S121.
41. BTS guidelines for the management of chronic obstructive pulmonary disease. The COPD Guidelines Group of the Standards of Care Committee of the BTS. Thorax 1997; 52 (suppl 5):S1–S28.
42. Siafakas NM, Vermeire P, Pride NB, Paoletti P, Gibson J, Howard P, Yernault JC, Decramer M, Higenbottam T, Postma DS. Optimal assessment and management of chronic obstructive pulmonary disease (COPD). The European Respiratory Society Task Force. Eur Respir J 1995; 8:1398–1420.
43. Barberà JA, Peces-Barba G, Agusti AGN, Izquierdo JL, Monsó E, Montemayor T, Viejo JL. Guía Clínica para el diagnóstico y el tratamiento de la enfermedad pulmonar obstructiva crónica. Arch Bronconeumol 2001; 37:297–316.
44. Pauwels RA, Buist AS, Calverley PM, Jenkins CR, Hurd SS. Global strategy for the diagnosis, management, and prevention of chronic obstructive pulmonary disease. NHLBI/WHO Global Initiative for Chronic Obstructive Lung Disease (GOLD) Workshop summary. Am J Respir Crit Care Med 2001; 163:1256–1276.
45. Karpel JP, Pesin J, Greenberg D, Gentry E. A comparison of the effects of ipratropium bromide and metaproterenol sulfate in acute exacerbations of COPD. Chest 1990; 98:835–839.
46. Ringsted CV, Eliasen K, Andersen JB, Heslet L, Qvist J. Ventilation-perfusion distributions and central hemodynamics in chronic obstructive pulmonary disease. Effects of terbutaline administration. Chest 1989; 96:976–983.
47. Barbera JA, Riverola A, Roca J, Ramirez J, Wagner PD, Ros D, Wiggs BR, Rodriguez-Roisin R. Pulmonary vascular abnormalities and ventilation-perfusion relationships

in mild chronic obstructive pulmonary disease. Am J Respir Crit Care Med 1994; 149:423–429.

48. Khoukaz G, Gross NJ. Effects of salmeterol on arterial blood gases in patients with stable chronic obstructive pulmonary disease. Comparison with albuterol and ipratropium. Am J Respir Crit Care Med 1999; 160:1028–1030.

49. Viegas CA, Ferrer A, Montserrat JM, Barbera JA, Roca J, Rodriguez-Roisin R. Ventilation-perfusion response after fenoterol in hypoxemic patients with stable COPD. Chest 1996; 110:71–77 (Erratum 1997; 111:258).

50. Ballester E, Reyes A, Roca J, Guitart R, Wagner PD, Rodriguez-Roisin R. Ventilation-perfusion mismatching in acute severe asthma: effects of salbutamol and 100% oxygen. Thorax 1989; 44:258–267.

51. Wong CS, Pavord ID, Williams J, Britton JR, Tattersfield AE. Bronchodilator, cardiovascular, and hypokalaemic effects of fenoterol, salbutamol, and terbutaline in asthma. Lancet 1990; 336:1396–1399.

52. Blanch L, Joseph D, Fernandez R, Mas A, Martinez M, Valles J, Diaz E, Baigorri F, Artigas A. Hemodynamic and gas exchange responses to inhalation of nitric oxide in patients with the acute respiratory distress syndrome and in hypoxemic patients with chronic obstructive pulmonary disease. Intensive Care Med 1997; 23:51–57.

53. Hopkins SR, Johnson EC, Richardson RS, Wagner H, De Rosa M, Wagner PD. Effects of inhaled nitric oxide on gas exchange in lungs with shunt or poorly ventilated areas. Am J Respir Crit Care Med 1997; 156:484–491.

54. Rennotte MT, Reynaert M, Clerbaux T, Willems E, Roeseleer J, Veriter C, Rodenstein D, Frans A. Effects of two inotropic drugs, dopamine and dobutamine, on pulmonary gas exchange in artificially ventilated patients. Intensive Care Med 1989; 15:160–165.

55. Guénard H, Castaing Y, Melot C, Naeije R. Gas exchange during acute respiratory failure in patients with chronic obstructive pulmonary disease. In: Derenne JP, Whitelaw WA, Similowski X, eds. Acute Respiratory Failure in Chronic Obstructive Pulmonary Disease. New York: Marcel Dekker, 1996:227–266.

56. Andrivet P, Chabrier PE, Defouilloy C, Brun-Buisson C, Adnot S. Intravenously administered atrial natriuretic factor in patients with COPD. Effects on ventilation-perfusion relationships and pulmonary hemodynamics. Chest 1994; 106:118–124.

57. Adnot S, Kouyoumdjian C, Defouilloy C, Andrivet P, Sediame S, Herigault R, Fratacci MD. Hemodynamic and gas exchange responses to infusion of acetylcholine and inhalation of nitric oxide in patients with chronic obstructive lung disease and pulmonary hypertension. Am Rev Respir Dis 1993; 148:310–316.

58. Castaing Y, Manier G, Varene N, Guenard H. [Effects of oral almitrine on the distribution of $\dot{V}_A/\dot{Q}$ ratio in chronic obstructive lung diseases (author's transl)]. Bull Eur Physiopathol Respir 1981; 17:917–932.

59. Melot C, Naeije R, Rothschild T, Mertens P, Mols P, Hallemans R. Improvement in ventilation-perfusion matching by almitrine in COPD. Chest 1983; 83:528–533.

60. Rossaint R, Falke KJ, Lopez F, Slama K, Pison U, Zapol WM. Inhaled nitric oxide for the adult respiratory distress syndrome. N Engl J Med 1993; 328:399–405.

61. Reyes A, Roca J, Rodriguez-Roisin R, Torres A, Ussetti P, Wagner PD. Effect of almitrine on ventilation-perfusion distribution in adult respiratory distress syndrome. Am Rev Respir Dis 1988; 137:1062–1067.

12

Radiology of Acute Exacerbations of Chronic Obstructive Pulmonary Disease

KATERINA MALAGARI

University of Athens
Athens, Greece

ARGYRO VOLOUDAKI

University Hospital of Heraklion
Heraklion, Crete, Greece

I. Introduction

A. Radiology in COPD: An Overview

Chronic obstructive pulmonary disease (COPD) is defined physiologically as a disorder characterized by a slowly progressive airflow obstruction, only partially reversible (1–3). Cigarette smoking is by far the main risk factor for COPD but genetic, environmental, and occupational risk factors also contribute. Most of the airflow limitation is due to varying combinations of emphysema and chronic bronchitis. The airway component consists mainly of decreased luminal diameters of the larger airways due to increased wall thickening and mucus gland hyperplasia as well as small airways inflammation, edema, fibrosis, and obliteration (4–8).

The severity of an acute exacerbation of COPD is strongly related to the severity of the underlying COPD (1,9). It is therefore mandatory to know what is expected from radiology in this context.

Imaging methods assess primarily morphological changes in the lung caused by COPD. Radiographic features of hyperinflation are the most reliable signs of emphysema, although chest radiography is insensitive for the detection of mild and moderate emphysema (10–16). On the contrary, CT, particularly high-resolution computed tomography (HRCT) and minimum intensity projection technique (MINIP) are the most accurate means of detecting emphysema in vivo (17–19).

CT-based grading and quantification of the severity and extent of emphysema either by subjective visual or objective methods using standard CT software have shown good correlation with pathology scores and pulmonary function tests (20–25). Recently, hyperpolarized noble gases have opened the way to functional imaging of pulmonary ventilation in emphysema using magnetic resonance imaging (MRI) techniques (26–29).

The majority of patients with *chronic bronchitis* have a normal chest radiograph. The most frequently reported radiographic features of chronic bronchitis—bronchial wall thickening and increased lung markings known as "dirty lung"—are quite subjective and not fully elucidated by HRCT (30). However, HRCT studies have shown bronchial wall thickening in 33% of smokers compared to 16% of ex-smokers and 18% of control subjects (31). CT measurements of both airway wall thickening and emphysema correlate with measurements of lung function (32).

B. Acute Exacerbation of COPD: Introductory Notes

A relative clinical stability is frequently interrupted by recurrent acute exacerbation of COPD (AECOPD), defined as sustained worsening of the patient's condition, from the stable state and beyond normal day-to-day variations, which is acute in onset and necessitates a change in regular medication (9,33). It may also be considered as an episode of worsening dyspnea and increased sputum purulence and production, the latter definition being more indicative of an infectious etiology (4). Slight differences of definitions of AECOPD as stated by several authors arise from the heterogeneous nature of etiology and pathophysiology, comorbid conditions and variable degree of severity of underlying COPD (1,2,33–35).

Conditions that may be confused with AECOPD include infection of tracheobronchial tree, pneumonia, air pollution, pneumothorax, pneumomediastinum, right or left heart failure, pulmonary artery hypertension, pulmonary embolism, and fatigue of the respiratory muscles. Most of them are now considered triggering factors or comorbidities that may provoke an exacerbation (1–4,9,34). However, there is an established causal association with bacterial and viral infections in approximately 50 to 70% and 20 to 30% of COPD exacerbations, respectively. Besides infectious association, response to steroids may imply other mechanisms as well (4,9).

This variety of infectious and noninfectious insult results in functional deterioration. However, these functional changes, despite their impact on gas exchange, produce no radiologically detectable findings. Therefore, the role of imaging in AECOPD reflected in the structure of this chapter is to (1) identify changes from previous imaging findings and address specific, potentially treatable, causes of symptoms; (2) assist in monitoring patients under noninvasive intermittent positive pressure ventilation (NIPPV) or mechanical ventilation; (3) provide early evidence-based recognition of complications; and (4) monitor comorbidities.

II. Imaging Modalities

A. Chest Radiography

Chest radiographs (posteroanterior and lateral) are seldom diagnostic in AECOPD but they are useful in identifying alternative diagnoses that can mimic the symptoms of an exacerbation. There are no dedicated studies reporting the performance of CXR in the diagnosis of AECOPD. However, chest radiography is established as an initial tool for the detection of conditions that mimic, provoke, or complicate AECOPD and its specific role in the diagnosis of each one of them is described in the following paragraphs.

In AECOPD, imaging patterns are distorted by the underlying emphysematous or chronic bronchitis changes. In patients with severe AECOPD admitted in the ICU, sequential film comparison may be of value (Fig. 1). Additional difficulties in film interpretation are associated with the considerable intra- and interobserver variation in relation to radiographic signs; the higher variation is observed in vascular signs compared to signs of hyperinflation. Moreover, heart failure and edema may result in a more rounded and elevated diaphragm as lung compliance falls. Provided that there is consistency of film technique, comparisons provide suggestive information for the diagnosis. Digital radiography allows consistency of images over a wide range of actual exposure factors (36,37) and may be at advantage for the radiographic recognition of AECOPD.

For practical purposes, it should be kept in mind that most studies report overall accuracy of CXR in the diagnosis of emphysema at 65 to 80% depending on sample size and selection criteria. However, although severe disease is diagnosed in more than 90%, miss rates for mild disease are well above 50% (38). To the contrary, specificity is good, especially for moderate or advanced disease with less than 5% false-positive diagnoses.

B. Computed Tomography

In contrast to the chest radiograph, computed tomography (CT) has proved very sensitive and specific in assessing emphysema (Fig. 1C) and recognizing alternative causes of AECOPD symptoms. Besides the patterns of the underlying COPD changes, CT can identify local consolidations, detect early pneumothorax or pneumomediastinum, small pleural effusions, pulmonary embolism, pleural effusions, and assess air-trapping bullae that compress adjacent lung parenchyma (39–41).

HRCT methods for the quantification of COPD described in the introduction of this chapter at the moment have no applications in AECOPD since there is substantial evidence that overestimation and moderate interobserver agreement may compromise subjective visual grading techniques while the more objective computer-aided methods need more improvement (23,25).

C. Magnetic Resonance Imaging

Magnetic resonance imaging (MRI) is not in clinical use in AECOPD.

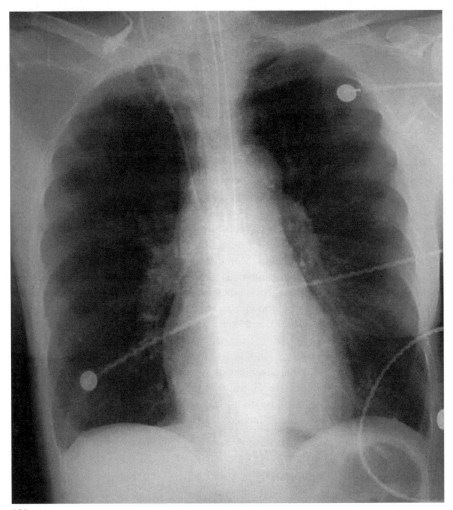

(A)

Figure 1   AECOPD. Sequential chest radiographs reveal impairment of overinflation in
(B) compared to (A) that was obtained a month earlier. HRCT (C) reveals no specific cause
for the exacerbation. Note the emphysematous parenchymal destruction with thin-wall
bullae, and bronchial wall thickening at the periphery, compatible with the coexisting
chronic bronchitis.

III.   Imaging Pathological Conditions Provoking, Precipitating, or Mimicking AECOPD

A.   Pneumonia

COPD related to lifetime smoking history has proved to be a major risk factor for
community-acquired pneumonia diagnosed either by general practitioners in the
community or upon hospital admission (42,43).

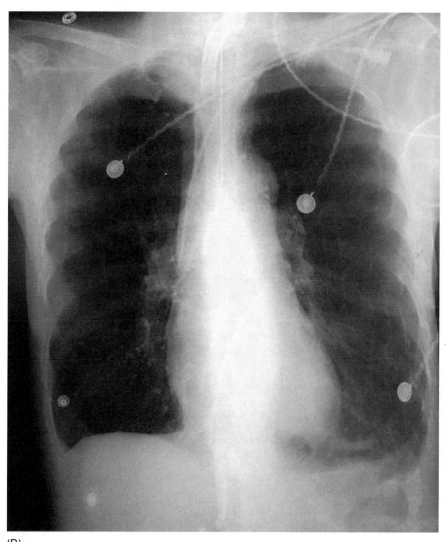

(B)

Figure 1 (*continued*)

Imaging has an important role in patients with suspected pulmonary infection. The chest radiograph is the method of choice for the detection of pneumonia and for the assessment of its location, extent, and complications such as abscess formation, pleural effusion, and empyema, as well as response to treatment. Review of previous radiographs, repeat chest radiographs, and different views may be helpful especially if other abnormalities such as pulmonary embolism, cardiogenic edema, or neoplasm coexist, as the progression and time course of various etiologies can be quite different (44).

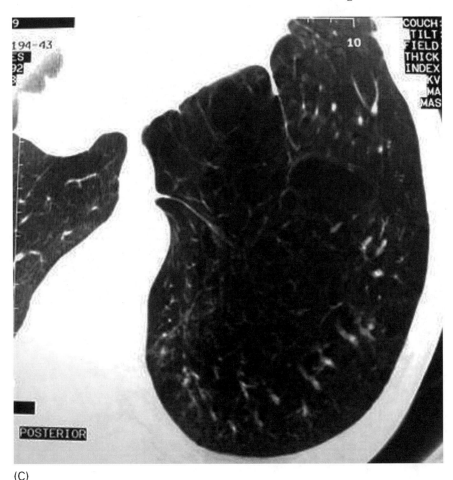

Figure 1 (*continued*)

CT is reserved for select cases showing radiographically complex images, suspicion of abscess, or loculated pleural fluid. An incidentally found carcinoma is not an unexpected finding. A 5% rate of stage I primary lung cancer was found incidentally on chest CT of patients selected for lung volume reduction surgery (45) and a 2% rate of unsuspected malignancy was diagnosed in patients undergoing HRCT 2 months after an episode of AECOPD (46).

Morphological patterns based on the chest radiographic appearances, bronchopneumonia, lobar pneumonia, and interstitial pneumonia are still widely used (47,48). In bronchopneumonia, which is the most common pattern, imaging findings consist of a nodular pattern, patchy consolidation, volume loss, and absence of air bronchograms. In lobar pneumonia, often homogeneous consolidation is bounded by fissures, with or without air bronchograms. It is the most common manifestation of community-acquired pneumonia. Finally, interstitial pneumonia corresponds to a radiographic pattern comprising extensive peribronchial thickening and reticulonodular shadowing. The most common causes are viral and *Mycoplasma pneumoniae* infections. Although the pattern depends to some extent on the causal agent, radiography—and to a lesser degree CT—are usually poor at predicting the specific infective organism because the same organism may produce several patterns and different patterns often overlap in the same patient (49,50). HRCT is superior to radiography in revealing acute infectious bronchiolitis, most often caused by mycoplasma, viral, and *Haemophilus influenzae* infection (51). The tree-in-bud sign corresponds to bronchiolar dilatation and filling by mucus, pus, or fluid, resulting in a pattern of centrilobular nodular, branching, or Y-shaped densities, usually visible in the lung periphery (52–54).

The awareness of unusual appearance of pneumonia in patients with emphysema is of great importance. If the emphysema is mild, the well-known patterns of air-space consolidation with or without air bronchograms may be expected. In the presence of severe emphysema, the radiographic appearance is atypical, ranging from inhomogeneous consolidation to a coarse reticular pattern mimicking interstitial edema or honeycombing, even for organisms that typically cause dense consolidation (Fig. 2) (50,55–57). Multiple radiolucencies resembling abscesses may be seen representing aerated emphysematous spaces outlined against the opacity of adjacent pulmonary consolidation rather than true areas of lung necrosis. In a series, 17 of 38 patients over the age of 40 demonstrated this atypical pattern (58). Comparison with previous radiographs or CT may be helpful in questionable cases.

B. Congestive Heart Failure, Pulmonary Hypertension, and Cor Pulmonale

Over 40% of patients with COPD may present comorbid conditions (59). Cardiovascular events such as congestive heart failure, pulmonary hypertension, and right heart failure are most frequent in this population and may provoke, precipitate, or mimic an exacerbation (1,2,60), contributing to the mortality associated with AECOPD. Cigarette smoking, raised plasma fibrinogen levels, elevation of pulmonary vascular resistance probably due to a combination of destruction of the capillary bed, hypecapnia, acidemia, erythrocytosis, hypervolemia, and reflex vasoconstriction due to hypoxia are all factors leading to increased cardiovascular risk in COPD (15,35,61,62).

It is important to be aware of the unusual appearances of congestive heart failure and pulmonary edema in COPD patients, especially those with emphysema. The accumulation of fluid in the airspaces and in the interstitial compartment reduces the radiability of emphysematous lung and decreases pulmonary compliance (63). Thus, the diaphragm tends to become more rounded and elevated since it cannot be driven to its usual low level by the less compliant lung. Comparison with previous films may give the wrong impression of improvement of hyperinflation rather than diagnosing that cardiac failure has supervened (47). Obliteration of the

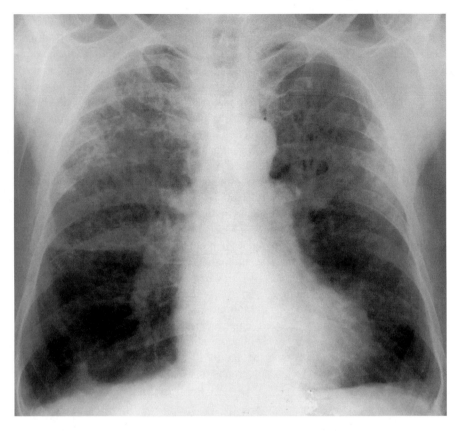

Figure 2   Pneumonia involving both upper lobes due to *Hemophilus influenzae* in an emphysematous patient, shows an interstitial pattern rather than the expected dense consolidation.

pulmonary vascular bed and redistribution of blood flow in the presence of pulmonary venous hypertension and pulmonary edema may produce bizarre radiographic patterns (Fig. 3) due to the nonuniform character of the capillary bed destruction of emphysematous lung which causes a "patchy" distribution of pulmonary edema (Fig. 4) (64).

Pulmonary arterial hypertension leading to right heart failure known as "cor pulmonale" is a recognized complication of emphysema and chronic bronchitis especially in hypoxic patients at the end of the spectrum (1,15,65). Although imaging methods cannot measure the pulmonary arterial pressure, they can depict the morphological changes due to pulmonary hypertension, which are right ventricular hypertrophy and dilatation of right ventricle, right atrium, vena cava, coronary sinus, and enlargement of the main and central pulmonary arteries with rapid tapering as they proceed distally (66). The distal vessels may be large, normal, or reduced in caliber but there is always a disparity in the relative size of the central

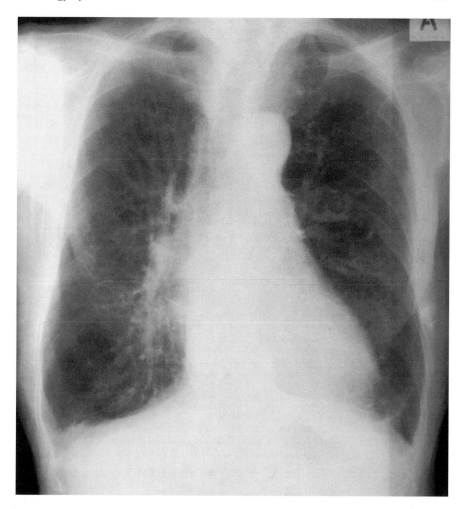

Figure 3 Pulmonary edema in a patient with emphysema, shows rather unilateral distribution evident on the right. Emphysematous left lung shows impressively less vascular engorgement probably due to variable degree of destruction of the capillary bed.

and peripheral vessels. The most widely used measurement of pulmonary artery on chest radiograph is that of the right descending pulmonary artery (67). Measurement of the transverse diameter at the midpoint of the right descending artery equal to 17 mm or greater is strongly indicative of dilatation. An increase in caliber, presuming to reflect worsening of pulmonary hypertension, is the only radiographic correlate of AECOPD. Radiographic changes are quite specific, but they are neither sensitive nor well correlated with the severity of the hypertension (15).

 CT provides more precise measurements of pulmonary arteries (68,69). A CT-determined main pulmonary artery diameter greater than 2.9 cm, measured at its

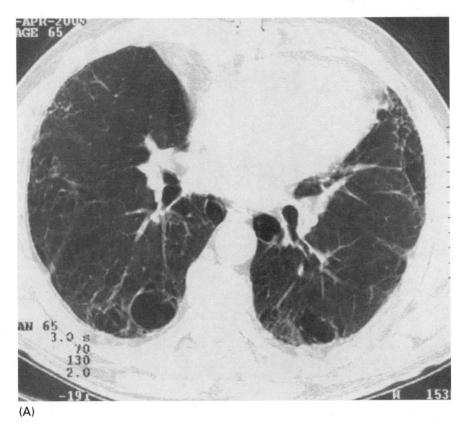

(A)

Figure 4 (A) HRCT shows emphysematous parenchymal changes and subpleural cysts bilaterally. (B) CT obtained 2 years later at the same level as (A) depicts pulmonary edema sparing emphysematous areas resulting in inhomogeneous lung involvement.

widest portion, has a positive predictive value of 0.97 for predicting pulmonary arterial hypertension in patients with parenchymal lung disease (70). A simple, practical rule based on the ratio of the diameter of the main pulmonary artery to the diameter of the aorta has been reported. If this ratio is greater than 1, pulmonary hypertension is likely, with a positive predictive value of 96%. However, a negative predictive value of 52% is low, and a nondilated main pulmonary artery in relation to the aorta does not exclude pulmonary arterial hypertension (71). Interestingly, pericardial thickening or effusion is a frequent CT finding in patients with severe pulmonary hypertension, although the pathophysiological mechanism is unclear (72).

Right ventricular volume, mass, and ejection fraction can be calculated quantitatively by MRI (73). Reasonable correlations have been found between pulmonary artery pressure estimated with right-sided heart catheterization and

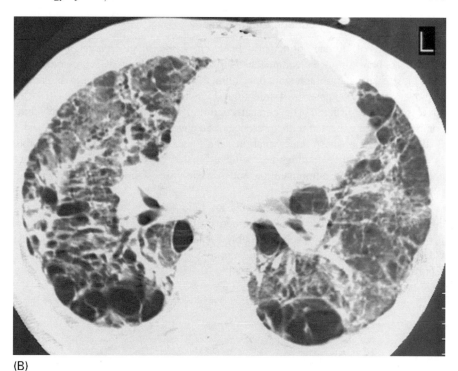

(B)

Figure 4 (*continued*)

MRI measures of pulmonary artery diameter, flow characteristics, and other variables based on several MR techniques (74–76). The ratio of the caliber of the main pulmonary artery to the mid-descending aorta using MR imaging is significantly higher in patients with pulmonary arterial hypertension (77). Velocity-encoded MR imaging demonstrates an inhomogeneous flow profile in the main pulmonary artery in cases with pulmonary hypertension (78), and can provide accurate pulmonary arterial blood-flow measurements (75).

The severity of pulmonary hypertension can be accurately assessed with pulsed Doppler echocardiography from the subxiphoid region, using a general purpose ultrasound device. This technique is considered a simple and reliable adjunct to the noninvasive evaluation of COPD and represents a satisfactory alternative to the classic parasternal approach preferred by cardiologists but often not suitable for emphysematous patients (78,79).

With the onset of heart failure, the heart and hilar and intermediate lung vessels become enlarged. Enlargement of vessels is present in all zones and affects particularly segmental vessels and a few divisions beyond giving the appearance of plethora (15,47,48,65).

C. Complicated Bullous Emphysema

Complications of bullae, principally *infection, hemorrhage, pneumothorax, and atelectasis*, may mimic or complicate AECOPD. Thickening of a previously thin wall on a plain radiograph and development of air–fluid levels into bullae are findings strongly suggestive of infection (Fig. 5). Differential diagnosis from an abscess may be difficult. The clinical condition of the patient is relatively mild compared to that expected in the presence of an abscess, the wall of the cystic lesion is thinner with a sharp inner margin, and there is less adjacent pneumonitis (48,80,81). The above findings are better estimated on CT. Therapeutic approach consists of antibiotic administration and occasionally of infected bullae drainage (81,82).

Hemorrhage into a bulla, seen as air–fluid level, is a much less common complication, which may be accompanied by hemoptysis. Following infection or hemorrhage, bullae often resolve probably because of collapse and scarring (15,83), although spontaneous regression of multiple emphysematous bullae has been reported (83).

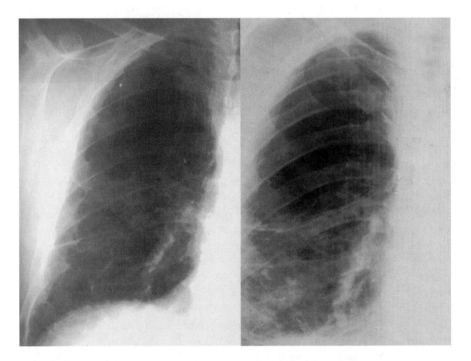

Figure 5   Chest radiographs of a COPD patient focused on the right lung, obtained with a time interval of 1 month. In the left image, emphysematous changes are obvious, especially at the upper lung zone where a translucent area with reduced vasculature is compatible with the presence of a bulla. In the right image, during an AECOPD event, thickening of the bulla wall and increased interstitial markings are suggestive of infection.

The presence of pneumothorax may be quite difficult to diagnose especially in cases of idiopathic giant bullous disease, an entity known as vanishing lung syndrome, involving predominantly the upper lobes (84). The diagnosis of giant bullous emphysema is made if the chest radiograph shows one or more bullae occuping at least one-third of a hemithorax and compressing surrounding lung parenchyma (85). Radiological distinction from pneumothorax may be difficult even with CT, which is advantageous over plain radiograph (Fig. 6) (86–90). In the study

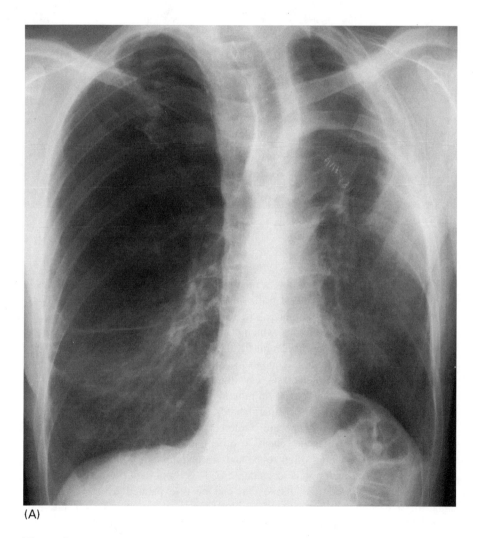

(A)

Figure 6 (A) Chest x-ray, in a patient with a left upper lobe bullectomy 5 years ago with rapid deterioration shows an avascular area displacing mediastinum and lung tissue, suggesting a possible pneumothorax. (B) CT reveals remnants of lung tissue pointing to expansion of a bulla rather than pneumothorax.

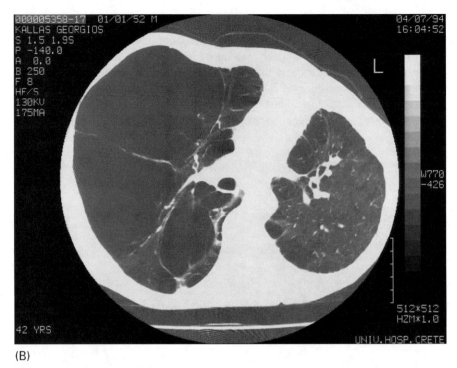

(B)

Figure 6   (*continued*)

of Waitches et al. (91), "the double wall sign," defined as air outlining both sides of the bulla wall parallel to the chest wall, was seen in all patients with pneumothorax and was absent in those without. Absence of this CT sign provides increased confidence against pneumothorax, which can prevent unnecessary chest tube placement and avoidance of bronchopleural fistula.

Bullae may become large enough to cause compression of the adjacent lung parenchyma, resulting in atelectasis, causing further impairment of lung function. Atelectatic lung may mimic a mass on radiological studies. The diagnosis should be suspected when central, sharply marginated, masslike opacities that are oblong, lenticular, or triangular in shape are bordered by severe bullous emphysema. CT often reveals subsegmental atelectasis in other lobes adjacent to the bullous lung (84,92,93). Atelectatic lung often re-expands in patients who undergo resection of bullous lung. If bullectomy is considered, CT is important in determining the presence of compressed lung tissue that can be re-expanded by removal of the bulla, in assessing the severity of emphysema in the remainder of the lung parenchyma, and may assist the surgeon in operative planning (94–96).

D. Pleural Effusion

Pleural fluid collections may mimic AECOPD and are readily recognized by imaging. The distribution of fluid within the pleural space depends primarily on gravity, elastic recoil of the lung, and the presence of pleural adhesions. In COPD patients, elastic recoil is definitely altered while the presence of pleural thickening from previous infections or pneumothorax increase the likelihood of loculation (97). For these reasons, atypical distribution of pleural fluid is not uncommon in COPD, and differential diagnosis from non–pleural effusion associated AECOPD may be difficult.

In posteroanterior (PA) and lateral chest radiographs obtained at TLC, pleural effusion is recognized if it is at least 175 mL in volume. However, fluid volume greater than 200 mL is usually necessary to cause posterior sulcus blunting. Lateral decubitus radiographs are considerably more sensitive in the detection of pleural effusions but are difficult to obtain for technical reasons. In AECOPD, blunting of the lateral or posterior sulcus may be difficult to differentiate from the wide costophrenic sulcus due to diaphragmatic flattening; film comparisons may be particularly useful (98). In the COPD setting, and given the flattening of the diaphragm, subpulmonic localization of fluid is recognized as "diaphragmatic elevation." Should this occur to the left, recognition is facilitated by the increase of the distance of the diaphragm apex to the fundus of the stomach, normally not exceeding 2 cm.

In the supine position, the most dependent pleural spaces are the posterobasal and the apices in which free fluid accumulates. This results in a posterior layering of pleural fluid that produces a homogeneous increase of density of the affected hemithorax without obscuration of the bronchovascular markings depending on the amount of the accumulation. However, the density of the opacity may be missed because of its uniformity; even moderately large effusions may go unde-tected, particularly if they are bilateral. Overall, supine chest radiographs have low diagnostic accuracy (<67%) in the detection of pleural effusion (47,99,100).

Ultrasonograply and computed tomography (CT), are more sensitive in the detection of small or loculated effusions and the distinction of effusions from pleural thickening. Ultrasonography has become a particularly useful tool available at bedside, for confirmation of pleural fluid, early recognition of internal septa, compartmentalization and image-guided aspiration. Prior to aspiration, ultrasono-graphy allows precise location and quantification of the amount of fluid within a pleural pocket.

CT is particularly useful in the presence of pleuroparenchymal disease; CT attenuation values between those of water (0 HU) and soft tissue (approximately 100 HU) are obtained in pleural effusions and allow differential diagnosis (97). Although measurement of the attenuation of pleural fluid per se is of limited value in differentiating transudates, exudates, and chylous effusions, with the occasional exception of hemothorax that is characterized by increased density, contrast enhancement may be of value to this end (101,102). Exudates are frequently associated with pleural enhancement and increased thickness of the extrapleural tissues that normally measure ≤ 2 mm (101). Moreover, contrast enhancement is necessary in the AECOPD patient for accurate assessment of complicated pleuro-parenchymal disease and for early detection of development of pleural thickening or pleural masses (101,103,104). Passive atelectasis of the lower lobe associated with pleural effusion has to be differentiated from true parenchymal consolidation.

Magnetic resonance imaging (MRI) is difficult to perform in the AECOPD setting since the respiratory gating motion artifacts cannot be eliminated in dyspneic patients and is only reserved for the evaluation of pleural masses.

E. Pulmonary Embolism

Pulmonary embolism (PE) may complicate or mimic AECOPD. Although there are no dedicated studies on the frequency of PE in COPD population or during AECOPD, COPD patient groups have been included in large studies designed for imaging evaluation of PE; in the PIOPED study, the incidence of PE reached 19% in COPD patients, while postmortem data indicate high prevalence ranging from 28 to 51% (105–107).

To safely establish or refute the diagnosis of PE in the COPD setting, objective diagnostic examinations are mandatory. The role of imaging in differential diagnosis of PE from a non-PE-related AECOPD is increased since pretest probability evaluation is hampered by the fact that clinical and ECG findings may be altered by the underlying disease and particularly right heart strain. For the general population, the examinations established for the diagnosis of PE include ventilation-perfusion (V-P) lung scanning, pulmonary angiography, spiral and electron-beam computed tomography (CT), and, perhaps in the near future, magnetic resonance (MR) angiography (108–112).

Since chest radiography has a low sensitivity and specificity (0.33 and 0.59, respectively) its principal role is to exclude other diagnoses that might mimic pulmonary embolism (pneumothorax, pneumonia, pleural effusion, rib fractures), and to assist in the interpretation of V-P scintigraphy.

The classic signs of pulmonary embolism without infarction on chest radiographs, notably oligemia of the lung beyond the occluded vessel (Westermark's sign), increase in the size of the main pulmonary artery, and elevation of a hemidiaphragm, are not recognized in the COPD patient since emphysema causes similar pulmonary vascular changes, and the position of the diaphragm is low from overinflation (113). Pulmonary infarction results in radiographically detectable consolidation assuming atypical shapes in severe emphysema. Cavitation within the infarct is rare. However, aseptic cavitation may occur in large infarcts (>4 cm). Pleural effusions (small and unilateral) may reach an incidence of 50% and may be the only manifestation of PE.

V-P scintigraphy in the AECOPD setting is difficult to perform, and less than 10% fall in the clear-cut categories of normal or high probability. Thus, the diagnosis of PE can only be resolved definitively by proceeding to spiral CT and/or angiography (108,111,112).

Spiral computed tomographic pulmonary angiography (herein referred to as spiral CT) has become an important imaging tool for the detection of PE. It is a rapid examination, safe for critically ill patients. Technical improvements in spiral CT (thinner sections, shorter scanning times, higher pitch, multiple detectors, and workstation viewing) have improved the diagnostic accuracy in the evaluation of PE. Moreover, reduced scanning time allows short breath-holds that COPD patients are able to perform, and markedly improves the visibility of the smaller arteries.

Signs of acute pulmonary embolism on spiral CT include central or eccentric filling defects producing a "railway track" sign in in-plane artery sections (Figs. 7, 8). Ancillary signs include pleural effusions or infarcts. On CT, the pleural-based location and wedge shape of infarcts are seen at better advantage (114).

Several recent studies have shown that contrast-enhanced spiral CT has sensitivity 90 to 92% and specificity 86 to 96% in the diagnosis of PE involving large or segmental vessels (Figs. 7–9). These levels of diagnostic accuracy surpass those of ventilation-perfusion (V-P) scintigraphy in the general population (72% sensitivity and 94% specificity) and certainly those in the COPD subgroups, since they also apply for the intermediate category scintigraphy results (115,116).

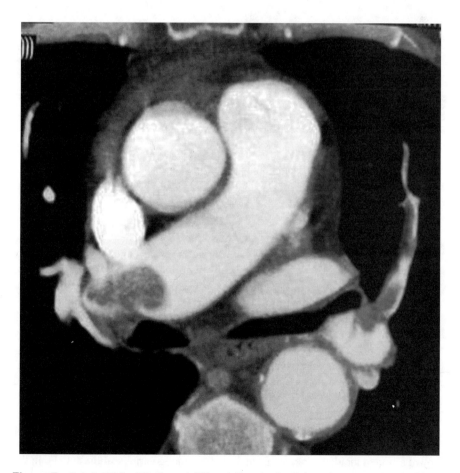

Figure 7 Spiral CT for PE. Central filling defects in the right pulmonary artery and in the left lingular branch imaged in-plane producing the railway track sign.

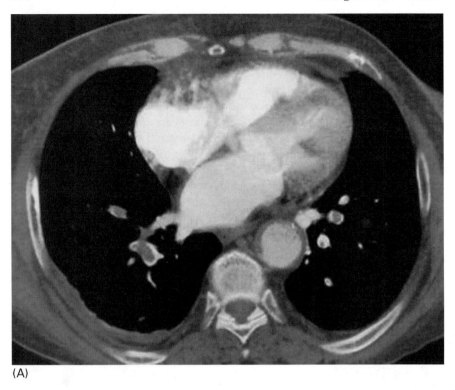

(A)

Figure 8 Spiral CT for PE. Central filling defects in segmental vessels seen in (A) axial plane and (B) longitudinally in reconstructed images. Small pleural effusions are noted bilaterally.

Reported negative predictive value of spiral CT for PE is 0.99, similar to the clinical predictive value of a negative scintigram (1.0) and a low-probability scintigram (0.97) (117). Garg et al. recently reported similar negative predictive values in patients with negative spiral CT scans (118). However, it has to be pointed out that in none of the large studies examining the accuracy of spiral CT in the diagnosis of PE a large number of COPD or AECOPD patients has been included, and therefore specially designed, controlled, prospective studies are necessary (119,120).

Spiral CT examination for PE may also provide important additional diagnostic information and may depict other conditions that have similar physiological sequelae with AECOPD such as pneumonia, atelectasis, pleural effusion, or pneumothorax, excluding at the same time PE (120).

Especially troubling is the limitation of spiral CT to reliably depict isolated small emboli. The incidence of this situation within patients with PE is not exactly known; reported incidence ranges from 6 to 30% among various studies (121). In the Prospective Investigation of Pulmonary Embolism Diagnosis (PIOPED) study, 17% of patients with low-probability scintigrams had clots limited to the subsegmental

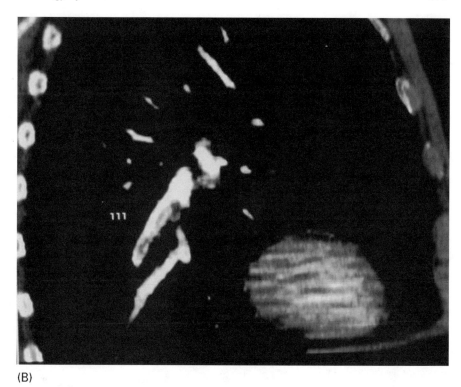

(B)

Figure 8 (*continued*)

vessels at angiography (106). More recent large series indicate that isolated subsegmental clots occur in 4 to 6% (120,123), whereas series with different patient samples show that subsegmental clots are more frequent (124,125). On the subsegmental level, when scanning in a caudocranial direction, the less adequately enhanced vessels are those of the upper lobes, and those running obliquely to the transverse scanning plane (middle lobe and lingular vessels) (125).

The physiological consequences of solitary small clots in subsegmental pulmonary arteries have been widely investigated with contradictory results; a prospective 3-month follow-up study showed that the prevalence of clinically apparent PE after a negative spiral CT scan was low (1.0%) and not significantly different from that after a normal V-P scan (0%) (126,127). Mayo et al. (128) followed 44 patients with negative spiral CT scans for 3 months, and none of these patients had a recurrence. In addition, the prevalence of PE after a negative spiral CT scan was slightly, but not significantly, lower than that after a low-probability V-P scan (3.1%), results that were in concordance with other studies (129). Other series with similar design report 2.7 to 4.9% rates of subsequent PE (130,131). Despite this controversy regarding the clinical importance of such isolated, small, nontreated peripheral clots, in the absence of central emboli in the general population

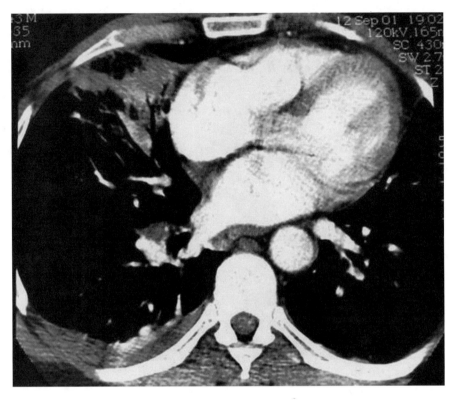

Figure 9 Large clot is seen at this level in a AECOPD treated for middle-lobe pneumonia. There is also ipsilateral pleural effusion.

(132,133), in patients with AECOPD—which present limited cardiopulmonary reserve—small emboli may become physiologically important or have prognostic relevance for the development of chronic pulmonary hypertension. There is no doubt that the goal is to increase the sensitivity of spiral CT in this respect; the development of faster imaging systems with submillimeter isotropic imaging are expected to improve imaging at the subsegmental level, with optimal spatial and temporal resolution, in the very near future.

It is generally agreed that the presence of pulmonary emboli is an important indicator for current deep venous thrombosis, which thus potentially heralds more severe embolic events. The combination of spiral CT of the chest for PE with CT venography thus emerged; CT venography is performed by scanning pelvic and leg veins immediately after spiral CT of the chest. This is achieved without additional contrast (indirect CT venography) and can demonstrate deep venous thrombosis in a single session in the CT suite prolonging the initial examination 3 to 4 min. Reported data indicate that indirect CT venography can detect DVT with high concordance with the standard examination, namely, ultrasound (134,135). In studies comparing indirect CT venography with ultrasound for deep venous thrombosis (DVT), Loud et al. (136) found sensitivity and specificity of 100% for both of them, while Shah et al. (137) found 94% agreement between the two examinations.

The addition of CT venography has been reported to increase the diagnosis of thromboembolism by 18% and may be preferred over algorithms that include US for DVT in institutions where it is available (134–138). Furthermore, for AECOPD patients who have a considerable lower belly distention, CT may be preferable to US for the detection of iliac vein thrombosis (incidence 22–30%) (138). Direct lower limb venography was the traditional standard to assure that no substantial clots reside in the femoropopliteal system but is no longer in routine use mainly because of its invasive nature. US has become the most commonly used diagnostic tool for the detection of DVT with a 97% sensitivity and specificity (139), also providing information for the exact morphology of the clots (floating, adhering to vein walls). Before a final agreement is settled on the exact algorithm for the detection of PE, especially in the AECOPD patient, further controlled studies are needed.

Indeterminate spiral CT studies range from 6 to 11% because of motion artifacts, poor contrast opacification, or poor signal-to-noise ratio. False-positive results are associated with hilar and bronchopulmonary lymph nodes, incomplete vessel opacification, or partial volume effect and are currently less than 6% (140).

Pulmonary angiography is recognized as the gold standard for the diagnosis of PE. Angiographic signs of acute pulmonary embolism include intraluminal filling defects, obstruction of a pulmonary artery branch, and delayed branch opacification (141). Both sensitivity and specificity rates exceed 95% in the hands of experienced operators (142). Nevertheless, pulmonary angiography is invasive and has been shown to have 4 to 6% morbidity and 0.2 to 0.5% mortality rates (143). Moreover, pulmonary artery pressures greater than 35 mmHg are a relative contraindication for angiography. Major complications of pulmonary angiography occur in approximately 1% of patients (143).

A frequently overlooked aspect of selective pulmonary arteriography is that it also has limitations in the diagnosis of subsegmental emboli, as demonstrated by the high interobserver variability reported at this level (144,145). In the PIOPED study, 20 patients who had small clots were missed at the initial pulmonary angiogram reading (146). Miss rates significantly increase in dyspneic patients (40,41).

For all the above reasons, pulmonary angiography should be reserved for selected patients with an unresolved diagnosis.

IV. Imaging Complications of AECOPD

In this section, complications of AECOPD diagnosed by imaging studies are described. These may complicate spontaneously breathing AECOPD patients or may be associated with barotrauma in assisted ventilation. Of the three ventilatory modes most widely used in AECOPD, pressure support ventilation is associated with the higher incidence of these complications.

A. Pneumothorax

Pneumothorax may mimic or complicate AECOPD. The radiological diagnosis can be made by the identification of the visceral pleural line. The latter is visualized as a sharply defined line of increased opacity associated with a negative Mach band (black) (Fig. 10A). The Mach effect is particularly useful in differentiation from the projection of skin folds (always associated with a positive Mach band) that constitute common pitfalls leading to false-positive diagnosis of pneumothorax (1) (Fig. 10B). The Mach effect may also be of value to differentiate a true pleural line from a peripheral bulla (147).

In the erect position, and in the absence of pleural adhesions, pneumothorax is seen at the apices. Recognition is facilitated by expiratory films. High-frequency enhancing algorithms used in digital radiographs demonstrate at better advantage the thin pleural line (148,149) (Fig. 11). Large bullae may resemble pneumothorax and CT is required for differential diagnosis (Fig. 12).

Atypical (non–gravity dependent) distributions of pneumothorax may be related to large bullae, pleural adhesions, atelectasis, and anatomical variations of

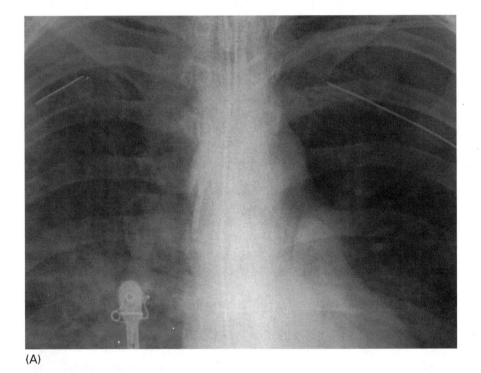

(A)

Figure 10 (A) Bilateral pneumothoraces complicating AECOPD. The thin pleural line on the left has a negative Mach band. Pneumomediastinum is also present, visualized as lucent stripes along mediastinal vessels. (B) In another patient, skin folds on the left are associated with a positive Mach band.

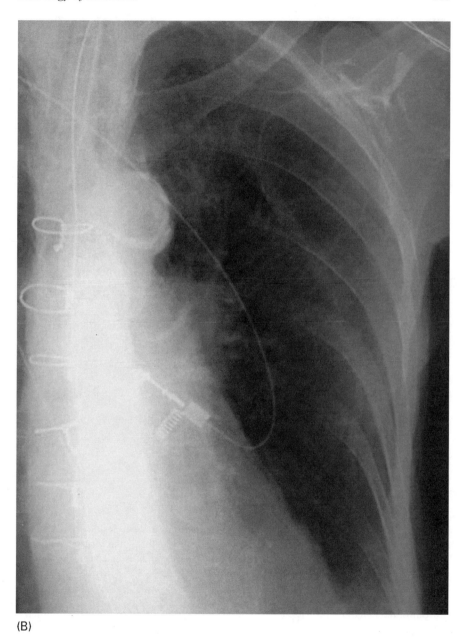

(B)

Figure 10   (*continued*)

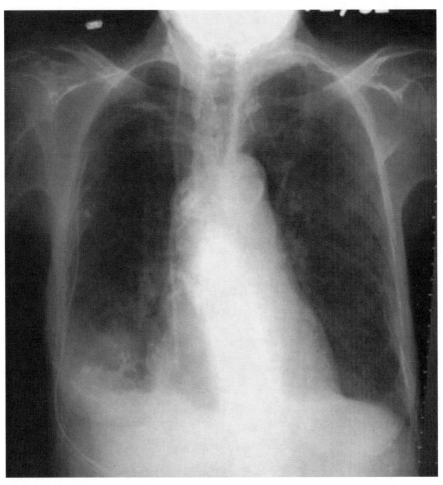

(A)

Figure 11 (A) Portable computed radiography in a semirecumbent position. (A) Low-
and (B) high-frequency-enhancing algorithms. The latter facilitates the visualization of
lines and interfaces (the pleural line of pneumothorax on the right is enhanced), while it
produces a pseudointerstitial parenchymal pattern.

the pulmonary ligament. Atypical distributions include subpulmonary, within the
pulmonary ligament, and paramediastinal locations and need to be distinguished
from bullae (CT is required). In particular, subpulmonic pneumothorax (Fig. 13) is
not infrequent in patients with chronic obstructive pulmonary disease and may be the
first sign of barotrauma especially during AECOPD. Localized pneumothorax of
paramediastinal distribution or pneumothorax within the pulmonary ligament can be
easily detected by CT and distinguished from pneumomediastinum and bullae. To
this end, inspiratory and expiratory CT is necessary.

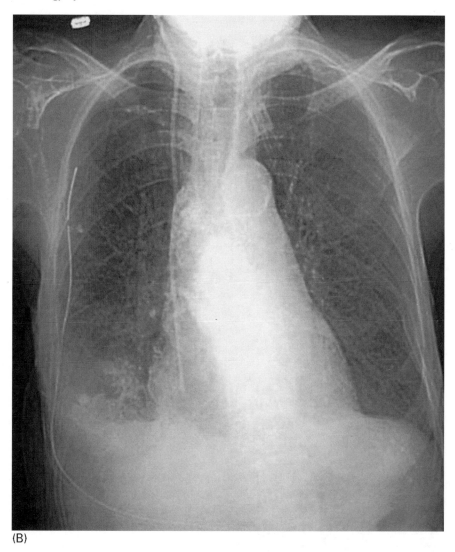

(B)

Figure 11 (*continued*)

Hydropneumothorax is easily recognized by the presence of an air–fluid level and differentiation from infected bullae is based on distribution and shape. In the supine position air–fluid levels cannot be demonstrated due to beam–fluid surface geometry and hydropneumothorax may only be suspected by the visualization of a pleural line surrounded by a band of increased homogeneous opacity.

In films obtained in the supine position—in the intensive care unit—pneumothorax is recognized by a number of radiological signs produced by the distribution of free air in the anteromedial, subpulmonic, or apicolateral pleural

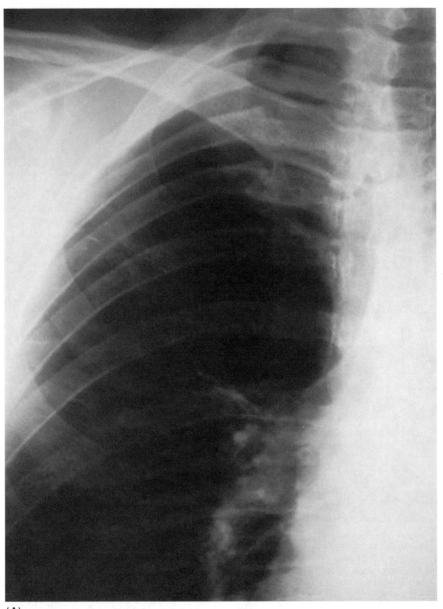

(A)

Figure 12   (A) Localized view of the chest at the right apex demonstrates an avascular area. (B,C) Continuous CT slices document the presence of a large bulla with tags of remaining lung parenchyma around it. This configuration virtually excludes pneumothorax.

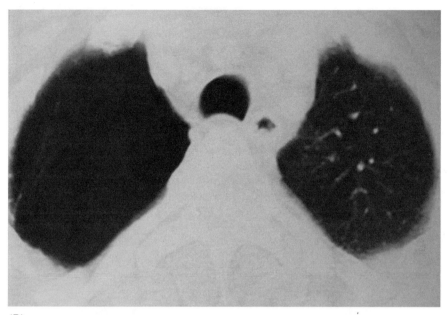

(B)

Figure 12 (*continued*)

spaces. However, more than one-third of pneumothoraces may be missed at supine chest films. Supine views have a sensitivity of only 37% in the detection of moderate pneumothorax (150). Portable computerized radiography with edge enhancement has slightly better results (148,149) (Fig. 11).

Notably, depending on the amount of pneumothorax, radiological signs in the supine position (Figs. 10,14,15) include (1) deep radiolucent costophrenic sulcus (deep sulcus sign); (2) increased lucency over the hemidiaphragms; (3) increased sharpness and enhancement of the negative Mach band of the cardiac boarder (air anteromedially); (4) collection of air within the minor fissure; (5) further depression and flattening of the ipsilateral hemidiaphragm; and (6) visualization of the anterior costophrenic sulcus seen as an interface outlining the dome of the ipsilateral hemidiaphragm (double diaphragm sign) (150,151). Recognition of these signs in the AECOPD setting requires comparisons of sequential films. Positive-pressure ventilation increases the risk of tension pneumothorax, which is visualized on chest radiographs as an excessive shift of the mediastinum associated with clinical signs of hemodynamic compromise.

CT is very sensitive, detecting even a few milliliters of air (Fig. 15); CT depiction may suggest early prophylactic chest-tube placement in patients under mechanical ventilation since one-third of them will develop tension pneumothorax if untreated. CT may also assist in revealing malpositioned chest tubes and residual pneumothorax.

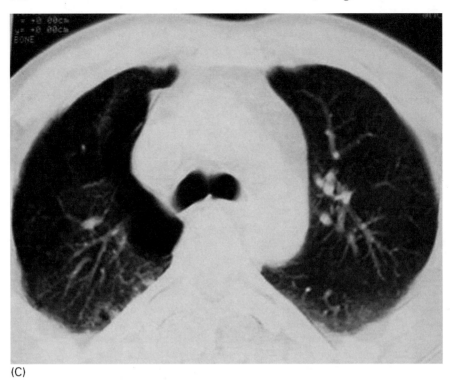

(C)

Figure 12   (*continued*)

B. Pneumomediastinum

Pneumomediastinum due to the Macklin effect may complicate AECOPD, resulting from ruptured alveoli and subsequent passage of air into the interstitium along the bronchovascular bundle to the hilum and mediastinum (152). The initially resulting interstitial emphysema and subsequent course of air along the peribronchovascular interstitium has been recently demonstrated by CT (153,154). From the mediastinal areolar tissue, air can leak peripherally and cause pneumothorax that is a common concurrent finding (154).

Imaging (chest radiographs or CT) reveals linear radiolucencies within the mediastinal structures, often extending into the neck. These lucencies (produced as air lifts the mediastinal pleura off the heart and the other mediastinal structures), outline the margins of the aortic knob, the descending aorta, and the extrapericardial parts of the pulmonary artery (Fig. 10A). CT is very sensitive in the detection of pneumomediastinum and can easily differentiate it from paramediastinal bullae or pneumothorax.

At chest radiographs, air interposed between the heart and the diaphragm allows visualization of the central portion of the diaphragm that is normally obscured by the heart producing the "continuous diaphragm sign" (155). The concurrent

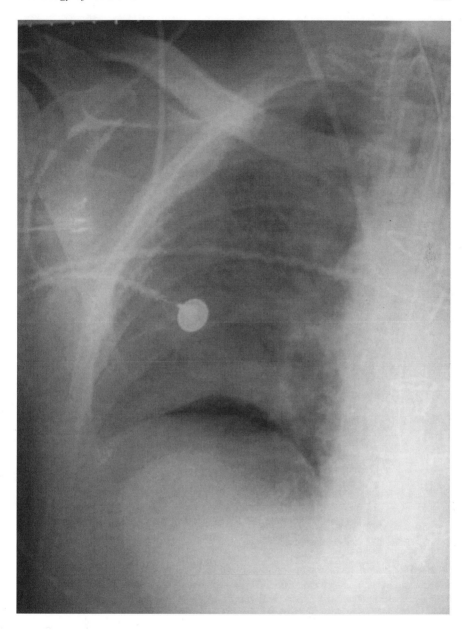

Figure 13 Subpulmonary lucency indicating small pneumothorax.

visualization of paraspinal and extrapleural supradiaphragmatic air described as "V sign" by Naclerio is another finding of pneumomediastinum (156). However, in plain films, the latter is difficult to distinguish from subpulmonary pneumothorax, or paramediastinal bullae, and CT is necessary.

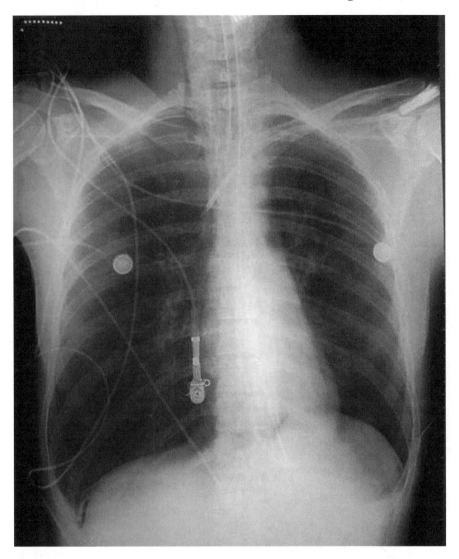

Figure 14   Pneumothorax complicating AECOPD. Chest roentgenogram in the supine
position demonstrates a deep sulcus on the right associated with increased transradiancy of
the ipsilateral hemidiaphragm. These findings are highly suggestive of pneumothorax.

C.   Pulmonary Aspiration

Pulmonary aspiration associated AECOPD may be observed in general anesthesia,
loss of consciousness, structural abnormalities of the pharynx and esophagus,
or neuromuscular disorders with deglutition abnormalities. The radiological manifestations depend on the aspirated material and have been described in detail
(157,158). However, underlying emphysema contributes in inhomogeneity of the

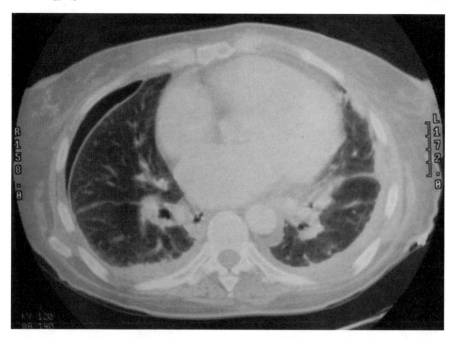

Figure 15 The small pneumothorax on the right and the visceral pleural line are readily visualized by CT.

consolidations (Fig. 16), while in COPD patients complication with pulmonary infection pneumonia, bronchopneumonia, lung abscess, and empyema is more likely.

In the supine patient, the posterior segment of the upper lobes and the superior segment of the lower lobes are the most commonly involved locations (Fig. 16). Computed tomography allows better evaluation of aspiration not visible on conventional chest radiographs, while in exogenous lipoid pneumonia images can be pathognomonic demonstrating negative attenuation values (159–161). Chronic endogenous accumulation of lipid material may mimic lung neoplasms (160,161).

In aspiration of gastric fluid, the extent of findings is directly related to the pH and volume of the aspirated material (162). Chest radiography reveals bilateral perihilar, ill-defined, alveolar consolidations or multifocal patchy infiltrates (Fig. 16). Aspiration of contaminated material from the oropharynx and gastrointestinal tract in patients with poor oral hygiene may result in severe necrotizing bronchopneumonia (163). Chest radiography and/or CT reveal focal or patchy, ill-defined lung consolidations and progressive abscess formation. The visualization of small lucencies within the consolidated area may represent early cavitation or preexisting emphysematous areas; comparison of sequential images is necessary for differential diagnosis (164).

There is evidence that a significant number of patients with chronic bronchitis have gastrointestinal reflux (165), and that an association between reflux and asthma (166) does exist. Moreover, gastroesophageal reflux and aspiration have been

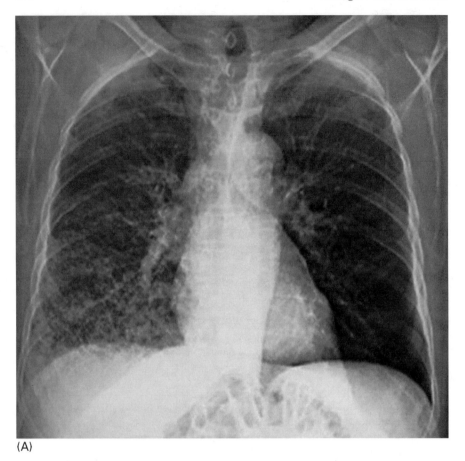

(A)

Figure 16 Aspiration in the right lower lobe. (A,B) Consolidation appears quite inhomogeneous due to the underlying emphysema, best depicted on HRCT (B).

considered predisposing factors in the development of obliterative bronchiolitis (167). High-resolution CT findings associated with obliterative bronchiolitis are demonstrated with inspiratory, expiratory sections and include bronchial dilatation, mosaic perfusion, bronchial wall thickening, and regional air trapping (168) that are virtually indistinguishable from the underlying COPD abnormalities. Barium studies or esophageal pH measurements may be of use for confirmation of gastroesophageal reflux.

V. Future Imaging Research

Improved methods for early detection, and identification of the most susceptible subjects may reduce the severity and improve the management of exacerbations.

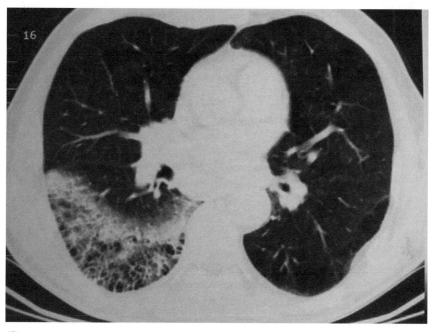

(B)

Figure 16 *(continued)*

Considerable research is currently underway for the use of MRI in the assessment of ventilation and perfusion globally and regionally (169–171). Moreover, standardized protocols with spiral CT as a major tool for the detection of pulmonary embolism in AECOPD, not including ventilation-perfusion scintigraphy, are going to be presented in the very near future.

References

1. Siafakas NM, Vermeire P, Pride NB, Paoletti P, Gibson J, Howard P, Yenault JC, Decramer M, Higenbottam T, Postma DS, Rees J. Optimal assessment and management of chronic obstructive pulmonary disease (COPD). The European Respiratory Society Task Force. Eur Respir J 1995; 8(8):1398–1420.
2. Standards for the diagnosis and care of patients with chronic obstructive pulmonary disease. American Thoracic Society. Am J Respir Crit Care Med 1995; 152(5 Pt 2): S77–S121.
3. British Thoracic Society guidelines for the management of chronic obstructive pulmonary disease. The COPD Guidelines Group of the Standards of Care Committee of the BTS. Thorax 1997; 52:S1–S28.
4. Senior RM, Anthonisen NR. Chronic obstructive pulmonary disease (COPD). Am J Respir Crit Care Med 1998; 157(4 Pt 2):S139–S147.

5. Gelb AF, Hogg JC, Muller NL, Schein MJ, Kuei J, Tashkin DP, Epstein JD, Kollin J, Green RH, Zamel N, Elliott WM, Hadjiaghai L. Contribution of emphysema and small airways in COPD. Chest 1996; 109(2):353–359.

6. Gelb AF, Schein M, Kuei J, Tashkin DP, Muller NL, Hogg JC, Epstein JD, Zamel N. Limited contribution of emphysema in advanced chronic obstructive pulmonary disease. Am Rev Respir Dis 1993; 147(5):1157–1161.

7. Shapiro SD Evolving concepts in the pathogenesis of chronic obstructive pulmonary disease. Chin Chest Med 2000; 21(4):621–632.

8. Calverley PM. COPD: early detection and intervention. Chest 2000; 117(5 suppl 2): 365S–371S.

9. Rodriguez-Roisin R. Toward a consensus definition for COPD exacerbations. Chest 2000; 117(5 suppl 2):398S–401S.

10. Pratt PC. Role of conventional chest radiography in diagnosis and exclusion of emphysema. Am J Med 1987; 82(5):998–1006.

11. Sutinen S, Christoforidis AJ, Klugh GA, Pratt PC. Roentgenologic criteria for the recognition of non-symptomatic pulmonary emphysema: correlation between roentgenologic findings and pulmonary radiology. Am Rev Respir Dis 1965; 91:69–76.

12. Thurlbeck WM, Simon G. Radiographic appearance of chest in emphysema. Am J Roentgenol 1978; 130(3):429–440.

13. Reich SB, Weinshelbaum A, Yee J. Correlation of radiographic measurements and pulmonary function tests in chronic obstructive pulmonary disease. Am J Roentgenol 1985; 144(4):695–699.

14. Webb R. Radiology of obstructive pulmonary disease. Am J Roentgenol 1997; 169: 637–647.

15. Takasugi JE, Godwin JD. Radiology of chronic obstructive pulmonary disease. Radiol Clin North Am 1998; 36(1):29–55.

16. Cleverley JR. Muller NL. Advances in radiologic assessment of chronic obstructive pulmonary disease. Clin Chest Med 2000; 21(4):653–663.

17. Remy-Jardin M, Remy J, Gosselin B, Copin MC, Wurtz A, Duhamel A. Sliding thin slab, minimum intensity projection technique in the diagnosis of emphysema: histopathologic-CT correlation. Radiology 1996; 200(3):665–671.

18. Klein JS, Gamsu G, Webb WR, Golden JA, Muller NL. High-resolution CT diagnosis of emphysema in symptomatic patients with normal chest radiographs and isolated low diffusing capacity. Radiology 1992; 182(3):817–821.

19. Gurney JW, Jones KK, Robbins RA, Gossman GL, Nelson KJ, Daughton D, Spurzem JR, Rennard SI. Regional distribution of emphysema: correlation of high-resolution CT with pulmonary function tests in unselected smokers. Radiology 1992; 183(2):457–463.

20. Stern EJ, Song JK, Frank MS. CT of the lungs in patients with pulmonary emphysema. Scmin Ultrasound CT MR 1995; 16(5):345 352.

21. Gevenois PA, Yernault JC. Can computed tomography quantify pulmonary emphysema? Eur Respir J 1995; 8(5):843–848.

22. Gevenois PA, De Vuyst P, Sy M, Scillia P, Chaminade L, de Maertelaer V, Zanen J, Yernault JC. Pulmonary emphysema: quantitative CT during expiration. Radiology 1996; 199(3):825–829.

23. Nishimura X, Murata K, Yamagishi M, Itoh H, Ikeda A, Tsukino M, Koyama H, Sakai N, Mishima M, Izumi T. Comparison of different computed tomography scanning methods for quantifying emphysema. J Thorac Imaging 1998; 13(3):193–198.

24. Kauczor HU, Heussel CP, Fischer B, Klamm R, Mildenberger P, Thelen M. Assessment of lung volumes using helical CT at inspiration and expiration: comparison with pulmonary function tests. Am J Roentgenol 1998; 171(4):1091–1095.
25. Bankier AA, De Maertelaer V, Keyzer C, Gevenois PA. Pulmonary emphysema: subjective visual grading versus objective quantification with macroscopic morphometry and thin-section CT densitometry. Radiology 1999; 211(3):851–858.
26. MacFall JR, Charles HC, Black RD, Middleton H, Swartz JC, Saam B, Driehuys B, Erickson C, Happer W, Cates GD, Johnson GA, Ravin CE. Human lung air spaces: potential for MR imaging with hyperpolarized He-3. Radiology 1996; 200(2):553–558.
27. Kauczor H, Surkau R, Roberts T. MRI using hyperpolarized noble gases. Eur Radiol 1998; 8(5):820–827.
28. Kauczor HU, Kreitner KF. MRI of the pulmonary parenchyma. Eur Radiol 1999; 9(9):1755–1764.
29. Kauczor HU, Kreitner KF. Contrast-enhanced MRI of the lung. Eur J Radiol 2000; 34(3):196–207.
30. Guckel C, Hansell DM. Imaging the 'dirty lung'—has high resolution computed tomography cleared the smoke? Clin Radiol 1998; 53(10):717–722.
31. Remy-Jardin M, Remy J, Boulenguez C, Sobaszek A, Edme JL, Furon D. Morphologic effects of cigarette smoking on airways and pulmonary parenchyma in healthy adult volunteers: CT evaluation and correlation with pulmonary function tests. Radiology 1993; 186(1):107–115
32. Nakano Y, Muro S, Sakai H, Hirai T, Chin K, Tsukino M, Nishimura K, Itoh H, Pare PD, Hogg JC, Mishima M. Computed tomographic measurements of airway dimensions and emphysema in smokers. Correlation with lung function. Am J Respir Crit Care Med 2000; 162(3 Pt 1):1102–1108.
33. Voelkel NF, Tuder R. COPD: exacerbation. Chest 2000; 117(5 suppl 2):376S–379S
34. Sherk PA, Grossman RF. The chronic obstructive pulmonary disease exacerbation. Clin Chest Med 2000; 21(4):705–721.
35. Wedzicha JA. The heterogeneity of chronic obstructive pulmonary disease. Thorax 2000; 55(8):631–632.
36. Schaefer-Prokop C, Eisenhuber E, Fuchsjager M, Puig S, Prokop M. Current developments in the area of digital thoracic radiography. Radiology 2001; 41(3):230–239.
37. Prokop M, Schaefer-Prokop CM. Digital image processing. Eur Radiol 1997; 21:73–82.
38. Sanders C. The radiologic diagnosis of emphysema. Radiol Clin North Am 1991; 29(5):1019–1030.
39. Fraser RsS, Muller NL, Colman N, Pare PD. Fraser's and Pare's Diagnosis of Diseases of the Chest. Philadelphia: WB Saunders, 1999.
40. Zompatori M, Fasano L, Battista G, Pacilli AM, Stopazzoni C, Cavina M. Role of emphysema in the etiology of functional impairment in patients with severe chronic obstructive pulmonary disease. Study with high resolution computerized tomography. Radiol Med (Torino) 1999; 97(1–2):26–32.
41. Mergo PJ, Williams WF, Gonzalez-Rothi R, Gibson R, Ros PR, Staab EV, Helmberger T. Three-dimensional volumetric assessment of abnormally low attenuation of the lung from routine helical CT: inspiratory and expiratory quantification. Am J Roentgenol 1998; 170(5):1355–1360.
42. Farr BM, Woodhead MA, Macfarlane JT, Bartlett CL, McCraken JS, Wadsworth J, Miller DL. Risk factors for community-acquired pneumonia diagnosed by general practitioners in the community. Respir Med 2000; 94(5):422–427.

43. Farr BM, Bartlett CL, Wadsworth J, Miller DL. British Thoracic Society Pneumonia Study Group. Risk factors for community-acquired pneumonia diagnosed upon hospital admission. Respir Med 2000; 94(10):954–963.
44. Henschke CI, Yankelevitz DF, Wand A, Davis SD, Shiau M. Accuracy and efficacy of chest radiography in the intensive care unit. Radiol Clin North Am 1996; 34 (1):21–31.
45. Rozenshtein A, White CS, Austin JH, Romney BM, Protopapas Z, Krasna MJ. Incidental lung carcinoma detected at CT in patients selected for lung volume reduction surgery to treat severe pulmonary emphysema. Radiology 1998; 207(2):487–490.
46. Gompertz S, O'Brien C, Bayley DL, Hill SL, Stockley RA. Changes in bronchial inflammation during acute exacerbations of chronic bronchitis. Eur Respir J 2001; 17(6):1112–1119.
47. Groskin SA. Heitzman's the lung. Radiologic–Pathologic Correlations, 3rd ed. St Louis: Mosby-Year Book, 1993.
48. Hansell D, Dee P. Infections of the lungs and pleura. In: Armstrong P, Wilson A, Dee P, Hansell D, eds. Imaging of Diseases of the Chest, 3rd ed. London: Mosby, 2000: 163–253.
49. Tew J, Calenoff L, Berlin BS. Bacterial or nonbacterial pneumonia: accuracy of radiographic diagnosis. Radiology 1977; 124:607–612.
50. Macfarlane JT, Miller AC, Roderick Smith WH, Morris AH, Rose DH. Comparative radiographic features of community acquired Legionnaires' disease, pneumococcal pneumonia, mycoplasma pneumonia, and psittacosis. Thorax 1984; 39(1):28–33.
51. Tanaka N, Matsumoto T, Kuramitsu T, Nakaki H, Ito K, Uchisako H, Miura G, Matsunaga N, Yamakawa K. High resolution CT findings in community-acquired pneumonia. J Comput Assist Tomogr 1996; 20(4):600–608.
52. Aquino SL, Gamsu G, Webb WR, Kee ST. Tree-in-bud pattern: frequency and significance on thin section CT. J Comput Assist Tomogr 1996; 20(4):594–599.
53. Hwang JH, Kim TS, Lee KS, Choi YH, Han J, Chung MP, Kwon OJ, Rhee CH. Bronchiolitis in adults: pathology and imaging. J Comput Assist Tomogr 1997; 21(6):913–919.
54. Takahashi M, Murata K, Takazakura R, Nakahara T, Shimizu K, Minese M, Itoh H. Bronchiolar disease: spectrum and radiological findings. Eur J Radiol 2000; 35(1): 15–29.
55. Hall FM, Levin DL. Emphysema and chronic obstructive pulmonary disease. Am J Roentgenol 1997; 169(5):1460–1461.
56. Ziskind MM, Schwarz MI, George RB, Weill H, Shames JM, Herbert SJ, Ichinose H. Incomplete consolidation in pneumococcal lobar pneumonia complicating pulmonary emphysema. Ann Intern Med 1970; 72(6):835–839.
57. Fujita J, Sato K, Irino S. Emphysematous modification of diffuse centrilobular lesions due to staphylococcal pneumonia. Am J Roentgenol 1991; 156:1322–1323.
58. Ziskind M, George B, Weill H. Acute localized and diffuse alveolar pneumonias. Semin Roentgenol 1967; 2:46–60.
59. O'Brien C, Guest PJ, Hill SL, Stockley RA. Physiological and radiological characterisation of patients diagnosed with chronic obstructive pulmonary disease in primary care. Thorax 2000; 55(8):635–642.
60. Bach PB, Brown C, Gelfand SE, McCrory DC. American College of Physicians-American Society of Internal Medicine; American College of Chest Physicians. Management of acute exacerbations of chronic obstructive pulmonary disease: a summary and appraisal of published evidence. Ann Intern Med 2001; 134(7):600–620.

61. Wedzicha JA, Seemungal TA, MacCallum PK, Paul EA, Donaldson GC, Bhowmik A, Jeffries DJ, Meade TW. Acute exacerbations of chronic obstructive pulmonary disease are accompanied by elevations of plasma fibrinogen and serum IL-6 levels. Thromb Haemost 2000; 84(2):210–215.

62. Matthay RA, Berger HJ. Cardiovascular function in cor pulmonale. Clin Chest Med 1983; 4(2):269–295.

63. Milne EN, Bass H. Roentgenologic and functional analysis of combined chronic obstructive pulmonary disease and congestive cardiac failure. Invest Radiol 1969; 4:129–147.

64. Hublitz UF, Shapiro JH. Atypical pulmonary patterns of congestive failure in chronic lung disease. The influence of pre-existing disease on the appearance and distribution of pulmonary edema. Radiology 1969; 93(5):995–1006.

65. Vandiviere HM. Pulmonary hypertension and cor pulmonale. South Med J 1993; 86(10):2S7–S10.

66. Walcott G, Burchell HB, Brown AL Jr. Primary pulmonary hypertension. Am J Med 1970; 49(1):70–79.

67. Chang CH. The normal roentgenographic measurement of the right descending pulmonary artery in 1085 cases. Am J Roentgenol 1962; (87):929–935.

68. Haimovici JB, Trotman-Dickenson B, Halpern EF, Dec GW, Ginns LC, Shepard JA, McLoud TC. Relationship between pulmonary artery diameter at computed tomography and pulmonary artery pressures at right-sided heart catheterization. Massachusetts General Hospital Lung Transplantation Program. Acad Radiol 1997; 4(5):327–334.

69. Edwards PD, Bull RK, Coulden R. CT measurement of main pulmonary artery diameter. Br J Radiol 1998; 71(850):1018–1020.

70. Tan RT, Kuzo R, Goodman LR, Siegel R, Haasler GB, Presberg KW. Utility of CT scan evaluation for predicting pulmonary hypertension in patients with parenchymal lung disease. Medical College of Wisconsin Lung Transplant Group. Chest 1998; 113(5): 1250–1256.

71. Ng CS, Wells AU, Padley SP. A CT sign of chronic pulmonary arterial hypertension: the ratio of main pulmonary artery to aortic diameter. J Thorac Imaging 1999; 14(4):270–278.

72. Baque-Juston MC, Wells AU, Hansell DM. Pericardial thickening or effusion in patients with pulmonary artery hypertension: a CT study. Am J Roentgenol 1999; 172(2):361–364.

73. Frank H, Globits S, Glogar D, Neuhold A, Kneussl M, Mlczoch J. Detection and quantification of pulmonary artery hypertension with MR imaging: results in 23 patients. Am J Roentgenol 1993; 161(1):27–31.

74. Bergin CJ, Hauschildt J, Rios G, Belezzuoli EV, Huynh T, Channick RN. Accuracy of MR angiography compared with radionuclide scanning in identifying the cause of pulmonary arterial hypertension. Am J Roentgenol 1997; 168(6):1549–1555.

75. Mousseaux E, Tasu JP, Jolivet O, Simonneau G, Bittoun J, Gaux JC. Pulmonary arterial resistance: noninvasive measurement with indexes of pulmonary flow estimated at velocity-encoded MR imaging—preliminary experience. Radiology 1999; 212(3): 896–902.

76. Laffon E, Laurent F, Bernard V, De Boucaud L, Ducassou D, Marthan R. Noninvasive assessment of pulmonary arterial hypertension by MR phase-mapping method. J Appl Physiol 2001; 90(6):2197–2202.

77. Murray TI, Boxt LM, Katz J, Reagan K, Barst RJ. Estimation of pulmonary artery pressure in patients with primary pulmonary hypertension by quantitative analysis of magnetic resonance images. J Thorac Imaging 1994; 9(3):198–204.
78. Kondo C, Caputo GR, Masui T, Foster E, O'Sullivan M, Stulbarg MS, Golden J, Catterjee K, Higgins CB. Pulmonary hypertension: pulmonary flow quantification and flow profile analysis with velocity-encoded cine MR imaging. Radiology 1992; 183(3):751–758.
79. Zompatori M, Battaglia M, Rimondi MR, Battista G, Stambazzi C. Hemodynamic estimation of chronic cor pulmonale by Doppler echocardiography. Clinical value and comparison with other noninvasive imaging techniques. Rays 1997; 22(1):73–93.
80. Richardson MS, Reddy VD, Read CA. New air-fluid levels in bullous lung disease: a reevaluation. Natl Med Assoc 1996; 88(3):185–187.
81. Mahler DA, D'Esopo ND. Peri-emphysematous lung infection. Clin Chest Med 1981; 2(1):51–57.
82. Kirschner LS, Stauffer W, Krenzel C, Duane PG. Management of a giant fluid-filled bulla by closed-chest thoracostomy tube drainage. Chest 1997; 111(6):1772–1774.
83. Satoh H, Suyama T, Yamashita YT, Ohtsuka M, Sekizawa K. Spontaneous regression of multiple emphysematous bullae. Can Respir J 1999; 6(5):458–460.
84. Stern EJ, Webb WR, Weinacker A, Muller NL. Idiopathic giant bullous emphysema (vanishing lung syndrome): imaging findings in nine patients. Am J Roentgenol 1994; 162(2):279–282.
85. Roberts L, Putman CE, Chen JTT, Goodman LR, Ravin CE. Vanishing lung syndrome: upper lobe bullous pneumonopathy. Radiol Inter Radiol 1987; 12:249–255.
86. Philips GD, Trotman-Dickenson B, Hodson ME, Geddes DM. Role of CT in the management of pneumothorax in patients with complex cystic lung disease. Chest 1997; 112(1):275–278.
87. Bourgouin P, Cousineau G, Lemire P, Hebert G. Computed tomography used to exclude pneumothorax in bullous lung disease. J Can Assoc Radiol 1985; 36(4):341–342.
88. Engdahl O, Toft T, Boe J. Chest radiograph—a poor method for determining the size of a pneumothorax. Chest 1993; 103(1):26–29.
89. Mitlehner W, Friedrich M, Dissmann W. Value of computer tomography in the detection of bullae and blebs in patients with primary spontaneous pneumothorax. Respiration 1992; 59(4):221–227.
90. Smit HJ, Wienk MA, Schreurs AJ, Schramel FM, Postmus PE. Do bullae indicate a predisposition to recurrent pneumothorax? Br J Radiol 2000; 73(868):356–359.
91. Waitches G, Stern G, Dubinsky T. Usefulness of the double-wall sign in detecting pneumothorax in patients with giant bullous emphysema. Am J Roentgenol 2000; 174:1765–1768.
92. Gierada DS, Glazer HS, Slone RM. Pseudomass due to atelectasis in patients with severe bullous emphysema. Am J Roentgenol 1997; 168(1):85–92.
93. Webb WR. High-resolution computed tomography of obstructive lung disease. Radiol Clin North Am 1994; 32(4):745–757.
94. Mehran RJ, Deslauriers J. Indications for surgery and patient work-up for bullectomy. Chest Surg Clin N Am 1995; 5(4):717–734.
95. Laros CD, Gelissen HJ, Bergstein PG, Van den Bosch JM, Vanderschueren RG, Westermann CJ, Knaepen PJ. Bullectomy for giant bullae in emphysema. J Thorac Cardiovasc Surg 1986; 91(1):63–70.
96. Carr DH, Pride NB. Computed tomography in pre-operative assessment of bullous emphysema. Chin Radiol 1984; 35(1):43–45.

97. Kuhlman JE, Singha NK. Complex disease of the pleural space: radiographic and CT evaluation. RadioGraphics 1997; 17:63–79.

98. Malagari K, Fraser RG. Imaging of the chest wall and diaphragm. In: Roussos C, ed. The Thorax. New York: Marcel Dekker, 1995: 1763–1837.

99. Bouros D, Plataki M, Antoniou KM. Parapneumonic effusion and empyema: best therapeutic approach. Monaldi Arch Chest Dis. 2001; 56(2):144–148.

100. Papiris S, Roussos Ch. Pleural Effusions in the Intensive Care Unit. New York: Marcel Dekker, in press.

101. Aquino SL, Webb WR, Gushiken BJ. Pleural exudates and transudates: diagnosis with contrast-enhanced CT Radiology 1994; 192:803–808.

102. Song JW, Im JG, Goo JM, Kim HY, Song CS, Lee JS. Pseudochylous pleural effusion with fat-fluid levels: report of six cases. Radiology 2000; 216:478–480.

103. Eibenberger KL, Dock WI, Ammann ME, Dorffner R, Hormann MF, Grabenwoger F. Quantification of pleural effusions: sonography versus radiography. Radiology 1994; 191:681–684.

104. Miller WT, Tino G Jr, Friedburg JS. Thoracic CT in the intensive care unit: assessment of clinical usefulness. Radiology 1998; 209:491–498.

105. Lesser BA, Leeper KV Jr, Stein PD, Saltzman HA, Chen J, Thompson BT, Hales CA, Popovich J Jr, Greenspan RH, Weg JG. The diagnosis of acute pulmonary embolism in patients with chronic obstructive pulmonary disease. Chest 1992; 102:17–22.

106. PIOPED Investigators. Value of the ventilation/perfusion scan in acute pulmonary embolism. JAMA 1990; 263:2753–2759.

107. Stebbings AEL, Kim TK. A patient with acute exacerbation of COPD who did not respond to conventional treatment. Chest 1998; 114(6):1759–1761.

108. Blachere H, Latrabe V, Montaudon M, Valli N, Couffinhal T, Raherisson C, Leccia F, Laurent F. Pulmonary embolism revealed on helical CT angiography comparison with ventilation—perfusion radionuclide lung scanning. Am J Roentgenol 2000; 174:1041–1047.

109. Schoepf UJ, Bruening R, Konschitzky H, Becker CR, Knez A, Weber J, Muehling O, Herzog P, Huber A, Haberl R, Reiser MF. Segmental and subsegmental pulmonary arteries: evaluation with electron-beam versus spiral CT. Radiology 2000; 214:433–439.

110. Goodman LR, Lipchik RJ. Diagnosis of acute pulmonary embolism: time for a new approach (editorial). Radiology 1996; 199:25–27.

111. Gerard SK, Hsu Te-C. Pulmonary embolism: diagnosis with spiral CT versus ventilation-perfusion scintigraphy. Radiology 1999; 210:576–577.

112. Goodman LR, Curtin JJ, Mewissen MW, Foley WD, Lipchik RJ, Crain MR, Sagar KB, Collier BD. Detection of pulmonary embolism in patients with unresolved clinical and scintigraphic diagnosis: helical CT versus angiography. Am J Roentgenol 1995; 164:1369–1374.

113. Worsley DF, Alavi A, Aronchick JM, Chen JT, Greenspan RH, Ravin CE. Chest radiographic findings in patients with acute pulmonary embolism: observations from the PIOPED study. Radiology 1993; 189:133–136.

114. Kuzo RS, Goodman LR. HCT evaluation of pulmonary embolism: technique and interpretation. Am J Roentgenol 1997; 169:959–965.

115. Kim KI, Müller NL, Mayo JR. Clinically suspected pulmonary embolism: utility of spiral CT. Radiology 1999; 210:693–697.

116. Kahn D, Bushnell DL, Dean R, Perlman SB. Clinical outcome of patients with a low probability of pulmonary embolism on ventilation-perfusion lung scan. Arch Intern Med 1989; 149:377–379.

117. Lee ME, Biello DR, Kumar B, Siegel BA. Low-probability ventilation-perfusion scintigrams: clinical outcomes in 99 patients. Radiology 1985; 156:497–500.
118. Garg K, Sieler H, Welsh CH, Johnston RJ, Russ PD. Clinical validity of helical HCT being interpreted as negative for pulmonary embolism: implications for patient treatment. Am J Roentgenol 1999; 172:1627–1631.
119. Ghali WA, Cornuz J, Perrier Λ. New methods for estimating pretest probability in the diagnosis of pulmonary embolism. Curr Opin Pulm Med 2001; 7(5):349–353.
120. Qanadli SD, Hajjam ME, Mesurolle B, Barre O, Bruckert F, Joseph T, Mignon F, Vieillard-Baron A, Dubourg O, Lacombe P. Pulmonary embolism detection: prospective evaluation of dual-section helical CT versus selective pulmonary arteriography in 157 patients. Radiology 2000; 217:447–455.
121. Cheely R, McCartney WH, Perry JR, Delany DJ, Bustad L, Wynia VH, Griggs TR. The role of noninvasive tests versus pulmonary embolism. Am J Med 1981; 70: 17–22.
122. Remy-Jardin M, Remy J, Deschildre F, Artaud D, Beregi JP, Hossein-Foucher C, Marchandise X, Duhamel A. Diagnosis of pulmonary embolism with spiral CT: comparison with pulmonary angiography and scintigraphy. Radiology 1996; 200: 699–706.
123. Stein PD, Henry JW, Gottschalk A. Reassessment of pulmonary angiography for the diagnosis of pulmonary embolism: relation of interpreter agreement to the order of the involved pulmonary arterial branch. Radiology 1999; 210:689–691.
124. Novelline R, Baltarowich O, Athanasoulis C, Greenfield A, McKusick K. The clinical course of patients with suspected pulmonary embolism and a negative pulmonary angiogram. Radiology 1978; 126:561–567.
125. Oser RF, Zuckerman DA, Gutierrez FR, Brink JA. Anatomic distribution of pulmonary emboli at pulmonary arteriography: implications for spiral and ultrafast helical CT. Radiology 1996; 199:31–35.
126. Goodman LR, Lipchik RJ, Kuzo RS, Liu Y, McAuliffe TL, O'Brien DJ. Subsequent pulmonary embolism: risk after a negative helical CT pulmonary angiogram—prospective comparison with scintigraphy. Radiology 2000; 215: 535–542.
127. Henry JW, Relyea B, Stein PD. Continuing risk of thromboemboli among patients with normal pulmonary angiograms. Chest 1995; 107:1375–137.
128. Mayo JR, Remy-Jardin M, Muller NL, Remy J, Worsley DF, Hossein-Foucher C, Kwong JS, Brown MJ. Pulmonary embolism: prospective comparison of spiral helical CT with ventilation-perfusion scintigraphy. Radiology 1997; 205:447–452.
129. Patriquin L, Khorasani R, Polak JF. Correlation of diagnostic imaging and subsequent autopsy findings in patients with pulmonary embolism. Am J Roentgenol 1998; 171:347–349.
130. Van Beck EJR, Philomeen MM, Schenk BE, Brandjes DPM, ten Cate JW, Büller HR. A normal perfusion lung scan in patients with clinically suspected pulmonary embolism. Chest 1995; 108:170–173.
131. Ferretti GR, Bosson JL, Bullaz PD, et al. Acute pulmonary embolism: role of helical HCT in 164 patients with intermediate probability at ventilation-perfusion scintigraphy and normal results at duplex US of the legs. Radiology 1997; 205:453–458.
132. Gurney JA. No fooling around: direct visualization of pulmonary embolism. Radiology 1993; 188:618–619
133. Ryu JH, Olson EJ, Pellikka PA. Clinical recognition of pulmonary embolism: problem of unrecognized and asymptomatic cases. Mayo Clin Proc 1998; 73:873–879.

134. Cham MD, Yankelevitz DF, Shaham D, Shah AA, Sherman L, Lewis A, Rademaker J, Pearson G, Choi J, Wolff W, Prabhu PM, Galanski M, Clark RA, Sostman HD, Henschke CI. Deep venous thrombosis: detection by using indirect CT venography. Radiology 216:744–751.

135. Garg K, Kemp JL, Wojcik D, Hoehn S, Johnston RJ, Macey LC, Barón, AE 2000; Thromboembolic disease: comparison of combined CT pulmonary angiography and venography with bilateral leg sonography in 70 patients. Am J Roentgenol 2000; 175: 997–1001.

136. Loud PA, Katz DS, Klippenstein DL, Shah RD, Grossman ZD. Combined CT venography and pulmonary angiography in suspected thromboembolic disease: diagnostic accuracy for deep venous evaluation. Am J Roentgenol 1998; 170:951–953.

137. Shah AA, Buckshee N, Yankelevitz DF, Henschke CI. Assessment of deep venous thrombosis using routine pelvic CT. Am J Roentgenol 1999; 173:659–663.

138. Yankelevitz DF, Gamsu G, Shah A, Rademaker J, Shaham D, Buckshee N, Cham MD, Henschke CI. Optimization of combined CT pulmonary angiography with lower extremity CT venography. Am J Roentgenol 2000; 174:67–69.

139. Baldt MM, Zontsich T, Stumpflen A, Fleischmann D, Schneider B, Minar E, Mostbeck GH. Deep venous thrombosis of the lower extremity: efficacy of spiral CT venography compared with conventional venography in diagnosis. Radiology 1996; 200:423–428.

140. Mandelli V, Schmid C, Zogno C, Morpurgo M. "False negatives" and "false positives" in acute pulmonary embolism: a clinical-postmortem comparison. Cardiologia 1997; 42:205–210.

141. Remy-Jardin M, Remy J. Spiral CT angiography of the pulmonary circulation. Radiology 1999; 212:615–636.

142. Stein PD, Athanasoulis C, Alavi A, Greenspan RH, Hales CA, Saltzman HA, Vreim CE, Terrin ML, Weg JG. Complications and validity of pulmonary angiography in acute pulmonary embolism. Circulation 1992; 85:462–468.

143. Zuckerman DA, Sterling KM, Oser RF. Safety of pulmonary angiography in the 1990s. J Vasc Interv Radiol 1996; 7:199–205.

144. Woodard PK. Pulmonary arteries must be seen before they can be assessed. Radiology 1997; 204:11–12.

145. Diffin DC, Leyendecker JR, Johnson SP, Zucker RJ, Grebe PJ. Effect of anatomic distribution of pulmonary emboli on interobserver agreement in the interpretation of pulmonary angiography. Am J Roentgenol 1998; 171:1085–1089.

146. Worsley DF, Alavi A. Comprehensive analysis of the results of the PIOPED study. J Nucl Med 1995; 36:2380–2387.

147. Chasen MH. Practical applications of Mach band theory in thoracic analysis. Radiology 2001; 219(3):596–610.

148. Carr JJ, Reed JC, Choplin RH, Pope Th O Jr. Case DL. Plain and computed radiography for detecting experimentally induced pneumothorax in cadavers: implications for detection in patients. Radiology 1992; 183:193–199.

149. Fajardo LL, Hillman BJ, Pond GD, Carmody RF, Johnson JE, Ferrell WR. Detection of pneumothorax: comparison of digital and conventional chest imaging. Am J Roentgenol 1989; 152:475–480.

150. Tocino IM, Miller MH, Fairfax WR. Distribution of pneumothorax in the supine and semirecumbent critically ill adult. Am J Roentgenol 1985; 144(5):901–905.

151. Swischuk L. Two lesser known but useful signs of neonatal pneumothorax. Radiology 1976; 127:623–627.

152. Macklin NT, Maclin CC. Malignant interstitial emphysema of lungs and mediastinum as important occult complications in many respiratory diseases and other conditions. Medicine 1994; 23:281–358.
153. Wintermark M, Wicky S, Schnyder P, Capasso P. Blunt traumatic pneumomediastinum using CT to reveal the Macklin effect. Am J Roentgenol 1999; 172(1):129–130.
154. Kemper AC, Steinberg KP, Stern EJ. Pulmonary interstitial emphysema: CT findings. Am J Roentgenol 1999; 172:1642–1644.
155. Levin B. The continuous diaphragm sign—a newly recognized sign of pneumomediastinum. Clin Radiol 1973; 24:337–338.
156. Naclerio EA. The "V" sign in the diagnosis of spontaneous rupture of the esophagus (an early clue). Am J Surg 1957; 93:291–294.
157. Marom EM, McAdams HP, Erasmus JJ, Goodman PC. The many faces of pulmonary aspiration. Am J Roentgenol 1999; 172:121–128.
158. Franquet T, Giménez A, Rosón N, Torrubia S, Sabaté JM, Pérez C. Aspiration diseases: findings, pitfalls, and differential diagnosis. Radiographics 2000; 20:673–685.
159. Gondouin A, Manzoni P, Ranfaing E, Brun J, Cadranel J, Sadoun D, Cordier JF, Depierre A, Dalphin JC. Exogenous lipoid pneumonia: a retrospective multicentre study of 44 cases in France. Eur Resp J 1996; 9:1463–1469.
160. Franquet T, Giménez A, Bordes R, Rodriguez-Arias JM, Castella J. The crazy-paving pattern in exogenous lipoid pneumonia: CT-pathologic correlation. Am J Roentgenol 1997; 170:315–317.
161. Lee KS, Müller NL, Hale V, Newell JDJ, Lynch DA, Im JG. Lipoid pneumonia: CT findings. J Comput Assist Tomogr 1995; 19:48–51.
162. Bynum LD, Pierce AK. Pulmonary aspiration of gastric contents. Am Rev Resp Dis 1976; 114:1129–1136.
163. DePaso WJ. Aspiration pneumonia. Clin Chest Med 1991; 12:269–284.
164. Groskin SA, Panicek DM, Ewing DK, Rivera F, Math K, Teixeira J, Heitzman ER, Markarian B. Bacterial lung abscess: a review of the clinical and radiographic features of 50 cases. J Thorac Imaging 1991; 6:62–67.
165. David P, Denis P, Nouvet G, Pasquis P, Lefrancois R, Morere P. Fonction respiratoire et reflux gastro-oesophagien au cours de la bronchite chronique. Bull Eur Physiopathol Respir 1982; 18:81–86.
166. Ayres JG, Miles JF. Oesophageal reflux and asthma. Eur Respir J 1996; 9:1073–1078.
167. Matsuse T, Oka T, Kida K, Fukuchi Y. Importance of diffuse aspiration caused by chronic occult aspiration in the elderly. Chest 1996; 110:1289–1293.
168. Arakawa H, Webb WR. Air trapping on expiratory high-resolution CT scans in the absence of inspiratory scan abnormalities: correlation with pulmonary function tests and differential diagnosis. Am J Roentgenol 1998; 170:1349–1353.
169. Kauczor HU, Chen XJ, van Beek EJ, Schreiber WG. Pulmonary ventilation imaged by magnetic resonance: at the door step of clinical application. Eur Respir J, 2001; 17(5):1008–1023.
170. Schreiber WG, Eberle B, Laukemper-Ostendorf S, Markstaller K, Weiler N, Scholz A, Burger K., Heussel CP, Thelen M, Kauczor HU. Dynamic (19)F-MR1 of pulmonary ventilation using sulfur hexafluoride (SF(6) gas. Magn Reson Med 2001; 45(4):605–613.
171. Kauczor HU, Markstaller K, Puderbach M, Lill J, Eberle B, Hanisch G, Grossman T, Heussel CP, Schreiber W, Thelen M. Volumetry of ventilated airspaces by 3He MRI: preliminary results. Invest Radiol 2001; 36(2):110–142.

13

Assessment of Severity of Acute Exacerbations of Chronic Obstructive Pulmonary Disease

CRAIG A. PIQUETTE and STEPHEN I. RENNARD

University of Nebraska Medical Center
Omaha, Nebraska, U.S.A.

I. Introduction

There are several reasons to assess the severity of COPD exacerbations. First, assessment of severity can be helpful clinically to triage the patient to the appropriate level of medical care. It helps the physician target the intensity of therapy and may help to prognosticate patient outcomes. Second, a severity assessment may be helpful from a health-care economic standpoint. In a single-payer health-care system, resources can be directed to areas based on the numbers and severity of exacerbations. In a third-party payer system, payment might be tied to the severity level of the exacerbation. Finally, assessment of the severity of an exacerbation could provide a standard by which various studies of exacerbation can be compared. This is important for evaluating new therapies and for examining the natural history of the disease.

COPD is a heterogeneous collection of conditions characterized by the progressive loss of lung function associated with the insidious limitation of physical activity and development of symptoms. Superimposed on this inexorable, but gradual, decline are exacerbations when a patient is acutely, but transiently, worse for a period of days to weeks. Not only is COPD heterogeneous, but exacerbations are as well. A diverse set of etiologies can lead to worsening, which can manifest a variety of clinical presentations and follow variable natural histories. Not surprisingly, no completely satisfactory definition of an exacerbation or a system to gauge exacerbation severity has emerged.

The situation, however, is not entirely hopelessly confused. Many, if not the majority, of exacerbations are characterized by increased inflammation of the lower respiratory tract, suggesting a set of measures for both classifying and for staging exacerbations. Exacerbations, despite the semantic difficulties, appear to be a robust clinical endpoint. A variety of clinical interventions have been demonstrated to affect measures of clinical status including health status, health-care resource utilization, and mortality. That various studies of exacerbations reveal similar results despite the difficulty of defining exacerbations suggests they are a highly relevant and robust clinical feature of COPD. Perhaps what is required is a better nosology reflecting the diversity of exacerbations rather than a single unifying definition and severity scale.

II. Definition of an Exacerbation

Exacerbations of COPD are well recognized by clinicians but opinions vary on what defines an exacerbation. A number of definitions have been offered for the exacerbation of COPD but currently there is no consensus (1). Most clinicians would agree that an exacerbation is a relatively sudden and prolonged worsening of symptoms in a patient with COPD. These patients are often older and have or are at risk for other comorbidities. The American Thoracic Society statement on COPD states that "Accurate diagnosis (of an acute exacerbation) in a patient experiencing rapid deterioration of respiratory function may be confounded by underlying myocardial ischemia, congestive heart failure, thromboemboli or recurrent aspiration, which can simulate an exacerbation of airway disease" (2). Clearly, the ability to diagnose the presence of an exacerbation depends on the assessment of the individual patient and knowledge of preexisting conditions. The European Respiratory Society Consensus Statement adds: "During exacerbations, the clinical findings depend on the degree of additional airflow limitation, the severity of the underlying COPD, and the presence of coexisting conditions" (3).

Many clinical studies investigating exacerbations of COPD have used a definition based on symptoms established by Anthonisen and colleagues for their landmark study on the use of antibiotics in exacerbations of COPD (4). They defined a type I exacerbation as the presence of increased sputum volume, increased sputum purulence, and increased dyspnea. A type II exacerbation was defined as the presence of two of the above symptoms. A type III exacerbation was defined as the presence of only one of these symptoms. This study identified a group of patients more likely to benefit from the use of antibiotics to treat their exacerbation. Others have extended Anthonisen's original definition of exacerbations by defining increased sputum volume, increased sputum purulence, and increased dyspnea as major symptoms and have included minor symptoms, such as increase in nasal discharge, wheeze, sore throat, cough, or fever in the definition (5). This expanded definition of an exacerbation required two of the three major symptoms or one of the

Table 1 Investigational Definitions of Exacerbation

Anthonisen[a]	*Seemungal*[b]

Two or more of the following symptoms
  Increased dyspnea
  Increased sputum volume
  Increased sputum purulence
	Major symptoms
	  Increased dyspnea
	  Increased sputum volume
	  Increased sputum purulence
	Minor symptoms
	  Nasal discharge/congestion
	  Wheeze
	  Cough
	  Sore throat
	  Fever
	Requires two major symptoms or one major
	  and one minor symptom

[a]Ref. 4
[b]Ref. 5

major symptoms and any one of the minor symptoms. Exacerbations based on different sets of symptoms, particularly if related to the nose and throat, may reflect different etiologies (see Table 1). This definition has not been standardized and consensus is required to advance the field of exacerbation research. Recently, a group of experts convened and arrived at a consensus definition (6). "An exacerbation is a sustained worsening of the patient's condition from the stable state and beyond normal day-to-day variations that is acute in onset and necessitates a change in regular medication in a patient with underlying COPD." Such a definition has operational validity. However, patients may be more or less likely to seek or receive new medications depending on many factors, including access to health care, local reimbursement practices, concurrent depression, and social support. Moreover, a definition requiring an increase in medication is likely to miss milder exacerbations as well as exacerbations in patients with less severe disease.

III. Definition of Severity

Several scales can be used to judge the severity of an exacerbation. As noted above, a staging system for severity of the exacerbation based on health-care utilization has been proposed (6). A mild exacerbation is defined as one in which the patient has an increased need for medication but can manage the exacerbation in the home environment; a moderate exacerbation is one in which the patient needs to seek additional medical assistance to manage the exacerbation, and a severe exacerbation requires hospitalization. This definition of severity is not ideal as it depends on the discretion of the patient to decide if symptoms are severe enough to seek medical attention. Until we have better means for patients to track the development of an exacerbation and its severity, however, this may be the best definition.

IV. Clinical Assessment

Worsening of symptoms and alterations in physiological homeostasis are key components of an exacerbation. Among the symptoms to assess at the time of presentation are cough, quantity and purulence of sputum, dyspnea, wheezing, chest tightness, fever, and the ability to perform activities of daily living (4, 7). Other nonspecific symptoms may be present, including malaise, depression, fatigue, insomnia, sleepiness, and confusion (8). The most important physical findings reflect the patient's work of breathing. This assessment includes observing the presence of a prolonged expiratory phase indicating worsening airway obstruction, the use of accessory muscles, respiratory rate, breathing pattern, and the presence of tripoding, a position assumed by using the arms or elbows to support a forward-leaning chest. A loud pulmonary component of the second heart sound or increasing peripheral edema may be a clue to worsening cor pulmonale and right heart failure (9). Diagnostic tests to assess the severity of the exacerbation should include pulmonary function tests, arterial blood gases, blood chemistry to include electrolytes, complete blood cell count, and a chest roentgenogram. The three latter tests help to elucidate any comorbid conditions that may be complicating or mimicking the presentation of an exacerbation. If the symptoms or the physiological derangements are severe enough or comorbidities complicate the therapy, admission to the hospital is advised. A number of published guidelines suggest indications for admission to the hospital (see Table 2) (2, 3, 8, 10).

V. Predicting Patient Outcomes

A. Risk Factors for Admission

The level of health-care utilization by a COPD patient experiencing sudden worsening of symptoms defines exacerbation severity using the proposal of Rodriguez-Roisin and colleagues. Factors that contribute to increased frequency of exacerbation and/or hospitalizations, will affect exacerbation severity. Several studies have addressed this issue. Among the factors that led to relapse or treatment failure of an exacerbation, in a study reported by Dewan and colleagues, were stage III COPD denoted by an $FEV_1 < 35\%$ of predicted normal value, use of home oxygen, the frequency of exacerbations over the previous 24 months, the average cumulative steroid dose over 24 months, history of previous pneumonia, and history of sinusitis (11). Individuals with these risk factors, therefore, are more likely to be hospitalized and, by the system of Rodriguez-Roisin, to have severe exacerbations.

Adams and colleagues, evaluating relapse at 2 weeks following treatment of an acute exacerbation, found that use of amoxicillin increased the rate of relapse while all other antibiotics decreased the risk of relapse (12). Coronary heart disease and active smoking both contributed to an increased risk of relapse in this study as well. Ball et al. reported that a history of greater than four chest infections per year and a history of cardiopulmonary disease were associated with an increased risk of relapse and cardiopulmonary disease was also associated with increased risk for admission

Table 2 Guidelines for Admission to Hospital and ICU

Indication	Guideline
Hospital admission	
Marked increase in intensity of symptoms (e.g., resting dyspnea, inability to perform activities of daily living)	ATS, BTS, ERS, GOLD
Failure to respond to outpatient management	ATS, BTS, ERS, GOLD
Onset of new physical signs (e.g., cyanosis, peripheral edema, cor pulmonale)	ATS, BTS, ERS, GOLD
Insufficient home support	ATS, BTS, GOLD
Altered mentation	ATS, BTS, ERS, GOLD
Significant comorbid conditions (e.g., older age, changes on CXR, steroid myopathy, compression fractures, planned procedure requiring sedation/analgesia)	ATS, BTS, GOLD
Severe background COPD (e.g., requires LTOT, etc.)	BTS, GOLD
pH < 7.35	BTS
Diagnostic uncertainty	GOLD
Newly occurring arrhythmias	GOLD
ICU admission[a]	
Severe dyspnea that responds adequately to initial emergency therapy	ATS, GOLD
Confusion, lethargy, coma or respiratory muscle fatigue (paradoxical abdominal motion)	ATS, ERS, GOLD
Persistent or worsening hypoxemia ($PaO_2 < 6.7$ kPa or < 50 mmHg) despite supplemental O_2 or severe/worsening hypercapnia ($PaCO_2 > 9.3$ kPa or 70 mmHg) or severe/worsening respiratory acidosis (pH < 7.30) despite supplemental O_2 and NIPPV	ATS, GOLD
Assisted mechanical ventilation is required (ETT or NIPPV)	ATS

ATS = American Thoracic Society; BTS = British Thoracic Society; ERS = European Respiratory Society; GOLD = Global Initiative for Chronic Obstructive Lung Disease.
[a]BTS did not provide guidelines on ICU admission.

to the hospital (13). Miravitlles and colleagues found that increasing age, severity of FEV_1 impairment, and the presence of chronic mucus hypersecretion were independently associated with the increased risk of having two or more acute exacerbations of COPD per year (14). They also found that FEV_1 impairment was associated with increased risk of hospital admission, as was the presence of comorbidity such as diabetes mellitus, congestive heart failure, or ischemic heart disease.

Kessler et al. evaluated 64 patients presenting for exacerbation of COPD for predictive factors of hospitalization (15). These patients were enrolled in the stable state and followed for at least 2.5 years. The criteria for hospitalization were those outlined by the ATS guidelines. They found that a low body mass index (BMI < 20 kg/m^2), a decreased PaO_2 and increased $PaCO_2$ and an increased mean pulmonary artery pressure were associated with significantly increasing rates of hospitalization at 1 year. Garcia-Aymerich et al. found that the most frequent risk factors for exacerbation were lack of pulmonary rehabilitation in the previous year and a poor working knowledge of metered-dose-inhaler technique (16). Thus, the severity of both the underlying COPD and comorbid conditions contribute to the risk of relapse following outpatient treatment and to the hospitalization rate.

B. Risk Factors for Mortality

Admission for an exacerbation indicates increased severity, but factors that predict mortality suggest extreme severity. One of the most comprehensive outcome studies for acute exacerbations of COPD is the SUPPORT trial (17). All patients enrolled in this trial were expected to have a 20 to 80% chance of dying in the following 6 months. Consequently, the COPD patients had to have breathlessness, respiratory failure, or change in mental status due to exacerbation and documentation of hypercapnia ($PaCO_2 \geq 50\,mmHg$) on the day of admission or within the previous week. There were eight variables that demonstrated a significant independent relationship to survival in a multivariate analysis. Those variables and differences were a 10-point difference in the acute physiological score (Apache III); a difference of 1 point in the Katz Activities of Daily Living (ADL) scale; a 5-kg/m^2 difference in the body mass index (BMI); a difference of 1 g/dL in albumin level; a 10-year difference in age; a 100-mm difference in the PaO_2/FiO_2 (P/F) ratio; the presence of cor pulmonale and congestive heart failure as a cause of the acute exacerbation. A lower acute physiology score, lower ADL score, lower age, higher BMI, higher albumin, higher P/F ratio, cor pulmonale, and CHF were all associated with higher survival.

In a smaller study of 270 patients exploring the role of comorbidity on mortality for COPD, Antonelli Incalzi and colleagues found that age, ECG signs of right ventricular failure or ischemic heart disease, and chronic renal failure were associated with an increased rate of death (18). Connors et al. did not find that a history of cardiac disease or the number of comorbid illnesses were associated with a higher death rate in patients admitted for exacerbation of COPD. These studies suggest that in older, less functional, and more malnourished patients without evidence of cardiac disease the risk of death is much higher. Consequently, these factors are indicative of the most severe exacerbations.

C. Symptoms

Symptom scores were measured in a group of 10 asthma and 61 COPD patients at baseline and during an exacerbation of their disease (19). Symptoms of wheeze or dyspnea, cough with mucus production, cough without mucus production, and awakening with dyspnea were recorded using a 4-point scale ranging from 0 to 3. The mean severity score at baseline was 0.6 and on the day of presentation for exacerbation rose to approximately 1.4 and returned to baseline at approximately day 10 or 11.

One-hundred-one COPD patients recorded changes in daily symptoms on diary cards in a study by Seemungal and colleagues (5). Major symptoms were dyspnea, sputum purulence, and sputum amount while minor symptoms were wheeze, sore throat, cough, and nasal congestion or discharge. Symptoms increased dramatically on the day of onset of exacerbation. Symptoms of dyspnea were part of the presentation in 64% of exacerbations, sputum purulence in 42%, wheeze in 35%, nasal congestion or discharge in 35%, sputum volume in 26%, cough in 20% and sore throat in 12%. Increased dyspnea and increased wheeze or cold symptoms were associated with a greater decrease in peak expiratory flow rate (PEFR). Presentations with dyspnea or cold symptoms (nasal congestion/discharge) were associated with longer recovery times while presentations with wheeze or sore throat had shorter recovery times. Prednisolone had no effect on recovery times of the symptom score. The median time to recovery of symptom scores was 7 days. Dyspnea was the greatest indicator symptom of severity, but this study also defined cold symptoms as having an impact on severity. However, symptoms alone do not provide a complete picture of exacerbation severity. Therefore, physiological measures of gas exchange must be made to contribute to the decision-making process for intensity of therapy.

VI. Physiological Measurements

A. Arterial Blood Gases

Arterial blood gases are recommended and frequently obtained at presentation of an acute exacerbation. Emerman and colleagues have demonstrated that spirometry cannot reliably predict results of arterial blood gases, but there was a moderate correlation between $PaCO_2$ and the FEV_1 and the percent predicted FEV_1 (20). Hypercapnia is felt to be a poor prognostic sign but it has been recognized that some patients with COPD develop hypercapnia only with acute exacerbations. Costello et al. investigated long-term outcomes of patients who have reversible hypercapnia (21). They found no significant difference in the $PaCO_2$ on room air or on low-flow oxygen obtained on admission from a patient who survived versus one who did not. Patients with irreversible hypercapnia had significantly worse survival over 5 years than did patients who were nonhypercapnic or those who had reversible hypercapnia. Also, patients with reversible hypercapnia did not progress to chronic hypercapnia over time. In this study, hypercapnia did not predict survival of an admission for COPD and this corroborates earlier work that determined that $PaCO_2$ independent of pH did not influence the prognosis during an acute exacerbation (22). Recent guidelines suggest that respiratory failure is present when $PaO_2 < 60$ mmHg or $SaO_2 < 90\%$ on room air and that pH < 7.30, $PaO_2 < 50$ mmHg and $PaCO_2 > 70$ mmHg indicate a life-threatening exacerbation requiring intensive monitoring (see Table 3) (8).

B. Measures of Cardiac Function

COPD patients presenting with symptoms of exacerbation should be evaluated for the presence of cor pulmonale and other signs of cardiac compromise. Data from the SUPPORT trial demonstrated that congestive heart failure as a cause of the exacerbation and cor pulmonale were predictive of longer survival in patients

Table 3 Physiological Signs of Exacerbation Severity

	Severity	
Sign	Moderate	Severe
pH	< 7.35	< 7.30
$PaCO_2$		> 70 mmHg
PaO_2		< 50 mmHg
ECG		S1, S2, S3
		P axis > +90°
Post-treatment FEV_1		< 40% predicted normal

predicted to have higher mortality, based on the entry criteria for the trial (17). Cor pulmonale was felt to be present if there were two or more of the following clinical signs: right ventricular hypertrophy or right atrial enlargement on electrocardiogram; enlarged pulmonary arteries on chest roentgenogram; pedal edema; jugular venous distention; or a mean pulmonary artery pressure > 20 mmHg, measured by pulmonary artery catheter. In this study, heart failure was felt to be the cause of exacerbation in 25.7% of patients, with arrhythmias accounting for 4.8% of exacerbations. This represents a relatively large proportion of exacerbations for which the etiology would be undetermined if cardiac function is not assessed.

In a study by Antonelli Incalzi and colleagues, patients with ECG signs of cor pulmonale were more likely to be younger, but with a longer length of hospital stay following an exacerbation, were more likely to have been on mechanical ventilation during their exacerbation, and more likely to have a history of systolic hypertension (23). Patients with cor pulmonale had a lower PaO_2 on room air and during oxygen therapy and had a higher $PaCO_2$ on room air. The ECG patterns with the strongest predictive factors for death included the S1, S2, S3 pattern and right atrial overload indicated by a P-wave axis of plus 90 degrees or more. A shorter survival occurred in patients who had at least one ECG sign of chronic cor pulmonale and an A-a gradient of > 48 mmHg. This increased mortality with chronic cor pulmonale contrasts with the SUPPORT trial, showing improved survival with cor pulmonale; however, SUPPORT used clinical signs rather than the specific ECG signs to define the presence of cor pulmonale.

Pulmonary artery catheterization is a much more accurate measure of pulmonary hypertension in patients with exacerbation of COPD. However, the use of pulmonary artery catheterization has recently come under scrutiny. Using a decision analysis model, Smith and Pesce determined that pulmonary artery catheterization in patients with exacerbation of COPD was not cost effective, even under conditions that favored the use of the pulmonary artery catheter (24). Noninvasive measures of pulmonary artery pressures are well correlated with the pulmonary artery catheter. However, echocardiograms done in COPD patients are often technically difficult because the Doppler-detected tricuspid regurgitation jet is often lacking (25). Measures of cardiac function at presentation with acute exacerbation of COPD may be helpful for predicting long-term outcome but not severity of the exacerbation itself.

C. Chest X-Ray

The chest radiograph (posterior/anterior plus lateral views) can be used to identify alternative diagnoses that simulate an acute exacerbation of COPD. They may also be predictive of airflow obstruction but cannot replace objective measurements of airflow (26). Evaluation of the chest radiograph has not been correlated with the severity of the exacerbation.

D. Pulmonary Function

Measures of airflow obstruction such as FEV_1 and peak expiratory flow rate (PEFR) are markers of severity of COPD and these measures worsen during an exacerbation. Emerman et al. demonstrated that a post-treatment FEV_1 of $< 40\%$ predicted normal, at the time of presentation with exacerbation, identified patients who either required hospital admission or subsequently relapsed (27). The sensitivity and specificity were 0.96 and 0.58, respectively, the positive predictive value was 0.73, and the overall accuracy of this measurement was 0.78. The area under the receiver operating characteristic curve using the post-treatment FEV_1 was 0.81. A post-treatment FEV_1 of $< 70\%$ of the baseline FEV_1 at initial presentation identified a later admission for relapse with a sensitivity of 0.83 and a specificity of 0.56. This study also demonstrated that physicians' estimates of lung function were poor and physicians tended to overestimate the FEV_1 (28). This suggests that an objective measure of lung function should be made on presentation with an exacerbation. Vitacca has shown that a discriminant equation including an index of nutritional status and FVC had a 76% accuracy rate, with a 64% positive predictive value to predict the need for mechanical ventilation in patients admitted for exacerbation of COPD (29). Thus FEV_1 and FVC may be important for evaluating the severity of the exacerbation.

The drop in lung function from baseline levels may also be predictive of the severity of the exacerbation. Sachs et al. measured PEFR in a group of 10 asthma and 61 COPD patients at baseline and during an exacerbation of their disease (19). At the time of presentation for exacerbation, PEFR had decreased approximately 20% from baseline. It was then measured daily through the course of the exacerbation. After 14 days, PEFR had risen to within 95% of the baseline values. In a similar study, Seemungal and colleagues followed 101 patients over two-and-a-half years to determine the time course of recovery of exacerbations (5). They demonstrated that a greater fall in PEFR, FEV_1, and forced vital capacity (FVC) was related to the respective recovery time of these parameters. On the day of presentation, PEFR had fallen by a median 8.6 L/min, FEV_1 fell by 24 mL, and FVC fell by 76 mL; all decreases were highly significant. The medium time to recover was 6 days, with 75.2% of exacerbations recovering within 35 days. The use of steroids increased the rate of recovery of PEFR. This corroborated previous findings (30, 31). Bhowmik et al., in a group of COPD patients who were part of the same cohort in the study by Seemungal et al., demonstrated a decrease in FEV_1, measured during stable conditions at 1.07 L down to 0.99 L at the time of exacerbation (32). PEFR fell from 239 L/min to 225 L/min at the time of exacerbation. The magnitude of the fall in lung function at the time of exacerbation is predictive of the time to recovery, and recovery is hastened by the use of steroids. Presumably this would be due to the downregulation of the inflammatory processes that are thought to play a role in many exacerbations.

VII. Biological Inflammatory Markers of Exacerbations

As we have seen from the discussion of the definition of an exacerbation, an increase in symptoms is an important determinant of when the exacerbation starts and its severity. The etiology of exacerbations has been reviewed elsewhere, but most exacerbations are caused by infection or some other mechanism that alters gas exchange homeostasis (3). Inflammation plays a key role in most exacerbations. Thus, many investigators have pursued measurements of inflammatory markers as a means of determining when an exacerbation is present and of assessing its severity. A noninvasive means of measuring these inflammatory markers is most readily applicable clinically. Hence, sputum and serum are the most frequently evaluated fluids. How to compare values obtained by such means among patients or in a given patient at different times, however, is unclear. Among the markers that have been evaluated are the absolute and relative numbers of inflammatory cells, the color of expectorated sputum, C-reactive protein, cytokines and their soluble receptors, proteins released from inflammatory cells, and the acute-phase reactants (see Table 4). A discussion of these follows.

A. Inflammatory Cells

Neutrophils have been found in large amounts in the airways of patients with chronic bronchitis and are retained in the lung for longer periods of time in patients with active symptoms of COPD (33, 34). Neutrophils have also been found in higher amounts in BAL and blood from patients with an exacerbation of chronic bronchitis versus patients under baseline conditions (35). The neutrophil plays an important role in the inflammation that develops during an exacerbation of COPD and there are increasing numbers in sputum and blood, an indication of ongoing and acute inflammation.

The eosinophil plays an important role in the airway inflammation that is present in patients with asthma but it may also contribute to the development of airway inflammation in chronic bronchitis. Eosinophils are present in the mucosa of the airways in chronic bronchitis and increase dramatically during exacerbations (36, 37). The numbers of the eosinophils in the sputum also increase during exacerbations compared with baseline.

In summary, in exacerbations of COPD there are airway neutrophilia and eosinophilia but the absolute numbers have not been correlated with the severity of the exacerbation. Such studies are urgently needed.

Table 4 Biological Markers of Exacerbation

Sputum, BAL, or Biopsy	Serum	Urine
Increased neutrophils	Increased neutrophils	Increased desmosine
Increased eosinophils	Increased eosinophils	Increased isodesmosine
Increased leukotriene B4	Increased fibrinogen	
Increased myeloperoxidase	Increased endothelin-1	
Increased eosinophil cationic protein	Increased C-reactive protein	
Increased elastase		Breath
Decreased SLPI		Increased nitric oxide
Increased α_1-protease inhibitor		
Increased endothelin-1		

Increased Cytokines/Cytokine Receptors		
GM-CSF	GM-CSF	
TNF-α	IL-6	
IL-6	TNF-R55	
IL-8	TNF-R75	
RANTES	IL-1RII	
	sFas	

B. Cytokines

Cytokines such as the interleukins (IL) mediate the inflammatory response in the airways. These intercellular signals are released in response to an inflammatory stimulus and initiate cellular mechanisms that amplify or modulate the inflammatory response. Cytokine levels can be measured in sputum and in serum and may be used to track the inflammatory response.

C. Tumor Necrosis Factor-α

Many cells in the airway release tumor necrosis factor-α (TNF-α) in response to infection or other stimulus. TNF-α release is one of the initial steps in the inflammatory pathway and levels are found to be elevated in sputum from patients with COPD exacerbation relative to baseline (38). In exacerbations caused by *Haemophilus influenza* and *Moraxella catarrhalis*, Aaron and colleagues found that mean concentrations of TNF-α rose from 404 pg/mL at baseline up to 1649 pg/mL at the time of the exacerbation and then fell back to baseline 1 month later. Sethi and colleagues found that TNF-α measured at the time of the exacerbation had a 25th/75th interquartile range (IQR) from 0 to 1250 pg/mL (39). In neither study was TNF-α measured throughout the time course of exacerbation, and was not evaluated for correlation with an assessment of severity of the exacerbation.

D. Granulocytes/Macrophage Colony-Stimulating Factor

Maturation of granulocytes and monocytes is under the control of several growth factors including granulocyte/macrophage colony-stimulating factor (GM-CSF). Balbi and colleagues measured serum levels of GM-CSF in patients with chronic bronchitis during an exacerbation and compared them with patients under baseline conditions (35). Bronchoalveolar lavage (BAL) levels were also measured. Serum levels of GM-CSF in patients with stable chronic bronchitis were 1.4 pg/mL and levels in BAL fluid were 25 pg/mL. When measured in patients during an exacerbation, GM-CSF levels in serum were 13 pg/mL and in BAL were 54 pg/mL. The levels of GM-CSF in this study were not evaluated for correlation with the severity of the exacerbation.

E. Interleukin-5 and RANTES

Interleukin-5 promotes maturation and survival of eosinophils and enhances their adherence to vascular endothelium. As noted above, eosinophilia is present during exacerbations of chronic bronchitis. Saetta and colleagues also evaluated the expression of IL-5 in patients with exacerbations of bronchitis and at baseline conditions (40). They found that although there were increased numbers of eosinophils in the bronchial biopsies of patients with chronic bronchitis during exacerbations compared to baseline, there was no increase in the number of IL-5-positive cells between chronic bronchitis patients at baseline and during an exacerbation. Zhu and colleagues demonstrated that there are increased numbers of eosinophils in the mucosa of patients with an exacerbation of chronic bronchitis compared to stable chronic bronchitis and control patients (37). They also demonstrated an increase in RANTES in chronic bronchitis patients during stable conditions and a further increase during exacerbation.

RANTES is another cytokine that promotes chemotaxis of inflammatory cells and viruses and bacteria increases its expression. An association was demonstrated between the number of eosinophils and the number of cells expressing RANTES in mucosal biopsies (37). This evidence suggests that RANTES and not IL-5 may be responsible for the eosinophilia seen in chronic bronchitis. Neither RANTES nor IL-5 levels have been evaluated for correlation with the severity of exacerbations of COPD.

F. Interleukin-6

This cytokine induces the production of many acute-phase reactants by the hepatocytes. Wedzicha and colleagues have demonstrated that IL-6 levels in plasma from patients with stable chronic bronchitis at baseline were approximately 4 pg/mL increasing to 6 pg/mL at the time of exacerbation and returning to baseline levels later (41). The levels in sputum demonstrated by Bhowmik and colleagues increased from stable levels of 65 pg/mL up to 122.7 pg/mL during an exacerbation (32). IL-6 levels were also found to correlate with frequency of exacerbations. Those patients with higher levels during stable periods were more likely to exacerbate more frequently. Cough and cold symptoms were associated with increased sputum IL-6 levels compared with sputum levels during the absence of those symptoms. There was no significant relationship between IL-6 levels and severity of exacerbation or the time to recovery of the peak expiratory flow to baseline values in these patients.

G. Interleukin-8

Interleukin-8 is a powerful chemotactic factor for neutrophils and, as neutrophils are present in greater numbers during exacerbations of COPD, it might be expected that interleukin-8 levels would precede this rise in neutrophil numbers. Two groups have recently demonstrated this. Aaron and colleagues demonstrated that IL-8 in sputum rose from 69.8 ng/mL at baseline to 127.3 ng/mL at the time of exacerbation, returning to 67.2 ng/mL when measured 1 month later (38). Sethi and his colleagues found IL-8 in sputum was elevated in patients with an exacerbation due to *Haemophilus influenza* and the 25th/75th interquartile range was from 11,000 pg/mL to 20,000 pg/mL (39). The levels of IL-8 in these two studies differ, but they were not evaluated for correlation with an assessment of the severity of exacerbation in individual patients or as a group. Therefore, it is difficult to extrapolate that higher IL-8 levels indicate a more severe exacerbation.

Stockley and colleagues found IL-8 levels in stable chronic bronchitis patients varied between 4.02 nM and 6.05 nM and in another study found that sputum IL-8 in COPD subjects during acute exacerbation was 10.4 nM versus 30.9 nM in COPD patients with α_1-antitrypsin (AAT) deficiency during exacerbation (42, 43). IL-8 levels, in sputum of COPD patients with AAT deficiency experiencing an exacerbation, dropped to baseline levels by day 7. The baseline in these patients was 12.6 nM and at resolution on day 28 was measured at 10.4 nM (42). Culpitt and colleagues found that inhaled steroids in stable COPD patients did not significantly decrease IL-8 levels (44). Patients with frequent exacerbations had IL-8 levels during stable conditions of 6694 pg/mL and those with infrequent exacerbations had a median IL-8 level of 1628 pg/mL (32). This same relationship was also demonstrated for IL-6. When the results for the frequent and infrequent exacerbators in this study were pooled, the median IL-8 levels in stable chronic bronchitis patients were 3953 pg/mL, increasing to 4085 pg/mL during exacerbation. These results contrast with those of Aaron and colleagues, who processed the sputum in a different manner but measured IL-8 using the same method (38). Fourteen COPD patients had mean IL-8 concentrations of 69.8 ± 26.1 ng/mL at baseline, increasing to 127.3 ± 46.2 ng/mL at the time of exacerbation. Kanazawa and colleagues found that IL-8 levels in serum correlated with the smoking index of emphysema patients but did not correlate with pulmonary function tests, although it was correlated with the degree of annual decrease in FEV_1 (45).

Levels of IL-8 in sputum are higher in patients who have more severe disease evidenced by more frequent exacerbations or earlier onset of emphysema and levels in serum correlate with the annual decline in lung function (45). Inhaled steroids had no effect on decreasing sputum IL-8 levels in stable patients, but data exist that suggest that inhaled steroids decrease exacerbation rates (46). Noting the response of

IL-8 during the evolution of an exacerbation would provide some interesting data and following the response to systemic steroids would complete the picture.

H. Cytokine Receptor Levels

During an acute inflammatory response, the levels of selected soluble cytokine receptors increase in the serum. These soluble receptors are thought to be part of the downregulation process for the acute inflammatory response. Dentener and colleagues recently measured IL-1-receptor II (IL-1RII), TNF-receptor 55 (TNF-R55), and TNF-receptor 75 (TNF-R75) levels during an exacerbation of COPD (47). They found that soluble TNF-R55 levels were higher in stable COPD patients than in healthy controls, and following exacerbations, there was a significant increase in TNF-R55 and TNF-R75 levels from day 1 to day 3 but a return to levels that were not different from day 1 at day 5 and day 7. Soluble IL-1RII levels continued to increase for 7 days following the start of the exacerbation. The exacerbations were characterized by higher $PaCO_2$ and lower PaO_2 than in the stable state and 9 of 13 patients had a bacterial infection. Presence of a positive bacterial culture was not associated with the levels of inflammatory mediators found in the serum. A significant improvement in FEV_1 was seen on days 3 and 7. The increase in soluble IL-1RII levels coincided with treatment of the exacerbation with corticosteroids and the authors suggest that "the continuous administration of corticosteroids is responsible for the increase in soluble IL-1RII levels and may thus contribute to the clinical improvement of these patients."

Schols and colleagues, investigating the relationship of resting energy expenditure (REE) to inflammatory mediators in patients with stable COPD found that soluble TNF-receptor 55 (sTNF-R55) levels were not significantly different in these patients compared with healthy subjects but sTNF-R75 levels were significantly higher in COPD patients (48). There was no significant difference in either soluble receptor level between patients with normal REE and those with high REE. Patients receiving theophylline had lower levels of both sTNF-R55 and sTNF-R75 than did patients not on theophylline. Given these data, it appears that sTNF-R and sIL-1RII levels may be correlated with therapy during an exacerbation. TNF-receptor levels, especially TNF-R75, may indicate the initial timeframe of the exacerbation, but do not appear to correlate with severity of the exacerbation.

I. Acute-Phase Reactants

One clinically important acute-phase reactant is C-reactive protein (CRP). Dev and colleagues demonstrated that CRP levels were elevated in all patients with an exacerbation associated with a recognized bacterial pathogen and in 62% of patients where no evidence of bacterial infection was present (49). Only one of the control patients had elevated CRP levels. The CRP levels correlated with the peripheral blood white-cell count and levels fell with adequate treatment of the exacerbation. Given that CRP levels were elevated in most patients who did not have evidence of a bacterial infection, the authors concluded that CRP might be a marker of COPD but not necessarily a marker for bacterial infections. Stockley and colleagues report that

CRP levels were significantly elevated in patients with an exacerbation with purulent sputum when compared to patients with an exacerbation having mucoid sputum (50). When evaluated in the stable clinical state, the CRP levels in the two groups were statistically significantly different. Hill and colleagues evaluated the time course of exacerbations in COPD patients deficient of α_1-antitrypsin (AAT) and found that CRP levels were elevated on presentation and continued to rise for the next 24 h, returning to baseline by day 3 (43) CRP levels in the AAT-deficient patients were not significantly higher than the control group (COPD patients without AAT deficiency) at the start of exacerbation. CRP levels are elevated in most exacerbations but this is not a consistent finding in individual patients and CRP levels fall as the exacerbation resolves.

Fibrinogen is also an acute-phase reactant and concentrations rise in response to infection. Wedzicha and colleagues measured fibrinogen levels in patients presenting with acute exacerbations of COPD and found a significant increase in fibrinogen levels during an exacerbation compared to the stable state (41). The fibrinogen level during an exacerbation was dependent on the level during the steady state and was higher if the exacerbation manifested with purulent sputum, increased cough, and the presence of a cold. Elevated fibrinogen levels have been found in some stable COPD patients and infection increases fibrinogen levels (51). A further increase in fibrinogen with an exacerbation increases the risk for cardiovascular events and possibly contributes to the comorbidity of the exacerbation.

J. Other Inflammatory Mediators

Leukotriene B_4 (LTB_4) is an important chemoattractant for neutrophils and is produced by the metabolism of arachidonic acid released during the acute inflammatory response. Crooks et al. studied eight patients admitted for an exacerbation of COPD and measured LTB_4 levels in the sol phase of sputum during an exacerbation and when clinically stable (≥ 2 weeks after the end of antibiotic therapy) (52). LTB_4 levels were 82.0 ± 20.8 nM at the start of the exacerbation and fell by the end of antibiotic treatment to 6.0 ± 3.1 nM. LTB_4 levels were significantly reduced at 5 days when compared to those at the onset of antibiotic treatment and rose again following cessation of antibiotic treatment. When measured during the stable period, LTB_4 levels were 10.2 ± 4.5 nM. Hill et al. compared LTB_4 levels in COPD patients at the start of exacerbation with levels in patients with alpha-1 antitrypsin deficiency experiencing an exacerbation of COPD. They found that LTB_4 levels were higher in the COPD patients with AAT deficiency, 15.9 ± 4.9 nM versus 33.2 ± 8.3 nM. They also found that LTB_4 levels in the AAT-deficient patients fell from the time of presentation after initiation of antibiotic therapy, reaching their lowest point at day 14 of antibiotics and then rose again to approximately 16 nM at day 28 (43). Gompertz et al. measured LTB_4 levels in two groups of COPD patients who were stratified by the frequency of exacerbations in 1 year. Frequent exacerbators were characterized as those having three or more exacerbations in the preceding 12 months; infrequent exacerbators had two or less in the previous year (53). There were no significant differences in the LTB_4 levels in these two groups of patients. These data suggest that although leukotriene levels in the sputum are elevated at the start of the exacerbation and fall with treatment, they do not correlate with the severity of the disease and no association with the severity of exacerbation has been demonstrated. LTB_4 levels in samples other than sputum have not been reported in this patient population.

K. Cellular Products of Neutrophils and Eosinophils

Myeloperoxidase and elastase are elaborated from neutrophils during the acute inflammatory process and the eosinophil cationic protein (ECP) is elaborated from eosinophils. Myeloperoxidase levels are higher in patients with stable COPD versus control patients and are markedly elevated at the time of an exacerbation and are not significantly different between frequent and infrequent exacerbators (53, 54). Myeloperoxidase is elevated at the time of exacerbation and decreases with treatment in COPD with or without AAT deficiency (43, 52). Stockley et al. have shown a correlation between the mean color of the sputum and the myeloperoxidase concentrations in patients with exacerbation (42). Although myeloperoxidase levels and sputum color have been shown to be associated with the onset of an exacerbation, they have not been evaluated for correlation with severity of the exacerbation.

Elastase activity has also been measured during exacerbations and found to increase at the time of presentation and decrease by day 5 (43, 52). Neutrophil elastase is also increased significantly in the presence of known respiratory pathogens, such as *Haemophilus influenza*, *Haemophilus parainfluenza*, and *Moraxella catarrhalis* (39). In this study by Sethi and colleagues, a clinical score was assessed at each visit and compared with the neutrophil elastase present in the sputum at that time. This showed a correlation between the free sputum elastase activity and the clinical score during each exacerbation. Stockley et al. demonstrated a correlation between elastase activity and myeloperoxidase (42). Thus, by inference, the myeloperoxidase levels should correlate with the severity of the exacerbation, given the results of these two studies, but this has not been evaluated directly.

Eosinophil cationic protein (ECP) is elevated in patients with stable COPD and further increased with acute exacerbation (54, 55). ECP has not been correlated with the severity of the exacerbation.

L. Sputum Antiprotease Levels

Secretory leukocyte protease inhibitor (SLPI) and α_1-protease inhibitor (α_1-PI), also known as AAT, are the most abundant antiproteases found in the airways. Stockley and colleagues found that the sputum α_1-PI concentration rose progressively through the course of an exacerbation and showed a positive relationship with the color of the sputum (50). In contrast, SLPI decreased with increasing purulence of the sputum. Gompertz found lower sputum SLPI concentrations in patients who experienced $\geq$ three exacerbations over the preceding 12 months, than those who had two or less exacerbations (53). Sputum levels of SLPI at the start of an exacerbation were lower in COPD patients with α_1-PI deficiency, compared with levels found in COPD patients. In the α_1-PI deficient patients, SLPI increased through the course of the exacerbation as elastase levels fell. The antiprotease levels were not examined in relationship to severity during the exacerbation (43).

M. Nitric Oxide

Nitric oxide is an important bronchodilator and vasodilator in the lung and is produced by the enzyme nitric oxide synthase (NOS). TNF-α increases the expression of the inducible form of this enzyme, resulting in increased nitric oxide levels during acute inflammation. Maziak measured exhaled nitric oxide in patients with chronic COPD under various conditions and in normal smokers (56). Nitric oxide levels were highest for those in the unstable COPD group, those experiencing an exacerbation, or those who had severe disease. Separating the group of 12 unstable COPD patients into those with exacerbation and those with severe disease did not demonstrate any statistically significant difference between nitric oxide levels. Agusti et al. demonstrated that nitric oxide exhaled from patients with COPD at admission for an exacerbation was higher than levels during stable conditions (57). Nitric oxide levels did not change significantly during the course of hospitalization despite the use of I.V. steroids. This is in agreement with previous studies (58). Nitric oxide levels, therefore, do not appear to correlate with the severity of the exacerbation, although it is likely that levels parallel the acute inflammation. Severity of inflammation may not correlate with the clinical symptomatology.

N. Desmosine and Isodesmosine

Degradation of mature lung elastin results in the excretion of peptides containing desmosine and isodesmosine in the urine (59). The urinary levels of these cross-linked amino acids are considered to represent the breakdown of total body elastin. Urinary desmosine levels are elevated in patients with COPD when compared to normal healthy smokers and urinary excretion of desmosine has been correlated with the decline in lung function over time (60, 61). In a recent study, Viglio et al. measured desmosine and isodesmosine levels in smokers with normal lung function, patients with stable COPD, and patients with COPD with an exacerbation (62). The levels in stable COPD were significantly elevated over those in smokers with normal lung function and were elevated even further in patients with exacerbations with COPD. Urinary desmosine and isodesmosine levels were stable over 3 days in patients with stable COPD. It is not known how these levels vary during the course of an exacerbation. The implication of these studies is that breakdown of elastin by elastases during times of chronic or acute inflammation is responsible for the decrement in lung function over time. The levels of desmosine and isodesmosine, however, have not been correlated with severity of the exacerbation.

O. Other Markers of Inflammation

Fas is a cell-surface protein that belongs to the TNF-α-receptor family and is designated as CD95. The binding of Fas ligand (Fas-L) to Fas induces apoptosis. Fas-L can be converted to a soluble form (sFas-L) by a matrix metalloproteinase and sFas-L can inhibit the binding of Fas-L to its receptor, thereby inhibiting apoptosis. Yasuda et al. recently demonstrated that plasma levels of sFas were significantly increased in severe COPD compared to mild-to-moderate COPD and healthy controls (63). In COPD patients, neither TNF-α nor IL-6 were correlated with sFas levels. Higher plasma sFas levels were associated with higher levels of dyspnea on a standardized exercise test. Patients were studied in a stable condition and correlations between sFas levels and exacerbations were not performed.

Endothelin-1 (ET-1) is a vasoconstrictive and bronchoconstrictive peptide that is produced by the bronchial epithelium, pulmonary endothelium, and alveolar macrophages. It is induced by hypoxia and viral infections, as well as by several cytokines, including TNF-α and IL-6. Roland et al., using a rolling cohort of COPD patients followed in the East London COPD study, reported an inverse correlation between stable plasma ET-1 levels and baseline FEV_1 and FVC (64). These levels were unrelated to the baseline PaO_2, $PaCO_2$, and exacerbation frequency of these patients. ET-1 levels increased significantly at exacerbation and the change in levels was universally related to the change in SaO_2, between baseline and exacerbation but not related to the symptom score. Levels of ET-1 in sputum were also measured during the stable state and during exacerbation and, with exacerbation, ET-1 levels significantly increased. The change in sputum ET-1 levels was related to the change in plasma ET-1 levels and in sputum IL-6 levels. The rise in sputum ET-1 levels was not related to the dose of inhaled corticosteroids and was not related to the symptom score.

VIII. Functional Measurements

A. Quality of Life

Health status, often termed "quality of life" is a measure that provides important information about many aspects of a COPD patient's state of health. Various instruments have been developed to investigate this parameter in COPD patients. These include general health and disease-specific measures. The most common include generic measures—the Medical Outcome Study Short Form-36, the Sickness Impact Profile, and the Nottingham Health Profile; and the disease-specific measures—the St. Georges's Respiratory Questionnaire (SGRQ) and the Chronic Respiratory Disease Questionnaire (CRQ). Current practice is to use both a disease-specific and a generic measure whenever possible (65). Ferrer and colleagues demonstrated that scores on a disease-specific measure of quality of life were associated with the categories of staging by FEV_1 as proposed by the ATS (66). Comorbid conditions contribute to the worsening of scores in the more severe stages of COPD and scores were more dependent on the severity of the COPD. Another interesting finding from this study was that in stage I disease patients with an

$FEV_1 > 50\%$ had a significant decrease in their health-related quality of life on the disease-specific measure, as compared to the normal reference group.

A severe exacerbation of COPD has been defined as one that requires admission to the hospital and two recent studies indicate that worsening health-related quality of life is associated with a greater risk for readmission to the hospital. Osman et al. administered the SGRQ to 266 patients admitted for exacerbations of COPD and found that patients who had higher scores were more likely to be readmitted or die within 12 months of the initial admission for exacerbation of COPD (67). A four-point difference in score on the SGRQ is felt to be clinically significant and this difference was achieved for all scores in this study except the activity subscore of the SGRQ (68). In a recent study of COPD patients with exacerbation randomized to hospital or home care, Davies et al. found that there was no difference in initial SGRQ scores between the two randomized groups (69). However, total scores were higher in the 32 patients who were readmitted within 3 months compared with the 58 who were not readmitted. This would suggest that the health status at the time of exacerbation reflects the severity of the disease and, consequently, the probability of admission to the hospital and severity of exacerbation.

The ISOLDE trial evaluated COPD patients with mild-to-severe disease receiving inhaled steroids or placebo and found that the rate of decline in health status was lower in the steroid-treated group (46). The mean change in the SGRQ score per year in the placebo group was 3.2 units compared with 2 units per year in the steroid-treated group. A four-point change in the SGRQ is clinically significant (68). Therefore, the time to a clinically significant change in health status was 15 months in the placebo group and 24 months in the steroid group. The rate of exacerbations was also reduced by 25% in the steroid group. This suggested that a higher exacerbation rate contributed to a decline in health status, but the relationship of exacerbation severity to this decline has not been investigated.

Seemungal and colleagues followed COPD patients closely with daily PEFR and daily respiratory symptoms for 1 year (7). The SGRQ was administered at the last clinic visit for the study. Exacerbations were diagnosed when patients reported deterioration in their symptoms compatible with an exacerbation, or a review of the diary cards revealed an unreported exacerbation. There were 184 exacerbations in 70 patients for which data were available, and the group was stratified into those with two or fewer exacerbations and those with three or more. There was strong correlation between the SGRQ total score and each of the subscores. Only 16% of the exacerbations required hospital admission and there was no relation between exacerbation frequency and hospital admission. Increased exacerbation frequency is associated with decreased health status, but health-status scores may not predict the severity of the exacerbation.

Pulmonary rehabilitation has been shown to improve scores on disease-specific health-status measures. A recent study by Behnke et al. demonstrates that, after an exacerbation of COPD, patients trained with a daily walking exercise regimen had improved health status measured by the CRQ over that of a control group (70). The CRQ was administered at baseline (during hospitalization), at 3 months, and at 6 months. This study is important in light of the findings of Garcia-Aymerich and colleagues who demonstrated in a group of patients admitted for exacerbation of COPD, that one of the most frequent risk factors for exacerbation was no pulmonary rehabilitation during the year preceding their exacerbation (16). This is indirect evidence that pulmonary rehabilitation with exercise training can improve health-status scores and may decrease exacerbations requiring hospitalization.

B. Functional Status

Functional status can be measured with physical testing or by questionnaire (71, 72). This has not been reported often in the setting of exacerbations of COPD but there are some data from the SUPPORT trial (17). Patients were asked to estimate their functional status 2 weeks prior to admission using the Katz Activities of Daily Living (ADL) Scale and the Duke Activity Status Index (DASI) (71, 72). There was a bivariable relationship to survival with both the ADL scale and the DASI. When subjected to multivariate analysis, only a lower ADL score was associated with longer survival.

In a study of nutritional support for patients hospitalized with COPD exacerbation, Saudny-Unterberger and colleagues demonstrated that respiratory muscle strength and handgrip strength were not improved with supplementation compared to controls (73). A general well-being score and FVC were improved in the treatment group. Muscle wasting as measured by nitrogen balance and handgrip strength was negatively correlated with the methylprednisolone dose. More research needs to be done before functional tests can be used to gauge the severity of an exacerbation.

IX. Summary

The severity of an exacerbation of COPD may be assessed for a variety of reasons. The clinician may want to adjust the intensity of therapy, the health economist may want to determine if quality care can be provided at a lower cost outside the hospital setting, and the researcher may want to compare results of one clinical trial with another. The scale of severity will differ based on the needs of the person making the assessment. Certain truths remain a constant, however. Acute changes in symptoms resulting in marked alterations in pH, oxygenation, hemodynamics or mental status will always require intensive therapy and monitoring. As more data become available, we may develop noninvasive tests, available clinically, which will indicate the severity of the pathophysiological mechanisms underlying the exacerbation. Then specific therapies to target those mechanisms can be used to modulate the clinical symptoms experienced by the patient during exacerbations and decrease the morbidity and mortality of this aspect of COPD.

References

1. Voelkel NF, Tuder R. COPD: exacerbation. Chest 2000; 117:376S–379S.
2. Standards for the diagnosis and care of patients with chronic obstructive pulmonary disease. American Thoracic Society. Am J Respir Crit Care Med 1995; 152:S77–121.
3. Siafakas NM, Vermeire P, Pride NB, et al. Optimal assessment and management of chronic obstructive pulmonary disease (COPD). The European Respiratory Society Task Force. Eur Respir J 1995; 8:1398–1420.
4. Anthonisen NR, Manfreda J, Warren CP, Hershfield ES, Harding GK, Nelson NA. Antibiotic therapy in exacerbations of chronic obstructive pulmonary disease. Ann Intern Med 1987; 106:196–204.
5. Seemungal TA, Donaldson GC, Bhowmik A, Jeffries DJ, Wedzicha JA. Time course and recovery of exacerbations in patients with chronic obstructive pulmonary disease. Am J Respir Crit Care Med 2000; 161:1608–1613.
6. Rodriguez-Roisin R. Toward a consensus definition for COPD exacerbations. Chest 2000; 117:398S–401S.
7. Seemungal TA, Donaldson GC, Paul EA, Bestall JC, Jeffries DJ, Wedzicha JA. Effect of exacerbation on quality of life in patients with chronic obstructive pulmonary disease. Am J Respir Crit Care Med 1998; 157:1418–1422.
8. Pauwels RA, Buist AS, Calverley PM, Jenkins CR, Hurd SS. Global strategy for the diagnosis, management, and prevention of chronic obstructive pulmonary disease. NHLBI/WHO Global Initiative for Chronic Obstructive Lung Disease (GOLD) Workshop summary. Am J Respir Crit Care Med 2001; 163:1256–1276.
9. Piquette CA, Rennard SI, Snyder GL. Chronic Bronchitis and Emphysema. In: Murray JF, Nadel JA, eds. Textbook of Respiratory Medicine. Vol. 2. Philadelphia: W.B. Saunders Co., 2000:1187–1245.
10. BTS guidelines for the management of chronic obstructive pulmonary disease. The COPD Guidelines Group of the Standards of Care Committee of the BTS. Thorax 1997; 52(Suppl 5):S1–28.
11. Dewan NA, Rafique S, Kanwar B, et al. Acute exacerbation of COPD: factors associated with poor treatment outcome. Chest 2000; 117:662–671.
12. Adams SG, Melo J, Luther M, Anzueto A. Antibiotics are associated with lower relapse rates in outpatients with acute exacerbations of COPD. Chest 2000; 117:1345–1352.
13. Ball P, Harris JM, Lowson D, Tillotson G, Wilson R. Acute infective exacerbations of chronic bronchitis. Q J Med 1995; 88:61–68.
14. Miravitlles M, Guerrero T, Mayordomo C, Sanchez-Agudo L, Nicolau F, Segu JL. Factors associated with increased risk of exacerbation and hospital admission in a cohort of ambulatory COPD patients: a multiple logistic regression analysis. The EOLO Study Group. Respiration 2000; 67:495–501.
15. Kessler R, Faller M, Fourgaut G, Mennecier B, Weitzenblum E. Predictive factors of hospitalization for acute exacerbation in a series of 64 patients with chronic obstructive pulmonary disease. Am J Respir Crit Care Med 1999; 159:158–164.
16. Garcia-Aymerich J, Barreiro E, Farrero E, Marrades RM, Morera J, Anto JM. Patients hospitalized for COPD have a high prevalence of modifiable risk factors for exacerbation (EFRAM study). Eur Respir J 2000; 16:1037–1042.
17. Connors AF, Jr., Dawson NV, Thomas C, et al. Outcomes following acute exacerbation of severe chronic obstructive lung disease. The SUPPORT investigators (Study to

Understand Prognoses and Preferences for Outcomes and Risks of Treatments). Am J Respir Crit Care Med 1996; 154:959–967.

18. Antonelli Incalzi R, Fuso L, De Rosa M, et al. Co-morbidity contributes to predict mortality of patients with chronic obstructive pulmonary disease. Eur Respir J 1997; 10:2794–2800.

19. Sachs AP, Koeter GH, Groenier KH, van der Waaij D, Schiphuis J, Meyboom de Jong B. Changes in symptoms, peak expiratory flow, and sputum flora during treatment with antibiotics of exacerbations in patients with chronic obstructive pulmonary disease in general practice. Thorax 1995; 50:758–763.

20. Emerman CL, Connors AF, Lukens TW, Effron D, May ME. Relationship between arterial blood gases and spirometry in acute exacerbations of chronic obstructive pulmonary disease. Ann Emerg Med 1989; 18:523–527.

21. Costello R, Deegan P, Fitzpatrick M, McNicholas WT. Reversible hypercapnia in chronic obstructive pulmonary disease: a distinct pattern of respiratory failure with a favorable prognosis. Am J Med 1997; 102:239–244.

22. Asmundsson T, Kilburn KH. Survival of acute respiratory failure. A study of 239 episodes. Ann Intern Med 1969; 70:471–485.

23. Incalzi RA, Fuso L, De Rosa M, et al. Electrocardiographic signs of chronic cor pulmonale: A negative prognostic finding in chronic obstructive pulmonary disease. Circulation 1999; 99:1600–1605.

24. Smith KJ, Pesce RR. Pulmonary artery catheterization in exacerbations of COPD requiring mechanical ventilation: a cost-effectiveness analysis. Respir Care 1994; 39:961–967.

25. Tramarin R, Torbicki A, Marchandise B, Laaban JP, Morpurgo M. Doppler echocardiographic evaluation of pulmonary artery pressure in chronic obstructive pulmonary disease. A European multicentre study. Working Group on Noninvasive Evaluation of Pulmonary Artery Pressure. European Office of the World Health Organization, Copenhagen. Eur Heart J 1991; 12:103–111.

26. Kilburn KH, Warshaw RH, Thornton JC. Do radiographic criteria for emphysema predict physiologic impairment? Chest 1995; 107:1225–1231.

27. Emerman CL, Effron D, Lukens W. Spirometric criteria for hospital admission of patients with acute exacerbation of COPD. Chest 1991; 99:595–599.

28. Emerman CL, Lukens TW, Effron D. Physician estimation of FEV_1 in acute exacerbation of COPD. Chest 1994; 105:1709–1712.

29. Vitacca M, Clini E, Porta R, Foglio K, Ambrosino N. Acute exacerbations in patients with COPD: predictors of need for mechanical ventilation. Eur Respir J 1996; 9:1487–1493.

30. Paggiaro PL, Dahle R, Bakran I, Frith L, Hollingworth K, Efthimiou J. Multicentre randomised placebo-controlled trial of inhaled fluticasone propionate in patients with chronic obstructive pulmonary disease. International COPD Study Group. Lancet 1998; 351:773–780.

31. Niewoehner DE, Collins D, Erbland ML. Relation of FEV(1) to clinical outcomes during exacerbations of chronic obstructive pulmonary disease. Department of Veterans Affairs Cooperative Study Group. Am J Respir Crit Care Med 2000; 161:1201–1205.

32. Bhowmik A, Seemungal TA, Sapsford RJ, Wedzicha JA. Relation of sputum inflammatory markers to symptoms and lung function changes in COPD exacerbations. Thorax 2000; 55:114–120.

33. Thompson AB, Daughton D, Robbins RA, Ghafouri MA, Oehlerking M, Rennard SI. Intraluminal airway inflammation in chronic bronchitis. Characterization and correlation with clinical parameters. Am Rev Respir Dis 1989; 140:1527–1537.

34. Selby C, Drost E, Lannan S, Wraith PK, MacNee W. Neutrophil retention in the lungs of patients with chronic obstructive pulmonary disease. Am Rev Respir Dis 1991; 143:1359–1364.
35. Balbi B, Bason C, Balleari E, et al. Increased bronchoalveolar granulocytes and granulocyte/macrophage colony-stimulating factor during exacerbations of chronic bronchitis. Eur Respir J 1997; 10:846–850.
36. Saetta M, Di Stefano A, Maestrelli P, et al. Airway eosinophilia in chronic bronchitis during exacerbations. Am J Respir Crit Care Med 1994; 150:1646–1652.
37. Zhu J, Qiu YS, Majumdar S, et al. Exacerbations of bronchitis: bronchial eosinophilia and gene expression for interleukin-4, interleukin-5, and eosinophil chemoattractants. Am J Respir Crit Care Med 2001; 164:109–116.
38. Aaron SD, Angel JB, Lunau M, et al. Granulocyte inflammatory markers and airway infection during acute exacerbation of chronic obstructive pulmonary disease. Am J Respir Crit Care Med 2001; 163:349–355.
39. Sethi S, Muscarella K, Evans N, Klingman KL, Grant BJ, Murphy TF. Airway inflammation and etiology of acute exacerbations of chronic bronchitis. Chest 2000; 118:1557–1565.
40. Saetta M, Di Stefano A, Maestrelli P, et al. Airway eosinophilia and expression of interleukin-5 protein in asthma and in exacerbations of chronic bronchitis. Clin Exp Allergy 1996; 26:766–774.
41. Wedzicha JA, Seemungal TA, MacCallum PK, et al. Acute exacerbations of chronic obstructive pulmonary disease are accompanied by elevations of plasma fibrinogen and serum IL-6 levels. Thromb Haemost 2000; 84:210–215.
42. Stockley RA, Bayley D, Hill SL, Hill AT, Crooks S, Campbell EJ. Assessment of airway neutrophils by sputum colour: correlation with airways inflammation. Thorax 2001; 56:366–372.
43. Hill AT, Campbell EJ, Bayley DL, Hill SL, Stockley RA. Evidence for excessive bronchial inflammation during an acute exacerbation of chronic obstructive pulmonary disease in patients with alpha(1)-antitrypsin deficiency (PiZ). Am J Respir Crit Care Med 1999; 160:1968–1975.
44. Culpitt SV, Maziak W, Loukidis S, Nightingale JA, Matthews JL, Barnes PJ. Effect of high dose inhaled steroid on cells, cytokines, and proteases in induced sputum in chronic obstructive pulmonary disease. Am J Respir Crit Care Med 1999; 160:1635–1639.
45. Kanazawa H, Kurihara N, Otsuka T, et al. Clinical significance of serum concentration of interleukin 8 in patients with bronchial asthma or chronic pulmonary emphysema. Respiration 1996; 63:236–240.
46. Burge PS, Calverley PM, Jones PW, Spencer S, Anderson JA, Maslen K. Randomised, double blind, placebo controlled study of fluticasone propionate in patients with moderate to severe chronic obstructive pulmonary disease: the ISOLDE trial. Br Med J 2000; 320:1297–1303.
47. Dentener MA, Creutzberg EC, Schols AM, et al. Systemic anti-inflammatory mediators in COPD: increase in soluble interleukin 1 receptor II during treatment of exacerbations. Thorax 2001; 56:721–726.
48. Schols AM, Buurman WA, Staal van den Brekel AJ, Dentener MA, Wouters EF. Evidence for a relation between metabolic derangements and increased levels of inflammatory mediators in a subgroup of patients with chronic obstructive pulmonary disease. Thorax 1996; 51:819–824.
49. Dev D, Wallace E, Sankaran R, et al. Value of C-reactive protein measurements in exacerbations of chronic obstructive pulmonary disease. Respir Med 1998; 92:664–667.

50. Stockley RA, O'Brien C, Pye A, Hill SL. Relationship of sputum color to nature and outpatient management of acute exacerbations of COPD. Chest 2000; 117:1638–1645.
51. Alessandri C, Basili S, Violi F, Ferroni P, Gazzaniga PP, Cordova C. Hypercoagulability state in patients with chronic obstructive pulmonary disease. Chronic Obstructive Bronchitis and Haemostasis Group. Thromb Haemost 1994; 72:343–346.
52. Crooks SW, Bayley DL, Hill SL, Stockley RA. Bronchial inflammation in acute bacterial exacerbations of chronic bronchitis: the role of leukotriene B4. Eur Respir J 2000; 5:274–280.
53. Gompertz S, Bayley DL, Hill SL, Stockley RA. Relationship between airway inflammation and the frequency of exacerbations in patients with smoking related COPD. Thorax 2001; 56:36–41.
54. Fiorini G, Crespi S, Rinaldi M, Oberti E, Vigorelli R, Palmieri G. Serum ECP and MPO are increased during exacerbations of chronic bronchitis with airway obstruction. Biomed Pharmacother 2000; 54:274–278.
55. Gibson PG, Woolley KL, Carty K, Murree-Allen K, Saltos N. Induced sputum eosinophil cationic protein (ECP) measurement in asthma and chronic obstructive airway disease (COAD). Clin Exp Allergy 1998; 28: 1081–1088.
56. Maziak W, Loukides S, Culpitt S, Sullivan P, Kharitonov SA, Barnes PJ. Exhaled nitric oxide in chronic obstructive pulmonary disease. Am J Respir Crit Care Med 1998; 157:998–1002.
57. Agusti AG, Villaverde JM, Togores B, Bosch M. Serial measurements of exhaled nitric oxide during exacerbations of chronic obstructive pulmonary disease. Eur Respir J 1999; 14:523–528.
58. Yates DH, Kharitonov SA, Robbins RA, Thomas PS, Barnes PJ. Effect of a nitric oxide synthase inhibitor and a glucocorticosteroid on exhaled nitric oxide. Am J Respir Crit Care Med 1995; 152:892–896.
59. Goldstein RA, Starcher BC. Urinary excretion of elastin peptides containing desmosin after intratracheal injection of elastase in hamsters. J Clin Invest 1978; 61:1286–1290.
60. Stone PJ, Gottlieb DJ, O'Connor GT, et al. Elastin and collagen degradation products in urine of smokers with and without chronic obstructive pulmonary disease. Am J Respir Crit Care Med 1995; 151:952–959.
61. Gottlieb DJ, Stone PJ, Sparrow D, et al. Urinary desmosine excretion in smokers with and without rapid decline of lung function: the Normative Aging Study. Am J Respir Crit Care Med 1996; 154:1290–1295.
62. Viglio S, Iadarola P, Lupi A, et al. MEKC of desmosine and isodesmosine in urine of chronic destructive lung disease patients. Eur Respir J 2000; 15:1039–1045.
63. Yasuda N, Gotoh K, Minatoguchi S, et al. An increase of soluble Fas, an inhibitor of apoptosis, associated with progression of COPD. Respir Med 1998; 92:993–999.
64. Roland M, Bhowmik A, Sapsford RJ, et al. Sputum and plasma endothelin-1 levels in exacerbations of chronic obstructive pulmonary disease. Thorax 2001; 56:30–35.
65. Engstrom CP, Persson LO, Larsson S, Sullivan M. Health-related quality of life in COPD: why both disease-specific and generic measures should be used. Eur Respir J 2001; 18:69–76.
66. Ferrer M, Alonso J, Morera J, et al. Chronic obstructive pulmonary disease stage and health-related quality of life. The Quality of Life of Chronic Obstructive Pulmonary Disease Study Group. Ann Intern Med 1997; 127:1072–1079.
67. Osman IM, Godden DJ, Friend JA, Legge JS, Douglas JG. Quality of life and hospital readmission in patients with chronic obstructive pulmonary disease. Thorax 1997; 52:67–71.

68. Jones PW, Quirk FH, Baveystock CM. The St George's Respiratory Questionnaire. Respir Med 1991; 85(Suppl B):25–31; discussion 33–37.
69. Davies L, Wilkinson M, Bonner S, Calverley PM, Angus RM. "Hospital at home" versus hospital care in patients with exacerbations of chronic obstructive pulmonary disease: prospective randomised controlled trial. Br Med J 2000; 321:1265–1268.
70. Behnke M, Taube C, Kirsten D, Lehnigk B, Jones RA, Magnussen H. Home-based exercise is capable of preserving hospital-based improvements in severe chronic obstructive pulmonary disease. Respir Med 2000; 94:1184–1191.
71. Katz S, Downs TD, Cash HR, Grotz RC. Progress in development of the index of ADL. Gerontologist 1970; 10:20–30.
72. Hlatky MA, Boineau RE, Higginbotham MB, et al. A brief self-administered questionnaire to determine functional capacity (the Duke Activity Status Index). Am J Cardiol 1989; 64:651–654.
73. Saudny-Unterberger H, Martin JG, Gray-Donald K. Impact of nutritional support on functional status during an acute exacerbation of chronic obstructive pulmonary disease. Am J Respir Crit Care Med 1997; 156:794–799.

14

Cardiopulmonary Interaction in Acute Exacerbations of Chronic Obstructive Pulmonary Disease

ZOHEIR BSHOUTY

University of Manitoba
Winnipeg, Manitoba, Canada

I. Introduction

The interaction between the heart and lungs, even under physiological conditions, is not surprising for several reasons:

1. The effects of transpulmonary pressure (P_{tp}, alveolar minus pleural pressure), on pulmonary vascular dimensions at all levels (alveolar and extra-alveolar), and hence, pulmonary vascular resistance (PVR).
2. The effects of pleural pressure (P_{pl}) and PVR on right- and left-ventricular preload and afterload.
3. The effect of changes in pleural and abdominal pressures on venous return (VR).

The assessment of pulmonary hemodynamics requires the measurement of pulmonary arterial pressure (P_{PA}), pulmonary capillary wedge pressure (PCWP), and cardiac output (CO) through right heart catheterization. Right heart catheterization is an invasive procedure that is not often employed in patients with COPD exacerbation even when mechanical ventilation is required. Also, assessment of right-ventricular function in COPD by echocardiography is confounded by increased retrosternal air space, secondary to hyperinflation, which interferes with sound-wave transmission making echocardiography difficult to interpret. In addition, factors that contribute to the development of worsening pulmonary arterial hypertension (PAH) in acute exacerbation of COPD are likely multifactorial and assessing the relative contribution of each factor is not always possible. Therefore, to better understand the effects of the various pathophysiological processes that occur during acute exacerbation of COPD on right- and left-ventricular performance, and the pulmonary circulation overall, one must rely on either indirect evidence or model predictions. In this section, we first examine the degree and the various factors that contribute to the development of PAH in stable COPD. We also examine the effect of PAH on RV function and the interaction between the right and left ventricles. We then extend our discussion to exacerbation of COPD. A basic knowledge of the interaction between CO and VR and the cardiac and vascular factors that affect this interaction is assumed.

II. PAH and RV Function in COPD

Preload is the force per unit cross-sectional area acting on the ventricular wall immediately prior to contraction (1). This force is directly related to ventricular end-diastolic pressure (P_{ED}) and volume (V_{ED}) and inversely related to ventricular wall thickness. In spite of a normal right-ventricular P_{ED} in most patients with COPD, a large variability in V_{ED} makes preload difficult to predict in this group of patients (2). Nevertheless, right-ventricular V_{ED} is an important determinant of RV function and stroke volume (SV) and, hence, is often substituted for preload.

Similarly, afterload is the force per unit cross-sectional area acting on the ventricular wall during active contraction (1). This force is directly related to ventricular systolic pressure (P_S) and volume, and inversely related to ventricular wall thickness. P_{PA} is an important determinant of right-ventricular P_S and is often used as an estimate of right-ventricular afterload.

Contractility is a measure of the ability of cardiac muscle to perform stroke work. Ventricular function (SV) is dependent on preload, afterload, and myocardial contractility and, hence, changes in ejection fraction (EF) do not always reflect changes in contractility. Adverse loading conditions can cause the ventricle to fail as a pump without depressed contractility, and ventricular pump function may be maintained by favorable loading conditions in spite of poor myocardial contractility. The independent assessment of myocardial contractility in COPD is especially important for two reasons. First, the large variability in preload and afterload in this group of patients and second, contractility is the best predictor of the ability of the right ventricle to handle large changes in preload and afterload without failing at rest, during exercise, or acute exacerbation of COPD. One measure of contractility is the relationship between end-systolic pressure (P_{ES}) and volume (V_{ES}) (3). Based on such measurements, several investigators have shown normal, if not supernormal, right-ventricular contractility in COPD patients (4, 5) even during exercise (6). For this discussion, we will assume that myocardial contractility is normal in most patients with COPD and that it remains normal in spite of large changes in preload and afterload (see also discussion under intrinsic positive end-expiratory pressure, iPEEP). This information is also very important for our model predictions (see below).

Most patients with stable COPD have normal P_{PA} (6–10) and CO (9–11) at rest and, hence, PVR. During exercise (9, 10, 12, 13) and exacerbation of COPD (14–20), P_{PA} may rise to abnormal levels. With the development of worsening airflow limitation, PAH may become evident at rest (2, 21, 22). However, even in patients with very severe airflow limitation with hypoxemia and hypercapnia, P_{PA} is only moderately elevated (23–29). In a study by Naeji et al. (24) of 74 patients with severe but clinically stable COPD, with FEV_1 25.7 ± 1% predicted (mean ± SD), the majority having hypoxemia and hypercapnia, mean P_{PA} (P_{PA}) was only 35 mmHg.

The progression of PAH in COPD is slow (29) and, therefore, its effect on right-ventricular dimensions and function is different from what is observed in acute pulmonary hypertension secondary to a massive pulmonary embolism (30) or in patients with primary pulmonary hypertension where P_{PA} is quite high (31). In COPD, the right ventricle has time to adapt to the modest increase in P_{PA} and right-ventricular end-diastolic pressure is normal in most patients at rest (2, 23, 32–34). However, the correlation between right-ventricular end-diastolic pressure and volume in COPD is poor and, hence, a normal pressure does not necessarily indicate a normal right-ventricular end-diastolic volume (2). Right-ventricular end-diastolic pressure and stroke work increase to abnormal levels with exercise due to a high P_{PA} (2).

III.   Right- and Left-Ventricular Interaction in COPD

The right and left ventricles share the interventricular septum and are both enclosed in the pericardial sac. As such, alterations in RV size and function may influence left-ventricular (LV) performance. LV systolic dysfunction is rare in COPD unless there is an associated history of heart disease. In a study by Boussuges et al. (35), standard indices of LV dimensions and systolic function (LV end-diastolic and end-systolic diameters, LV mass, EF, and fractional shortening) at rest were not different between patients with stable COPD and control subjects in spite of enlarged RV dimensions (RV end-systolic and end-diastolic diameters) in the former group.

In another study by Slutsky et al. (36), 10 normal subjects were compared to 12 patients with COPD and without coronary artery disease at rest and during exercise. In the COPD group, LV end-diastolic and end-systolic volumes and SV decreased significantly during exercise, whereas in the normal subjects LV end-diastolic volume did not change, while LV end-systolic volume decreased, thus increasing SV. As a result, when considering heart rate, CO rose by only 41% at maximal exercise in the COPD group compared with 137% in normal subjects. Exercise capacity (% predicted) was not stated in this study and, therefore, commenting on whether the attenuated rise in CO was exercise limiting in this group of patients is not possible. The authors hypothesized that the drop in LV end-diastolic volume (decreased preload) in COPD patients was due to the development of pulmonary hypertension, and hence increased pressure load on the RV causing

RV dilatation and possible encroachment on LV filling. The effects of hyperventilation and the possible development of iPEEP and the contribution of the latter to the decrease in LV end-diastolic and end-systolic volumes were not explored in this study.

IV. Factors Contributing to the Development of PAH in COPD

Several factors have been implicated in the development of PAH in COPD patients. The relative contribution of each factor to the development of PAH is not known. These factors will be discussed individually below. Model predictions will be used to assess the severity of an abnormality required to induce PAH at levels seen in severe COPD.

A. Changes in Arterial Blood Gases

It is well established that acute hypoxia increases P_{PA} in normal subjects (37–40) without a change in pulmonary capillary wedge pressure (40) suggesting that the rise in P_{PA} is the result of pulmonary arterial constriction. Also, a negative correlation between P_{PA} and arterial saturation (S_aO_2) has been reported by many investigators (41–48) in COPD patients. Similarly, a positive correlation between arterial carbon dioxide (P_aCO_2) and P_{PA} has been described (44, 49), although the rise in P_{PA} with hypercapnia may not be due to vasoconstriction but a rise in CO (50, 51). Decreasing pH by infusing hydrochloric acid (53, 54) or by the oral administration of ammonium chloride (55) had inconsistent effects on P_{PA} in patients with COPD. However, acidemia potentiated hypoxic vasoconstriction (52). The contribution of pulmonary vascular constriction to the development of PAH in COPD patients will be further examined.

B. Loss of Capillary Bed

In COPD patients with hypoxemia, the acute administration of oxygen, even in high concentrations, often produces a trivial drop in P_{PA} (44, 56–58). This suggests that the mechanisms for the rise in P_{PA} in COPD include other irreversible factors besides simple vasoconstriction. It has long been thought that the development of PAH in COPD patients is the result of destruction of small pulmonary vessels and capillary bed. This occurs because of small vessel thrombosis (59) and alveolar destruction, respectively, and hence, is irreversible. However, it is well known that emphysema patients with significant vessel destruction do not develop PAH until late in their disease course (60). The lack of correlation between right-ventricular hypertrophy and total alveolar surface area (61), reflecting the size of the capillary bed, suggests that loss of capillary bed per se is not a major determinant of the development of PAH. Structural changes in peripheral pulmonary arteries of COPD patients, presumed to be the result of persistent hypoxemia, have been documented (62–66). Not only does the luminal surface area of these resistive vessels diminish, but also the distensibility of each vessel diminishes (i.e., becomes more stiff, less distension for an equivalent transmural pressure compared with normal). The contribution of these two factors to the development of PAH will be examined.

C. Intrinsic Positive End-Expiratory Pressure (iPEEP)

The increase in lung volume, above functional residual capacity (FRC), at end-expiration is termed dynamic hyperinflation. Dynamic hyperinflation cannot occur without a concomitant increase in P_{tp} unless lung compliance changes. This increase in P_{tp} infers that alveolar pressure (P_{al}) remains positive throughout expiration. At end-expiration, this positive pressure is termed auto PEEP or iPEEP (67, 68). The development of iPEEP with dynamic hyperinflation is an important consequence of increased minute ventilation in COPD such as occurs during exercise or acute exacerbation (69). Also, the presence of dynamic hyperinflation infers that the inspiratory muscles must generate sufficient force to overcome iPEEP to initiate a breath. This results in more negative swings in P_{pl} during inspiration (70, 71). Various, and at times opposing, hemodynamic effects may occur as direct or indirect consequences of iPEEP and dynamic hyperinflation. Increasing lung volume, for example, has opposing effects on alveolar and extra-alveolar vessels. Whereas pulmonary capillary resistance may increase (72) through derecruitment with increasing P_{al}, resistance of extra-alveolar vessels actually decreases (73). The end result will ultimately depend on the relationship between pressure and resistance of the individual compartment and the contribution of each vascular bed to total PVR. It has been hypothesized that iPEEP ultimately increases PVR (72) and that this increase is further enhanced during exercise or acute exacerbation of COPD (69, 72, 74). At the same time, the increase in lung volume may impede VR directly through compression of the vena cava (71) and the right heart (76), or indirectly through an increase in right atrial pressure (P_{RA}) and, hence, a decrease in the pressure gradient for VR (77). On the other hand, the pressure gradient for VR may increase due to a drop in P_{RA} because of the large negative swings in P_{pl} and a concomitant rise in abdominal pressure (P_{abd}) due to diaphragmatic descent during inspiration or the activation of abdominal muscles during expiration. This potential increase in VR, however, may be limited as it may lie in the flat portion of the VR curve (78). The relationship between P_{RA}, atmospheric pressure (P_{atm}), and P_{abd} in determining VR has been described by Takata et al. (79, 80). An increase in P_{abd} would enhance VR when P_{RA} exceeds P_{atm} (abdominal zone III conditions, similar to pulmonary zone III of West). However, when P_{RA} decreases below P_{atm}, large veins collapse as they enter the thorax producing a Starling resistor effect (abdominal zone II conditions). In a study by Dhainaut et al. (17), in 10 spontaneously breathing COPD patients, pulmonary hemodynamics and dimensional changes in the RV and inferior vena cava (IVC) were simultaneously assessed. During inspiration, RV end-diastolic diameter increased while IVC collapsed, suggesting an increase in VR and RV preload. Settle et al. (81) and Jardin et al. (82), studying stable and mild acute exacerbation of COPD, respectively, further showed that the increase in RV dimensions during inspiration is associated with a reduction in LV dimensions and, hence, LV preload.

However, in the study of Dhainaut et al. (17), right-ventricular EF and right-ventricular and pulmonary artery pressures did not rise.

D. Other Factors

Other factors that may contribute to increased PVR are pulmonary thrombosis (59) through loss of vascular bed, and polycythemia, through its effect on viscosity, and hence, resistance under laminar flow conditions ($R = 8\pi\mu l/A^2$).

Given this complex relationship between iPEEP, preload, and afterload, and the importance of preload and afterload in determining SV and, hence, CO, it is not surprising that results in the literature are inconsistent. Several important questions remain. Is RV function preserved in COPD, and is the RV able to accommodate changes in preload and afterload during an exacerbation? And does CO eventually rise or fall during an exacerbation? Also, what is the effect of iPEEP and dynamic hyperinflation alone (i.e., without changes in preload and CO), on total PVR? The answers to these questions have significant impact on the degree of interaction between the cardiac and pulmonary systems and eventually determine the outcome during an exacerbation. It is quite reasonable to expect that not all patients with COPD will respond in the same way. Patients with mild COPD may have quite a different response from patients with very severe COPD. In the next section, using a multibranched model of the pulmonary circulation, we will attempt to answer some of these questions. Assumptions will be made based on clinical evidence where possible.

V.   Model Predictions

A.   Multibranched Model of the Pulmonary Circulation

The details of the multibranched model (Fig. 1) have been previously described (83, 84). In brief, starting from the pulmonary artery, the model bifurcates sequentially to eight capillary levels and converges on the venous side to end in the left atrium (LA). The behavior of the extra-alveolar vessels (both arteries and veins) is based on data obtained by Smith and Mitzner (73) and the behavior of the capillary bed is based on the model of Fung and Sobin (85). The model accounts for various factors including the effect of gravity, independent changes in alveolar and pleural pressures, and lung compliance. For individual vessels within the model, resistance, smooth muscle tone, and the characteristic behavior of each vessel can be determined. Cardiac output and LA pressure (LAP) are entered and the computer iterates until a stable solution for the model is reached. The model has been based on data obtained in the dog and model predictions have been previously validated. The agreement between model predictions and animal data was striking both qualitatively and quantitatively (83, 84). There is no reason to believe that model predictions are not applicable to humans, at least qualitatively.

Using the multibranched model of the pulmonary circulation described above, it is possible to examine the various pathophysiological processes that contribute to PAH in COPD. The severity of each process required to induce a significant rise in

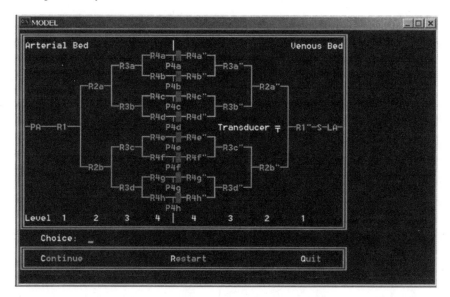

Figure 1 Multibranched model. Starting at the pulmonary artery (PA), the arterial bed bifurcates sequentially up to eight parallel channels that converge and reunite, on the venous side, to end in the left atrium (LA). Separating the two vascular beds are eight capillary sheets (rectangles) representing the capillary bed. By assigning the model a certain height, gravity effects are included in the simulations.

P_{PA} can be examined individually or in combination with other processes. Model predictions can be extended to exercise and acute exacerbation of COPD by raising or lowering CO, increasing the swings in pleural pressure between inspiration and expiration, with and without the development of iPEEP.

To establish baseline (normal) conditions, we assumed a lung height (LH) of 30 cm (assuming an erect position), lung compliance (C_L) of 0.25 L/cmH$_2$O, mean P_{al} (P_{al}) of 0 cmH$_2$O, mean P_{pl} (P_{pl}) of -5 cmH$_2$O, left atrial pressure (LAP) of 2 mmHg, and a CO of 5 L/min. All pressures are referenced to the LA. Total PVR was adjusted to yield a P_{PA} of 17.93 mmHg. Under these conditions, total PVR was 3.19 mmHg/L/min distributed almost equally between upstream (arterial bed), capillary bed, and downstream (venous bed) (1.14, 0.95, and 1.10 mmHg/L/min, respectively). Flow in the capillary bed at the lung apices (through vessels R4a) was 2% of total flow and, hence, most of the capillary bed at the lung apices was considered derecruited.

As a first step, we examined the effect of raising lung compliance alone (simulating worse COPD) on pulmonary arterial pressure. Raising compliance from 0.25 to 0.50 L/cmH$_2$O caused P_{PA} to rise minimally from 17.93 to 18.38 mmHg. This increase was considered insignificant and unlikely to explain the higher pulmonary arterial pressures seen with disease progression and, therefore, for the rest of the simulations lung compliance was left at 0.25 L/cmH$_2$O.

The increase in P_{PA} secondary to alveolar hypoxia is mainly due to constriction of pulmonary arteries that are smaller than $1000\,\mu m$ in diameter (86, 87). To test whether vasoconstriction alone could contribute to the development of PAH in COPD at rest, we added smooth muscle tone evenly to the precapillary level (level 4, vessels R4a through R4h) in increasing amounts to achieve a P_{PA} of approximately $35\,mmHg$. A smooth muscle tone of $35\,mmHg$ resulted in a mean P_{PA} of $36.32\,mmHg$. In a $100\,\mu m$ diameter vessel, with a muscular layer of $5\,\mu m$, this pressure translates to a stress of approximately $1 \times 10^6\,dyne/cm^2$. Under these conditions, derecruitment occurred in capillary beds a, b, and c (equivalent to 37.5% derecruitment). Eliminating smooth muscle tone from vessel R4h caused a drop in P_{PA} to $32.07\,mmHg$ in spite a rise in derecruitment to 50% (vessels a, b, c, and d). Eliminating smooth muscle tone in vessels R4g and R4h caused P_{PA} to drop to $26.87\,mmHg$ in spite a further rise in derecruitment to 75% (vessels a, b, c, d, e, and f). These findings suggest that, in order for smooth muscle tone alone to induce a rise in P_{PA} to levels seen in COPD at rest, vasoconstriction has to be applied diffusely and in significant amounts. Furthermore, derecruitment alone is unlikely to cause PAH at rest if the remainder of the pulmonary circulation remains intact. When capillary beds a, d, f, and h (randomly selected) were destroyed (50% destruction) leaving capillary beds b, c, e, and g intact, P_{PA} rose from 17.93 to $22.29\,mmHg$ at rest. A smooth muscle tone of $29\,mmHg$ applied to the remainder of the vessels was needed to raise P_{PA} to $36.54\,mmHg$. When capillary beds a, c, d, f, g, and h were destroyed (75% destruction), P_{PA} rose to $31.69\,mmHg$ and a smooth muscle tone of $15\,mmHg$ caused P_{PA} to further rise to $36.12\,mmHg$. This suggests that even in the presence of significant (50%) vessel destruction, an almost equivalent amount of smooth muscle tone (29 vs. $35\,mmHg$) is still needed in the remainder of the vessels to cause a significant rise in P_{PA}. However, when more than 75% of the vessels are destroyed, lower, but not insignificant, levels of smooth muscle tone ($15\,mmHg$ vs. $35\,mmHg$) were still needed to cause P_{PA} to rise to levels seen in COPD.

To simulate vessel narrowing, the cross-sectional area of vessels R4b, R4c, R4e, and R4g in the first example (50% destruction) and vessels R4b and R4e in the second example (75% destruction) were reduced by half. In the first example, a smooth muscle tone of only $15\,mmHg$ caused P_{PA} to rise to $36.43\,mmHg$, whereas in the second example, without any smooth muscle tone, P_{PA} rose to $39.37\,mmHg$. These findings suggest that the mechanisms for the development of PAH in COPD patients at rest must be multifactorial. The contribution of each factor to the development of PAH may vary and depend on the degree of alveolar destruction and, hence, severity of COPD.

During exercise, CO and minute ventilation rise with the possible development of iPEEP. Depending on the severity of COPD, desaturation with or without CO_2 retention and worsening acidemia may also develop. As mentioned above, worsening hypoxemia is likely to cause more vasoconstriction, which is further potentiated by acidemia (52), and the rise in CO_2 causes an increase in CO (50, 51). The effects of vasoconstriction have already been described. To examine the effects of increasing CO on P_{PA}, realizing that the mechanisms contributing to PAH are multifactorial, we doubled CO (from 5 to 10 L/min) in four conditions; normal lungs (condition 1), mild, severe, and very severe COPD (conditions 2, 3, and 4, respectively) (Table 1). Condition 2 had 25% vessel destruction (vessels R4b and R4g) and 7.5 mmHg vasoconstriction in the remainder of the vessels at level 4 without other vessel narrowing. Condition 3 had 50% vessel destruction (vessels R4a, R4d, R4f, and R4h), 15 mmHg smooth muscle tone, and 50% reduction in cross-sectional area in the remaining vessels at level 4. Condition 4 had 75% vessel destruction (vessels R4a, R4c, R4d, R4f, R4g, and R4h) without added smooth muscle tone but with 50% reduction in cross-sectional area in the remaining vessels. Smooth muscle tone was removed from the last condition to explore whether, in very severe COPD with most vessels being destroyed, PAH would occur without added smooth muscle tone. Raising CO from 5 to 10 L/min caused P_{PA} to rise from 17.93 to 25.72 (7.79 mmHg, 43.4%) in condition 1, from 20.67 to 29.15 mmHg (8.48 mmHg, 41%) in condition 2, from 36.43 to 46.83 mmHg (10.4 mmHg, 28.5%) in condition 3, and from 39.37 to 54.19 mmHg (14.82 mmHg, 37.6%) in condition 4. These findings confirm that although PAH may not be apparent at rest in COPD, P_{PA} does rise to significant levels during exercise. Furthermore, P_{PA} is quite sensitive to changes in CO even in mild COPD if vasoconstriction is present and in very severe COPD without vasoconstriction. Notice that it is the absolute rise, and not the percent rise, in P_{PA} that correlates with the severity of disease.

To simulate the effect of large swings in alveolar and pleural pressures on pulmonary hemodynamics, we divided the respiratory cycle into inspiratory (I) and expiratory (E) phases with an I : E ratio of 1 : 2. P_{al} during inspiration was decreased from 0 (C1) to -10 (C2) to -20 (C3) and P_{pl} was decreased from -5 to -15 to -25 cmH$_2$O, respectively (Table 2). During expiration, P_{al} was increased from 0 to $+5$ to $+10$ and P_{pl} from -5 to 0 to $+5$ cmH$_2$O, respectively. Notice that P_{tp} under these conditions was kept constant (5 cmH$_2$O), thus simulating large swings in alveolar and pleural pressures without the development of dynamic hyperinflation. The degree of variation in alveolar and pleural pressures between inspiration and expiration therefore varied from 0 (C1) to 15 (C2) to 30 cmH$_2$O (C3). Although these swings may be considered large, they enabled us to explore extreme conditions such as occur during exercise and acute exacerbation of COPD. We also reasoned

Table 1 Details of Vessel Destruction, Smooth Muscle Tone, and Vessel Narrowing Simulating Normal Lungs and Patients with Mild, Severe, and Very Severe COPD

Condition	% Vessel destruction	Vessels destructed	Smooth muscle tone in remainder of vessels	Narrowing in remainder of vessels
1	0	None	None	None
2	25	R4b, R4g	7.5 mmHg	None
3	50	R4a, R4d, R4f, R4h	15.0 mmHg	50%
4	75	R4a, R4c, R4d, R4f, R4g, R4h	None	50%

Table 2 The Effects of Large Swings in Alveolar and Pleural Pressure, Without the Development of iPEEP and at a Fixed CO, on P_{PA} During Inspiration, Expiration, and Averaged Over the Whole Respiratory Cycle with an I : E of 1 : 2

			I	E	I P_{PA}	E P_{PA}	Mean P_{PA}
Normal lungs	C1	P_{al}	0	0	17.93	17.93	17.93
		P_{pl}	−5	−5			
	C2	P_{al}	−10	+5	13.97	20.61	18.40
		P_{pl}	−15	0			
	C3	P_{al}	−20	+10	11.55	24.65	20.28
		P_{pl}	−25	+5			
Severe COPD	C1	P_{al}	0	0	36.43	36.43	36.43
		P_{pl}	−5	−5			
	C2	P_{al}	−10	+5	30.17	39.88	36.64
		P_{pl}	−15	0			
	C3	P_{al}	−20	+10	24.92	43.64	37.40
		P_{pl}	−25	+5			
Very severe COPD	C1	P_{al}	0	0	39.37	39.37	39.37
		P_{pl}	−5	−5			
	C2	P_{al}	−10	+5	33.33	42.79	39.64
		P_{pl}	−15	0			
	C3	P_{al}	−20	+10	29.14	46.55	40.75
		P_{pl}	−25	+5			

that by examining extremes we were likely to cover intermediate situations. This was done under three conditions; healthy lungs, severe and very severe COPD (conditions 1, 3, and 4 as described in Table 1, respectively). Table 2 shows the effects on P_{PA} assuming a constant CO of 5 L/min and Table 3 shows the effects on CO assuming a constant P_{PA} of 17.93 mmHg for normal lungs, 36.43 mmHg for severe COPD, and 39.37 mmHg for very severe COPD. From Table 2 it is evident that, at a fixed CO, large swings in alveolar and pleural pressures between inspiration and expiration will cause large swings in P_{PA} (in healthy subjects and in patients with severe and very severe COPD), in a direct relation, without a change in mean P_{PA} when averaged over the whole respiratory cycle. It is also evident from Table 3 that a constant P_{PA}, as described by Dhainaut et al. (17), will cause large swings in CO between inspiration and expiration without a change in overall CO compared to baseline. These large swings in CO may be the result of large swings in VR which, in turn, are the result of the effects of P_{pl} on right atrial pressure. We conclude that, during an exacerbation, the large swings in alveolar and pleural pressures per se, although they may cause large swings in P_{PA} and CO between inspiration and expiration, do not affect CO and P_{PA} overall.

With the development of iPEEP and dynamic hyperinflation, P_{al} may increase significantly as does lung volume with P_{pl} increasing to a lesser extent. Changes in

Table 3 The Effects of Large Swings in Alveolar and Pleural Pressure, Without the Development of iPEEP and at a Fixed P_{PA}, on CO During Inspiration, Expiration, and Averaged Over the Whole Respiratory Cycle with an I : E of 1 : 2

			I	E	I CO	E CO	Mean CO
Normal lungs	C1	P_{al}	0	0	5.0	5.0	5.0
		P_{pl}	−5	−5			
	C2	P_{al}	−10	+5	7.5	3.7	5.0
		P_{pl}	−15	0			
	C3	P_{al}	−20	+10	9.5	2.3	4.8
		P_{pl}	−25	+5			
Severe COPD	C1	P_{al}	0	0	5.0	5.0	5.0
		P_{pl}	−5	−5			
	C2	P_{al}	−10	+5	7.75	3.8	5.11
		P_{pl}	−15	0			
	C3	P_{al}	−20	+10	10.35	2.73	5.27
		P_{pl}	−25	+5			
Very severe COPD	C1	P_{al}	0	0	5.0	5.0	5.0
		P_{pl}	−5	−5			
	C2	P_{al}	−10	+5	6.75	4.1	4.98
		P_{pl}	−15	0			
	C3	P_{al}	−20	+10	8.1	3.2	4.83
		P_{pl}	−25	+5			

P_{al}, P_{pl}, and lung volume have independent effects on alveolar and extra-alveolar vessels (73, 85). To examine the effects of iPEEP with dynamic hyperinflation on P_{PA}, we raised P_{al} from 0 to 10 and then to 20 cmH$_2$O while raising P_{pl} from −5 to 0 and then to +5 cmH$_2$O, respectively. Resting lung volume under these conditions increased from 1.35 to 2.6 and then to 3.85 L. We examined this effect in conditions 1, 3, and 4, as described in Table 1. The results are shown in Table 4. From Table 4, it is evident that the combination of a rise in CO and the development of iPEEP and hyperinflation cause a significant rise in P_{PA} even in normal lungs. However, the rise in P_{PA} is higher with worsening COPD as previously hypothesized.

In conclusion, given the distensibility of the pulmonary circulation, a substantial amount of smooth muscle tone, applied diffusely at the precapillary level, is needed to increase P_{PA} to levels seen in COPD at rest. Similarly, a large degree of alveolar vascular destruction with vascular narrowing in the remainder of the pulmonary circulation is needed to induce such an increase in P_{PA}. Under these conditions, no additional vascular tone is needed. However, during an exacerbation with worsening hypoxemia and acidosis, further vasoconstriction may occur thus worsening P_{PA}. Furthermore, with the development of iPEEP and the concomitant increase in CO, P_{PA} may rise to very high levels. The clinical outcome under these conditions will highly depend on whether the RV can accommodate such acute

Table 4 The Effects of iPEEP and Rise in CO on P_{PA} in Normal Lungs, Severe, and Very Severe COPD

		P_{al}	P_{pl}	CO = 5 P_{PA}	CO = 10 P_{PA}
Normal lungs	C1	0	−5	17.93	25.72
	C2	+10	0	22.03	29.69
	C3	+20	+5	27.76	35.96
Severe COPD	C1	0	−5	36.43	46.83
	C2	+10	0	40.12	50.79
	C3	+20	+5	44.09	55.22
Very severe COPD	C1	0	−5	39.37	54.19
	C2	+10	0	44.45	59.36
	C3	+20	+5	49.78	65.14

changes which in turn depends on the acuity and severity of the derangement and the status of the myocardium.

References

1. Goerke J, Mines AH. Cardiovascular Physiology. New York: Raven Press, 1988; 99–152.
2. Khaja F, Parker JO. Right and left ventricular performance in chronic obstructive lung disease. Am Heart J 1971; 82:319–327.
3. Sagawa K. The end-systolic pressure volume relation of the ventricle: definition, modifications and clinical use. Circulation 1981; 63:1223–1227.
4. MacNee W, Wathen CG, Hanna WJ, Flenley DC, Muir AL. Effects of pirbuterol and sodium nitroprusside on pulmonary haemodynamics in hypoxic cor pulmonale. Br Med J 1983; 287:1169–1172.
5. Burghuber OC, Bergmann H. Right ventricular contractility in chronic obstructive pulmonary disease. A combined radionuclide and haemodynamic study. Respiration 1988; 53:1–12.
6. Biernacki W, Flenley DC, Muri AL, MacNee W. Pulmonary hypertension and right ventricular function in patients with COPD. Chest 1988; 94:1169–1175.
7. MacNee W. Pathophysiology of cor pulmonale in chronic obstructive pulmonary disease. Am J Respir Crit Care Med 1994; 150:833–852.
8. Mounsey JPD, Ritzman LW, Selverstone NH, Briscoe WA, McLemore GA. Circulatory changes in severe pulmonary emphysema. Br Heart J 1952; 14:153–172.
9. Oswald-Mammosser M, Kessler R, Massard G, Wihlm JM, Weitzenblum E, Lonsdorfer J. Effect of lung volume reduction surgery on gas exchange and pulmonary hemodynamics at rest and during exercise. Am J Respir Crit Care Med 1998; 158:1020–1025.
10. Kubo K, Koizumi T, Fujimoto K, Matsuzawa Y, Yamanda T, Haniuda M, Takahashi S. Effects of lung volume reduction surgery on exercise pulmonary hemodynamics in severe emphysema. Chest 1998; 114:1575–1582.
11. Niederman MS, Matthay RA. Cardiovascular function in secondary pulmonary hypertension. Heart Lung 1986; 15:341–351.

12. Matthay RA, Berger HJ, Davies RA, Loke RA, Mahler DA, Gottschalk A. Right and left ventricular performance in chronic obstructive pulmonary disease: radionuclide assessment. Ann Intern Med 1983; 88:234–239.

13. Mahler DA, Brent BN, Loke J, Zaret BL, Matthay RA. Right ventricular performance and central circulatory hemodynamics during upright exercise in patients with chronic obstructive pulmonary disease. Am Rev Respir Dis 1984; 130:722–729.

14. Lemaire F, Tebul J-L, Cinotti L, et al. Acute left ventricular dysfunction during unsuccessful weaning from mechanical ventilation. Anesthesiology 1988; 69:171–179.

15. Tebull J-L, Abrouk F, Lemaire F. Right ventricular function in COPD patients during weaning from mechanical ventilation. Intens Care Med 1988; 14:483–485.

16. Fishman A. Chronic cor pulmonale. Am Rev Respir Dis 1976; 114:775–794.

17. Dhainaut JF, Brunet F, Armaganidis A. Phasic changes of right ventricular ejection in acute exacerbation of COPD. Am Rev Respir Dis 1987; 135:A113.

18. Dhainaut JF, Brunet F. Phasic changes of right ventricular ejection fraction in patients with acute exacerbation of chronic obstructive pulmonary disease. Intens Care Med 1987; 12:214–215.

19. Marangoni S, Scalvini S, Schena M, Vitacca M, Quadri A, Levi G. Right ventricular diastolic function in chronic obstructive lung disease. Eur Respir J 1992; 5:438–443.

20. Richard C, Tebul J-L, Archambaud F, Hebert J-L, Michaut P, Auzepy P. Left ventricular function during weaning of patients with chronic obstructive pulmonary disease. Intens Care Med 1994; 20:181–186.

21. Jezek V, Schrijen F, Sadoul P. Right ventricular function and pulmonary haemodynamics during exercise in patients with chronic obstructive bronchopulmonary disease. Cardiology 1973; 58:20–31.

22. Light RW, Mintz HM, Linden GS, Brown SE. Hemodynamics of patients with severe chronic obstructive pulmonary disease during progressive upright exercise. Am Rev Respir Dis 1984; 130:391–395.

23. Boushy SF, North LB. Haemodynamic changes in chronic obstructive pulmonary disease. Chest 1977; 72:565–570.

24. Naeije R. Should pulmonary hypertension be treated in chronic obstructive pulmonary disease? In: Weir EK, Archer SL, Reeves JT, eds. The Diagnosis and Treatment of Pulmonary Hypertension. New York: Futura Publishing, 1992; 209–239.

25. Sadoul P, Schrijen F, Uffholz H, Pham QT. Evolution clinique de 195 pulmonares soumis a un catheterisme du coeur droit entre 1957 et 1965. Bull Eur Physiopathol Respir 1968; 4:255–240.

26. Schrijen F, Uffholtz H, Polu JM, Poincelot F. Pulmonary and systemic hemodynamic evaluation in chronic bronchitis. Am Rev Respir Dis 1978; 117:25–31.

27. Weizenblum E, Hirth C, Parini JP, Rasaholinjanahary J, Oudet P. Clinical, function and pulmonary haemodynamic course of patients with COPD followed up over 3 years. Respiration 1978; 36:1–9.

28. Weizenblum E, Loiseau A, Hirth C, Mirhom R, Rasaholinjanahary J. Course of pulmonary haemodynamics in patients with chronic obstructive pulmonary disease. Chest 1979; 75:656–662.

29. Weitzenblum E, Sautejeau A, Ehrhart M, Mammosser M, Pettetier A. Long-term course of pulmonary arterial pressure in chronic obstructive pulmonary disease. Am Rev Respir Dis 1984; 130:993–998.

30. Stein PD, Sabbah NH, Anbe DT, Marzilli M. Performance of the failing and nonfalling right ventricle of patients with pulmonary hypertension. Am J Cardiol 1979; 44:1050–1055.

31. Wagenvoort CA, WagenVoort N. Primary pulmonary hypertension; a pathological study of the lung vessels in 156 clinically diagnosed cases. Circulation 1970; 42:1163–1184.

32. Fishman AP. State of the art: chronic cor pulmonale. Am Rev Respir Dis 1976; 114:775–794.

33. Burrows B, Strauss RH, Nider AH. Chronic obstructive lung disease. III. Interrelationships of pulmonary function data. Am Rev Respir Dis 1965; 91:861–868.

34. Burrows B, Kettel LJ, Niden AH, Rabinowitz M, Dierer CF. Patterns of cardiovascular dysfunction in chronic obstructive lung disease. N Engl J Med 1972; 286:912–918.

35. Boussuges A, Pinet C, Molenat F, Burnet H, Ambrosi P, Badier M, Sainty JM, Orehek J. Left atrial and ventricular filling in chronic obstructive pulmonary disease. Am J Respir Crit Care Med 2000; 162:670–675.

36. Slutsky R, Hooper W, Ackerman W, Ashburn W, Gerber K, Moser K, Karliner J. Evaluation of left ventricular function in chronic pulmonary disease by exercise gated equilibrium radionuclide angiography. Am Heart J 1981; 101:414–420.

37. Matthay RA, Niederman MS, Wiedemann HP. Cardiovascular pulmonary interaction in chronic obstructive pulmonary disease with special reference to the pathogenesis and management of cor pulmonale. Med Clin North Am 1990; 74:571–617.

38. Weber K, Janicki J, Shroff SG, Likoff MJ, St John Sutton MG. The right ventricle: physiology and pathophysiologic consideration. Crit Care Med 1983; 11:323–328.

39. Fritts HW, Odell JE, Harris P, Braunwald EW, Fishman AO. Effects of acute hypoxia on the volume of blood in the thorax. Circulation 1960; 22:216–219.

40. Harris P, Bishop JM, Segel N. The influence of guanethidine on hypoxic pulmonary hypertension in normal man. Clin Sci 1961; 21:295–300.

41. Harvey RM, Ferrer MI, Richards DW, Cournand A. Influence of chronic pulmonary disease on the heart and circulation. Am J Med 1951; 10:719–738.

42. Emirgil C, Sobol BJ, Herbert WH. Routine pulmonary function studies as a key to the status of the lesser circulation in chronic obstructive pulmonary disease. Am J Med 1971; 5:191–199.

43. Fowler NO, Westcott RN, Scott RG, Hess E. The cardiac output in chronic cor pulmonale. Circulation 1952; 6:888–893.

44. Horsfield K, Segal N, Bishop JM. The pulmonary circulation in chronic bronchitis at rest and during exercise breathing air and 80% oxygen. Clin Sci 1968; 34:473–483.

45. Millard J, Reid L. Right ventricular hypertrophy and its relationship to chronic bronchitis and emphysema. Br J Dis Chest 1974; 68:103–110.

46. Williams JF, Behuke RH. The effect of pulmonary emphysema upon cardiopulmonary hemodynamics at rest and during exercise. Ann Intern Med 1964; 60:824–842.

47. Yu PN, Lovejoy FW, Joos HA, Nye RE, McCann WS. Studies of pulmonary hypertension. I. Pulmonary circulatory haemodynamics in patients with pulmonary emphysema at rest. J Clin Invest 1953; 32:130–137.

48. Bishop JM, Cross KW. Use of other physiological variables to predict pulmonary arterial pressure in patients with chronic respiratory disease—a multicentre study. Eur Heart J 1981; 2:509–517.

49. Aber GM, Bayley TJ, Bishop JM. Inter-relationships between renal and cardiac function and respiratory gas exchange in obstructive airways disease. Clin Sci 1963; 25:159–170.

50. Kilburn KR, Asmundsson T, Britt RC, Cardon R. Effects of breathing 10% carbon dioxide on the pulmonary circulation of human subjects. Circulation 1969; 39:639–653.

51. Rokseth R. The effect of altered blood carbon dioxide tension and pH on the human pulmonary circulation. Scand J Clin Lab Invest 1966; 18(Suppl):90–94.

52. Enson Y, Guitini C, Lewis ML, Morris TQ, Ferrer MI, Harvey RM. The influence of hydrogen in concentration and hypoxia on the pulmonary circulation. J Clin Invest 1964; 43:1146–1162.

53. Harvey RM, Enson Y, Betti R, Lewis ML, Rochester DF, Ferrer MI. Further considerations of the causes of pulmonary hypertension in cor pulmonale. Bull Eur Physiopathol Respir 1967; 3:623–632.

54. Housley EE, Clarke SW, Hedworth-Whitty RB, Bishop JM. Effect of acute and chronic acidaemia and associated hypoxia on the pulmonary circulation of patients with chronic bronchitis. Cardiovasc Res 1970; 4:482–489.

55. Campbell EJM, Short DS. The cause of oedema in "cor pulmonale." Lancet 1960; 1:1184–1186.

56. Wilson RH, Houseth W, Dempsey MG. The effects of breathing 99.6% oxygen on pulmonary vascular resistance and cardiac output in patients with pulmonary emphysema and chronic hypoxia. Ann Intern Med 1955; 42:629–637.

57. Kitchen AJ, Lowther CP, Matthews MD. The effects of exercise and breathing oxygen-enriched air on the pulmonary circulation in emphysema. Clin Sci 1961; 21:93–106.

58. Aber GM, Harris AM, Bishop JM. Effect of acute changes in inspired oxygen concentration on cardiac, respiratory, and renal function in patients with chronic obstructive airways disease. Clin Sci 1964; 26:133–143.

59. Bignion J, Khoury F, Even P, Andre J, Brouet G. Morphometric study in chronic obstructive broncho-pulmonary disease. Pathologic, clinical and physiologic correlations. Am Rev Respir Dis 1969; 99:669–695.

60. Thurlbeck WM, Henderson JA, Fraser RG, Bates DV. Chronic obstructive lung disease. A comparison between clinical, roentgenologic, functional and morphologic criteria in chronic bronchitis, emphysema, asthma and bronchiectasis. Medicine 1970; 49:81–145.

61. Hicken P, Brewer D, Heath D. The relation between the weight of the right ventricle of the heart and the internal surface area and the number of alveoli in the human lung in emphysema. J Pathol Bacteriol 1966; 92:529–546.

62. Haselton PS, Heath D, Brewer DB. Hypertensive pulmonary vascular disease in states of chronic hypoxia. J Pathol Bacteriol 1968; 95:431–440.

63. Wilkinson M, Langhorn CA, Heath D, Barer GR, Howard P. A pathophysiological study of 10 cases of hypoxic cor pulmonale. Q J Med 1988; 66:65–85.

64. Wright JL, Lawson L, Pare PD, Hooper RO, Peretz DI, Nelems JM, Schulzer M, Hogg JC. The structure and function of pulmonary vasculature in mild chronic obstructive pulmonary disease; the effect of oxygen on exercise. Am Rev Respir Dis 1983; 128:702–707.

65. Magee F, Wright JL, Wiggs BR, Pare PD, Hogg JC. Pulmonary vascular structure and function in chronic obstructive pulmonary disease. Thorax 1988; 43:183–189.

66. Dunnill MS. Fibrinoid necrosis in the branches of the pulmonary artery and chronic non-specific lung disease. Br J Dis Chest 1960; 54:355–360.

67. Pepe PE, Marini JJ. Occult positive end-expiratory pressure in mechanically ventilated patients with airflow obstruction; the auto-PEEP effect. Am Rev Respir Dis 1982; 126:166–170.

68. Rossi A, Gottfried SB, Higgs BD, et al. Measurement of static compliance of the total respiratory system in patients with acute respiratory failure during mechanical ventilation. Am Rev Respir Dis 1985; 131:672–677.

69. Kimball WR, Leith DE, Robins AG. Dynamic hyperinflation and ventilatory dependence in chronic obstructive pulmonary disease. Am Rev Respir Dis 1982; 126:991–995.

70. Smith TC, Marini JJ. Impact of PEEP on lung mechanics and work of breathing in severe airflow obstruction. J Appl Physiol 1988; 65:1488–1499.

71. Petrof BJ, Legare M, Goldberg P, Milic-Emili J, Gottfried SB. Continuous positive airway pressure reduces work of breathing and dyspnea during weaning from mechanical ventilation in severe chronic obstructive pulmonary disease. Am Rev Respir Dis 1990; 141:281–289.

72. Harris P, Segel N, Green J, Housley E. The influence of the airways resistance and alveolar pressure on the pulmonary vascular resistance in chronic bronchitis. Cardiovasc Res 1968; 2:84–94.

73. Smith, JC and W Mitzner. Analysis of pulmonary vascular interdependence in excised dog lobes. J Appl Physiol 1980; 48(3):450–467.

74. Lockhart A, Nader F, Tzareva M, Schrijen F. Comparative effects of exercise and isocapnic voluntary hyperventilation on pulmonary haemodynamics in chronic bronchitis and emphysema. Eur J Clin Invest 1970; 1:69–76.

75. Nakhjavan FK, Palmer WH, McGregor M. Influence of respiration on venous return in pulmonary emphysema. Circulation 1966; 33:8–16.

76. Brookhart JM, Boyd TE. Local differences in intrathoracic pressure and their relation to cardiac filling pressure in the dog. Am J Physiol 1947; 148:434–444.

77. Pinsky MR. Determinants of pulmonary artery flow variation during respiration. J Appl Physiol 1984; 56:1237–1245.

78. Guyton AC, Lindsey AW, Abernathy B. Venous return at various right arterial pressures and the normal venous return curve. Am J Physiol 1957; 189:609–615.

79. Takata M, Wise RA, Robotham JL. Effects of abdominal pressure on venous return: abdominal vascular zone conditions. J Appl Physiol 1990; 69:1961–1972.

80. Takata M, Robotham JL. Effects of inspiratory diaphragmatic descent on inferior vena caval venous return. J Appl Physiol 1992; 72:597–607.

81. Settle HP, Engel PJ, Fowler NO. Echocardiographic study of the paradoxical arterial pulse in chronic obstructive lung disease. Circulation 1980; 62:1297–1307.

82. Jardin F, Gueret P, Prost JF, Farcot JC, Ozier Y, Bourdarias JP. Two-dimensional echocardiographic assessment of left ventricular function in chronic obstructive pulmonary disease. Am Rev Respir Dis 1984; 129:135–142.

83. Bshouty Z, Younes M. Distensibility and pressure-flow relationship of the pulmonary circulation. I. Single-vessel model. J Appl Physiol 1990; 68(4):1501–1513.

84. Bshouty Z, Younes M. Distensibility and pressure-flow relationship of the pulmonary circulation. II. Multibranched model. J Appl Physiol 1990; 68(4):1514–1527.

85. Fung YC, Sobin SS. Pulmonary alveolar blood flow. Circ Res 1972; 30:470–490.

86. Al-Tinawi A, Krenz GS, Rickaby DA, Linehan JH, Dawson CA. Influence of hypoxia and serotonin on small pulmonary vessels. J Appl Physiol 1994; 76:56–64.

87. Hillier SC, Graham JA, Hanger CC, Godbey PS, Glenny RW, Wagner WW Jr. Hypoxic vasoconstriction in pulmonary arterioles and venules. J Appl Physiol 1997; 82(4):1084–1090.

15

Skeletal Muscles in Acute Exacerbations of Chronic Obstructive Pulmonary Disease

THIERRY TROOSTERS, RIK GOSSELINK, GHISLAINE GAYAN-RAMIREZ, MARTIJN A. SPRUIT, and MARC DECRAMER

Katholieke Universiteit Leuven
Leuven, Belgium

I. Introduction: Relevance of Skeletal Muscles in COPD

During the last decade, impaired skeletal muscle function has been identified as an independent contributor to both morbidity and mortality in COPD. We showed that patients with recurrent hospitalizations and high medical consumption were characterized by muscle weakness rather than impaired pulmonary function (1). In addition, exacerbations may have devastating effects on skeletal muscle function in patients with COPD. This chapter will deal with both these aspects.

First, skeletal muscle weakness and, more generally, deconditioning, will be discussed as risk factors for exacerbations in COPD. Second, mechanisms that may contribute to reduced skeletal muscle function during and after an exacerbation will be reviewed. A special section is devoted to respiratory muscle function during exacerbations. The relevance of this section is illustrated by the observation that respiratory muscle weakness was associated with impaired survival in a large cohort of COPD patients (2).

Although this chapter will discuss several hypotheses in support of the presence of muscle dysfunction during exacerbations, research investigating the direct impact of acute exacerbations on skeletal muscle function is scarce. Recent unpublished data from our lab, however, support a decline in handgrip force during the first week of a hospitalization for an acute exacerbation ($-5\pm6\%$; $p = 0.01$). A study by Vermeeren (3) clearly demonstrates that patients with COPD admitted to a hospital have an elevated resting energy expenditure and reduced calorie intake, resulting in a negative energy balance. Although this study (3) does not present prospective data on weight loss during exacerbation, the authors report a 1.6-kg weight gain at discharge compared to a follow-up visit 3 months later. This suggests that COPD patients may indeed actively lose weight and possibly muscle mass during a severe acute exacerbation.

II. Deconditioning and Exacerbations

When COPD patients with frequent exacerbations are compared to patients with less frequent exacerbations requiring hospitalization, they are characterized by overt skeletal muscle weakness (1). Although in a more general population pulmonary function was shown to be a strong predictor of hospitalization (4), it was essentially identical between both our COPD patient populations (1). Taken all together, skeletal muscle weakness should be regarded as an independent risk factor for hospitalization. Quadriceps force expressed as a percentage of the predicted value is related to the number of hospital admissions, the number of hospital days, and to the number of outpatient consultations. Intriguingly, FEV_1 was not significantly related to utilization of health-care recourses in the cohort of patients we studied (Fig. 1). Along tne same lines, Kessler et al. (5) showed that—apart from gas exchange limitation and pulmonary hemodynamics—a low body mass index (BMI) and a poor 6-min walking distance (6 MWD) were strong predictors of hospital admission. Muscle strength was not measured in this trial, but we showed that 6 MWD was strongly related to skeletal muscle strength in COPD patients (6). Further indirect

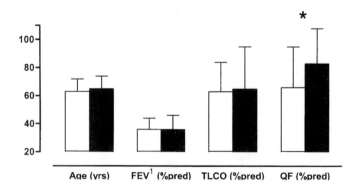

Figure 1   Differences between consecutive patients with high medical consumption (> 2 hospital admissions in the year preceding the study; $n = 23$ number of hospital days 30 ± 16), and low medical consumption (no admissions, $n = 34$). Data for lung function [(FEV_1) and diffusion capacity (TL, CO) are displayed], expressed as % of the predicted variable, were not different. Quadriceps force (QF), expressed as a % of predicted value, was significantly lower in the patients with high medical consumption. (Adapted from Ref. 1.)

evidence pointing to a protective effect of preserved skeletal muscle function and, hence, good physical condition on exacerbation control is summarized below.

The absence of a pulmonary rehabilitation program showed to be a risk factor for hospitalization in a large cohort of patients studied in Spain (7). Since pulmonary rehabilitation generally improves skeletal muscle force and deconditioning (8, 9), this study may provide indirect evidence that when patients are deprived of interventions improving skeletal muscle function they may be at risk for having exacerbations. More direct evidence comes from the study by Griffiths et al., who showed that patients after pulmonary rehabilitation had fewer hospitalizations related to the deterioration of their COPD over a 1-year follow-up period (10). In addition, we showed that pulmonary rehabilitation initiated after an acute exacerbation requiring hospitalization improved survival in these patients with high mortality risk (11).

It is well accepted that, from a physiological point of view, pulmonary rehabilitation has significant impact on skeletal muscle properties (muscle strength, muscle endurance, muscle bioenergetics, and exercise capacity) without significant impact on pulmonary function. Therefore, if there is any relation between reduction of medical consumption and pulmonary rehabilitation, the mediator of this relation may well be (directly or indirectly) improved peripheral and/or respiratory muscle function.

To our knowledge, no direct prospective evidence has been reported to relate skeletal muscle dysfunction to increased risk for hospitalizations in COPD, but one may speculate that deconditioning may make COPD patients more vulnerable for exacerbations. In healthy, deconditioned elderly subjects, participation in exercise training programs has been suggested to slow down the age-related deterioration of the immune response (12) and therefore may protect these frail subjects from infections. It is of note, however, that this is not a universal finding (13). The most important effects of exercise training in COPD are improved exercise tolerance and skeletal muscle force, improved functional exercise capacity, and enhanced health-related quality of life. Whether exercise training may protect COPD patients from infections needs to be confirmed in large, well-controlled clinical trials. Unfortunately, since there is overwhelming evidence that exercise training is beneficial to patients with COPD, the setup of such a controlled trial would be ethically unacceptable.

III. Factors Affecting Skeletal Muscle Relevant to Exacerbations

The exacerbation of COPD can result in impaired skeletal muscle functioning, and may induce muscle weakness. The environment in which the muscle has to function clearly compromises muscle contractile properties (hypercapnia, hypoxia, electrolyte disturbance, and substrate depletion). These factors are discussed in Sec. III.B. Moreover, the overwhelming inflammatory response during the exacerbation, the increased oxidative stress, bed rest, and medication (corticosteroids, muscle relaxants) may impact the integrity of the muscle itself favoring muscle damage, apoptosis, and, eventually, myopathy.

A. Factors That May Induce Muscle Atrophy or Myopathy

Bed Rest

Bed rest is devastating for skeletal muscle function. Even after a few days of bed rest, general skeletal muscle atrophy sets in. Models for deconditioning using bed rest show a negative protein balance (14), a rapid and impressive loss of skeletal muscle mass, and generalized muscle fiber atrophy (15). In little as 1 week, hindlimb unloading, for example, showed, significantly reduced fiber size and force of rat soleus muscle (16). The reduction in muscle mass is, in humans, accompanied by a disproportionately greater ($\approx 30\%$) reduction in muscle strength (17, 18). The latter is the net result of the inactivity (bed rest), since these changes are not observed in the upper limb muscles, which remain more active during bed rest (19, 20). Fiber-type transformation from slow-twitch to fast-twitch fibers has been documented in animal models of deconditioning. In human models, fiber-type transition has not been documented. Andersen et al., however, showed that there were more mismatched fibers after 6 weeks of bed rest. These so-called mismatched fibers express myosin heavy chain mRNA of the type IIa or IIx, whereas the muscle fiber itself is stained at the protein level, as a fiber type I or IIa, respectively. This mismatching, therefore, may indicate that the muscle fiber is in transition from type I to type IIa or from type IIa to type IIx, and that longer term bed rest may indeed provoke changes in fiber type distribution in favor of fiber type IIa and IIx (15). Interestingly, the same authors reported that coexpression of different myosin heavy chain types was increased in the elderly (21). Therefore, in that age group, typical for COPD patients, the effects of bed rest on fiber type distribution could be even more pronounced than in younger subjects. Older animal populations, indeed, seemed to be more susceptible to unloading than young animals on the single-muscle-cell level (especially in fiber type I) (22). This hypothesis needs confirmation in COPD patients.

Human and animal models show rapid decrease in myofibrillary protein synthesis and increase in protein degradation through the ATP-dependent ubiquitin proteosome pathway (23). Besides bed rest, this pathway is further stimulated by malnutrition, sepsis, and inflammation (see Sec. III.A). Loss of skeletal muscle mass due to deconditioning is further characterized by changes in muscle regulatory factors (MRF), upregulated myostatin (24), and progressive denervation of muscle fibers. The exact contribution of each of these factors, however, is far from elucidated. Although clean human and animal models of muscle unloading exist, during an acute exacerbation of COPD the deleterious effects of bed rest should be seen within the context of the acute exacerbation where all these factors act simultaneously and probably amplify each other.

Medication

In the treatment of acute exacerbations of COPD, corticosteroids are administered in relatively high doses. These have modest, but statistically significant, short-term effects on pulmonary function (25–27) and may reduce hospital stay (28).

Continuous use of oral corticosteroids or repeated bursts of corticosteroids may, however, have deleterious effects on muscle function and induce steroid myopathy (29, 30). Schols and coworkers even showed a dose-dependent inverse relation between corticosteroid use and survival (31). In patients, this steroid-induced myopathy is characterized by a general myopathy affecting all fiber types, slightly more marked in fiber types IIb and IIa and by the presence of necrotic fibers (32). Strength of all skeletal muscles is reduced (33) in COPD patients, but no systematic studies of the impact of corticosteroids on different skeletal muscles with different fiber type distribution are present in humans. In animal models, corticosteroid-induced myopathy showed to be more pronounced after treatment with fluorinated corticosteroids, and myopathy was more confined to type IIb fibers (34). These histological changes in the rat diaphragm and gastrocnemius after such treatment were clearly different than those observed after nutritional depletion, where more generalized atrophy was observed (35). Note that, in these models, animals were treated with massive doses of corticosteroids for short periods. This may not be representative for COPD patients, where longer term treatment with substantially lower doses is applied. This may account for the differences observed between the animal models resulting in acute steroid-induced myopathy and the clinical picture, where changes are induced by more chronic, continuous, or repetitive bursts, or steroid abuse (32). Growth factors may play an important role in the etiology of steroid-induced myopathic changes. We recently showed that insulin-like growth factor (IGF)-I and, to a lesser extend, IGF-II were downregulated in the diaphragm and gastrocnemius of rats treated with high-doses of corticosteroids for 5 days (36). Administration of IGF could not facilitate the recovery after steroid-induced atrophy (37). Observations by Kanda et al. (38) and Chysis et al. (39) showed that administration of IGF-I together with the dexamethasone treatment may partially prevent the catabolic effects of administered corticosteroids in rats. These studies, however, were not entirely conclusive. It remains an appealing area of research to investigate the effects on the autocrine IGF-production in the skeletal muscle when corticosteroids are administered in patients during an acute exacerbation of COPD. The protective effect of IGF-I may result from its inhibition of the corticosteroid-induced increase in glutamine synthetase (40) and through its downregulation of the activated components of the ubiquitin pathway (39). It is interesting that exercise was reported to induce the same protective effect (41, 42). In a randomized controlled trial, Braith et al. reported that resistance training was able to counteract glucocorticoid-induced changes in heart transplant patients (43). It is unclear whether exercise training during an acute exacerbation of COPD, treated with corticosteroids may have similar beneficial effects. In contrast to exercise training, bed rest seems to attenuate the catabolic response to increased cortisol levels. Ferrando et al. showed in six healthy male subjects that the devastating catabolic effects of hypercortisolemia were attenuated by 14 days of strict bed rest (44).

It is our clinical opinion (supported by findings in rats treated with corticos-teroids) that patients with frequent exacerbations, who are repeatedly treated with bursts of corticosteroids, are equally prone to developing corticosteroid-induced myopathy. Although muscle weakness in COPD is clearly multifactorial in nature,

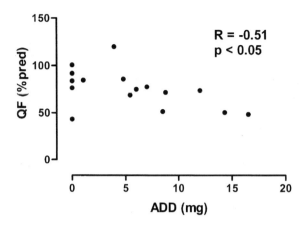

Figure 2   Relation between average daily dose of corticosteroids over 6 months (ADD) expressed as mg methylprednisolone equivalents, and quadriceps force (QF), expressed as percentage of the predicted value, in a cohort of COPD patients admitted to an outpatient pulmonary rehabilitation program in our facilities.

the average daily dose of oral corticosteroid use (expressed as methylprednisolone equivalents per day) showed to be one of the variables related to muscle weakness in COPD patients. Figure 2 illustrates the relationship of this variable to quadriceps strength in a sample of COPD patients studied in our center. Observations by Saundy-Unterberger of a close relation between corticosteroid dose during an acute exacerbation of COPD and the degree of negative nitrogen balance (an indirect index of muscle wasting) (45) run along these lines.

In very severe exacerbations or life-threatening status asthmaticus, mechanical ventilation in combination with neuromuscular blocking agents (NMBAs: pancuronium, vecuronium, or atracurium) may be required as a life-saving treatment. It is clear, however, that the administration of NMBAs should be well considered. A study by Behbehani et al. indicated that in patients with acute asthma the odds ratio to develop acute myopathy increased by 2.1 (95% CI 1.4–3.2) for each day of muscle relaxation (46).

The Role of Oxidative Stress

COPD patients are subjected to increased oxidative stress (47). As potential sources for oxidative stress in COPD, cigarette smoke, inflammation, infections, and hypoxia have been identified (48,49). During exacerbations, more reactive oxygen species are formed, causing disturbances in the oxidant/antioxidant status (50). Recently, oxidative stress during viral infections—such as influenza—received attention (51). Besides the skeletal muscle cells, immune cells activated by the inflammation can play a potential role during exacerbation. In addition, TNF-α, produced by monocytes and macrophages, may induce oxidative stress in myocytes (52). Although most research on oxidative stress has focused on the lung, this imbalance may make the skeletal muscle vulnerable, particularly during the first days of the acute exacerbation. The protection against reactive oxygen species seems to be poorest during an acute exacerbation (53). Even when stable, the muscle redox potential showed to be lower in COPD, compared to normal subjects (54). In a study with smaller sample size, Rabinovich et al. could not confirm these findings (55). However, these authors confirmed that patients with COPD, especially those with low BMI, might be vulnerable to oxidative stress induced by high-intensity endurance training. Reactive oxygen species have impressive harmful effects on the skeletal muscle, reducing its contractility and leading to apoptosis, and may play a role in skeletal muscle dysfunction in COPD (56). Further research, however, is warranted to investigate the role of excessive oxidative stress during exacerbations on muscle function.

The Role of Systemic Inflammation on Muscle Function During Exacerbation

Acute exacerbations of COPD are associated with increased circulating proinflammatory cytokines and inflammatory mediators. In pulmonary stable, but weight-losing COPD patients, increased plasma levels of proinflammatory cytokines (especially TNF-α) have been reported (57, 58). In addition, increased inflammatory cytokines including TNF-α, interleukin-2 (IL-2), and interleukin-6 (IL-6) have also been reported in patients with chronic hypoxia (59) and increased C-reactive protein (CRP) levels (60). It is generally accepted that these proinflammatory cytokines contribute to reduced fat-free mass, reduced muscle function, and impaired response to nutritional interventions (61). In mouse-derived C1C12 cell line, Li et al. showed a direct effect of exogeneous TNF-α on muscle protein loss through close interaction with NF-κB (62). During acute exacerbations, circulating inflammatory markers were increased in COPD (63).

The presence of systemic inflammation during COPD exacerbations has been demonstrated by Wedzicha et al. who showed increased plasma IL-6 levels (64). In a more recent study, Dentener et al. (65) confirmed an increase of several inflammatory markers. This was accompanied by a temporary rise (first 3 days) of soluble TNF-α and IL-1 receptors. It is still open to discussion whether this systemic inflammation may impact on the skeletal muscle in COPD. The involvement of the inflammatory response in the onset of anorexia (a strong correlate of skeletal muscle weakness in COPD) (66) after an exacerbation became evident from the work of Creutzberg et al. (63). These authors showed a negative relation between soluble TNF receptors and energy balance (dietary intake/resting energy expenditure) during an exacerbation. Similar observations were made by Nguyen et al. (67), showing a close relation between circulating plasma TNF-α and resting energy expenditure in stable COPD patients. In models with profound inflammation (burn, endotoxin, sepsis), significant increases in TNF-α were reported. However, administration of TNF binding protein could not prevent the loss of muscle protein content (68). The authors suggest an important role in these models may be allotted to increased myostatin activity (muscle growth and differentiation factor 8, a member of the TGF-β family). This factor promotes fiber IIa and IIb atrophy (24). Consequently, knock-out of the myostatin gene results in dramatic increase in muscle mass. The myostatin upregulation seems to be enhanced by administration of dexamethasone (68). The latter may be relevant in the patient with COPD, treated with high-dose corticosteroids.

B. Factors Affecting Proper Functioning of the Muscle During Exacerbations

The conditions in which skeletal muscles have to work may be compromised in patients during an acute exacerbation. Depletion of substrates, hypoxia, and uncompensated hypercapnia resulting in acidemia contribute to an environment in which the contractile properties of the skeletal muscle are compromised. The effect of this unfavorable environment in which the skeletal muscles have to work is illustrated in Figure 3. From this older work of Gertz and colleagues, it is obvious that the skeletal muscle is deprived from ATP and phosphocreatine, both immediately available energy stores. Moreover, intramuscular lactate concentration was increased in the acute phase. These abnormalities gradually returned to normal COPD values as the extracellular environment recovered (69).

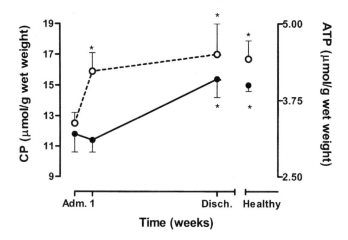

Figure 3 Concentrations of metabolites: creatinine phosphate (CP, open circles, dashed line) and ATP (closed circles, solid line) in quadriceps muscle samples from patients admitted to the hospital with acute respiratory failure requiring ICU admission. (Mechanical ventilation was initiated in 30% of the patients). Samples were taken on admission (Adm.), after 1 week of treatment, and at discharge (Disch.). For comparison, values obtained in healthy controls are displayed. Significant lactic acid production was observed in the skeletal muscle at rest on admission (data not shown). (Data obtained from Ref. 69.)

Hypoxia

The lack of oxygen in the skeletal muscle causes task failure. Glycolytic processes will take over ATP supply for the force-generating processes, but this results in inevitable decrease in intracellular pH and early task failure. In stable patients with COPD, there has been debate as to whether peak exercise is dependent on reduced oxygen supply. Data from Richardson et al. (70) are in favor of an O_2 supply dependence in these patients. Administering supplemental oxygen indeed showed an improvement in muscle bioenergetics (71) in hypoxic (PaO_2 57 ± 3 mmHg) and moderately hypercapnic $PaCO_2$ (47 ± 3 mmHg) patients. Other studies showed that acute relief of chronic hypoxia improved maximum strength of adductor pollicis, vastus lateralis, and diaphragm muscle (72). From these studies, however, it is difficult to deduce the impact of acute hypoxia on skeletal muscle performance, since the impact on oxygen delivery to the skeletal muscle may not be altered dramatically. During acute exacerbations of COPD, hypoxia may be present, predominantly because of increased resting oxygen consumption and moderately increased ventilation/perfusion mismatching (73). In a recent study, Gonzàlez-Alonso et al. studied the effects of acute hypoxia on leg O_2 delivery. Despite a significant reduction of the PaO_2 (105 ± 3 to 47 ± 3 mmHg), leg O_2 delivery did not change significantly due to a concomitant rise in leg blood flow (74). In COPD patients, the reduction in oxygen saturation, in combination with the poor capillarization (75), may lead to reduction in oxygen delivery to the skeletal muscle. Notwithstanding the maintained oxygen delivery, it has been shown that hypoxemia results in tissue hypoxia and even reduced mitochondrial VO_2 (76). Therefore, it is not surprising that exercise at isowork under acute hypoxic conditions increases glycolysis and, hence, lactate concentration (77). This increased lactate concentration in addition to hypoxia will result in a higher ventilatory demand. The latter may cause problems to the respiratory pump, which, during an acute exacerbation, already has to work against increased resistance (see Sec. V). It is of note that intermittent hypoxia, followed by relative hyperoxia when oxygen is administered, may result in a boost of free radicals (reactive oxygen species) known as reperfusion injury and may cause additional muscle damage (78). In addition, it has been shown that even short-term hypoxia leads to increased circulating leptin levels (79). Through this pathway, intermittent (or continuous) hypoxia may contribute to loss of appetite, protein imbalance, and loss of skeletal muscle mass.

Hypercapnia

Hypercapnia and especially the associated respiratory acidosis (80) may result in lower mitochondrial efficiency and early onset of fatigue. Mador et al. (81) reported a significant reduction of twitch force of the abductor pollicis muscle when healthy subjects were breathing a CO_2-enriched mixture resulting in $PaCO_2$ similar to that observed during acute exacerbations ($FICO_2$ 8% with $PaCO_2$ of $\cong 60$ mmHg). Similar findings were observed in other human (82) and animal studies (83). It remains unclear whether modest CO_2 retention is capable of increasing intracellular pH. While Sahlin et al. (84) found no short-term effect (10 min) of CO_2 breathing on resting intracellular pH. Results obtained from muscle biopsies in patients with respiratory failure pointed out that skeletal muscle pH was indeed lower (69, 85). Fiaccadori et al. reported a close relationship between arterial PCO_2 and intracellular pH in patients with acute respiratory failure just before intubation (85).

During mild exercise, however, Sahlin et al. showed a clear rise in intramuscular CO_2 content (84) and an abnormal energy metabolism. The authors concluded that the increased H^+ compromises the force-generating capacity and induces early muscle fatigue (83).

Depletion of Substrates and Electrolytes

Few studies investigated the fuel-content of skeletal muscles during exacerbations. In stable but hypoxic and hypercapnic (severe) COPD patients, Jakobsson et al. reported that skeletal muscles had significantly lower glycogen and phosphocreatine content, compared to COPD patients without respiratory failure (86, 87). In addition, the muscle glycogen content was related both to resting PaO_2 ($R = 0.70$; $p < 0.0001$) and to resting $PaCO_2$ ($R = -0.50$; $p < 0.05$). It should be pointed out that treatment with corticosteroids during the exacerbation may interfere with the glucose uptake in skeletal muscles during exercise. In the earlier mentioned study by Fiaccadori (85), the authors report significant derangement of the intramuscular electrolyte and acid base equilibrium. This derangement undoubtedly adds to impaired muscle function in patients with COPD admitted to the intensive care unit for intubation.

IV. Respiratory Muscles in Exacerbation

Respiratory muscle adaptations should be approached differently from other skeletal muscles in COPD patients suffering from acute exacerbations. Evidently the environment in which the muscle has to contract (hypoxic, hypercapnic, treated with corticosteroids, etc.) is largely comparable to the other skeletal muscles. However, the mechanical disadvantage (hyperinflation), reduced dynamic pulmonary compliance and increased airway resistance, all of which increase the work of breathing, leads to overuse rather than deconditioning. Especially during acute exacerbations requiring hospitalization, the work of breathing is increased (88). This, accelerated by the impaired gas exchange during exacerbations, leads to excess ventilatory demands (89), which may lead to respiratory muscle failure. In experimental conditions, sudden increase of respiratory resistance showed that glycogen depletion may contribute to task failure (90). In the end-stage, respiratory muscle pump failure argues for (invasive or noninvasive) mechanical ventilation as a life-saving strategy for these patients (91, 92). Applying noninvasive ventilation on such occasions reduced the work imposed on the inspiratory muscles (93).

In stable patients with COPD, specific adaptations are seen in the diaphragm muscle (Table 1). These adaptations are believed to compensate for hyperinflation and chronically increased inspiratory resistance. Briefly, the adaptations consist of a reduction of sarcomeres in series, and a relatively increased oxidative capacity of the diaphragm with higher proportion of slow (oxidative) fiber types (94–96). On a

Table 1 Summary of Adaptations in the Diaphragm of Stable COPD Patients

	Property	Compared to normal
Macroscopic level	Radius of the diaphragm	↑
	Zone of apposition	↓
	Energetic demand	↑
	Pressure-generating capacity (PGC)	↓
	PGC corrected for operating lung volume	=
Fiber level	Myosin heavy chain (MHC) fiber 1 proportion	↑
	Intrinsic muscle fiber strength	=
	Microvascular PO$_2$	↓
	Capillary density	=
	Number of sarcomeres in series	↓
Subcellular level	Mitochondrial concentration	↑
	Oxidative potential (citrate synthase)	↑
	Glycogen stores	=
	Sarcomere length	↓

subcellular level, Orozco et al. (95) reported that, in steroid-free, normally nourished COPD patients, reduced sarcomere length and increased mithochondrial density was inversely related to the airflow obstruction. From these observations it can be understood that the diaphragm of stable patients with COPD lost the absolute ability to generate negative pleural pressure because of mechanical disadvantages. However, it adapts to the best of its possibilities to prevent respiratory failure (97). It should be noted that most COPD patients die from respiratory failure, most of them during an acute exacerbation of their disease. Hence, during acute exacerbations, the adaptations of the diaphragm may be insufficient to meet the increased demands. During exacerbations, the work of breathing increases considerably. The total resistive work per liter of ventilation was reported threefold higher in COPD patients suffering from an acute exacerbation compared to normal subjects (88). Dynamic hyperinflation forces the respiratory muscles to operate at a shorter length, which again reduces their force-generating capacity (98, 99). As a result, the maximal pressure that can be generated is reduced and the relative load (PI/PI$_{max}$) may increase up to 0.30, or sixfold the normal value (100). As a consequence of the high resistance to expiratory flow, low elastic recoil, high ventilatory demands, and relatively short expiratory time, inspiration starts when there is still a positive recoil pressure [intrinsic positive end expiratory pressure (iPEEP)] (101). An additional load to the respiratory muscles is imposed by this iPEEP since the inspiratory muscles have to overcome this pressure, ranging from 6 to 13 cmH$_2$O in a classic study by Fleury et al. (102), even before inspiratory flow can start.

In an attempt to avoid task failure, the breathing pattern shifts to a rapid and shallow breathing pattern in order to reduce the duty cycle of the inspiratory muscles. Because of the excess in deadspace ventilation, however, this strategy generally results in hypercapnia, and assisted ventilation may be required (103). Although in healthy subjects, stable COPD patients, or animals, intermittent periods of loaded breathing (using inspiratory resistance) generally result in a training effect (104), the situation of an acute exacerbation may resemble a model of overtraining rather than a model of training. In animal models of chronic overload, Reid et al. (105) showed the presence of diaphragm injury. The same investigators showed that the abnormal diaphragm area (defined as fibers with central nuclear, small angulated fibers, lipofuscin pigmentation, and some inflammation) ranges from 3 to 34% in patients undergoing thoracotomy. This abnormal diaphragm area was inversely related to the FEV_1 (106). In addition, Zhu et al. (107) demonstrated significant— and predominantly fiber type—muscle damage after 4 days of intermittent resistive breathing. However, it is not clear whether this muscle damage initiates the processes necessary for muscle adaptation to increased load, or if they contribute to the task failure preceding the onset of respiratory failure. It is of note that similar findings of diaphragm injury have been demonstrated in patients who died from fatal asthma (108). Because of these abnormalities, the respiratory muscles may be well prepared to deal with slightly increased work, but in the case of long-term overload (acute exacerbation) it may be very slow in its recovery. The increased work of breathing, and the predominance of oxidative fibers, renders the diaphragm vulnerable to oxidative stress caused by free radical production as a spin-off of the electron chain. Borzone et al. showed that large quantities of free radicals were indeed produced in the diaphragm when resistive loading was applied in rats until respiratory pump failure (109, 110). Interesting investigations by Poole et al. highlighted that in experimentally induced emphysema, pulmonary microvascular oxygen content (and therefore probably intramuscular oxygen availability) is reduced, despite increased capillary-to-fiber contacts (111, 112). The authors calculated that in the diaphragm the microvascular O_2 content of the diaphragm falls twofold more than the arterial O_2 content. Therefore, the O_2 and substrate extraction reserve of the diaphragm in emphysema is greatly reduced, which impacts on the force-generating capacity and reduces the resistance to fatigue. In the context of hypoxia and increased work of breathing during an acute exacerbation, the latter may become clinically important.

Treatment of a failing respiratory muscle pump is generally considered to be complete or partial rest. The most typical, and most accepted form, is controlled (full rest) or assisted (partial rest) ventilation (113). Several other strategies have been propagated. Breathing control, or diaphragmatic breathing, has been proposed as a way to increase tidal volume and reduce breathing frequency in patients with COPD (114). Different studies, however, showed that diaphragmatic breathing increased the work of breathing in patients with COPD (115, 116), and therefore should not be a preferred strategy in treating the failing ventilatory pump. Breathing gas mixtures with low density reduced the work of breathing in COPD patients through a reduction of the resistance to gas flow (117). Therefore, breathing these low-density gas mixtures or assisted ventilation with these mixtures may be beneficial to the respiratory muscles (118, 119). The effects of HELIOX breathing, however, showed to be inferior to the effects of noninvasive ventilation with normal air. The combination of noninvasive ventilation and HELIOX showed the greatest effect on hypercapnia and work of breathing (118). During exacerbations, care should be taken that the nutritional status of the patients is improved, or at least maintained. Improvements in nutritional status were shown to coincide with improved respiratory muscle function (120), while nutritional depletion was related to respiratory and skeletal muscle dysfunction (121). Lastly, poor respiratory muscle function is a significant predictor of hospitalizations (1). Therefore, training the respiratory muscles may be an effective strategy to prevent acute respiratory failure during acute exacerbations. When properly controlled, training of the inspiratory muscles consistently increased inspiratory muscle strength and hence improved the PI/PI_{max} ratio. It is of note, however, that inspiratory muscle training is restricted to stable patients, and should not be applied during acute exacerbations.

Acknowledgments

This work has been supported by grants Fonds voor Wetenschappelijk Onderzoek Vlaanderen, Grant # G.0237.01 and # G.0175.99, and Levenslijn grant # 7.0007.00.

References

1. Decramer M, Gosselink R, Troosters T, Verschueren M, Evers G. Muscle weakness is related to utilization of health care resources in COPD patients. Eur Respir J 1997; 10:417–423.
2. Gray-Donald K, Gibbons L, Shapiro SH, Macklem PT, Martin JG. Nutritional status and mortality in chronic obstructive pulmonary disease. Am J Respir Crit Care Med 1996; 153:961–966.
3. Vermeeren MA, Schols AM, Wouters EF. Effects of an acute exacerbation on nutritional and metabolic profile of patients with COPD. Eur Respir J 1997; 10:2264–2269.
4. Vestbo J, Rasmussen FV. Respiratory symptoms and FEV1 as predictors of hospitalization and medication in the following 12 years due to respiratory disease. Eur Respir J 1989; 2:710–715.
5. Kessler R, Faller M, Fourgaut G, Mennecier B, Weitzenblum E. Predictive factors of hospitalization for acute exacerbation in a series of 64 patients with chronic obstructive pulmonary disease. Am J Respir Crit Care Med 1999; 159:158–164.
6. Gosselink R, Troosters T, Decramer M. Peripheral muscle weakness contributes to exercise limitation in COPD. Am J Respir Crit Care Med 1996; 153:976–980.
7. Garcia-Aymerich J, Barreiro E, Farrero E, Marrades RM, Morera J, Anto JM. Patients hospitalized for COPD have a high prevalence of modifiable risk factors for exacerbation (EFRAM study). Eur Respir J 2000; 16:1037–1042.
8. O'Donnell DE, McGuire M, Samis L, Webb KA. General exercise training improves ventilatory and peripheral muscle strength and endurance in chronic airflow limitation. Am J Respir Crit Care Med 1998; 157:1489–1497.

9. Troosters T, Gosselink R, Decramer M. Short- and long-term effects of outpatient rehabilitation in patients with chronic obstructive pulmonary disease: a randomized trial. Am J Med 2000; 109:207–212.

10. Griffiths TL, Burr ML, Campbell IA, Lewis-Jenkins V, Mullins J, Shiels K, et al. Results at 1 year of outpatient multidisciplinary pulmonary rehabilitation: a randomised controlled trial. Lancet 2000; 355:362 368.

11. Troosters T, Gosselink R, De Paepe K, Decramer M. Pulmonary rehabilitation improves survival after a severe acute exacerbation in COPD patients. Am J Respir Crit Care Med 2002; 65:A16(abstr).

12. Paw MJ, de Jong N, Pallast EG, Kloek GC, Schouten EG, Kok FJ. Immunity in frail elderly: a randomized controlled trial of exercise and enriched foods. Med Sci Sports Exerc 2000; 32:2005–2011.

13. Bruunsgaard H, Pedersen BK. Special feature for the Olympics: effects of exercise on the immune system: effects of exercise on the immune system in the elderly population. Immunol Cell Biol 2000; 78:523–531.

14. Ferrando AA, Lane HW, Stuart CA, Davis-Street J, Wolfe RR. Prolonged bed rest decreases skeletal muscle and whole body protein synthesis. Am J Physiol 1996; 270:E627–E633.

15. Andersen JL, Gruschy-Knudsen T, Sandri C, Larsson L, Schiaffino S. Bed rest increases the amount of mismatched fibers in human skeletal muscle. J Appl Physiol 1999; 86:455–460.

16. McDonald KS, Fitts RH. Effect of hindlimb unloading on rat soleus fiber force, stiffness, and calcium sensitivity. J Appl Physiol 1995; 79:1796–1802.

17. Vandenborne K, Elliott MA, Walter GA, Abdus S, Okereke E, Shaffer M, et al. Longitudinal study of skeletal muscle adaptations during immobilization and rehabilitation. Muscle Nerve 1998; 21:1006–1012.

18. Berg HE, Larsson L, Tesch PA. Lower limb skeletal muscle function after 6 weeks of bed rest. J Appl Physiol 1997; 82:182–188.

19. Desplanches D, Hoppeler H, Mayet MH, Denis C, Claassen H, Ferretti G. Effects of bedrest on deltoideus muscle morphology and enzymes. Acta Physiol Scand 1998; 162:135–140.

20. Gea JG, Pasto M, Carmona MA, Orozco-Levi M, Palomeque J, Broquetas J. Metabolic characteristics of the deltoid muscle in patients with chronic obstructive pulmonary disease. Eur Respir J 2001; 17:939–945.

21. Andersen JL, Terzis G, Kryger A. Increase in the degree of coexpression of myosin heavy chain isoforms in skeletal muscle fibers of the very old. Muscle Nerve 1999; 22:449–454.

22. Thompson LV, Johnson SA, Shoeman JA. Single soleus muscle fiber function after hindlimb unweighting in adult and aged rats. J Appl Physiol 1998; 84:1937–1942.

23. Mitch WE, Goldberg AL. Mechanisms of muscle wasting. The role of the ubiquitin-proteasome pathway. N Engl J Med 1996; 335:1897–1905.

24. Reardon KA, Davis J, Kapsa RM, Choong P, Byrne E. Myostatin, insulin-like growth factor-1, and leukemia inhibitory factor mRNAs are upregulated in chronic human disuse muscle atrophy. Muscle Nerve 2001; 24:893–899.

25. Niewoehner DE, Erbland ML, Deupree RH, Collins D, Gross NJ, Light RW, et al. Effect of systemic glucocorticoids on exacerbations of chronic obstructive pulmonary disease. Department of Veterans Affairs Cooperative Study Group. N Engl J Med 1999; 340:1941–1947.

26. Albert RK, Martin TR, Lewis SW. Controlled clinical trial of methylprednisolone in patients with chronic bronchitis and acute respiratory insufficiency. Ann Intern Med 1980; 92:753–758.

27. Thompson WH, Nielson CP, Carvalho P, Charan NB, Crowley JJ. Controlled trial of oral prednisone in outpatients with acute COPD exacerbation. Am J Respir Crit Care Med 1996; 154:407–412.

28. Davies L, Angus RM, Calverley PM. Oral corticosteroids in patients admitted to hospital with exacerbations of chronic obstructive pulmonary disease: a prospective randomised controlled trial. Lancet 1999; 354:456–460.

29. Decramer M, Lacquet LM, Fagard R, Rogiers P. Corticosteroids contribute to muscle weakness in chronic airflow obstruction. Am J Respir Crit Care Med 1994; 150:11–16.

30. Gayan-Ramirez G, Bisschop A, Decramer M. Repetitive burst methylprednisolone treatment affects rat diaphragm more than continuous dose treatment. Am J Respir Crit Care Med 1995; 151:A812.

31. Schols AM, Wesseling G, Kester AD, de Vries G, Mostert R, Slangen J, et al. Dose dependent increased mortality risk in COPD patients treated with oral glucocorticoids. Eur Respir J 2001; 17:337–342.

32. Decramer M, de Bock V, Dom R. Functional and histologic picture of steroid-induced myopathy in chronic obstructive pulmonary disease. Am J Respir Crit Care Med 1996; 153:1958–1964.

33. Gosselink R, Troosters T, Decramer M. Distribution of muscle weakness in patients with stable chronic obstructive pulmonary disease. J Cardiopulm Rehabil 2000; 20:353–360.

34. Dekhuijzen PN, Gayan-Ramirez G, de Bock, V, Dom R, Decramer M. Triamcinolone and prednisolone affect contractile properties and histopathology of rat diaphragm differently. J Clin Invest 1993; 92:1534–1542.

35. Dekhuijzen PN, Gayan-Ramirez G, Bisschop A, de Bock V, Dom R, Decramer M. Corticosteroid treatment and nutritional deprivation cause a different pattern of atrophy in rat diaphragm. J Appl Physiol 1995; 78:629–637.

36. Gayan-Ramirez G, Vanderhoydonc F, Verhoeven G, Decramer M. Acute treatment with corticosteroids decreases IGF-1 and IGF-2 expression in the rat diaphragm and gastrocnemius. Am J Respir Crit Care Med 1999; 159:283–289.

37. Gayan-Ramirez G, Houtmeyers E, Decramer M. Insulin-like growth factor-1 treatment combined or not with growth hormone does not improve corticosteroid-induced effects on rat diaphragm. Am J Respir Crit Care Med 1998; 157:A668.

38. Kanda F, Takatani K, Okuda S, Matsushita T, Chihara K. Preventive effects of insulin-like growth factor-1 on steroid-induced muscle atrophy. Muscle Nerve 1999; 22:213–217.

39. Chrysis D, Underwood LE. Regulation of components of the ubiquitin system by insulin-like growth factor 1 and growth hormone in skeletal muscle of rats made catabolic with dexamethasone. Endocrinology 1999; 140:5635–5641.

40. Kimura K, Kanda F, Okuda S, Chihara K. Insulin-like growth factor 1 inhibits glucocorticoid-induced glutamine synthetase activity in cultured L6 rat skeletal muscle cells. Neurosci Lett 2001; 302:154–156.

41. Falduto MT, Young AP, Hickson RC. Exercise inhibits glucocorticoid-induced glutamine synthetase expression in red skeletal muscles. Am J Physiol 1992; 262:C214–C220.

42. Willoughby DS, Priest JW, Jennings RA. Myosin heavy chain isoform and ubiquitin protease mRNA expression after passive leg cycling in persons with spinal cord injury. Arch Phys Med Rehabil 2000; 81:157–163.

43. Braith RW, Welsch MA, Mills RM, Jr., Keller JW, Pollock ML. Resistance exercise prevents glucocorticoid-induced myopathy in heart transplant recipients. Med Sci Sports Exerc 1998; 30:483–489.

44. Ferrando AA, Stuart CA, Sheffield-Moore M, Wolfe RR. Inactivity amplifies the catabolic response of skeletal muscle to cortisol. J Clin Endocrinol Metab 1999; 84:3515–3521.

45. Saudny-Unterberger H, Martin JG, Gray-Donald K. Impact of nutritional support on functional status during an acute exacerbation of chronic obstructive pulmonary disease. Am J Respir Crit Care Med 1997; 156:794–799.

46. Behbehani NA, Al Mane F, D'yachkova Y, Pare P, Fitzgerald JM. Myopathy following mechanical ventilation for acute severe asthma: the role of muscle relaxants and corticosteroids. Chest 1999; 115:1627–1631.

47. Maller P, Loft S, Lundby C, Olsen NV. Acute hypoxia and hypoxic exercise induce DNA strand breaks and oxidative DNA damage in humans. FASEB J 2001; 15:1181–1186.

48. Corbucci GG, Menichetti A, Cogliati A, Ruvolo C. Metabolic aspects of cardiac and skeletal muscle tissues in the condition of hypoxia, ischaemia and reperfusion induced by extracorporeal circulation. Int J Tissue React 1995; 17:219–225.

49. Repine JE, Bast A, Lankhorst I. Oxidative stress in chronic obstructive pulmonary disease. Oxidative Stress Study Group. Am J Respir Crit Care Med 1997; 156:341–357.

50. Pratico D, Basili S, Vieri M, Cordova C, Violi F, Fitzgerald GA. Chronic obstructive pulmonary disease is associated with an increase in urinary levels of isoprostane F2alpha-III, an index of oxidant stress. Am J Respir Crit Care Med 1998; 158:1709–1714.

51. Peterhans E. Oxidants and antioxidants in viral diseases: disease mechanisms and metabolic regulation. J Nutr 1997; 127:962S–965S.

52. Buck M, Chojkier M. Muscle wasting and dedifferentiation induced by oxidative stress in a murine model of cachexia is prevented by inhibitors of nitric oxide synthesis and antioxidants. EMBO J 1996; 15:1753–1765.

53. Rahman I, Skwarska E, MacNee W. Attenuation of oxidant/antioxidant imbalance during treatment of exacerbations of chronic obstructive pulmonary disease. Thorax 1997; 52:565–568.

54. Engelen MP, Schols AM, Does JD, Deutz NE, Wouters EF. Altered glutamate metabolism is associated with reduced muscle glutathione levels in patients with emphysema. Am J Respir Crit Care Med 2000; 161:98–103.

55. Rabinovich RA, Ardite E, Troosters T, Carbò N, Alonso J, Gonzalez De Suso JM, et al. Reduced muscle redox capacity after endurance training in patients with chronic obstructive pulmonary disease. Am J Respir Crit Care Med 2001; 164:1114–1118.

56. Skeletal muscle dysfunction in chronic obstructive pulmonary disease. A statement of the American Thoracic Society and European Respiratory Society. Am J Respir Crit Care Med 1999; 159:S1–S4.

57. Di Francia M, Barbier D, Mege JL, Orehek J. Tumor necrosis factor-alpha levels and weight loss in chronic obstructive pulmonary disease. Am J Respir Crit Care Med 1994; 150:1453–1455.

58. de Godoy I, Donahoe M, Calhoun WJ, Mancino J, Rogers RM. Elevated TNF-alpha production by peripheral blood monocytes of weight-losing COPD patients. Am J Respir Crit Care Med 1996; 153:633–637.

59. Takabatake N, Nakamura H, Abe S, Inoue S, Hino T, Saito H, et al. The relationship between chronic hypoxemia and activation of the tumor necrosis factor-alpha system in

patients with chronic obstructive pulmonary disease. Am J Respir Crit Care Med 2000; 161:1179–1184.

60. Schols AM, Buurman WA, Staal van den Brekel AJ, Dentener MA, Wouters EF. Evidence for a relation between metabolic derangements and increased levels of inflammatory mediators in a subgroup of patients with chronic obstructive pulmonary disease. Thorax 1996; 51:819–824.

61. Creutzberg EC, Schols AM, Weling-Scheepers CA, Buurman WA, Wouters EF. Characterization of nonresponse to high caloric oral nutritional therapy in depleted patients with chronic obstructive pulmonary disease. Am J Respir Crit Care Med 2000; 161:745–752.

62. Li YP, Schwartz RJ, Waddell ID, Holloway BR, Reid MB. Skeletal muscle myocytes undergo protein loss and reactive oxygen-mediated NF-kappaB activation in response to tumor necrosis factor alpha. FASEB J 1998; 12:871–880.

63. Creutzberg EC, Wouters EF, Vanderhoven-Augustin IM, Dentener MA, Schols AM. Disturbances in leptin metabolism are related to energy imbalance during acute exacerbations of chronic obstructive pulmonary disease. Am J Respir Crit Care Med 2000; 162:1239–1245.

64. Wedzicha JA, Seemungal TA, MacCullum PK, Paul EA, Donaldson GC, Bhowmik A, et al. Acute exacerbations of chronic obstructive pulmonary disease are accompanied by elevations of plasma fibrinogen and serum IL-6 levels. Thromb Haemost 2000; 84:210–215.

65. Dentener MA, Creutzberg EC, Schols AM, Mantovani A, van't Veer C, Buurman WA, et al. Systemic anti-inflammatory mediators in COPD: increase in soluble interleukin 1 receptor II during treatment of exacerbations. Thorax 2001; 56:721–726.

66. Engelen MP, Schols AM, Does JD, Wouters EF. Skeletal muscle weakness is associated with wasting of extremity fat-free mass but not with airflow obstruction in patients with chronic obstructive pulmonary disease. Am J Clin Nutr 2000; 71:733–738.

67. Nguyen LT, Bedu M, Caillaud D, Beaufrere B, Beaujon G, Vasson M, et al. Increased resting energy expenditure is related to plasma TNF-alpha concentration in stable COPD patients. Clin Nutr 1999; 18:269–274.

68. Lang CH, Silvis C, Nystrom G, Frost RA. Regulation of myostatin by glucocorticoids after thermal injury. FASEB J 2001; 15:1807–1809.

69. Gertz I, Hedenstierna G, Hellers G, Wahren J. Muscle metabolism in patients with chronic obstructive lung disease and acute respiratory failure. Clin Sci Mol Med 1977; 52:396–403.

70. Richardson RS, Sheldon J, Poole DC, Hopkins SR, Ries AL, Wagner PD. Evidence of skeletal muscle metabolic reserve during whole body exercise in patients with chronic obstructive pulmonary disease. Am J Respir Crit Care Med 1999; 159: 881–885.

71. Payen JF, Wuyam B, Levy P, Reutenauer H, Stieglitz P, Paramelle B, et al. Muscular metabolism during oxygen supplementation in patients with chronic hypoxemia. Am Rev Respir Dis 1993; 147:592–598.

72. Zattara-Hartmann MC, Badier M, Guillot C, Tomei C, Jammes Y. Maximal force and endurance to fatigue of respiratory and skeletal muscles in chronic hypoxemic patients: the effects of oxygen breathing. Muscle Nerve 1995; 18:495–502.

73. Barbera JA. Chronic obstructive pulmonary disease. In: Roca J, Rodriguez-Roisin R, Wagner PD, eds. Pulmonary and peripheral gas exchange in health and disease. New York: Marcel Dekker, 2000:229–262.

74. Gonzalez-Alonso J, Richardson RS, Saltin B. Exercising skeletal muscle blood flow in humans responds to reduction in arterial oxyhaemoglobin, but not to altered free oxygen. J Physiol 2001; 530:331–341.

75. Jobin J, Maltais F, Doyon JF, LeBlanc P, Simard PM, Simard AA, et al. Chronic obstructive pulmonary disease: capillarity and fiber-type characteristics of skeletal muscle. J Cardiopulm Rehabil 1998; 18:432–437.

76. Richardson RS, Leigh JS, Wagner PD, Noyszewski EA. Cellular PO2 as a determinant of maximal mitochondrial O(2) consumption in trained human skeletal muscle. J Appl Physiol 1999; 87:325–331.

77. Parolin ML, Spriet LL, Hultman E, Hollidge-Horvat MG, Jones NL, Heigenhauser GJ. Regulation of glycogen phosphorylase and PDH during exercise in human skeletal muscle during hypoxia. Am J Physiol Endocrinol Metab 2000; 278:E522–E534.

78. Rubin BB, Romaschin A, Walker PM, Gute DC, Korthuis RJ. Mechanisms of postischemic injury in skeletal muscle: intervention strategies. J Appl Physiol 1996; 80:369–387.

79. Tschop M, Strasburger CJ, Hartmann G, Biollaz J, Bartsch P. Raised leptin concentrations at high altitude associated with loss of appetite. Lancet 1998; 352: 1119–1120.

80. Spriet LL, Matsos CG, Peters SJ, Heigenhauser GJ, Jones NL. Effects of acidosis on rat muscle metabolism and performance during heavy exercise. Am J Physiol 1985; 248:C337–C347.

81. Mador MJ, Wendel T, Kufel TJ. Effect of acute hypercapnia on diaphragmatic and limb muscle contractility. Am J Respir Crit Care Med 1997; 155:1590–1595.

82. Vianna LG, Koulouris N, Lanigan C, Moxham J. Effect of acute hypercapnia on limb muscle contractility in humans. J Appl Physiol 1990; 69:1486–1493.

83. Sahlin K, Edstrom L, Sjoholm H. Fatigue and phosphocreatine depletion during carbon dioxide-induced acidosis in rat muscle. Am J Physiol 1983; 245:C15–C20.

84. Sahlin K, Freyschuss U, Hultman E, Sjoholm H. Effect of short-term CO_2 breathing on the CO_2 content and intracellular pH in skeletal muscle of man. Clin Physiol 1981; 1:495–502.

85. Fiaccadori E, Del Canale S, Arduini U, Antonucci C, Coffrini E, Vitali P, et al. Intracellular acid-base and electrolyte metabolism in skeletal muscle of patients with chronic obstructive lung disease and acute respiratory failure. Clin Sci (Colch) 1986; 71:703–712.

86. Jakobsson P, Jorfeldt L, Brundin A. Skeletal muscle metabolites and fibre types in patients with advanced chronic obstructive pulmonary disease (COPD), with and without chronic respiratory failure. Eur Respir J 1990; 3:192–196.

87. Hughes RL, Katz H, Sahgal V, Campbell JA, Hartz R, Shields TW. Fiber size and energy metabolites in five separate muscles from patients with chronic obstructive lung diseases. Respiration 1983; 44:321–328.

88. Fleury B, Murciano D, Talamo C, Aubier M, Pariente R, Milic-Emili J. Work of breathing in patients with chronic obstructive pulmonary disease in acute respiratory failure. Am Rev Respir Dis 1985; 131:822–827.

89. Barbera JA, Roca J, Ferrer A, Felez MA, Diaz O, Roger N, et al. Mechanisms of worsening gas exchange during acute exacerbations of chronic obstructive pulmonary disease. Eur Respir J 1997; 10:1285–1291.

90. Namiot Z, Giedrojc J, Gorski J. The effect of increased respiratory resistance on glycogen and triglyceride levels in the respiratory muscles of the rat. Eur J Appl Physiol Occup Physiol 1985; 54:432–435.

91. Brochard L, Mancebo J, Wysocki M, Lofaso F, Conti G, Rauss A, et al. Noninvasive ventilation for acute exacerbations of chronic obstructive pulmonary disease. N Engl J Med 1995; 333:817–822.

92. Plant PK, Owen JL, Elliott MW. Early use of non-invasive ventilation for acute exacerbations of chronic obstructive pulmonary disease on general respiratory wards: a multicentre randomised controlled trial. Lancet 2000; 355:1931–1935.

93. Girault C, Chevron V, Richard JC, Daudenthun I, Pasquis P, Leroy J, et al. Physiological effects and optimisation of nasal assist-control ventilation for patients with chronic obstructive pulmonary disease in respiratory failure. Thorax 1997; 52:690–696.

94. Levine S, Kaiser L, Leferovich J, Tikunov B. Cellular adaptations in the diaphragm in chronic obstructive pulmonary disease. N Engl J Med 1997; 337:1799–1806.

95. Orozco-Levi M, Gea J, Lloreta JL, Felez M, Minguella J, Serrano S, et al. Subcellular adaptation of the human diaphragm in chronic obstructive pulmonary disease. Eur Respir J 1999; 13:371–378.

96. Mercadier JJ, Schwartz K, Schiaffino S, Wisnewsky C, Ausoni S, Heimburger M, et al. Myosin heavy chain gene expression changes in the diaphragm of patients with chronic lung hyperinflation. Am J Physiol 1998; 274:L527–L534.

97. Similowski T, Yan S, Gauthier AP, Macklem PT, Bellemare F. Contractile properties of the human diaphragm during chronic hyperinflation. N Engl J Med 1991; 325:917–923.

98. De Troyer A, Blair Pride N. The chest wall and respiratory muscles in chronic obstructive pulmonary disease. In: Roussos C, ed. The Thorax. New York: Marcel Dekker, 1995:1975–2069.

99. Polkey MI, Kyroussis D, Hamnegard CH, Mills GH, Green M, Moxham J. Diaphragm strength in chronic obstructive pulmonary disease. Am J Respir Crit Care Med 1996; 154:1310–1317.

100. Begin P, Grassino A. Inspiratory muscle dysfunction and chronic hypercapnia in chronic obstructive pulmonary disease. Am Rev Respir Dis 1991; 143:905–912.

101. Pepe PE, Marini JJ. Occult positive end-expiratory pressure in mechanically ventilated patients with airflow obstruction: the auto-PEEP effect. Am Rev Respir Dis 1982; 126:166–170.

102. Fleury B, Murciano D, Talamo C, Aubier M, Pariente R, Milic-Emili J. Work of breathing in patients with chronic obstructive pulmonary disease in acute respiratory failure. Am Rev Respir Dis 1985; 131:822–827.

103. Roussos C, Zakynthinos S. Ventilatory failure and respiratory muscles. In: Roussos C, ed. The Thorax. New York: Marcel Dekker, 1995:2071–2100.

104. Lötters F, Van Tol B, Kwakkel G, Gosselink R. Effects of controlled inspiratory muscle training in patients with COPD: a meta-analysis. Eur Respir J 2002; 20:570–576.

105. Reid WD, Huang J, Bryson S, Walker DC, Belcastro AN. Diaphragm injury and myofibrillar structure induced by resistive loading. J Appl Physiol 1994; 76:176–184.

106. Macgowan NA, Evans KG, Road JD, Reid WD. Diaphragm injury in individuals with airflow obstruction. Am J Respir Crit Care Med 2001; 163:1654–1659.

107. Zhu E, Petrof BJ, Gea J, Comtois N, Grassino AE. Diaphragm muscle fiber injury after inspiratory resistive breathing. Am J Respir Crit Care Med 1997; 155:1110–1116.

108. Douglass JA, Tuxen DV, Home M, Scheinkestel CD, Weinmann M, Czarny D, et al. Myopathy in severe asthma. Am Rev Respir Dis 1992; 146:517–519.

109. Borzone G, Zhao B, Merola AJ, Berliner L, Clanton TL. Detection of free radicals by electron spin resonance in rat diaphragm after resistive loading. J Appl Physiol 1994; 77:812–818.

110. Borzone G, Julian MW, Merola AJ, Clanton TL. Loss of diaphragm glutathione is associated with respiratory failure induced by resistive breathing. J Appl Physiol 1994; 76:2825–2831.

111. Poole DC, Mathieu-Costello O. Effect of pulmonary emphysema on diaphragm capillary geometry. J Appl Physiol 1997; 82:599–606.

112. Poole DC, Kindig CA, Behnke BJ. Effects of emphysema on diaphragm microvascular oxygen pressure. Am J Respir Crit Care Med 2001; 163:1081–1086.

113. Georgopoulos D, Brochard L. Ventilatory strategies in acute exacerbations of chronic obstructive pulmonary disease. In: Roussos C, ed. Mechanical Ventilation from Intensive Care to Home Care. Sheffield: European Respiratory Society, 1998:12–44.

114. Sackner MA. Diaphragmatic breathing exercises. Therapy in chronic obstructive pulmonary disease. JAMA 1975; 231:295–296.

115. Gosselink RA, Wagenaar RC, Rijswijk H, Sargeant AJ, Decramer ML. Diaphragmatic breathing reduces efficiency of breathing in patients with chronic obstructive pulmonary disease. Am J Respir Crit Care Med 1995; 151:1136–1142.

116. Vitacca M, Clini E, Bianchi L, Ambrosino N. Acute effects of deep diaphragmatic breathing in COPD patients with chronic respiratory insufficiency. Eur Respir J 1998; 11:408–415.

117. Swidwa DM, Montenegro HD, Goldman MD, Lutchen KR, Saidel GM. Helium-oxygen breathing in severe chronic obstructive pulmonary disease. Chest 1985; 87:790–795.

118. Jaber S, Fodil R, Carlucci A, Boussarsar M, Pigeot J, Lemaire F, et al. Noninvasive ventilation with helium-oxygen in acute exacerbations of chronic obstructive pulmonary disease. Am J Respir Crit Care Med 2000; 161:1191–1200.

119. Manthous CA, Hall JB, Caputo MA, Walter J, Klocksieben JM, Schmidt GA, et al. Heliox improves pulses paradoxus and peak expiratory flow in nonintubated patients with severe asthma. Am J Respir Crit Care Med 1995; 151:310–314.

120. Schols AM, Soeters PB, Mostert R, Pluymers RJ, Wouters EF. Physiologic effects of nutritional support and anabolic steroids in patients with chronic obstructive pulmonary disease. A placebo-controlled randomized trial. Am J Respir Crit Care Med 1995; 152:1268–1274.

121. Engelen MP, Schols AM, Baken WC, Wesseling GJ, Wouters EF. Nutritional depletion in relation to respiratory and peripheral skeletal muscle function in out-patients with COPD. Eur Respir J 1994; 7:1793–1797.

16

Water–Electrolyte Imbalances in Acute Exacerbations of Chronic Obstructive Pulmonary Disease

**MAURIZIO MORETTI and
LEONARDO M. FABBRI**

ENRICO CLINI

University of Modena and
  Reggio Emilia
Modena, Italy

Hospital Villa Pineta
Modena, Italy

I. Introduction

COPD is often associated with acute episodes of disease exacerbations (AECOPD). An exacerbation of mild-to-moderate COPD is most frequently associated with increased breathlessness, often accompanied by increased cough and sputum production, and only rarely with acute respiratory failure. The need for medical intervention intensifies as the airflow limitation worsens.

Exacerbations of severe COPD are associated with both exacerbation of respiratory symptoms and symptoms correlated with the acute respiratory failure. The patient with severe acute exacerbation complains marked dyspnea, is usually bedridden, and visibly tachypneic. Coughing is exacerbated and sputum production is increased. Fever may be present if the episode has been precipitated or aggravated by an infectious process. On examination, the patient displays tachypnea with prominent use of the accessory muscles of respiration, cyanosis, and tachycardia. When hypoxemia is associated with a severe decompensated hypercapnia, patients may exhibit confusion, agitation, or lethargy and marked fatigue.

Severe acute exacerbations of COPD often require hospital admission. Up to 20% of hospital admissions for COPD exacerbation may result in acute respiratory failure (i.e., severe hypoxemia with or without hypercapnia) requiring mechanical ventilation (1–3). Acute hypoxemia has been shown to have multifactorial origin due to intrapulmonary and extrapulmonary pathophysiological mechanisms (2). Gas exchange worsening during exacerbation is mainly due to the worsening of ventilation/perfusion (VA/Q) inequality that results from increased perfusion in poorly ventilated areas with low VA/Q ratios. This pathophysiological mechanism is consistent with airway narrowing by bronchial inflammation, bronchospasm, and mucus hypersecretion, and possibly involvement of the pulmonary arteries in the inflammatory process. Other extrapulmonary factors contribute to increased hypoxemia during an exacerbation of COPD. The most important is the increase of oxygen consumption resulting from an increased oxygen demand by the respiratory muscles. The increase of cardiac output, when possible, may partially compensate for the effect that increased oxygen consumption by the respiratory muscles has on mixed venous oxygen pressure.

The mechanisms of acute hypercapnia are not fully understood. Patients with advanced COPD may develop CO_2 retention both because of abnormalities in the gas exchange and of mechanical properties of the lung. In addition, acute exacerbations of COPD cause air trapping and lung hyperinflation resulting in muscle fatigue and acute hypercapnic respiratory failure (4).

A severe exacerbation of COPD is often associated with a significant increase in pulmonary artery mean pressure. In this clinical setting, the right ventricle cannot increase the stroke work without a significant increase of the right heart filling pressure. The patient develops the signs and symptoms of right ventricular failure if not present earlier. If it was chronically present before the exacerbation, it will markedly worsen. The patient gains weight with clinical evidence of fluid retention as pleural effusions, some degree of ascites, and dependent edema. The liver is enlarged and tender to palpation and it may pulsate reflecting the presence of a tricuspid insufficiency. Similarly, the neck veins are distended and may show the pressure waves characteristic of tricuspid insufficiency and increased right atrial contraction.

Hypoxemia and/or hypercapnia are believed to be the primary causes of acid–base imbalance, electrolyte abnormalities, and water retention that occur both during acute respiratory failure induced by exacerbations of COPD and chronic respiratory failure in severe COPD patients (i.e., cor pulmonale).

This chapter will focus on the acute changes of acid–base balance, electrolytes, and water retention that occur during acute exacerbations; a comparison will be done with findings occurring during chronic respiratory failure in severe COPD patients, and particularly in the presence of cor pulmonale.

II. Pathophysiology of Acid–Base, Water, and Electrolyte Imbalance

A. Acid–Base Imbalance

The acute carbon dioxide retention that causes arterial hypercapnia results in respiratory acidosis characterized by reduced pH. The retention of carbon dioxide causes an increased acidity of the blood and of the extracellular fluid and, as an adaptive response, of plasma bicarbonates (5). It has been estimated that an increase of 10 mmHg $PaCO_2$ is associated with an increase of approximately 1 mEq/L of bicarbonate concentration. The acute buffer response to hypercapnia is completed within a few minutes of the increase in $PaCO_2$, and it is caused primarily by the buffer response of the tissues and blood, considering that the renal adaptation mechanisms require more time (6). Hemoglobin is the predominant nonbicarbonate buffer. Bicarbonate concentration increases within minutes after acute change in $PaCO_2$ because of a fraction of the hydrogen ions, released by the dissociation of the carbonic acid, combines with nonbicarbonate buffer, thereby producing new bicarbonate ions (7). This acute rise in plasma bicarbonate concentration is largely due to the chloride shift via a Cl^-/HCO_3^- exchanger at the erythrocyte membrane. The increase of plasma bicarbonate concentration is associated with minor but still significant changes of serum potassium. The concentration of potassium increases by only 0.1 mEq/L for each 0.1-unit decrement in pH in acute respiratory acidosis (8). In acute acidosis, there is an increased internal transmembrane flux of H^+ ion and potassium release from the intracellular compartment via a K^+/H^+ exchanger mediated by the increase of extracellular H^+ concentration. Respiratory acidosis is also associated with minor adaptive, almost undetectable, changes (e.g., decrease of lactates, increase of phosphorus and sodium) (6). The "anion gap" and the concentration of the other serum electrolytes are essentially within normal limits. The concentration of chloride does not change significantly during acute respiratory failure, whereas it decreases markedly during chronic hypercapnia.

Furthermore, hypercapnia per se promotes sodium retention throughout an increase of tubular sodium exchange. Renal adaptive mechanisms exert an impact on plasma composition after 12 to 24 h of hypercapnia, but the full effect takes about 3 to 5 days during which there is a rise in the systemic pH toward the normal. The elevated $PaCO_2$ induces the renal secretion of hydrogen ions, which are electrochemically balanced by the reabsorption of sodium (9). Thus, in patients with hypercapnia, more sodium than normal is reabsorbed (10), and this mechanism may contribute to the formation of peripheral edema (Fig. 1).

B.   Water and Electrolyte Imbalance

Right Ventricular Failure

A simple hypothesis has been proposed for the development of cor pulmonale and edema: pulmonary hypertension → right ventricular hypertrophy and dilatation → right ventricular failure → venous engorgement → edema (11).

COPD patients experience episodes of acute right heart failure during exacerbation of the disease and these episodes are accounted for by a worsening of pulmonary hypertension. During severe exacerbation of COPD with pronounced peripheral edema, the acute increase of pulmonary arterial pressure (12–14) causes right ventricular failure documented by elevated right ventricular filling pressure (14). In an acute exacerbation, right ventricular contractility may be significantly depressed, although the cardiac output is preserved or even increased.

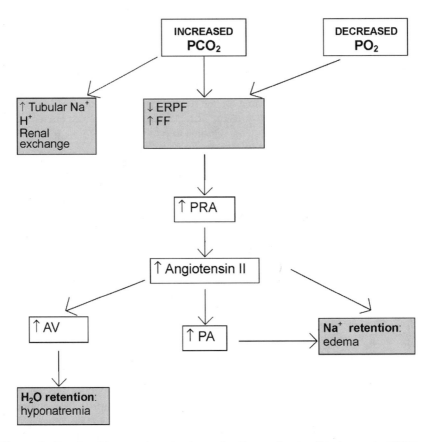

Figure 1 Renal and hormonal mechanisms of sodium and water disturbances in COPD patients. ERPF = effective renal plasma flow; FF = filtration fraction; PRA = plasma renin activity; AV = arginin vasopressin; PA = plasma aldosterone. (Modified from Ref. 10.)

The occurrence of true right ventricular failure during exacerbation of COPD has been recently questioned. In fact, a variable percentage of patients with AECOPD have marked peripheral edema without hemodynamic signs of right ventricular failure (14–16), suggesting that peripheral edema is not synonymous with right ventricular failure (17).

Sixteen COPD patients were investigated hemodynamically in the stable phase of the disease and during exacerbation (14). Nine of 16 patients with marked peripheral edema had hemodynamic signs of right ventricular failure. In these patients, pulmonary arterial pressure increased significantly between baseline and the episode of AECOPD associated with the occurrence of peripheral edema. This increase of pulmonary arterial pressure was accounted for by a marked worsening of arterial blood gases during exacerbation. The authors conclude that right ventricular failure and peripheral edema are effectively present in at least some patients with COPD when the acute exacerbation is associated with a significant increase of pulmonary arterial pressure from baseline.

Renal Failure and Hormonal Imbalance

Pathophysiology of water and electrolyte imbalances in patients with AECOPD is also characterized by the interaction of different promoting or protecting mechanisms, as documented by recent experimental evidence (i.e., reduction in renal blood flow and hormonal changes).

Renal Failure

Renal function in patients with COPD has been studied since the early 1950s (17) and it is clearly impaired in the advanced stage of the disease (18). There is evidence of a 60% reduction in effective renal plasma flow (ERPF) in COPD patients with peripheral edema, especially during exacerbation, as compared to healthy subjects (15, 19, 20). The reduction of ERPF is a major cause for impaired excretion of water and sodium retention.

Several studies have also shown both a decrease of renal functional reserve in severe stable patients (21), and a reduction in glomerular filtration rate and increase of filtration fraction in decompensated patients (15). The mechanism that causes the fall in renal perfusion in COPD is likely to differ from congestive heart failure as both right and left ventricular function and output are well maintained in most of the patients (22, 23). The decrease in renal perfusion is due to a rise in reno-vascular resistance. The combination of reduced ERPF and increased filtration fraction, which favors enhanced reabsorption of fluids and electrolytes from the proximal tubule, also points to an increased resistance in renal afferent arterioles (24). The mechanism whereby hypoxemia affects renal hemodynamics is not fully understood. Changes in ERPF might be caused by (1) a reflex mechanism that is partially independent on the sympathetic afferent nerves to the kidney and chemoreceptor stimulation (25, 26) or (2) by a disturbance in the nitric oxide pathway (27). The role of basal production and release of nitric oxide in actively regulating basal vascular tone of the systemic and pulmonary circulation has been investigated recently (28). In severe COPD patients with cor pulmonale, it has been shown to be impaired (29), probably due to a reduced endothelial synthase activity (30).

In acute hypoxemic COPD patients, there is evidence of a significant reno-vascular responsiveness to controlled O_2 therapy; this effect is blunted in the presence of hypercapnia. Furthermore, renal blood flow improves with oxygen and dopamine in stable hypoxiemic but not in hypercapnic COPD patients (20), suggesting a difference in reno-vascular control between normocapnic and hypercapnic patients. These findings indicate that (1) oxygen acts as an acute renal vasodilator in hypoxemic patients; and (2) carbon dioxide levels play a pivotal role in determining the renal hemodynamic response to changes in arterial blood gases. Hypercapnia can influence renal hemodynamics by direct and indirect mechanisms. Hypercapnia can cause direct renal vasoconstriction (31) and stimulate noradrenaline release by direct action on the sympathetic nervous system (15). Indirectly, hypercapnia causes systemic vasodilatation activating the baroreceptors with a subsequent release of noradrenaline, leading to a fall in ERPF (11, 15, 32). These findings indicate why controlled oxygen therapy does not decrease reno-vascular resistance when hypercapnia is present.

Furthermore, there is evidence of a parasympathetic autonomic dysfunction (diminution of vagal parasympathetic function) in hypoxemic COPD with preservation of sympathetic tone (33). These patients with autonomic dysfunction are more likely to be edematous, excreting much less urine and sodium.

Hormonal Imbalance

In severe AECOPD with respiratory failure, peripheral edema may also be induced by changes of hormonal homeostasis with particular regard to arginin vasopressin, renin acivity, and aldosterone plasma levels (10). Hyperaldosteronism may contribute to sodium retention and an increase of arginin vasopressin may cause water retention and hyponatremia.

As hypoxemia and hypercapnia decrease renal plasma flow, this results in a decreased delivery of sodium to the cells of *macula densa* which causes plasma renin secretion (10). The activation of the renin–aldosterone system causes peripheral edema.

Plasma renin activity and aldosterone plasma levels are increased in some of COPD patients with acute hypercapnic respiratory failure and peripheral edema (15, 34). Faber (34) showed the increase of sodium and water excretion and weight loss with 6-day conventional therapy of oxygen and antibiotics in those COPD patients without renin–aldosterone abnormalities. On the contrary, patients who failed to respond to the same treatment had aldosterone, renin, and arginin vasopressin significantly above the upper limits. Patients referred to as unresponders in the Faber study (34) had a significant positive correlation betweeen plasma renin or aldosterone and the impaired ability to excrete sodium. These data indicate that increased activity of the renin system is responsible of the disturbance in sodium and water metabolism with peripheral edema. In AECOPD with water retention, the inhibition of angiotensin-converting enzyme (ACE) has proven to be therapeutically useful (35).

Arginin vasopressin (often referred to as antidiuretic hormone) is increased in patients with COPD and edema (15); arginin vasopressin release is stimulated by activation of the renin–angiotensin system, specifically by angiotensin II (36). However, the arginin vasopressin level was found to vary a great deal in AECOPD with peripheral edema (10). Increased concentration of arginin vasopressin was inversely correlated with solute-free water excretion and positively correlated with the presence of hyponatremia (10). The effective role of the renin–aldosterone system and arginin vasopressin on sodium and water retention in each single COPD patient is conditioned by the concomitant presence of other mechanisms promoting or inhibiting water balance.

Norepinephrine plasma levels are increased in COPD patients with acute respiratory failure and fluid retention (15). The increased sympathetic activity is due to hypoxemia and hypercapnia and may contribute to sodium and water retention by different mechanisms: reduction in renal blood flow, renin release from the kidney, nonosmotic release of arginin vasopressin (32).

Atrial natriuretic peptide has been shown to be elevated in COPD patients, particularly during exacerbation with peripheral edema (24, 37); atrial natriuretic peptide has a number of beneficial effects in opposing the neuroendocrine edema-promoting factors in COPD patients with peripheral edema (see above). The general view is that atrial stretch is the major stimulus to the release of atrial natriuretic peptide (38). Its activity includes natriuretic and diuretic effect, depression of plasma rennin activity, inhibition of angiotensin II-mediated aldosterone production, and pulmonary vasodilatation (32, 39). The high levels of atrial natriuretic peptide may be the reason that not all patients who present with hypoxic-hypercapnic respiratory failure develop peripheral edema. The concomitant decrease of atrial natriuretic peptide level and peripheral edema with treatment confirms the strong relationship between high plasma atrial natriuretic peptide level and volume overload. Further, there is evidence of a positive correlation between atrial natriuretic peptide levels and right ventricular end-diastolic volume (37). Interestingly, the same study (37) has shown the fall of atrial natriuretic peptide level after 3 days during treatment in exacerbated COPD with peripheral edema; the fall highly correlated ($r = 0.85$) with the change in body weight. The atrial natriuretic peptide concentration increases according to disease severity, showing a positive correlation with $PaCO_2$ (24). In patients with severe COPD, baseline secretion of atrial natriuretic peptide is markedly elevated, but is no longer sensitive to acute variations of volemia experimentally induced by salt and water infusion (24). It seems that the volume regulatory role of atrial natriuretic peptide is lost in patients with severe COPD because of a limited atrial natriuretic peptide reserve that would prevent the appropriate increase of the hormone in response to elevated cardiac filling pressure. Indeed, infusion of atrial natriuretic peptide results in natriuresis in patients with hypoxic COPD, suggesting that the kidney is still responsive to atrial natriuretic peptide (40).

Dopamine is another peptide that could potentially prevent edema formation in hypoxic COPD. Circulating L-dopa enters renal tubular cells and is converted by L-dopa decarboxylase to dopamine able to promote natriuresis and diuresis. Dopamine also inhibits plasma renin activity (32). Dopamine seems to produce a natriuresis by three mechanisms: action on the renal tubules via dopamine receptors; (2) by vasodilation of the renal vasculature, thus increasing glomerular filtration rate; and possibly by (3) inhibiting renin release (41, 42).

Thus, dopamine may protect against edema formation. Although studies in normal subjects indicate that acute hypoxia is able to reduce renal dopamine production, the same hormone is of normal level (or indeed higher in association with edema or respiratory failure) during exacerbations of COPD (37). Renal hemodynamics improve with dopamine in hypoxic but not in hypercapnic COPD; these findings provide evidence of a different reno-vascular control between normocapnic and hypercapnic patients (20).

III. Edema Formation in COPD

A. COPD Without Peripheral Edema

The progression of pulmonary arterial hypertension in patients with COPD is slow and allows the right ventricle to adapt to the increase in outflow pressure; this process slowly leads to right ventricular hypertrophy and dilatation, also named cor pulmonale (43). Hypoxemic–hypercapnic COPD patients with cor pulmonale, without chronic peripheral edema, have a decreased (< 40 to 45%) right ventricular ejection fraction as a consequence of an increased afterload, but the right ventricular contractility and cardiac output remain normal (16, 44). Hypoxemic COPD patients have a reduced renal functional reserve that represents an early index of renal impairment (21). Further, hypercapnic patients without clinical evidence of renal disease have an impaired water and sodium excretion, a decreased glomerular filtration rate, higher levels of plasma renin activity, and plasma aldosterone and atrial natriuretic peptide when compared with hypoxemic COPD patients or with normal subjects (24, 45). The renal hemodynamics improve with oxygen and dopamine in hypoxic but not hypercapnic COPD patients, suggesting a different reno-vascular control due to hypercapnia (Table 1).

Table 1 Cardiac Hemodynamics, Renal and Hormonal Imbalances in COPD Patients

	Severe COPD hypoxemic-hypercapnic[a]	Severe COPD with cor pulmonale and peripheral edema[b]	Severe COPD with acute exacerbation and peripheral edema[c]
PAP	↑	↑↑/↑↑↑	↑↑↑
CI	Normal	Normal	Normal/↑
RVEF	↓	↓/↓↓	↓↓↓
RVEDP	Normal	↑↑	↑/↑↑↑
Edema	–	±	++
Renal plasma flow	Normal/↓	↓↓	↓↓↓
Filtration fraction	Normal/↑	↑↑	↑↑↑
Water excretion	Normal/↓	↓↓	↓↓↓
Sodium excretion	Normal/↓	↓↓	↓↓
Plasma renin activity	Normal/↑	↑	↑↑
Plasma aldosterone	Normal/↑	↑	↑↑
Arginin vasopressin	Normal	↑	↑↑↑
Atrial natriuretic peptide	Normal/↑	↑	↑↑↑

PAP: mean pulmonary artery pressure; CI: cardiac index; RVEF: right ventricular ejection fraction; RVEDP: right ventricular end-diastolic pressure.
[a]Refs. 27, 44, 45.
[b]Refs. 10, 16, 33, 44.
[c]Refs. 14–16.

B. COPD with Chronic Peripheral Edema

Although the progression of pulmonary hypertension in COPD is slow, a minority of patients exhibit a marked worsening of pulmonary hypertension during follow-up. These patients did not differ from the others at onset, but they are characterized by a progressive deterioration of PaO_2 and $PaCO_2$ (46). This rapid worsening of pulmonary hypertension can favor the development of right ventricular failure associated with the clincal signs of hemodynamic impairment: neck vein distension, liver enlargement, peripheral edema. Right heart failure is documented by the presence of elevated right ventricular filling pressures as right atrial pressure and right ventricular end-diastolic pressure.

• On the contrary, a variable percentage of COPD patients have peripheral edema with a mild degree of pulmonary hypertension and no signs of right heart failure. These patients show a significant decline in renal blood flow and glomerular filtration rate with an increase of filtration fraction. The impairment of renal function causes a reduction in sodium and water excretion associated with an increased fractional sodium reabsorption. Plasma aldosterone and vasopressin levels are significantly increased when compared to nonedematous COPD patients (33) contributing to sodium and water retention. At least some patients have a para-sympathetic autonomic dysfunction with preservation of sympathetic tone that could impair sodium and water homeostasis (33).

These data show that peripheral edema in COPD patients has multifactorial mechanisms—hormonal, renal, and cardiogenic, individually or in combination—and can contribute to sodium and water retention.

C. Acute Exacerbation of COPD

Some patients with acute exacerbation of COPD may show an abrupt worsening of baseline pulmonary hypertension due to a severe hypoxemia and hypercapnia with clinical signs of right heart failure. Pulmonary hemodynamics show a significant increase of right ventricular end-diastolic pressure > 12 mmHg as sign of right ventricular failure. In these patients, cardiac output is normal, while systemic vascular resistance and arterial blood pressure are low (14, 15).

On the contrary, most of COPD patients with acute exacerbation and peripheral edema have no hemodynamic signs of right ventricular failure and stable pulmonary arterial pressure. However, these patients have severe retention of salt and water, reduction in renal blood flow, and glomerular filtration, activation of renin–angiotensin–aldosterone system, increase in norepinephrine, atrial natruretic and arginin vasopressin peptides similar to those seen in stable COPD patients with peripheral edema syndrome (15). Although the renal and hormonal mechanisms of edema formation are similar in the two groups, the changes are quantitatively more significant in the acute exacerbation.

In summary, many patients with advanced COPD will never develop right heart failure; some COPD patients may experience episodes of right ventricular failure, particularly during exacerbation, and these episodes are accounted for by a worsening of pulmonary arterial pressure from baseline. Besides cardiogenic factors, other mechanisms cause sodium and water retention showing a pivotal role in edema formation during acute exacerbation.

IV. Therapeutic Implications

On the basis of the complex interactions between advanced COPD and water imbalance both in acute and chronic situations, a rational therapeutic approach may be as important as treating the airway obstruction. Overall, the strategy should be directed to reduce pulmonary hypertension and to improve salt–water imbalance.

The first, conservative approach to acute respiratory acidosis is to reduce $PaCO_2$ if possible. The physician should determine rapidly whether large airway obstruction is present and relieve it as promptly as possible. Immediate pharmacological treatment should be instituted to relieve ventilatory impairment. If this first, conservative approach fails to correct hypercapnia, ventilatory mechanical assistance is mandatory.

Renal generation of new bicarbonate is central to adaptation to chronic hypercapnia; thus the expected adaptive response does not occur in patients with severe renal failure. As a result, severe acidemia persists with sustained hypercapnia and survival is limited.

Given the body's slight buffer response to acute hypercapnia, some authors have advocated intravenous bicarbonate administration when severe respiratory acidemia occurs (pH < 7.10) (47, 48). It is difficult to agree with the intravenous bicarbonate administration in severe respiratory acidosis not complicated by metabolic acidosis. In fact, bicarbonate therapy entails the risk of volume overload and consecutive pulmonary congestion due to fluid accumulation. Further, bicarbonate administration might contribute to posthypercapnic alkalosis when $PaCO_2$ rapidly decreases with mechanical ventilation.

Rapid reduction in arterial $PaCO_2$ to normal levels after a vigorous ventilatory treatment in patients with moderate or severe chronic respiratory acidosis or in patients with combined metabolic alkalosis and respiratory acidosis may produce severe, life-threatening alkalemia. Even if sufficient plasma chloride is available, several hours may elapse before the elevated bicarbonate concentration is reduced by movement of hydrogen ion from cells, by renal excretion of bicarbonate, and by a decrease in renal acid excretion.

However, if water–ion complications are present such as a reduction in effective blood volume, or if the patient is hypokalemic or has a low chloride intake, the capacity of the kidney to reabsorb bicarbonate remains increased and alkalosis may be perpetuated (49). Posthypercapnic alkalosis may be corrected with careful administration of saline and potassium chloride or the administration of the diuretic acetozolamide, which inhibits carbonic anhydrase activity and impairs bicarbonate reabsorption by the kidney. In fact, acetozolamide results in sodium bicarbonate diuresis, favoring the decrease in pH and extracellular fluid volume.

Several drugs have been used experimentally in treating COPD with pulmonary hypertension, especially during the steady-state condition. Great enthusiasm for the use of vasodilators (i.e., calcium blockers and ACE inhibitors) arose from their apparent beneficial effect in patients with primary pulmonary hypertension (50). However, many of them did not sustain their acute effect over the long term, nor did they show any significant effect on improved survival. Finally, most of them showed no selective pulmonary vasodilation. In this light, only inhaled nitric oxide (51, 52) may be promising, although there is limited clinical experience to support this.

In an acute situation, in decompensated edematous exacerbation of COPD, where aldosterone levels are high, ACE inhibitors might prove therapeutically useful by reducing the production of angiotensin II. ACE inhibitors may interfere with the hormonal regulation of renal blood flow and also may improve the hypoxic vasoconstriction (53) that contributes to pulmonary hypertension. In an acute case-control study, a single 25-mg dose of captopril slightly improved sodium excretion in a group of hypoxemic COPD patients with peripheral edema (35). On the contrary, in the chronic management of edematous cor pulmonale, ACE inhibitors failed to improve sodium load excretion (54). Perindropil reduced plasma aldosterone level in the edematous patient to levels seen in nonedematous COPD patients (54). Despite this significant fall in aldosterone levels, there was no improvement in the excretion of saline load.

Short-term acute studies with other intravenous vasodilators such as atrial natriuretic peptide have shown positive effects on pulmonary pressure levels and diuresis (40), but the oral derivatives of this agent are still lacking.

Up to now, the long-term administration of oxygen seemed to be the most appropriate method of treating advanced-stage COPD patients (55), both in the stable state and the acute exacerbation of the disease.

Oxygen represents a new therapeutic opportunity in the impaired water–salt retention associated with AECOPD (56, 57). In acute exacerbation of COPD with hypoxemia, renovascular resistance decreases (20) and improves urinary sodium excretion (58) when hyperoxemia is given to obtain a oxygen saturation between 90% and 95%; this effect is blunted in the presence of hypercapnia (20). This raises the question of whether the simultaneous correction of gas abnormalities (such as noninvasive ventilation plus oxygen) might be more effective in the treatment of water retention in cor pulmonale than oxygen therapy alone.

Dopamine hydrochloride intravenously infused at a low dose ($2\,g/kg/min$) increases renal blood flow and promotes diuresis and natriuresis acting as an acute renal vasodilator in hypoxemic normocapnic COPD patients (20).

V. Conclusions

Water and electrolyte imbalance occurring in AECOPD suggests a complex interaction between pulmonary hemodynamics, acid–base balance, and hormonal and renal mechanisms. Further studies are required to (1) investigate the contribution of different mechanisms in edema formation; (2) select COPD patients at risk of developing chronic right ventricular failure; and (3) define more effective therapeutic approaches in preventing edema formation.

Acknowledgments

Work is supported by the Associazione Studio Tumori e Malattie Polmonari, Padova, and a Special Grant from AstraZeneca, Milan, Italy.

References

1. Curtis JR, Hudson LD. Emergent assessment and management of acute respiratory failure in COPD. Clin Chest Med 1994; 15:481–500.
2. Barbera JA, Roca J, Ferrer A, Felez MA, Diaz O, Roger N, Rodriguez-Roisin R. Mechanisms of worsening gas exchange during acute exacerbations of chronic obstructive pulmonary disease. Eur Respir J 1997; 10:1285–1291.
3. Plant PK, Owen JL, Elliott MW. One year period prevalence study of respiratory acidosis in acute exacerbations of COPD: implications for the provision of non-invasive ventilation and oxygen administration. Thorax 2000; 55:550–554.
4. Zakynthinos S, Roussos C. Hypercapnic respiratory failure. Respir Med 1993; 87:409–411.
5. Westenfelder C, Nascimento L. Respiratory acidosis and alkalosis. Semin Nephrol 1981; 1:220–231.
6. Bracket NC, Jorgan JC, Schwartz WB. Carbon dioxide tritation curve of normal man. N Engl J Med 1965; 272:6–12.
7. Madias NE, Wolf CJ, Cohen JJ. Regulation of acid-base equilibrium in chronic hypercapnia. Kidney Int 1985; 27:538–543.
8. Adrogue HJ, Madias NE. Changes in plasma potassium concentration during acute acid-base disturbances. Am J Med 1981; 71:456–467.
9. Schwartz WB, Hays RM, Polak A, Haynie GD. Effect of chronic hypercapnia on electrolyte and acid-base equilibrium. II. Recovery, with special reference to the influence of chloride intake. J Clin Invest 1965; 127:754–762.
10. Farber MO, Roberts LR, Weinberger MH, Robertson GL, Fineberg NS, Manfredi F. Abnormalities of sodium and H_2O handling in chronic obstructive lung disease. Arch Intern Med 1982; 142:1326–1330.
11. MacNee W. Pathophysiology of cor pulmonale in chronic obstructive pulmonary disease. I. Am J Respir Crit Care Med 1994; 150:833–852.
12. Abraham AS, Cole RB, Green ID, Hedworth-Whitty RB, Clarke SW, Bishop JM. Factors contributing to the reversible pulmonary hypertension of patients with acute respiratory failure studies by serial observations during recovery. Circ Res 1969; 24:51–60.
13. Weitzenblum E, Hirth C, Parini JP, Rasaholinjanahary J, Oudet P. Clinical, functional and pulmonary hemodynamic course of patients with chronic obstructive pulmonary disease followed-up over 3 years. Respiration 1978; 36:1–9.
14. Weitzenblum E, Apprill M, Oswald M, Chaouat A, Imbs JL. Pulmonary hemodynamics in patients with chronic obstructive pulmonary disease before and during an episode of peripheral edema. Chest 1994; 105:1377–1382.
15. Anand IS, Chandrashekhar Y, Ferrari R, Sarma R, Guleria R, Jindal SK, Wahi PL, Poole-Wilson PA, Harris P. Pathogenesis of congestive state in chronic obstructive pulmonary disease. Studies of body water and sodium, renal function, hemodynamics, and plasma hormones during edema and after recovery. Circulation 1992; 86:12–21.

16. MacNee W, Wathen CG, Flenley DC, Muir AD. The effects of controlled oxygen therapy on ventricular function in patients with stable and decompensated cor pulmonale. Am Rev Respir Dis 1988; 137:1289–1295.

17. Davies CE. Renal cirution in cor pulmonale. Lancet 1951; 2:1052–1057.

18. Kilburn KH, Dowell AR. Renal function in respiratory failure. Effects of hypoxia, hyperoxia, and hypercapnia. Arch Intern Med 1971; 127:754–762.

19. Baudouin SV, Bott J, Ward A, Deane C, Moxham J. Short term effect of oxygen on renal haemodynamics in patients with hypoxaemic chronic obstructive airways disease. Thorax 1992; 47:550–554.

20. Howes TQ, Deane CR, Levin GE, Baudouin SV, Moxham J. The effects of oxygen and dopamine on renal and aortic blood flow in chronic obstructive pulmonary disease with hypoxemia and hypercapnia. Am J Respir Crit Care Med 1995; 151:378–383.

21. Sharkey RA, Mulloy EM, Kilgallen IA, O'Neill SJ. Renal functional reserve in patients with severe chronic obstructive pulmonary disease. Thorax 1997; 52:411–415.

22. Richens JM. Oedema in cor pulmonale. Clin Sci 1982; 62:255–259.

23. Harris P. Are pulmonary haemodinamics important to survival in chronic obstructive lung disease? Eur Respir J 1989; 2(Suppl 7):674s–677s.

24. Adnot S, Sediame S, Defouilloy C, Andrivet P, Viossat I, Brun-Buisson C, Chabrier PE, Laurent D. Role of atrial natriuretic factor in impaired sodium excretion of normocapnic and hypercapnic patients with chronic obstructive lung disease. Am Rev Respir Dis 1993; 148:1049–1055.

25. Honig A, Wedler B, Zingler C, Ledderhos C, Schmidt M. Kidney function during arterial chemoreceptor stimulation. III. Long-lasting inhibition of renal tubular sodium reabsorption due to pharmacologic stimulation of the peripheral arterial chemoreceptors with almitrine bismesylate. Biomed Biochim Acta 1985; 44:1659–1672.

26. Sharkey RA, Mulloy EM, O'Neill SJ. Acute effects of hypoxaemia, hyperoxaemia and hypercapnia on renal blood flow in normal and renal transplant subjects. Eur Respir J 1998; 12:653–657.

27. Howes TQ, Keilty SE, Maskrey VL, Deane CR, Baudouin SV, Moxham J. Effect of L-arginine on renal blood flow in normal subjects and patients with hypoxic chronic obstructive pulmonary disease. Thorax 1996; 51:516–519.

28. Griffith TM, Edwards DH, Davies RL, Harrison TJ, Evans KT. EDRF coordinates the behaviour of vascular resistance vessels. Nature 1987; 329:442–445.

29. Clini E, Cremona G, Campana M, Scotti C, Pagani M, Bianchi L, Giordano A, Ambrosino N. Production of endogenous nitric oxide in chronic obstructive pulmonary disease and patients with cor pulmonale. Correlates with echo-Doppler assessment. Am J Respir Crit Care Med 2000; 162:446–450.

30. Giaid A, Saleh D. Reduced expression of endothelial nitric oxide synthase in the lungs of patients with pulmonary hypertension. N Engl J Med 1995; 333:214–221.

31. Sharkey RA, Mulloy EM, O'Neill SJ. The acute effects of oxygen and carbon dioxide on renal vascular resistance in patients with an acute exacerbation of COPD. Chest 1999; 115:1588–1592.

32. MacNee W. Pathophysiology of cor pulmonale in chronic obstructive pulmonary disease. Part two. Am J Respir Crit Care Med 1994; 150:1158–1168.

33. Stewart AG, Waterhouse JC, Billings CG, Baylis PH, Howard P. Hormonal, renal, and autonomic nerve factors involved in the excretion of sodium and water during dynamic salt and water loading in hypoxaemic chronic obstructive pulmonary disease. Thorax 1995; 50:838–845.

34. Farber MO, Weinberger MH, Robertson GL, Fineberg NS, Manfredi F. Hormonal abnormalities affecting sodium and water balance in acute respiratory failure due to chronic obstructive lung disease. Chest 1984; 85:49–54.
35. Farber MO, Weinberger MH, Robertson GL, Fineberg NS. The effects of angiotensin-converting enzyme inhibition on sodium handling in patients with advanced chronic obstructive pulmonary disease. Am Rev Respir Dis 1987; 136:862–866.
36. Robertson GL. Diseases of the posterior pituitary. In: Felig P, Baxter J, Broadus AE, Frohman LA, eds. Endocrinology and Metabolism. New York: McGraw-Hill, 1981; 251–277.
37. Skwarski K, Lee M, Turnbull L, MacNee W. Atrial natriuretic peptide in stable and decompensated chronic obstructive pulmonary disease. Thorax 1993; 48:730–735.
38. Raine AE, Erne P, Burgisser E, Muller FB, Bolli P, Burkart F, Buhler FR. Atrial natriuretic peptide and atrial pressure in patients with congestive heart failure. N Engl J Med 1986; 315:533–537.
39. Rogers TK, Sheedy W, Waterhouse J, Howard P, Morice AH. Haemodynamic effects of atrial natriuretic peptide in hypoxic chronic obstructive pulmonary disease. Thorax 1994; 49:233–239.
40. Adnot S, Andrivet P, Chabrier PE, Piquet J, Plas P, Braquet P, Roudot-Thoraval F, Brun-Buisson C. Atrial natriuretic factor in chronic obstructive lung disease with pulmonary hypertension. Physiological correlates and response to peptide infusion. J Clin Invest 1989; 83:986–993.
41. Ball SG, Lee MR. The effect of carbidopa administration on urinary sodium excretion in man. Is dopamine an intrarenal natriuretic hormone? Br J Clin Pharmacol 1977; 4:115–119.
42. Lee MR. Dopamine and the kidney: ten years on. Clin Sci (Lond) 1993; 84:357–375.
43. Chronic cor pulmonale. Report of an expert committee. Circulation 1963; 27:594–615.
44. Burghuber OC. Right ventricular contractility is preserved and preload increased in patients with chronic obstructive pulmonary disease and pulmonary artery hypertension. In: Jezek V, Morpurgo M, Tramarin R, eds. Current Topics in Rehabilitation. Right Ventricular Hypertrophy and Function in Chronic Lung Disease. Berlin: Springer-Verlag, 1992; 135–141.
45. Farber MO, Kiblawi SS, Strawbridge RA, Robertson GL, Weinberger MH, Manfredi F. Studies on plasma vasopressin and the renin-angiotensin-aldosterone system in chronic obstructive lung disease. J Lab Clin Med 1977; 90:373–380.
46. Weitzenblum E, Sautegeau A, Ehrhart M, Mammosser M, Hirth C, Roegel E. Long-term course of pulmonary arterial pressure in chronic obstructive pulmonary disease. Am Rev Respir Dis 1984; 130:993–998.
47. Mithoefer JC. Indication for the use of sodium bicarbonate in the treatment of intractable asthma. N Engl J Med 1965; 272:1200.
48. Lakashminarayan S. Bicarbonate therapy in severe acute respiratory acidosis. Scand J Respir Dis 1973; 28:317.
49. Schwartz WB, Bracket NC, Cohen JJ. The response of extracellular hydrogen ion concentration to graded degrees of chronic hypercapnia: the physiologic limits of the defense of pH. J Clin Invest 1961; 40:1238–1249.
50. Reeves JT. Hope in primary pulmonary hypertension. N Engl J Med 1980; 302:112–113.
51. Pepke-Zaba J, Higenbottam TW, Dinh-Xuan AT, Stone D, Wallwork J. Inhaled nitric oxide as a cause of selective pulmonary vasodilatation in pulmonary hypertension. Lancet 1991; 338:1173–1174.

52. Kouyoumdjian C, Adnot S, Levame M, Eddahibi S, Bousbaa H, Raffestin B. Continuous inhalation of nitric oxide protects against development of pulmonary hypertension in chronically hypoxic rats. J Clin Invest 1994; 94:578–584.

53. Burke CM, Harte M, Duncan J, Connolly HM, Horgan JH, Theodore J, Callaghan B. Captopril and domiciliary oxygen in chronic airflow obstruction. Br Med J (Clin Res Ed) 1985; 290:1251.

54. Stewart AG, Waterhouse JC, Billings CG, Baylis P, Howard P. Effects of angiotensin converting enzyme inhibition on sodium excretion in patients with hypoxaemic chronic obstructive pulmonary disease. Thorax 1994; 49:995–998.

55. Continuous or nocturnal oxygen therapy in hypoxemic chronic obstructive lung disease: a clinical trial. Nocturnal Oxygen Therapy Trial Group. Ann Intern Med 1980; 93:391–398.

56. Adnot S, Andrivet P, Chabrier PE, Defouilloy C, Viossat I, Braquet P, Atlan G, Brun-Buisson C. Plasma levels of atrial natriuretic factor, renin activity, and aldosterone in patients with chronic obstructive pulmonary disease. Response to O_2 removal and to hyperoxia. Am Rev Respir Dis 1990; 141:1178–1184.

57. Mannix ET, Dowdeswell I, Carlone S, Palange P, Aronoff GR, Farber MO. The effect of oxygen on sodium excretion in hypoxemic patients with chronic obstructive lung disease. Chest 1990; 97:840–844.

58. Skwarski KM, Morrison D, Barratt A, Lee M, MacNee W. Effects of hypoxia on renal hormonal balance in normal subjects and in patients with COPD. Respir Med 1998; 92:1331–1336.

17

Metabolism and Nutrition in Acute Exacerbations of Chronic Obstructive Pulmonary Disease

ROELINKA BROEKHUIZEN, EVA C. CREUTZBERG,
and ANNEMIE M. W. J. SCHOLS

University Hospital Maastricht
Maastricht, The Netherlands

I. Introduction

Weight loss is common in patients with chronic obstructive pulmonary disease (COPD). Reported prevalence rates range from 20% in clinically stable outpatients (1) up to 50% in patients with acute respiratory failure (ARF) (2). Involuntary weight loss and, in particular, loss of fat-free mass (FFM), as an indirect measure of muscle mass, have many adverse clinical consequences. Independently of lung function, they have been associated with impaired exercise performance (3) and weakening of peripheral skeletal muscles (1) and respiratory muscles (4). Moreover, fat-free mass–depleted patients have worse scores on quality-of-life questionnaires compared to nondepleted patients (5, 6). Furthermore, loss of body mass is associated with increased mortality (7–9).

In addition, weight loss negatively affects the prevalence and outcome of acute disease exacerbations of COPD. Kessler et al. have reported an increased risk of hospitalization in patients with a low body mass index (BMI) (body weight/ height^2) $\leq 20 \, \text{kg/m}^2$) (10). Weight loss during hospitalization and low body weight on admission are associated with early nonelective readmission (11). Nutritional depletion has also been associated with an increased risk for the need for mechanical ventilation (12). In addition, in patients on mechanical ventilation, nutritional depletion has a deleterious effect on the weaning-off process (13). Furthermore, involuntary weight loss is associated with increased risk for nosocomial pneumonia (14).

Low BMI negatively affects survival time after hospitalization as well. According to Connors et al., only 40% of the patients with a BMI $< 18\,kg/m^2$ survived 350 days after hospitalization for AECOPD, compared to 70% of patients with BMI $> 22\,kg/m^2$ (15).

Nutritional deprivation has been shown to suppress immune function (16, 17). In fact, it has been associated with death from infectious disease (18). Therefore, low BMI is a predictor of morbidity and mortality. Low BMI may be caused by nutritional deprivation itself, failing to provide enough nutrients for optimal immune function. Another possible explanation is the decreased amount of fat mass and coinciding decreased levels of leptin. This will be explained elsewhere in this chapter.

Weight loss is a consequence of either a decreased intake or an increased energy expenditure, or a combination of both, resulting in a negative energy balance. Loss of fat-free mass, however, is a more complex process involving imbalances in protein synthesis and breakdown, which results in negative protein balance.

Tissue depiction (i.e., loss of FFM) does not necessarily coincide with loss of fat mass (FM). In fact, in 16% of patients with emphysema and in 8% of COPD patients without emphysema, lean mass depletion was found despite a normal body weight (19). This suggests that more than one process influences metabolism to different degrees, resulting in different patterns of depletion.

To be able to reverse the process of weight loss and tissue depletion, knowledge of the course and contributing factors is important. In this chapter, we will try to unravel at least some of the factors contributing to weight loss and muscle wasting in AECOPD. More specifically, an overview will be given on the energy and protein balance during AECOPD relative to clinically stable periods of COPD, and the factors that contribute to the imbalances in energy and protein metabolism during both periods.

II. Clinically Stable Periods

A. Energy Balance

Dietary Intake

Clinically stable patients with COPD have a normal to elevated dietary intake compared to predicted energy requirements (20, 21). The subgroup of weight-losing patients, however, has a lower dietary intake as compared to weight-stable patients, both in absolute terms, and when expressed as a percentage of measured resting energy expenditure (REE) (21). Patients who fail to gain weight after nutritional therapy, the so-called "nonresponders," have a lower habitual dietary intake as compared to patients who do respond (22). Others reported that hypoxemic patients are at increased risk for a decreased dietary intake compared to basal energy expenditure (21–23).

Energy Expenditure

On the other side of the energy spectrum, energy expenditure, and in particular resting energy expenditure, is elevated in clinically stable COPD patients. REE is the energy needed to support the body in a resting state when no energy is needed for digestion [diet-induced thermogenesis (DIT)], nor for maintaining body temperature or activities. In sedentary people, total daily energy expenditure (TDEE) is composed mainly of REE, the rest being energy needed for diet-induced thermogenesis and activities (24).

Different studies have investigated REE in patients with COPD, revealing an increased REE compared to healthy subjects (25–27). Moreover, Schols et al. showed that weight-losing patients have a significantly higher REE than weight-stable patients with COPD (25). The prevalence of hypermetabolism at rest in COPD patients has been shown to be 26% based on adjustment for FFM. Based on Harris and Benedict (HB) equations, this percentage amounts to 54% (27). The difference in outcome can be attributed to the fact that the HB equations do not take FFM into account, which is the most important determinant of REE, thus overestimating prevalence of hypermetabolism. This could also explain the reported higher prevalence in increased REE in weight-losing patients by Schols et al. (25).

There have been few studies that have investigated TDEE in patients with COPD. In contrast to Hugli et al. (28), who found no increased TDEE in patients with COPD, Baarends et al. have previously reported a higher TDEE in patients with COPD compared to matched healthy subjects (29). Hugli et al., however, assessed TDEE in a metabolic chamber, having limited room for activities, while Baarends et al. used the doubly labeled water technique in free-living conditions, reflecting all activities that subjects perform during a 2-week period. In addition, Hugli et al. report lower activity in their patients than in healthy controls (28). This suggests that patients with COPD compensate for their increased resting energy expenditure by decreasing their activity patterns, thus resulting in equal TDEEs between patients and controls. Baarends et al. studied TDEE and activity patterns in patients at a rehabilitation center, involving standardized daily exercise. They showed an increased TDEE compared to healthy controls, while having equal to decreased activity levels. REE was comparable between groups, suggesting that increased TDEE is due to the nonresting component of TDEE (29). A subsequent study of Baarends et al. reported no differences in TDEE between patients with normal and elevated REE. They also reported that REE and FFM did not significantly contribute to the variation in TDEE, suggesting that underlying mechanisms for an increased REE are not involved in increasing TDEE in COPD (30).

Data on a complete energy balance are difficult to assess because of methodological limitations. In clinical practice, therefore, REE is used more often to have a simple and standardized measure for energy expenditure. However, increases in REE seem to reflect increased levels of systemic inflammation (31), while TDEE in relation to dietary intake reflects true energy balance. Because of adaptation in activity levels, differences in relatively increased TDEE are difficult to assess without data on physical activity.

B. Substrate Metabolism

Protein

Depletion of FFM is a result of negative protein balance. Protein metabolism is composed of protein intake and protein turnover, which is protein synthesis and protein breakdown. Negative nitrogen balance is the result of net protein breakdown. This could be due to decreased intake, decreased synthesis, or increased protein breakdown. However, net negative protein balance can also be due to an elevated protein turnover (i.e., synthesis and breakdown both being increased, while breakdown exceeds synthesis).

The consequences of net nitrogen balance can be quite extensive. For example, a net nitrogen loss of around 6 g/per day, as reported by Saudny-Unterberger et al., can lead to a loss of approximately 37 g of protein per day. When nitrogen balances are not restored, this can eventually lead to a 1.3 kg loss of lean tissue per week (32).

Besides an imbalance in energy intake, there are also indications for imbalances in protein metabolism in a subgroup of stable COPD patients. Especially in patients with selective FFM depletion (33), a negative protein balance is likely, even independently of energy balance. Low protein intakes due to lower dietary intake (21–23), as well as a reduced protein synthesis rate in underweight patients with emphysema have been reported (34). Weight-stable COPD patients have been shown to have an increased whole-body protein synthesis and breakdown, without a net negative protein balance, indicating an increased protein turnover (33).

It is hypothesized that, comparable to increased inflammation in sepsis, a shift in distribution of body protein takes place. As the liver increases its production of acute phase protein, protein requirements go up. To meet with the enhanced protein demands of the liver, peripheral muscle protein breakdown is increased (35). However, more research is needed to confirm this hypothesis and to elucidate the contribution of tissue-specific protein turnover to the elevated whole-body turnover in COPD.

Protein turnover is assumed to contribute to 20% of REE in normal adults (36) and thus may contribute to increased metabolism at rest in patients with COPD. This could also be an indirect relation caused by increased systemic inflammation, as inflammation increases both REE and protein turnover.

As protein is built from amino acids (AA), disturbances in amino acid metabolism could also be present. Indeed, several studies have shown that plasma amino acid profiles in patients with COPD differ from healthy controls (37, 38). Engelen et al. have reported a decreased level of branched chain amino acids (BCAA), in particular, leucine, in patients with COPD (38). This could be due to hyperinsulinemia, as insulin has been shown to increase BCAA uptake in muscle in cirrhotic patients (39). Indeed, in patients with severe hypoxemia, increased insulin concentrations are reported (40). Another possible explanation could be the increased systemic inflammation, reported in COPD (31), which has been shown to decrease BCAA levels in plasma (41, 42).

In addition, decreased levels of glutamate have been found in muscles of patients with emphysema (43). Glutamate is an important precursor for glutathione, an important intracellular antioxidant that protects tissue from damage caused by oxidative stress.

Carbohydrate and Fat

Not much is known about carbohydrate and fat metabolism in patients with COPD. Glucose metabolism in healthy subjects is improved by hypoxemia through stimulation of glucose transport and uptake (44, 45). In chronic and acute disease, insulin resistance is often observed (46, 47). However, in COPD patients with severe hypoxemia, increased insulin concentrations are reported, while in normoxemic patients glucose metabolism seems to be normal (40), suggesting a different mechanism in this disease. Fat metabolism seems to be different in patients with COPD as well. Lipolysis is blunted after administration of a β_2-agonist, compared to healthy subjects (48), which could contribute to the relative conservation of adipose tissue in patients with COPD.

Micronutrients

Most research on micronutrient metabolism in COPD has been done in the field of antioxidants. Antioxidants are oxygen-radical scavengers, which may protect lungs and tissues against oxidative stress. Oxidative stress is caused by free radicals, generated either exogenously (e.g., air pollution or smoking) or endogenously, such as antioxidants released from phagocytes or intracellular oxidants from mitochondrial electron transport (49). Oxidative stress occurs when the level of oxidants exceeds the level of antioxidants. The human body has a series of defense mechanisms against free radicals. The most important endogenous mechanism is composed of antioxidant enzymes like catalase, superoxide dismutase, and glutathione peroxidase. Another important antioxidant system is derived from food (50). Water-soluble vitamin C, fat-soluble vitamin E, and beta-carotene are well known antioxidants derived mainly from vegetables, fruits, and margarine and vegetable oils.

There is growing evidence that oxidant/antioxidant imbalances play a role in COPD (49, 51). Increased oxidative stress in the lungs has been linked to COPD (52). In tissues, however, not much research on antioxidants has been done. Engelen et al. have shown that, in muscle tissue, intracellular glutathione is decreased, impairing the antioxidant/oxidant balance (43). Rahman et al. have reported a decreased antioxidant capacity in plasma of smokers and patients with COPD, indicating increased systemic oxidative stress (53). Moreover, there is some epidemiological evidence that consumption of antioxidants might decrease the risk of getting COPD (54–56). However, no firm conclusions can be drawn on the relation between food antioxidants and COPD. For a review on this subject, see Ref. 57.

III. AECOPD

In the majority of patients, weight loss appears to develop gradually, indicating a chronic imbalance between dietary intake and energy expenditure. In a subgroup of patients, however, weight loss follows a stepwise pattern presumably related to AECOPD, suggesting additional factors that aggravate the imbalance during stable periods.

A. Energy Balance

Dietary Intake

Limited data are available on dietary intake during AECOPD. Two studies have investigated the effect of AECOPD on the nutritional and metabolic profile of patients with COPD. They have shown that the majority of patients have a dramatically decreased intake directly before hospitalization (Fig. 1). During the first days of hospitalization, a very low dietary intake is reported, improving quickly during the remaining hospital period. At discharge, dietary intake was even higher than habitual intake (58, 59) and is stabilized at habitual levels after 3 months of follow-up (59).

Energy Expenditure

Patients who are admitted to the hospital for acute exacerbation have been shown to have an increased REE. During the first few days of hospitalization, REE remains elevated, decreasing thereafter (59). A subgroup of patients, however, seems to have another pattern of REE during exacerbation. In this group, REE does not decrease during hospitalization, remaining high at discharge. Moreover, these patients have an even higher REE at admission than the patients who have the decreasing pattern of REE during admission. This group, which remained hypermetabolic at discharge, was characterized by a low BMI (59). Creutzberg et al. also found an increased REE

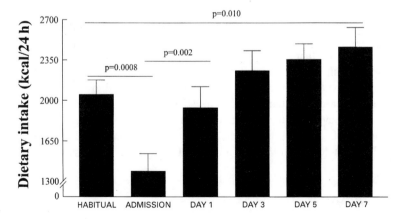

Figure 1   Habitual dietary intake and dietary intake in COPD patients during AECOPD. Data express mean dietary intake in kcal per 24 h (SEM). (Adapted from Ref. 58.)

during AECOPD, decreasing during hospitalization. Patients, however, remained hypermetabolic until day 7 (58).

Energy Balance

At hospital discharge for AECOPD, the dietary intake/REE ratio has been shown to increase to levels equal to TDEE corrected for REE in stable COPD patients. This indicates that energy balance was restored to normal (29, 58). A subgroup of patients, with a high risk of nonelective readmission to the hospital for AECOPD, has been shown to lose weight during admission, while patients with low risk for readmission were weight stable (11). This suggests that, at least for a subgroup of patients, a negative energy balance is present which contributes to the stepwise pattern of weight loss.

B. Substrate Metabolism

Protein

A decreased daily protein intake has been reported prior to and during the first few days of hospitalization, gradually increasing thereafter (59). In addition, during AECOPD, negative nitrogen balance has been reported, indicating muscle wasting. This negative nitrogen balance was strongly correlated with the dose of glucocorticosteroids (32).

Nitrogen balance is an indirect measure for protein metabolism, which does not reflect actual protein synthesis and protein breakdown. More information can be drawn from research with stable isotopes. However, during AECOPD, no such research has been done so far. Negative protein balance can result in an increased loss of fat-free mass due to aggravated imbalances during AECOPD. Because periods of AECOPD are usually not very long, weight loss and especially loss of fat-free mass are difficult to assess. However, a few periods of AECOPD can have their effect in the long run, which may explain the stepwise pattern of weight loss seen in some patients.

Carbohydrates

Carbohydrate intake is low prior to and during the first few days of hospitalization for AECOPD in absolute terms. However, it seems that the proportion of carbohydrates is increased on day 1 compared to habitual (53% vs. 44%) (59). This could reflect an adaptation, as carbohydrates have a lower gastric-emptying time compared to fats (60) and thus have a relatively low impact on complaints of bloating, abdominal discomfort, and early satiety (61). The proportion of carbohydrates subsequently decreases during hospitalization to percentages comparable to habitual (59). This is probably due to normalization of fat and protein intake. In absolute terms, however, there is an increase in carbohydrate intake at discharge, when compared to day 1. This is explained by the observed increased dietary intake (59).

Insulin resistance seems to play a role during AECOPD (58). Creutzberg et al. reported an elevated level of plasma glucose on day 1, decreasing during hospitalization to values comparable to healthy subjects. Insulin concentration was high on day 1, and remained elevated compared to healthy volunteers. This pattern in glucose and insulin levels could be related to the tapering off of the systemic prednisolone treatment (58), suggesting an induction of glucose and insulin by prednisolone. Other possible explanations will be described later in this chapter.

Fat

Fat intake is low prior to and during the first days of hospitalization, but increases fast during the days following. At discharge, absolute fat intake is higher than habitual fat intake, while proportional to total intake both are equal (59). This suggests that at discharge fat increase is due to increase in total dietary intake rather than to adaptation.

Micronutrients

During AECOPD, an increased oxidant/antioxidant imbalance has been found (62, 63). During the first days of AECOPD, the lipid peroxidation product malondialdehyde (MDA), which is a marker of oxidative stress, is increased, returning back to normal during the course of treatment (64). This suggests an even higher need for antioxidants, caused either by increased oxidative stress or by decreased antioxidant capacity. Further research needs to be done to elucidate the role of antioxidants during AECOPD.

IV. Contributing Factors and Mechanisms

A. Symptoms

The increase in symptoms during AECOPD has its effects on energy balance. A decrease in appetite has been reported during the first few days of AECOPD (59), having its impact on dietary intake. Vermeeren et al. hypothesize that, besides the decrease in appetite, the inability to eat due to increased dyspnea and fatigue is largely responsible for the low dietary intake prior to and during the first few days of hospitalization for AECOPD. At discharge, the dyspnea and fatigue improve, as well as the dietary intake and appetite (Fig. 2) (59). The increased sensation of dyspnea has also been found to be associated with the changes in REE, indicating a possible contribution of an increased oxygen cost of ventilation to increased REE during AECOPD (Fig. 3) (59).

Furthermore, during the first few days of hospitalization, a very low fat intake is reported, which could be related to the reported early feeling of satiety, together with decreased appetite and intake (59). This spontaneous change in macronutrient intake is in contrast with the long-held belief that a low-carbohydrate, high-fat meal

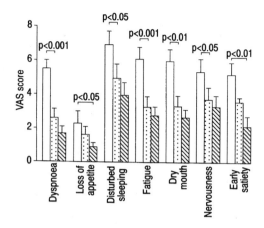

Figure 2 Disease symptoms (VAS scores) on admission (□), at day 5 (▨) and at discharge from the hospital (▨). Results are mean ± SEM. (From Ref. 59.)

would be beneficial to patients with COPD during metabolic stress because of the assumed increase in CO_2 load. In stable patients, however, no fluctuations in PCO_2 are seen during either high-carbohydrate or high-fat meals (65). In addition, consumption of a fat-rich food supplement increased feelings of dyspnea more than consumption of isocaloric, high-carbohydrate supplements (61). During AECOPD, no data are available on this subject.

At discharge, dietary intake was higher than habitual intake, which could be related to the improvements in symptoms like dyspnea, loss of appetite, and early satiety. This could also be compensation for energy deficits that had risen during the

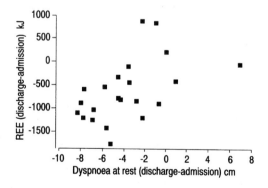

Figure 3 Significant relationship between the changes in resting energy expenditure (REE) and dyspnea sensation during the total hospitalization period ($r = 0.52$, $p = 0.004$). (From Ref. 59.)

first few days of AECOPD (59). Another explanation could be appetite-stimulating effects of high-dosage glucocorticosteroid treatment during AECOPD (66).

B. Leptin

Leptin is a hormone produced by adipose tissue that regulates energy homeostasis through a feedback mechanism by signaling the brain about the amount of fat stored in the body (67). Administration of leptin in animals results in a reduction of food intake (68) and an increase in energy expenditure (69). These effects seem to be mediated by a leptin-induced decrease of the hypothalamic biosynthesis and release of neuropeptide Y, a hormone that potently stimulates appetite and food intake and reduces energy expenditure (70–72).

In clinically stable, depleted patients with COPD, plasma leptin is indeed associated with fat mass. Leptin divided by fat mass is inversely related to dietary intake and body weight change (73). This is in accordance with the regular feedback mechanism in healthy subjects. However, as some patients have low fat mass, leptin levels can drop to very low levels (73). Research has shown that leptin might be an important factor in the regulation of the immune system. Lord et al. have shown that administration of leptin to mice reversed the immunosuppressive effects of starvation, indicating a key role for leptin (74). So the increased morbidity and mortality could be, at least partially, caused by a decreased level of leptin. Increased morbidity and AECOPD have, in turn, adverse effects on nutritional status in COPD patients, creating a negative vicious circle.

During AECOPD it was shown that plasma leptin, corrected for FM, is elevated compared to healthy subjects, decreasing gradually throughout the exacerbation but remaining higher than in healthy subjects (58). In addition, on day 1 of AECOPD, no correlation between plasma leptin and FM or dietary intake was found, indicating a disturbance in the normal leptin feedback mechanism controlling energy balance. This correlation is restored on day 7 of AECOPD, even though levels are still high (58).

This increase in leptin level could be caused by a flare-up of the systemic inflammatory response of AECOPD. Indeed, leptin levels are correlated to soluble tumor necrosis factor receptor 55 (sTNFr-55), which is a marker for systemic inflammation (73). In addition, leptin levels during acute illness have been shown to be increased (75, 76). This raises the question of whether leptin is a mediator or merely a marker in the whole process of AECOPD and weight loss. Nevertheless, the increased level of leptin does explain the temporary loss of appetite in patients during the first few days of AECOPD (58, 59). A possible explanation for the lack of effect of leptin on dietary intake on the first day of AECOPD could be an increased "leptin resistance," caused by the increase in inflammation. However, this hypothesis is only suggested as an explanatory mechanism for the etiology of obesity and therefore is never studied in this context (77).

The increased levels of leptin during AECOPD, together with the state of catabolism and increased proteolysis, could aggravate the already existing negative energy balance and thus accelerate weight loss and muscle wasting.

C. Systemic Inflammation

In the past, more and more evidence has emerged about the occurrence of an increased systemic inflammation in patients with COPD, along with local inflammation of the lungs. Evidence for this is given by several studies, reporting increased concentrations of proinflammatory cytokines and acute phase proteins in clinically stable patients with COPD (31, 78–81). This increased systemic inflammatory response is related to hypermetabolism at rest (REE) (31).

In particular tumor necrosis factor-α (TNF-α), a proinflammatory cytokine, has been associated with weight loss (79, 82, 83). In addition, depleted patients who do not respond to high-caloric nutritional therapy, have higher levels of soluble TNF receptors (sTNF-Rs) in peripheral blood than patients who do respond (22). This could be mediated through the action of leptin.

Inflammatory cytokines have been shown to increase circulating leptin (84, 85). In patients with emphysema, leptin is positively correlated with the proinflammatory sTNF-R55 independently of FM. Moreover, sTNF-R55 is related to both dietary intake as well as weight loss and REE (58, 73). In addition, TNF-α or interleukin-1α (IL-1α) infusion in cancer patients increases serum leptin concentration (86, 87). This suggests that the influence of leptin on energy balance might be under the control of the systemic inflammatory response, while the higher level of systemic inflammation could be causally related to involuntary weight loss (31).

Indeed, in animal models, several inflammatory cytokines can induce various features of cachexia. Exposure to lipopolysaccharide (LPS), IL-1, or TNF-α induces weight loss and anorexia in rats (88, 89). Chronic treatment of rats with TNF-α results in depletion of body protein, anorexia, weight loss, and tissue inflammation (90, 91). Moreover, high concentration of TNF-α increases amino acid release from mouse diaphragms (92). In humans, infusion of TNF-α into weight-stable cancer patients resulted in increased amino acid release and thus stimulated proteolysis (93, 94). This could cause a net negative nitrogen balance, resulting in selective FFM wasting.

During AECOPD, the elevated systemic inflammatory response seems to be even higher than during clinically stable periods. This flare-up of the chronic inflammatory process decreases during the period of hospitalization. Compared to stable patients, C-reactive protein (CRP) concentration is higher in patients with AECOPD, but declines during treatment (80, 95). Because CRP levels are elevated in most patients with AECOPD, including those without apparent bacterial infection as assessed by sputum culture, CRP has been suggested as a clinical marker for AECOPD (95). In contrast to CRP, our group found that sTNF-Rs levels are not increased during AECOPD (58, 80). An explanation for this phenomenon might be the suggestion that the sTNF-Rs represent a buffer system that slows the effects of TNF-α by forming a "slow-release reservoir." Therefore, sTNF-Rs are more likely to be markers for a proinflammatory response (96). However, the increased REE found during AECOPD points to an increased systemic inflammatory response (58, 59, 97).

D. Heart Rhythm

Contrary to Dallongeville, who hypothesizes that human leptin levels increase following dietary intake and are not influenced by circadian rhythm (98), Sinha et al. state that circulating leptin levels do have an ultradian and circadian variation that peaks during the night (99, 100). Takabatake et al. have shown that in COPD patients with a fat mass lower than 20%, circadian rhythm seems to be absent, as opposed to patients with FM > 20% and healthy controls. Moreover, very low frequency (VLF) of heart rhythm variability (HRV) showed identical fluctuations, with no circadian rhythm in patients with low FM. The authors state that leptin influences the VLF values of HRV. The VLF component of HRV is being considered to represent neuroendocrine and thermoregulatory influences of the heart. Because the VLF component carries a high predictive value of mortality and patients with low FM show reduced values of VLF, more support is said to be found for the fact that fat mass depletion is an independent risk factor of mortality (101).

However, Goldberger et al. state that in this study correlations are weak and, according to the international Task Force on Heart Rate Variability, VLF assessed in the short term is a dubious measure (102), questioning the relevance of the suggested mechanism. This hypothesis has not yet been investigated during AECOPD.

E. Hypoxemia

Another explanation for increased leptin concentration in patients with AECOPD might be hypoxemia. In volunteers at high altitudes, where oxygen pressure is low, an elevated concentration of leptin has been found, associated with a decrease in appetite (103). Dietary intake is lowest in COPD patients suffering from chronic hypoxemia (21, 23). In addition, desaturation has been shown to increase during eating in a subgroup of patients with COPD (65). This suggests that increases in leptin due to low oxygen saturation might contribute to less appetite and a limited dietary intake.

During AECOPD, hypoxemia is even more pronounced than during clinically stable periods (10, 15, 58, 80), possibly increasing leptin (58) contributing to the feeling of dyspnea and thus decreasing appetite (59). Hypoxemia has been shown to increase the in vitro release of the inflammatory cytokines IL-1 and TNF-α (104, 105). In COPD, low PaO_2 has been found to correlate with increased levels of TNF-α and the sTNF-Rs (79), which could, in turn, induce leptin production.

The increased IL-1 and TNF-α production could be due to a hypoxemia-induced decreased synthesis of prostaglandin H synthase-2 (PGHS-2), and thus decreased synthesis of prostaglandin E_2 (PGE_2). PGE_2 inhibits the expression of IL-1 and TNF-α genes (104). Another explanation for the increased levels of TNF-α and IL-1 is the enhanced expression of nuclear factor kappa B (NF-κB), a transcription factor that is thought to regulate the expression of inflammatory cytokines, like TNF-α (106). The expression of NF-κB could be activated by reactive oxygen species formed during acute hypoxia (106, 107). In addition, a profound oxidant–antioxidant imbalance has been found during AECOPD (62, 63), resulting in increased oxidative stress.

Hypoxemia has been shown to influence glucose metabolism in healthy subjects, increasing glucose concentration and stimulating glucose transport even in insulin-resistant skeletal muscle (44, 45). In hypoxemic COPD patients, however, increased insulin resistance has been reported, while this was normal in normoxemic patients with COPD (40). This effect is contrary to the effect hypoxemia has in healthy subjects. In addition, during AECOPD, when hypoxemia is even more pronounced than during clinically stable periods (10, 15, 58, 80), increased insulin resistance has been reported (58). Thus, hypoxemia may induce insulin resistance, which could induce leptin, thereby decreasing appetite during AECOPD.

F. Medication

Systemic Glucocorticosteroids

High-dose oral or intravenous glucocorticosteroids are often used as anti-inflammatory agents in the treatment of AECOPD, even though efficacy has not as yet been established. In contrast to treatment of asthma, inhalation of budisone or oral treatment with prednisolone does not affect the inflammatory profile of patients with COPD (108). Systemic glucocorticosteroids may stimulate appetite, as has been previously reported in patients with cancer (66). The high-dosage glucocorticosteroids administered during AECOPD could explain the increase in appetite seen during hospitalization (58, 59).

Unfortunately, treatment with glucocorticosteroids is known to have many adverse events, like catabolic effects on respiratory and peripheral muscles and bone mass (109–111). Indeed, a negative correlation has been reported between methylprednisolone intake and nitrogen balance during AECOPD intake (32). The catabolic effects of corticosteroids and the increased levels of inflammatory mediators may exceed the positive effects of increased appetite caused by glucocorticosteroids (32), creating a net negative nitrogen balance.

The reported increase in insulin resistance during AECOPD could be related to the systemic prednisolone treatment (58), suggesting an induction of glucose and insulin by prednisolone. This is partly in accordance with the effects seen by Tataranni et al. in healthy individuals. However, they found no acute effects of prednisolone on insulin (112). Acute administration of methylprednisolone in healthy men did increase fasting plasma glucose, while prolonged methylprednisolone administration increases fasting plasma insulin, indicating an induction of insulin resistance (112). However, in stable, normoxemic COPD patients, insulin resistance does not seem to play a role, while during AECOPD, with acute administration of prednisolone, insulin resistance is increased (58). More research is needed to elucidate the effects of glucocorticosteroids on glucose metabolism.

Reports concerning the effects of glucocorticosteroids on leptin are contradictory. The course of plasma leptin seems to follow the dose of glucocorticosteroids administered during AECOPD (58). Indeed, glucocorticosteroids are reported to induce leptin gene expression in rats (113). Furthermore, dexamethasone has been shown to induce leptin and leptin mRNA in healthy subjects (114, 115). Tataranni et al., however, did not find an increase in leptin concentration after administration of methylprednisolone (112).

Another possible mechanism to explain the observed relation between glucocorticosteroids and leptin is by means of TNF-α-induced insulin resistance. TNF-α has been shown to induce insulin resistance both in vitro as well as in rodents (116, 117). Since prolonged increases of insulin can induce leptin expression (118), the observed increase in leptin after administration of glucocorticosteroids could be an indirect effect. The induction of insulin resistance by TNF-α could be explained by a TNF-α-induced inhibition of intracellular signaling in the insulin receptor (116, 117). Another possible explanation of the induction of insulin resistance by TNF-α can be sought in the reduction of the expression of mRNA encoding for glucose transporters (GLUT-4 and GLUT-1) (119). However, no relation was found between the use of glucocorticosteroids and the level of sTNF-Rs, suggesting that the observed correlation is probably mere coincidence instead of a causal relation (73).

Overall, the effects of glucocorticosteroids on leptin metabolism and insulin resistance are debatable. Data are inconclusive, but it now seems that observed correlations are not causal. The increase in insulin resistance observed could also be due to an AECOPD-related catabolic state of the body. Catabolic hormones, like epinephrine, glucagon, and cortisol result in lipolysis, gluconeogenesis, and catabolism of body protein (120). Stress hormones are also known to induce insulin resistance, resulting in hyperglycemia, hyperinsulinemia, and elevated hepatic glucose production (47).

Other Medication

Salbutamol, a β_2-sympaticomimetic drug, has been shown to induce an increase in REE of 4% in patients with COPD. Even though the increase is 11% in healthy young subjects, REE only increases 6% in elderly subjects, which is comparable with COPD patients. This slight induction of REE by salbutamol cannot fully explain the rise in REE in patients with COPD. Furthermore, the use of salbutamol was comparable between hypermetabolic and normometabolic patients at rest, thus indicating a limited effect on the rise in REE (121–123).

Theophylline and ipratroprium bromide are reported not to have effect on REE in patients with COPD (124). Dash et al. reported an increase in resting oxygen consumption on heart rate after oral theophylline treatment. However, this did not alter the metabolic response to acutely inhaled salbutamol (125).

V. Therapy

A. Clinically Stable Periods

Because refeeding already malnourished patients is very difficult and because it takes high-energy intake to improve lean body mass in older people (126), prevention of loss of body mass is important. In addition, it is important because low body mass and low fat-free mass are associated with an increased risk for morbidity and mortality in COPD.

The main goal of nutritional therapy is to restore energy balance without overfeeding patients. Vermeeren et al. have shown that small portions several times a day are preferred to larger portions. This is due to increased metabolic and ventilatory response and increased satiety after the bigger portions. In addition, they have shown that consumption of high-carbohydrate supplements is preferable to isocaloric fat-rich supplements, because the latter causes a higher increase in feelings of dyspnea (61).

Another important focus should be restoring protein balance to prevent (further) loss of fat-free mass. To reverse catabolism, protein supplementation is needed as well as anabolic stimulation. During stable periods of COPD, nutritional therapy, containing sufficient amounts of calories as well as macronutrients, together with anabolic stimulation, like training, is effective in reversing the weight-loss process and can result in improving body composition (22, 127, 128). Furthermore, anabolic steroid supplementation has been shown to improve body composition and health status and to counteract the deleterious effects of systemic glucocorticosteroids (127, 129).

B. AECOPD

Little is known about the effects of nutritional therapy during AECOPD. Saudny-Unterberger et al. have investigated the effects of 2 weeks of nutritional therapy during AECOPD. A significant improvement of forced vital capacity (FVC) was found in the treatment group. However, no improvements were found in body composition or nitrogen balance. This could be due to the short intervention period. In addition, a negative correlation was found between nitrogen balance and methylprednisolone intake, suggesting a catabolic effect of this glucocorticosteroid. Thus, another explanation could be inadequate protein supplementation that does not meet the increased requirements due to the inflammatory, catabolic process (32). However, the main focus during AECOPD should be stabilization of catabolism as well as stabilization of negative energy and protein balances. After AECOPD, catabolism should be reversed into anabolism, with increased energy and protein intakes and, hopefully, eventually resulting in weight gain as well as increased fat-free mass. To accomplish this, anabolic stimulation is required (22, 127, 128).

For this reason, Vermeeren et al. suggest that, during AECOPD, no additional nutritional therapy is indicated as long as patients adequately respond within a few days to the medical therapy in terms of appetite and energy balance. It is, however, indicated to increase protein intake (1.5 g/kg/day) during AECOPD and its recovery phase in order to optimize conditions for protein synthesis (59). From a caloric point of view, nutritional support should be targeted to meet 1.3 times the (estimated or measured) resting energy expenditure, thus avoiding overfeeding in this still unstable period.

C. Other Possibilities

Since the current anti-inflammatory therapy (i.e., prescription of systemic glucocorticosteroids) has shown limited effects on the systemic inflammatory response and resulting systemic consequences, research needs to be done to find other anti-inflammatory agents. In other chronic diseases that involve inflammation and/or cachexia, like cancer, inflammatory bowel disease, and rheumatoid arthritis, encouraging effects have been found with the anti-inflammatory effects of n-3 polyunsaturated fatty acids (PUFA) (130–135, 136). The current hypothesis on the mechanism involved is that, instead of arachidonic acid, n-3 PUFA are incorporated in cell membranes competing with each other for metabolization. The n-3 PUFA are metabolized into milder eicosanoids than arachidonic acid, for example, from leukotriene B4 (LTB4) to leukotriene B5 (LTB5), which decreases chemotactic and inflammatory activity (137, 138). In COPD, this anti-inflammatory effect of n-3 PUFA is currently under investigation, as is other pharmacological anti-inflammatory modulation like anti-TNF-α.

A possible role for antioxidant therapy has not yet been fully explored. It has been shown, however, that the use of the antioxidant N-acetylcysteine (NAC) reduces the number and severity of AECOPD (139, 140). NAC acts like an antioxidant as it provides cysteine for the production of glutathione (141). Research is currently ongoing to elucidate the effectiveness of antioxidants as an anti-inflammatory agent (142).

VI. Conclusion

Prior to and during AECOPD, the risk for weight loss is increased, worsening an often already-impaired situation. Energy and protein balances are negative, related to an increase in symptoms, acute (partial) respiratory failure, and a flare-up of systemic inflammation. Loss of FM and FFM in particular are associated with increases in risk for exercise performance, AECOPD, and mortality, creating a viscious circle. Therefore, prevention of weight loss and tissue depletion and immediate treatment is of the utmost importance. During AECOPD, besides optimal medical intervention, the focus of nutritional intervention should be aimed at preventing or limiting weight loss and loss of fat-free mass by targeting energy intake to approximately 1.3 times the (measured or estimated) resting metabolic rate and protein intake to 1.5 g/kg body weight. Sometimes nutritional supplements are indicated to reach these goals. Nutritional support after hospitalization may be more aggressive if combined with an exercise program aimed at improvement of fat-free mass and functional capacity.

References

1. Engelen MPKJ, Schols AMWJ, Baken WC, Wesseling GJ, Wouters EFM. Nutritional depletion in relation to respiratory and peripheral skeletal muscle function in out-patients with COPD. Eur Respir J 1994; 7:1793–1797.
2. Driver AG, McAlevy MT, Smith JL. Nutritional assessment of patients with chronic obstructive pulmonary disease and acute respiratory failure. Chest 1982; 82:568–571.
3. Schols AM, Mostert R, Soeters PB, Wouters EF. Body composition and exercise performance in patients with chronic obstructive pulmonary disease. Thorax 1991; 46:695–699.

4. Rochester DF, Braun NM. Determinants of maximal inspiratory pressure in chronic obstructive pulmonary disease. Am Rev Respir Dis 1985; 132:42–47.

5. Mostert R, Goris A, Weling-Scheepers C, Wouters EF, Schols AM. Tissue depletion and health related quality of life in patients with chronic obstructive pulmonary disease. Respir Med 2000; 94:859–867.

6. Shoup R, Dalsky G, Warner S, et al. Body composition and health-related quality of life in patients with obstructive airways disease. Eur Respir J 1997; 10:1575–1580.

7. Schols AM, Slangen J, Volovics L, Wouters EF. Weight loss is a reversible factor in the prognosis of chronic obstructive pulmonary disease. Am J Respir Crit Care Med 1998; 157:1791–1797.

8. Wilson DO, Rogers RM, Wright EC, Anthonisen NR. Body weight in chronic obstructive pulmonary disease. The National Institutes of Health Intermittent Positive-Pressure Breathing Trial. Am Rev Respir Dis 1989; 139:1435–1438.

9. Landbo C, Prescott E, Lange P, Vestbo J, Almdal TP. Prognostic value of nutritional status in chronic obstructive pulmonary disease. Am J Respir Crit Care Med 1999; 160:1856–1861.

10. Kessler R, Faller M, Fourgaut G, Mennecier B, Weitzenblum E. Predictive factors of hospitalization for acute exacerbation in a series of 64 patients with chronic obstructive pulmonary disease. Am J Respir Crit Care Med 1999; 159:158–164.

11. Pouw EM, Ten Velde GP, Croonen BH, Kester AD, Schols AM, Wouters EF. Early non-elective readmission for chronic obstructive pulmonary disease is associated with weight loss. Clin Nutr 2000; 19:95–99.

12. Vitacca M, Clini E, Porta R, Foglio K, Ambrosino N. Acute exacerbations in patients with COPD: predictors of need for mechanical ventilation. Eur Respir J 1996; 9:1487–1493.

13. Laaban JP, Kouchakji B, Dore MF, Orvoen-Frija E, David P, Rochemaure J. Nutritional status of patients with chronic obstructive pulmonary disease and acute respiratory failure. Chest 1993; 103:1362–1368.

14. Gorse GJ, Messner RL, Stephens ND. Association of malnutrition with nosocomial infection. Infect Control Hosp Epidemiol 1989; 10:194–203.

15. Connors AF, Jr., Dawson NV, Thomas C, et al. Outcomes following acute exacerbation of severe chronic obstructive lung disease. The SUPPORT investigators (Study to Understand Prognoses and Preferences for Outcomes and Risks of Treatments). Am J Respir Crit Care Med 1996; 154:959–967.

16. Cason J, Ainley CC, Wolstencroft RA, Norton KR, Thompson RP. Cell-mediated immunity in anorexia nervosa. Clin Exp Immunol 1986; 64:370–375.

17. Chandra RK. 1990 McCollum Award lecture. Nutrition and immunity: lessons from the past and new insights into the future. Am J Clin Nutr 1991; 53:1087–1101.

18. Shears P. Epidemiology and infection in famine and disasters. Epidemiol Infect 1991; 107:241–251.

19. Engelen MP, Schols AM, Lamers RJ, Wouters EF. Different patterns of chronic tissue wasting among patients with chronic obstructive pulmonary disease. Clin Nutr 1999; 18:275–280.

20. Hunter AM, Carey MA, Larsh HW. The nutritional status of patients with chronic obstructive pulmonary disease. Am Rev Respir Dis 1981; 124:376–381.

21. Schols AMWJ, Soeters PB, Mostert R, Saris WH, Wouters EFM. Energy balance in chronic obstructive pulmonary disease. Am Rev Respir Dis 1991; 143:1248–1252.

22. Creutzberg EC, Schols AM, Weling-Scheepers CA, Buurman WA, Wouters EF. Characterization of nonresponse to high caloric oral nutritional therapy in depleted

patients with chronic obstructive pulmonary disease. Am J Respir Crit Care Med 2000; 161:745–752.

23. Fiaccadori E, Del Canale S, Coffrini E, et al. Hypercapnic-hypoxemic chronic obstructive pulmonary disease (COPD): influence of severity of COPD on nutritional status. Am J Clin Nutr 1988; 48:680–685.

24. Ravussin E, Lillioja S, Anderson TE, Christin L, Bogardus C. Determinants of 24-hour energy expenditure in man. Methods and results using a respiratory chamber. J Clin Invest 1986; 78:1568–1578.

25. Schols AMWJ, Fredrix EW, Soeters PB, Westerterp KR, Wouters EFM. Resting energy expenditure in patients with chronic obstructive pulmonary disease. Am J Clin Nutr 1991; 54:983–987.

26. Goldstein S, Askanazi J, Weissman C, Thomashow B, Kinney JM. Energy expenditure in patients with chronic obstructive pulmonary disease. Chest 1987; 91:222–224.

27. Creutzberg EC, Schols AM, Bothmer-Quaedvlieg FC, Wouters EF. Prevalence of an elevated resting energy expenditure in patients with chronic obstructive pulmonary disease in relation to body composition and lung function. Eur J Clin Nutr 1998; 52:396–401.

28. Hugh O, Schutz Y, Fitting JW. The daily energy expenditure in stable chronic obstructive pulmonary disease. Am J Respir Crit Care Med 1996; 153:294–300.

29. Baarends EM, Schols AMWJ, Pannemans DL, Westerterp KR, Wouters EFM. Total free living energy expenditure in patients with severe chronic obstructive pulmonary disease. Am J Respir Crit Care Med 1997; 155:549–554.

30. Baarends EM, Schols AMWJ, Westerterp KR, Wouters EFM. Total daily energy expenditure relative to resting energy expenditure in clinically stable patients with COPD. Thorax 1997; 52(9):780–785.

31. Schols AM, Buurman WA, Staal van den Brekel AJ, Dentener MA, Wouters EF. Evidence for a relation between metabolic derangements and increased levels of inflammatory mediators in a subgroup of patients with chronic obstructive pulmonary disease. Thorax 1996; 51:819–824.

32. Saudny-Unterberger H, Martin JG, Gray-Donald K. Impact of nutritional support on functional status during an acute exacerbation of chronic obstructive pulmonary disease. Am J Respir Crit Care Med 1997; 156:794–799.

33. Engelen MP, Deutz NE, Wouters EF, Schols AM. Enhanced levels of whole-body protein turnover in patients with chronic obstructive pulmonary disease. Am J Respir Crit Care Med 2000; 162:1488–1492.

34. Morrison WL, Gibson JN, Scrimgeour C, Rennie MJ. Muscle wasting in emphysema. Clin Sci 1988; 75:415–420.

35. O'Leary MJ, Ferguson CN, Rennie MJ, Hinds CJ, Coakley JH, Preedy VR. Sequential changes in in vivo muscle and liver protein synthesis and plasma and tissue glutamine levels in sepsis in the rat. Clin Sci (Lond) 2001; 101:295–304.

36. Waterlow JC. Whole-body protein turnover in humans—past, present, and future. Annu Rev Nutr 1995; 15:57–92.

37. Pouw EM, Schols AM, Deutz NE, Wouters EF. Plasma and muscle amino acid levels in relation to resting energy expenditure and inflammation in stable chronic obstructive pulmonary disease. Am J Respir Crit Care Med 1998; 158:797–801.

38. Engelen MP, Wouters EF, Deutz NE, Menheere PP, Schols AM. Factors contributing to alterations in skeletal muscle and plasma amino acid profiles in patients with chronic obstructive pulmonary disease. Am J Clin Nutr 2000; 72:1480–1487.

39. Munro HN, Fernstrom JD, Wurtman RJ. Insulin, plasma aminoacid imbalance, and hepatic coma. Lancet 1975; 1:722–724.
40. Hjalmarsen A, Aasebo U, Birkeland K, Sager G, Jorde R. Impaired glucose tolerance in patients with chronic hypoxic pulmonary disease. Diabetes Metab 1996; 22:37–42.
41. Andus T, Bauer J, Gerok W. Effects of cytokines on the liver. Hepatology 1991; 13: 364–375.
42. Nawabi MD, Block KP, Chakrabarti MC, Buse MG. Administration of endotoxin, tumor necrosis factor, or interleukin 1 to rats activates skeletal muscle branched-chain alpha-keto acid dehydrogenase. J Clin Invest 1990; 85:256–263.
43. Engelen MP, Schols AM, Does JD, Deutz NE, Wouters EF. Altered glutamate metabolism is associated with reduced muscle glutathione levels in patients with emphysema. Am J Respir Crit Care Med 2000; 161:98–103.
44. Brooks GA, Butterfield GE, Wolfe RR, et al. Increased dependence on blood glucose after acclimatization to 4300 m. J Appl Physiol 1991; 70:919–927.
45. Azevedo JL, Jr., Carey JO, Pories WJ, Moms PG, Dohm GL. Hypoxia stimulates glucose transport in insulin-resistant human skeletal muscle. Diabetes 1995; 44: 695–698.
46. Wolfe RR. Substrate utilization/insulin resistance in sepsis trauma. Baillieres Clin Endocrinol Metab 1997; 11:645–657.
47. Waldhausl WK, Gasic S, Bratusch-Marrain P, Komjati M, Korn A. Effect of stress hormones on splanchnic substrate and disposal after glucose ingestion in healthy humans. Diabetes 1987; 36:127–135.
48. Schifelers SL, Blaak EE, Baarends EM, et al. beta-Adrenoceptor-mediated thermogenesis and lipolysis in patients with chronic obstructive pulmonary disease. Am J Physiol Endocrinol Metab 2001; 280:E357–E364.
49. MacNee W, Rahman I. Is oxidative stress central to the pathogenesis of chronic obstructive pulmonary disease? Trends Mol Med 2001; 7:55–62.
50. Halliwell B. Antioxidants in human health and disease. Annu Rev Nutr 1996; 16:33–50.
51. Repine JE, Bast A, Lankhorst I. Oxidative stress in chronic obstructive pulmonary disease. Oxidative Stress Study Group. Am J Respir Crit Care Med 1997; 156: 341–357.
52. Cantin A, Crystal RG. Oxidants, antioxidants and the pathogenesis of emphysema. Eur J Respir Dis Suppl 1985; 139:7–17.
53. Rahman I, Swarska E, Henry M, Stolk J, MacNee W. Is there any relationship between plasma antioxidant capacity and lung function in smokers and in patients with chronic obstructive pulmonary disease? Thorax 2000; 55:189–193.
54. Miedema I, Feskens EJ, Heederik D, Kromhout D. Dietary determinants of long-term incidence of chronic nonspecific lung diseases. The Zutphen Study. Am J Epidemiol 1993; 138:37–45.
55. Strachan DP, Cox BD, Erzinclioglu SW, Walters DE, Whichelow MJ. Ventilatory function and winter fresh fruit consumption in a random sample of British adults. Thorax 1991; 46:624–629.
56. Rautalahti M, Virtano J, Haukka J, et al. The effect of alpha-tocopherol and betacarotene supplementation on COPD symptoms. Am J Respir Crit Care Med 1997; 156: 1447–1452.
57. Smit HA, Grievink L, Tabak C. Dietary influences on chronic obstructive lung disease and asthma: a review of the epidemiological evidence. Proc Nutr Soc 1999; 58:309–319.
58. Creutzberg EC, Wouters EF, Vanderhoven-Augustin IM, Dentener MA, Schols AM. Disturbances in leptin metabolism are related to energy imbalance during acute

exacerbations of chronic obstructive pulmonary disease [In Process Citation]. Am J Respir Crit Care Med 2000; 162:1239–1245.

59. Vermeeren MA, Schols AM, Wouters EF. Effects of an acute exacerbation on nutritional and metabolic profile of patients with COPD. Eur Respir J 1997; 10:2264–2269.

60. Akrabawi SS, Mobarhan S, Stoltz RR, Ferguson PW. Gastric emptying, pulmonary function, gas exchange, and respiratory quotient after feeding a moderate versus high fat enteral formula meal in chronic obstructive pulmonary disease patients. Nutrition 1996; 12:260–265.

61. Vermeeren MA, Wouters EF, Nelissen LH, van Lier AA, Hofman Z, Schols AM. Acute effects of different nutritional supplements on symptoms and functional capacity in patients with chronic obstructive pulmonary disease. Am J Clin Nutr 2001; 73:295–301.

62. Rahman I, Morrison D, Donaldson K, MacNee W. Systemic oxidative stress in asthma, COPD, and smokers. Am J Respir Crit Care Med 1996; 154:1055–1060.

63. Rahman I, Skwarska E, MacNee W. Attenuation of oxidant/antioxidant imbalance during treatment of exacerbations of chronic obstructive pulmonary disease. Thorax 1997; 52:565–568.

64. Sahin U, Unlu M, Ozguner F, Sutcu R, Akkaya A, Delibas N. Lipid peroxidation and glutathione peroxidase activity in chronic obstructive pulmonary disease exacerbation: prognostic value of malondialdehyde. J Basic Clin Physiol Pharmacol 2001; 12: 59–68.

65. Schols AMWJ, Mostert R, Cobben N, Soeters P, Wouters EFM. Transcutaneous oxygen saturation and carbon dioxide tension during meals in patients with chronic obstructive pulmonary disease. Chest 1991; 100:1287–1292.

66. Bruera E, Roca E, Cedaro L, Carraro S, Chacon R. Action of oral methylprednisolone in terminal cancer patients: a prospective randomized double-blind study. Cancer Treat Rep 1985; 69:751–754.

67. Campfield LA, Smith FJ, Burn P. The OB protein (leptin) pathway—a link between adipose tissue mass and central neural networks. Horm Metab Res 1996; 28:619–632.

68. Seeley RJ, van Dijk G, Campfield LA, et al. Intraventricular leptin reduces food intake and body weight of lean rats but not obese Zucker rats. Horm Metab Res 1996; 28: 664–668.

69. Hwa JJ, Ghibaudi L, Compton D, Fawzi AB, Strader CD. Intracerebroventricular injection of leptin increases thermogenesis and mobilizes fat metabolism in ob/ob mice. Horm Metab Res 1996; 28:659–663.

70. Friedman JM. The alphabet of weight control. Nature 1997; 385:119–120.

71. Dryden S, Frankish H, Wang Q, Williams G. Neuropeptide Y and energy balance: one way ahead for the treatment of obesity? Eur J Clin Invest 1994; 24:293–308.

72. Stephens TW, Basinski M, Bristow PK, et al. The role of neuropeptide Y in the antiobesity action of the obese gene product. Nature 1995; 377:530–532.

73. Schols AM, Creutzberg EC, Buurman WA, Campfield LA, Saris WH, Wouters EF. Plasma leptin is related to proinflammatory status and dietary intake in patients with chronic obstructive pulmonary disease. Am J Respir Crit Care Med 1999; 160: 1220–1226.

74. Lord GM, Matarese G, Howard JK, Baker RJ, Bloom SR, Lechler RI. Leptin modulates the T-cell immune response and reverses starvation-induced immunosuppression. Nature 1998; 394:897–901.

75. Bornstein SR, Licinio J, Tauchnitz R, et al. Plasma leptin levels are increased in survivors of acute sepsis: associated loss of diurnal rhythm, in cortisol and leptin secretion. J Clin Endocrinol Metab 1998; 83:280–283.

76. Torpy DJ, Bornstein SR, Chrousos GP. Letpin and interleukin-6 in sepsis. Horm Metab Res 1998; 30:726–729.
77. Auwerx J, Staels B. Leptin. Lance 1998; 351:737–742.
78. Takabatake N, Nakamura H, Abe S, et al. Circulating leptin in patients with chronic obstructive pulmonary disease. Am J Respir Crit Care Med 1999; 159:1215–1219.
79. Takabatake N, Nakamura H, Abe S, et al. The relationship between chronic hypoxemia and activation of the tumor necrosis factor-alpha system in patients with chronic obstructive pulmonary disease. Am J Respir Crit Care Med 2000; 161:1179–1184.
80. Dentener MA, Creutzberg EC, Schols AM, et al. Systemic anti-inflammatory mediators in COPD: increase in soluble interleukin 1 receptor II during treatment of exacerbations. Thorax 2001; 56:721–726.
81. Diez-Ruiz A, Tilz GP, Zangerle R, Baier-Bitterlich G, Wachter H, Fuchs D. Soluble receptors for tumor necrosis factor in clinical laboratory diagnosis. Eur J Haematol 1995; 54:1–8.
82. Di Francia M, Barbier D, Mege JL, Orehek J. Tumor necrosis factor-alpha levels and weight loss in chronic obstructive pulmonary disease. Am J Respir Crit Care Med 1994; 150:1453–1455.
83. de Godoy I, Donahoe M, Calhoun WJ, Mancino J, Rogers RM. Elevated TNF-alpha production by peripheral blood monocytes of weight-losing COPD patients. Am J Respir Crit Care Med 1996; 153:633–637.
84. Grunfeld C, Zhao C, Fuller J, et al. Endotoxin and cytokines induce expression of leptin, the ob gene product, in hamsters. J Clin Invest 1996; 97:2152–2157.
85. Sarraf P, Frederich RC, Turner EM, et al. Multiple cytokines and acute inflammation raise mouse leptin levels: potential role in inflammatory anorexia. J Exp Med 1997; 185:171–175.
86. Zumbach MS, Boehme MW, Wahl P, Stremmel W, Ziegler R, Nawroth PP. Tumor necrosis factor increases serum leptin levels in humans. J Clin Endocrinol Metab 1997; 82:4080–4082.
87. Janik JE, Curti BD, Considine RV, et al. Interleukin 1 alpha increases serum leptin concentrations in humans. J Clin Endocrinol Metab 1997; 82:3084–3086.
88. Fong Y, Moldawer LL, Marano M, et al. Cachectin/TNF or IL-1 alpha induces cachexia with redistribution of body proteins. Am J Physiol 1989; 256:R659–R665.
89. Michie HR, Sherman ML, Spriggs DR, Rounds J, Christie M, Wilmore DW. Chronic TNF infusion causes anorexia but not accelerated nitrogen loss. Ann Surg 1989; 209: 19–24.
90. Tracey KJ, Wei H, Manogue KR, et al. Cachectin/tumor necrosis factor induces cachexia, anemia, and inflammation. J Exp Med 1988; 167:1211–1227.
91. Pomposelli JJ, Flores EA, Bistrian BR. Role of biochemical mediators in clinical nutrition and surgical metabolism. J Parenter Enteral Nutr 1988; 12:212–218.
92. Mahony SM, Beck SA, Tisdale MJ. Comparison of weight loss induced by recombinant tumour necrosis factor with that produced by a cachexia-inducing tumour. Br J Cancer 1988; 57:385–389.
93. Warren RS, Starnes HF, Jr., Gabrilove JL, Oettgen HF, Brennan MF. The acute metabolic effects of tumor necrosis factor administration in humans. Arch Surg 1987; 122: 1396–1400.
94. Starnes HF, Jr., Warren RS, Jeevanandam M, et al. Tumor necrosis factor and the acute metabolic response to tissue injury in man. J Clin Invest 1988; 82:1321–1325.
95. Dev D, Wallace E, Sankaran R, et al. Value of C-reactive protein measurements in exacerbations of chronic obstructive pulmonary disease. Respir Med 1998; 92:664–667.

96. Mantzoros CS, Moschos S, Avramopoulos I, et al. Leptin concentrations in relation to body mass index and the tumor necrosis factor-alpha system in humans. J Clin Endocrinol Metab 1997; 82:3408–3413.

97. Schols AM. TNF-alpha and hypermetabolism in chronic obstructive pulmonary disease. Clin Nutr 1999; 18:255–257.

98. Dallongeville J, Hecquet B, Lebel P, et al. Short term response of circulating leptin to feeding and fasting in man: influence of circadian cycle. Int J Obes Relat Metab Disord 1998; 22:728–733.

99. Sinha MK, Ohannesian JP, Heiman ML, et al. Nocturnal rise of leptin in lean, obese, and non-insulin-dependent diabetes mellitus subjects. J Clin Invest 1996; 97:1344–1347.

100. Sinha MK, Sturis J, Ohannesian J, et al. Ultradian oscillations of leptin secretion in humans. Biochem Biophys Res Commun 1996; 228:733–738.

101. Takabatake N, Nakamura H, Minamihaba O, et al. A novel pathophysiologic phenomenon in cachexic patients with chronic obstructive pulmonary disease. The relationship between the circadian rhythm of circulating leptin and the very low-frequency component of heart rate variability. Am J Respir Crit Care Med 2001; 163:1314–1319.

102. Goldberger AL. Heartbeats, hormones, and health: is variability the spice of life? Am J Respir Crit Care Med 2001; 163:1289–1290.

103. Tschop M, Strasburger CJ, Hartmann G, Biollaz J, Bartsch P. Raised leptin concentrations at high altitude associated with loss of appetite [letter]. Lancet 1998; 352:1119–1120.

104. Hempel SL, Monick MM, Hunninghake GW. Effect of hypoxia on release of IL-1 and TNF by human alveolar macrophages. Am J Respir Cell Mol Biol 1996; 14:170–176.

105. Ghezzi P, Dinarello CA, Bianchi M, Rosandich ME, Repine JE, White CW. Hypoxia increases production of interleukin-1 and tumor necrosis factor by human mononuclear cells. Cytokine 1991; 3:189–194.

106. Leeper-Woodford SK, Detmer K. Acute hypoxia increases alveolar macrophage tumor necrosis factor activity and alters NF-kappaB expression. Am J Physiol 1999; 276:L909–L916.

107. Schreck R, Rieber P, Baeuerle PA. Reactive oxygen intermediates as apparently widely used messengers in the activation of the NF-kappa B transcription factor and HIV-1. EMBO J 1991; 10:2247–2258.

108. Keatings VM, Jatakanon A, Worsdell YM, Barnes PJ. Effects of inhaled and oral glucocorticoids on inflammatory indices in asthma and COPD. Am J Respir Crit Care Med 1997; 155:542–548.

109. Eastell R, Boyle IT, Compston J, et al. Management of male osteoporosis: report of the UK Consensus Group. QJM 1998; 91:71–92.

110. van Balkom RH, Dekhuijzen PN, Folgering HT, Veerkamp JH, Fransen JA, van Herwaarden CL. Effects of long-term low-dose methylprednisolone on rat diaphragm function and structure. Muscle Nerve 1997; 20:983–990.

111. Decramer M, Lacquet LM, Fagard R, Rogiers P. Corticosteroids contribute to muscle weakness in chronic airflow obstruction [see comments]. Am J Respir Crit Care Med 1994; 150:11–16.

112. Tataranni PA, Pratley R, Maffei M, Ravussin E. Acute and prolonged administration of glucocorticoids (methylprednisolone) does not affect plasma leptin concentration in humans. Int J Obes Relat Metab Disord 1997; 21:327–330.

113. De Vos P, Saladin R, Auwerx J, Staels B. Induction of ob gene expression by corticosteroids is accompanied by body weight loss and reduced food intake. J Biol Chem 1995; 270:15958–15961.

114. Dagogo-Jack S, Selke G, Melson AK, Newcomer JW. Robust leptin secretory responses to dexamethasone in obese subjects. J Clin Endocrinol Metab 1997; 82:3230–3233.

115. Larsson H, Ahren B. Short-term dexamethasone treatment increases plasma leptin independently of changes in insulin sensitivity in healthy women. J Clin Endocrinol Metab 1996; 81:4428–4432.

116. Lang CH, Dobrescu C, Bagby GJ. Tumor necrosis factor impairs insulin action on peripheral glucose disposal and hepatic glucose output. Endocrinology 1992; 130: 43–52.

117. Feinstein R, Kanety H, Papa MZ, Lunenfeld B, Karasik A. Tumor necrosis factor-alpha suppresses insulin-induced tyrosine phosphorylation of insulin receptor and its substrates. J Biol Chem 1993; 268:26055–26058.

118. Malmstrom R, Taskinen MR, Karonen SL, Yki-Jarvinen H. Insulin increases plasma leptin concentrations in nonnal subjects and patients with NIDDM. Diabetologia 1996; 39:993–996.

119. Stephens JM, Pekala PH. Transcriptional repression of the GLUT4 and C/EBP genes in 3T3-L1 adipocytes by tumor necrosis factor-alpha. J Biol Chem 1991; 266: 21839–21845.

120. Smeets HJ, Kievit J, Harinck HI, Frolich M, Hermans J. Differential effects of counter-regulatory stress hormones on serum albumin concentrations and protein catabolism in healthy volunteers. Nutrition 1995; 11:423–427.

121. Creutzberg EC, Schols AM, Bothmer-Quaedvlieg FC, Wesseling G, Wouters EF. Acute effects of nebulized salbutamol on resting energy expenditure in patients with chronic obstructive pulmonary disease and in healthy subjects. Respiration 1998; 65:375–380.

122. Burdet L, de Muralt B, Schutz Y, Fitting JW. Thermogenic effect of bronchodilators in patients with chronic obstructive pulmonary disease. Thorax 1997; 52:130–135.

123. Amoroso P, Wilson SR, Moxham J, Ponte J. Acute effects of inhaled salbutamol on the metabolic rate of normal subjects. Thorax 1993; 48:882–885.

124. Mosier K, Renvall MJ, Ramsdell JW, Spindler AA. The effects of theophylline on metabolic rate in chronic obstructive lung disease patients. J Am Coll Nutr 1996; 15:403–407.

125. Dash A, Agrawal A, Venkat N, Moxham J, Ponte J. Effect of oral theophylline on resting energy expenditure in normal volunteers. Thorax 1994; 49:1116–1120.

126. Shizgal HM, Martin MF, Gimmon Z. The effect of age on the caloric requirement of malnourished individuals. Am J Clin Nutr 1992; 55:783–789.

127. Schols AM, Soeters PB, Mostert R, Pluymers RJ, Wouters EF. Physiologic effects of nutritional support and anabolic steroids in patients with chronic obstructive pulmonary disease. A placebo-controlled randomized trial. Am J Respir Crit Care Med 1995; 152:1268–1274.

128. Wilson DO, Rogers RM, Sanders MH, Pennock BE, Reilly JJ. Nutritional intervention in malnourished patients with emphysema. Am Rev Respir Dis 1986; 134:672–677.

129. Creutzberg FC, Wouters EF, Mostert R, Pluymers RJ, Schols AM. Effects of anabolic steroids incorporated in a pulmonary rehabilitation program on body composition, functional capacity and quality of life in patients with COPD. Am J Respir Crit Care Med 2000; 161:A255.

130. Falconer JS, Fearon KL Ross JA, Carter DC. Polyunsaturated fatty acids in the treatment of weight-losing patients with pancreatic cancer. World Rev Nutr Diet 1994; 76: 74–76.

131. Wigmore SJ, Ross JA, Falconer JS, et al. The effect of polyunsaturated fatty acids on the progress of cachexia in patients with pancreatic cancer. Nutrition 1996; 12:S27–S30.

132. Wigmore SJ, Fearon KC, Maingay IP, Ross JA. Down-regulation of the acute-phase response in patients with pancreatic cancer cachexia receiving oral eicosapentaenoic acid is mediated via suppression of interleukin-6. Clin Sci (Colch) 1997; 92:215–221.

133. Belluzzi A, Boschi S, Brignola C, Munarini A, Cariani G, Miglio F. Polyunsaturated fatty acids and inflammatory bowel disease. Am J Clin Nutr 2000; 71:339S–342S.

134. Beck SA, Smith KL, Tisdale MJ. Anticachectic and antitumor effect of eicosapentaenoic acid and its effect on protein turnover. Cancer Res 1991; 51:6089–6093.

135. Belch JJ, Hill A. Evening primrose oil and borage oil in rheumatologic conditions. Am J Clin Nutr 2000; 71:352S–356S.

136. Kremer JM. Effects of modulation of inflammatory and immune parameters in patients with rheumatic and inflammatory disease receiving dietary supplementation of n-3 and n-6 fatty acids. Lipids 1996; 31(suppl):S243–S247.

137. Furst P, Kuhn KS. Fish oil emulsions: what benefits can they bring? Clin Nutr 2000; 19:7–14.

138. James MJ, Gibson RA, Cleland LG. Dietary polyunsaturated fatty acids and inflammatory mediator production. Am J Clin Nutr 2000; 71:343S–348S.

139. Pela R, Calcagni AM, Subiaco S, Isidori P, Tubaldi A, Sanguinetti CM. N-acetylcysteine reduces the exacerbation rate in patients with moderate to severe COPD. Respiration 1999; 66:495–500.

140. Poole PJ, Black PN. Oral mucolytic drugs for exacerbations of chronic obstructive pulmonary disease: systematic review. BMJ 2001; 322:1271–1274.

141. Moldeus P, Cotgreave IA, Berggren M. Lung protection by a thiol-containing antioxidant: N-acetylcysteine. Respiration 1986; 50:31–42.

142. Cuzzocrea S, Riley DP, Caputi AP, Salvemini D. Antioxidant therapy: a new pharmacological approach in shock, inflammation, and ischemia/reperfusion injury. Pharmacol Rev 2001; 53:135–159.

18

End-Stage Disease and Acute Exacerbations of Chronic Obstructive Pulmonary Disease

VICTOR M. PINTO-PLATA and BARTOLOME R. CELLI

Tufts University School of Medicine
St. Elizabeth's Medical Center
Boston, Massachusetts, U.S.A.

I. Introduction

Chronic obstructive pulmonary disease (COPD) is the fourth leading cause of death in the United States for people over age 45 and the fourth cause of death in the world (1, 2). Its mortality rate continues to rise as death from other causes continue to decline. The recent Global Burden of Disease Study (2) predicts that COPD will be the third leading cause of death and the fifth cause of morbidity in the entire world by the year 2020. The cost of COPD is staggering, reaching $31.9 billion annually in the United States alone. An important portion consists of direct expenditures due to recurrent exacerbations that lead to emergency visits and hospitalizations. Several factors have been associated with frequent exacerbations, including decreased scores in patient's perception of health status and reported daily cough, wheeze, and sputum production (3). In addition, 1-year mortality increases in patients admitted with an exacerbation, particularly if the $PaCO_2$ is elevated (4).

Morbidity due to COPD increases with age and is greater in men than women (1). Large population studies have shown that the frequency of the exacerbations seems to be related to the severity of the disease. A randomized, double-blind, placebo-controlled study of fluticasone propionate in patients with moderate-to-severe COPD (5) showed that patients with FEV_1 of 50% of predicted had 0.99 to

1.32 exacerbations per year. Paggiaro et al. (6), in a multinational study involving 281 patients with better pulmonary function (FEV$_1$ 60%) demonstrated that only one-third of the patients suffered at least one exacerbation. Anthonisen and co-workers (7) studied 173 patients with a mean FEV$_1$ of 34%, followed them for 3 years, and determined that only 25% of the cohort did not have an exacerbation. The median for the whole group was 1.3 ± 1.5 exacerbations per year.

Unfortunately, there are some limitations that restrict our ability to compare these studies. The definitions of COPD exacerbation differed among studies and, in addition, there is also a wide variation in the number of exacerbations, with some patients having more than three exacerbations per year despite similar physiological characteristics. What seems evident is that AECOPD is particularly prevalent in end-stage lung disease. In this chapter, we will review the possible mechanisms associated with this observation.

II. Pathophysiology of COPD

COPD is a disease state characterized by the presence of airflow obstruction due to emphysema or intrinsic airway inflammatory disease classically typified by chronic bronchitis. The airflow limitation is generally progressive, may be accompanied by airway hyperactivity, and may be partially reversible. Emphysema is defined pathologically as an abnormal permanent enlargement of the airspaces distal to the terminal bronchioles, accompanied by destruction of their walls, without fibrosis. Enlargement of the airspace to a large diameter (>1 cm) is defined as a bullae. The pathological spectrum of bullae is large, ranging from asymptomatic subpleural lesions to giant ones that may compress otherwise normal parenchyma. In most patients with emphysema, the airspace enlargement is variable with uneven distribution in the site and extent of these bullous changes (8, 9). On the other hand, chronic bronchitis is defined clinically as the presence of chronic productive cough for 3 months in each of two successive years in patients in whom other causes of chronic cough have been excluded. In most patients there is a variable degree of airway inflammation, mucous gland hypertrophy, and in up to 30% of them airways hyperreactivity. In most patients both processes coexist simultaneously. The disease does not affect all portions of the lung to the same degree. This uneven distribution influences the physiological behavior of different parts of the lung.

Biopsy studies from the large airways of patients with COPD reveal the presence of a large number of neutrophils (10). This neutrophilic predominance is more manifest in smoking patients who develop airflow obstruction compared to smoking patients without airflow limitation (11). Interestingly, biopsies of smaller bronchi reveal the presence of a large number of lymphocytes, especially of the CD8+ type (12). The same type of cells, as well as macrophages, have been shown to increase in biopsies that include lung parenchyma (12, 13). Taken together, these findings suggest that cigarette smoking induces an inflammatory process characterized by intense interaction and accumulation of cells, which are capable of releasing many cytokines and enzymes that may cause injury. Indeed, the level of interleukin-8 (IL-8) is increased in the secretions of patients with COPD (14). This is also true for tumor necrosis factor (TNF) (15) and markers of oxidative stress (16). In addition, the release of enzymes known to be capable of destroying lung parenchyma such as neutrophilic elastase and metalloproteinases (MMPs) by many of these activated cells has been documented in patients with COPD (17, 18).

A. Airflow Limitation

The resistance to flow is given by the interaction of air molecules with each other and with the internal surface of the airways. Therefore, airflow resistance depends on the physical property of the gas and the length and diameter of the airways. For a constant diameter, flow is proportional to the applied pressure. This relationship holds true in normal individuals for inspiratory flow measured at fixed lung volume, as shown in Figure 1. In contrast, expiratory flow is linearly related to the applied pressure only during the early portion of the maneuver. Beyond a certain point, flow does not increase despite further increase in driving pressure. This flow limitation is due to the dynamic compression of airways as force is applied around them during forced expirations. This can be readily understood in the commonly determined flow–volume expression of the vital capacity. The left panel of Figure 2 shows the flow–volume loop of a normal individual. It is clear that, as effort increases, expiratory flow increases up to a certain point (outer envelope) beyond which further efforts result in no further increase in airflow. During tidal breathing (inner tracing), only a small fraction of the maximal flow is used, and therefore flow is not limited under these circumstances.

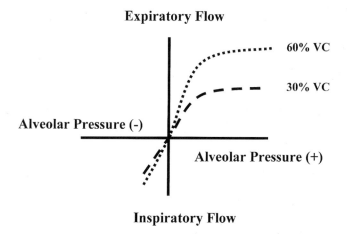

Figure 1 At a given lung volume (expressed as percent of vital capacity [VC]), inspiratory flow is proportional to inspiratory pressure. In contrast, expiratory flow does not increase with increased expiratory pressure because the airways are dynamically compressed by the increased pressure.

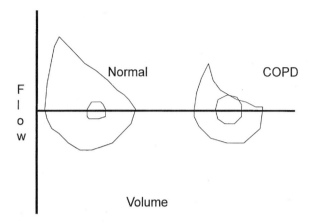

Figure 2   Flow–volume loop of a normal individual (left) and a patient with chronic obstructive pulmonary disease (COPD) (right). Notice the concave shape of the maximal flow volume envelope in the patient with airflow obstruction. As in this case, patients with COPD may reach their maximal airflow even during tidal breathing.

In contrast, the flow–volume loop of patients with COPD is markedly different as shown also in the right panel in Figure 2. The expiratory portion of the curve is carved out. This shape is due to the smaller diameter of the intrathoracic airways, which decreases even more as pressure is applied around them. The flow limitation can be severe enough that maximal flow may be reached even during tidal breathing, as represented in this diagram. A patient with this degree of obstruction (a not-uncommon finding in clinical practice) cannot increase flow with increased ventilatory demand. As we shall review later, increased demands can only be met by increasing respiratory rate, which in turn is detrimental to the expiratory time, a significant problem in patients with COPD.

The precise reason for the development of airflow obstruction in COPD is not entirely clear, but it may very likely be multifactorial. In pure emphysema, destruction of the tissue around the airways will decrease the forces that act to keep the airways open (19). In those patients with a component of airway inflammation, the problem is compounded by intrinsic narrowing of the airways (20).

Because airflow obstruction is physiologically evident during exhalation, COPD has been thought to be a problem of "expiration." Unfortunately, inspiration is also affected because inspiratory resistance is also increased and, more important, the inability to expel the inhaled air coupled with parenchymal destruction leads to hyperinflation (21).

B. Hyperinflation

As the parenchymal destruction of many patients with COPD progresses, the distal airspaces enlarge. The loss of the lung elastic recoil resulting from this destruction increases resting lung volume. In a pervasive way, the loss of elastic recoil and airway attachments narrows even more the already constricted airways. The decrease in airway diameter increases resistance to airflow and worsens the obstruction. Decreased lung elastic recoil, therefore, is a major contributor of airway narrowing in emphysema (21–23). Because in most patients the distribution of emphysema is not uniform, portions of lung with low elastic recoil may coexist with portions with more normal elastic recoil property. It follows that ventilation to each one of those portions will not be uniform. This helps explain some of the differences in gas exchange. It also explains why reduction of the uneven distribution of recoil pressures by procedures that resect more afflicted lung areas results in better ventilation of the remainder of the lung and improved gas exchange.

Increased breathing frequency worsens hyperinflation (24, 25) because the expiratory time decreases, even if patients simultaneously shorten their inspiratory time. The resulting "dynamic" hyperinflation is very detrimental to lung mechanics and helps explain many of the findings associated with higher ventilatory demand, such as acute exacerbation.

C. Alteration in Gas Exchange

The uneven distribution of airway disease and emphysema help explain the change in blood gases. The lungs of patients with COPD can be considered as consisting of two portions: one more emphysematous and the other one more normal. The pressure–volume curve of the emphysematous portion is displaced up and to the left compared to that of the more normal lung (Fig. 3). At low lung volume, the emphysematous (more compliant) portion undergoes greater volume changes than

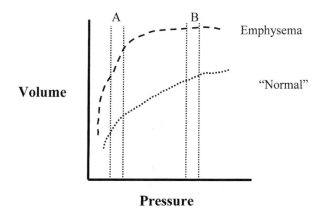

Figure 3 Volume–pressure relationship in portions of the lung with "normal" and "emphysema" behavior. At low volume (A), a small charge in pressure results in a larger volume increase in the emphysematous portion. At higher lung volume (B), a similar change in pressure results in minimal charge in volume in the emphysema portion, which now behaves as a stiff lung.

the more normal lung. In contrast, at higher lung volume, the emphysematous lung is overinflated and accepts less volume change per unit of pressure change than the normal lung. Therefore, the distribution of ventilation is nonuniform and, overall, the emphysematous areas of the lung are underventilated compared with the more normal lung. Because perfusion is even more compromised than ventilation in the emphysematous areas, they have a high ventilation/perfusion ratio and behave as dead space. Indeed, this wasted portion of ventilation (VD/VT) corresponding to approximately 0.3 to 0.4 of the tidal breath of a normal person has been measured to be much higher in patients with severe emphysema (26). At the same time, narrower bronchi in other areas may not allow appropriate ventilation to reach relatively well-perfused areas of the lung. This low ventilation perfusion ratio will contribute to venous admixture (V/Q) and hypoxemia (27, 28). The overall result is the simultaneous coexistence of high VD/VT regions with regions of low V/Q match. Both increase the ventilatory demand, thereby taxing even more the respiratory system of these patients.

As ventilatory demand increases, so does the work of breathing, and thus the patient with COPD must attempt to increase ventilation in order to maintain an adequate delivery of oxygen. Alveolar ventilation must also be sufficient to eliminate the produced CO_2. If this does not occur, $PaCO_2$ will increase. Indeed, the arterial blood gas changes over time in patients with COPD parallel this sequence. Initially PaO_2 progressively decreases, but is compensated by increased ventilation. When the ventilation is insufficient, the $PaCO_2$ rises (29, 30). This is consistent with the observation that patients with COPD who develop severe hypoxemia and hypercarbia have a very poor prognosis (31).

Therefore, an increasing body of evidence indicates that the anatomical alterations of COPD, such as airway inflammation and dysfunction as well as parenchymal destruction, could result from altered cellular interactions triggered by external agents such as cigarette or environmental smoke.

It follows that patients with severe or end-stage COPD have very little respiratory reserve left. Any worsening of the chronic persistent inflammatory condition of the airways results in inability of the system to cope with the increased ventilatory demand. In addition, recent evidence (32) has began to accumulate that COPD exacerbation is associated with a systemic inflammatory response that can result in severe respiratory demands that cannot be met by the most obstructed patients.

III. Pathophysiology During AECOPD

There is limited information regarding the pathophysiological events of AECOPD. The majority of studies have focused on the etiology and the response to diverse treatment modalities, including corticosteroids and antibiotics (33–35), or to measure the incidence of AECOPD on a large cohort of patients treated with different drug regimens (5, 6, 36). An important factor is that the follow-up of patients enrolled in these studies has been done mostly in the outpatient setting, limiting the capacity for closer observation and description of the physiological events during an episode of AECOPD.

A. Airflow Limitation During AECOPD

During an AECOPD, there seems to be a component of airway inflammation that worsens the already-compromised airway anatomy of these patients. Pulmonary function tests done on the first day after the enrollment in a study evaluating the effect of corticosteroids on the clinical course of AECOPD (33) reveal a worsening of FEV_1. Those patients treated with corticosteroids showed an improvement of approximately 0.2 L in FEV_1 during the first 3 days compared to patients not treated with this medication, whose FEV_1 improved by approximately 0.13 L. A smaller study by Thompson et al. (34) showed an 18% improvement in FEV_1 on day 3 in 13 patients with AECOPD treated with corticosteroids compared to -1.6% in patients not receiving this medication. Other studies have shown less important changes in spirometry during an AECOPD. However, they all show some worsening in the degree of obstruction. Seemungal et al. (37) reported in a cohort of 101 outpatients a change 0.024 L in FEV_1 and 0.008 L in peak expiratory flow rate (PEFR) on day 1 of an exacerbation. When patients manifested symptoms of dyspnea or increased wheeze, they also found greater changes in PEFR and a correlation of -0.12 between symptoms and lung function change. In our lab, we have also seen more modest changes in FEV_1 patients admitted and followed daily during an episode of AECOPD (38). The FEV_1 changed by 0.05 L while in the hospital (first 4 days) and by 0.29 L or 6% (relative change) after discharge (39).

Based on these findings, it is clear that there is a variable degree of worsening of airway obstruction during an acute exacerbation of COPD in outpatient and hospitalized patients (Table 1). The degree of obstruction seems to improve during the hospitalization period, but it takes a long time to completely resolve, with noticeable variation during the recovery period as well. Using PEFR measurements, Seemungal et al. (37) reported that 75% of the patients have a complete resolution of the obstruction at 35 days and 7% are not back to baseline even 91 days after the onset of the exacerbation. On the other hand, Niewoehner and coworkers (33) reported a faster peak FEV_1 recovery at 15 days postexacerbation. The reason for the difference in the rate of spirometric resolution between these two studies is not clear. It may relate primarily to the intensity of therapy (hospitalized versus outpatient

Table 1 Baseline Pulmonary Function Values and Changes During Acute AECOPD

Ref.	FEV_1 (L)$\pm$SD	Change in FEV_1 (L) during AE
33	0.76 ± 0.28	0.1
34	1.04 ± 0.36	0.05
37	1.10 ± 0.50	0.024
38	0.79 ± 0.32	0.05

treatment) and/or severity of the exacerbation, since the degree of airflow limitation was similar in both groups.

What is evident from all of these studies is that AECOPD is particularly prevalent in patients with end-stage disease. Patients enrolled in the above-mentioned studies had severe or very severe disease. The mean FEV_1 reported was 50% (5), 42% (37), 40% (3), 33% (7), or less than 1.0 L (4).

B. Hyperinflation During AECOPD

Dynamic hyperinflation (DH) is defined as the failure of the lungs to reach FRC at the end of exhalation. During an AECOPD, patients develop airway inflammation, bronchoconstriction, and mucus secretion that generates higher airways resistance with expiratory airflow limitation. The resulting increase in respiratory rate shortens the time of expiration and likely results in the development of DH (Fig. 4). We tested this hypothesis in our lab (38, 39), where we performed daily measurements of patients admitted with the diagnosis of COPD exacerbation. Pulmonary function tests, including inspiratory capacity (IC) and peak inspiratory pressure (PI_{max}) were obtained. The IC, an indirect measurement of DH, and the PI_{max} showed significant progressive increases during the hospitalization and after recovery compared to changes in FEV_1 (Table 2). Likewise, there was a significant decrease in respiratory rate which represents improvement in the level of DH. Very important for the patient is that the changes were associated with improvement in dyspnea.

C. Alteration of Gas Exchange

The underlying abnormalities in gas exchange during the stable phase in patients with COPD worsen during an exacerbation. The nonuniform distribution of emphysematous lung causes areas with different ventilation/perfusion ratios. During

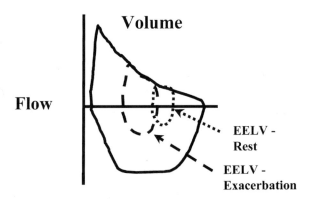

Figure 4 Flow–volume envelope of a patient with severe COPD. The small dotted line shows the end expiratory lung volume (EELV) at rest. As the respiratory rate increases and the expiratory time shortens during an acute exacerbation, there is a displacement of the tidal volume envelope to the left, signifying an increase in the EELV or "air trapping."

Table 2 Change Over Time in Vital Signs, Dyspnea, VAS, and Spirometric Measurements

Measurements	Day 1	Day 2	Day 3	Day 4	Recovery
Respiratory rate (b/min)	28 ± 5^a	27 ± 4^a	23 ± 4^a	23 ± 3^a	20 ± 5^a
Pulse (b/min)	98 ± 16^b	94 ± 13^b	90 ± 12^b	87 ± 11^b	82 ± 12^b
VAS (cm)	7.1 ± 1.8^c	6.1 ± 1.9^c	4.8 ± 2.3^c	3.1 ± 1.7^c	2.2 ± 2.3^c
FEV$_1$ (L)	0.79 ± 0.32	0.83 ± 0.34	0.80 ± 0.33	0.83 ± 0.33	1.08 ± 0.41
FVC (L)	1.87 ± 0.64^d	1.89 ± 0.54^d	1.86 ± 0.52^d	1.90 ± 0.65^d	2.11 ± 0.61^d
IC (L)	1.43 ± 0.54^e	1.36 ± 0.50^e	1.47 ± 0.47^e	1.66 ± 0.53^e	1.86 ± 0.59^e
PI$_{max}$ (cmH$_2$O)	43 ± 19^f		53 ± 31^f		63 ± 25^a

VAS = visual analog scale (measurement of dyspnea); FEV$_1$ = forced expiratory volume in 1 s; FVC = forced vital capacity; IC = inspiratory capacity.
By ANOVA $^a = p < 0.00001$; $^b = p < 0.0001$; $^c = p < 0.000001$; $^d = p < 0.05$; $^e = p < 0.01$; $^f = p < 0.02$.

an exacerbation, the increase in respiratory demand generates areas with more hyperinflation, particularly the more emphysematous portion of the lung which has higher compliance compared to that of the more normal lung. The hyperdynamic state coupled with the uneven hyperinflation also creates changes in lung perfusion that affect the gas-exchange process. According to the degree of the underlying lung disease, patients may only develop hypoxemia but, the abnormalities are more severe, patients may develop hypercapnia and ventilatory failure. Barbera and colleagues (40) studied 13 patients with severe disease (FEV$_1$ < 0.91 L) on admission with AECOPD and after discharge. Ventilation/perfusion (VA/Q) relationship was assessed using the inert gas technique. They found an increased Va/Q inequality during exacerbation due to greater perfusion in poorly ventilated alveoli, amplified by the decrease in mixed oxygen tension that results from greater oxygen consumption.

To correct these abnormalities, particularly in hypercapnic patients, invasive and noninvasive ventilation has been used. The latter avoids the complications of endotracheal intubation, preserves the airways defense mechanism, and allows the patient to eat and speak. It decreases the need for invasive ventilation, reduces mortality, complication rates, and hospital stays compare to standard care (41).

Intuitively, we would think that noninvasive positive pressure ventilation (NIPPV) improves gas-exchange abnormalities by correcting abnormalities in Va/Q. However, subsequent work by Diaz et al. (42) proved it wrong. They studied the affect of NIPPV on pulmonary gas exchange and hemodynamics during hypercapnic AECOPD. Using the same inert gas technique reported previously (40), patients were evaluated while breathing spontaneously, 15 and 30 min on NIPPV and 15 min after withdrawal. They found that the use of NIPPV significantly increased the PaO$_2$ and decreased the PaCO$_2$ and cardiac output, with no substantial changes in Va/Q mismatching. They concluded that the improvement in respiratory blood gases during NIPPV was due to improvement in alveolar ventilation and not to improvement in Va/Q relationships. These results suggest that respiratory muscle fatigue is a more important factor in hypercapnic respiratory failure than ventilation perfusion changes. Regardless of the mechanism, the data also support the notion that the most obstructed patients (those with end-stage disease) will more likely develop symptomatic exacerbation because they have minimal, if any, respiratory reserve.

IV. Mortality

Several authors have studied the association between AECOPD and mortality. Fuso and coworkers (43) reported in a retrospective study of 590 patients admitted with AECOPD a mortality of 14% and identified several factors as independent predictors of mortality: age, alveolar-arterial oxygen gradient, and cardiac arrhythmias. Subsequently, Incalzi et al. (44) studied 270 patients with severe disease (FEV_1: $34 + 16\%$) discharged from a University hospital with the diagnosis of AECOPD. The median survival was 3.1 years. A multivariate survival analysis showed that age, electrocardiogram (ECG) signs of right ventricular hypertrophy and myocardial infarction or ischemia, chronic renal failure, and $FEV_1 < 0.59\,L$ were all associated with increased mortality. A model using these variables predicted 5-year mortality with 63% sensitivity and 77% specificity.

When a patient's condition requires admission to the intensive care unit (ICU), the mortality is even higher. A multicenter study (45) involving 40 U.S. centers and 362 patients admitted to the ICU for AECOPD showed a hospital mortality of 24%. In those patients 65 years or older, the mortality doubled in 1 year from 30 to 59%. A nonrespiratory organ system dysfunction was the major predictor of hospital mortality (60% total explanatory power) and respiratory system abnormalities were more strongly associated with 180-day mortality (22% total explanatory power). Interestingly, after adjusting for severity of illness, mechanical intubation was not associated either with hospital mortality or with subsequent survival. Nevins and Epstein (46) studied 166 patients admitted to the hospital with a diagnosis of COPD who required mechanical ventilation. The in-hospital mortality rate for the entire cohort was 28%, but fell to 12% for those patients admitted with an AECOPD and no comorbidities. Multiple regression analysis showed that higher APACHE score at 6 h onset of mechanical intubation, malignancy, comorbidities, and need of mechanical ventilation over 72 h are associated with worse prognosis.

Connors and the Support investigators (4) also reported outcomes in a prospective cohort of 1016 patients from five hospitals admitted with an AECOPD and $PaCO_2$ of 50 mmHg. Their hospital mortality was lower (11%), but the 1- and 2-year mortality was as high as 43 and 49%, respectively. Survival time was independently related to severity of illness, body mass index, age, prior functional status, PaO_2/FiO_2, and serum albumin. The presence of cor pulmonale and congestive heart failure were associated with longer survival.

All these studies taken together point to the severity of pulmonary involvement as one important factor in the predisposition to develop more frequent and more severe exacerbations.

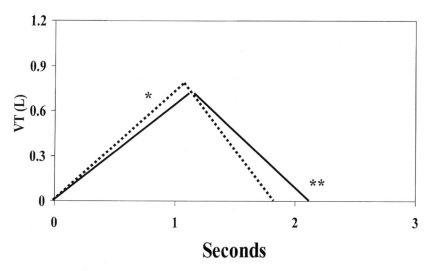

Figure 5 Average respiratory cycle during hospitalization (dotted line) and after discharge (solid line). Inspiratory time (Ti) is represented by the ascending limb of the schematic spirogram and expiratory time (Te) is represented by the descending one. Vt/Ti is represented by the slope of the ascending limb. $^* = p < 0.05$ (inspiratory time); $^{**} = p < 0.001$ (expiratory time).

V. Conclusion

Exacerbation of COPD tends to occur more frequently and with more severity in patients with end-stage pulmonary disease. This is even more distressing and has worse consequences in patients with other underlying systemic diseases.

It is likely that patients with end-stage airflow limitation have no reserve to compensate for the consequence of local airway and systemic inflammation. The only way to increase ventilation is to increase respiratory rate, which in turn shortens expiratory time and promotes hyperinflation. The dire consequences of this situation in patients with other system involvement is the development of ventilatory failure that requires life-saving interventions. Perhaps, as we develop a better and deeper understanding of the mechanism leading to this state, we can further enhance our already effective therapeutic armamentarium.

References

1. National Heart, Lung and Blood Institute, Morbidity and Mortality: 1998 Chart Book on Cardiovascular, Lung and Blood Diseases. Bethesda, MD: NHLBI, 1998.
2. Murray CJL, Lopez AD, eds. The global burden of disease: a comprehensive assessment of mortality and disability from diseases, injuries and risk factors in 1990 and projected to 2020. Cambridge, MA: Harvard University Press, 1996.

3. Seemungal TAR, Donaldson GC, Paul EA, Bestall JC, Jeffries DJ, Wedzicha JA. Effect of exacerbation on quality of life in patients with chronic obstructive pulmonary disease. Am J Respir Crit Care Med 1998; 157: 1418–1422.

4. Connors AF, Dawson NV, Thomas C, Harrell FE Jr., Desbiens N, Fulkerson WJ, Kussin P, Bellamy P, Goldman L, Knaus WA. Outcomes following acute exacerbation of severe chronic obstructive lung disease. Am J Respir Crit Care Med 1996; 154:959–967.

5. Burge PS, Calverley PMA, Jones PW, Spencer S, Anderson JA, Maslen TK. Randomized, double blind, placebo controlled study of fluticasone propionate in patients with moderate to severe chronic obstructive pulmonary disease: the ISOLDE trial. Br Med J 2000; 320:1297–1303.

6. Paggiaro PL, Dahle R, Bakran I, Frith L, Hollingworth K, Efthimiou J. Multicentre randomized placebo-controlled trial of inhaled fluticasone propionate in patients with chronic obstructive pulmonary disease. Lancet 1998; 351:773–780.

7. Anthonisen NR, Manfreda J, Warren CPW, Hershfield ES, Harding GKM, Nelson NA. Antibiotic therapy in exacerbations of chronic obstructive pulmonary disease. Ann Intern Med 1987; 106:196–204.

8. Mitchell RS, Stanford RE, Johnson JM, et al. The morphologic features of the bronchi, bronchioles and alveoli in chronic airway obstruction. Am Rev Respir Dis 1976; 114:137–145.

9. Thurlbeck WM. Pathophysiology of chronic obstructive pulmonary disease. Clin Chest Med 1990; 11:389–403.

10. Jeffrey PK. Structural and inflammatory changes in COPD: a comparison with asthma. Thorax 1998; 53:129–136.

11. Keatings VM, Barnes PJ. Granulocyte activation markers in induced sputum: comparison between chronic obstructive pulmonary disease, asthma and normal subjects. Am J Respir Crit Care 1997; 155:449–453.

12. Saetta M, Di Stefano A, Turato G. CD8+ T-lymphocytes in peripheral airways of smokers with chronic obstructive pulmonary disease. Am J Respir Crit Care Med 1998; 157:822–826.

13. Finkeistein R, Fraser RS, Ghezzo H, Cosio MG. Alveolar inflammation and its relation to emphysema in smokers. Am J Respir Crit Care Med 1995; 152:1666–1672.

14. Yamamoto C, Yoneda T, Yoshikawa M, Fu A, Tokuyama T, Tsukaguchi, K, Narita N. Airway inflammation in COPD assessed by sputum level of interleukin-8. Chest 1997; 112:505–510.

15. Barnes PJ. New therapies for chronic obstructive pulmonary disease. Thorax 1998; 53:137–147.

16. Pratico D, Basili S, Vieri M, et al. Chronic obstructive pulmonary disease is associated with an increase in urinary levels of isoprostane F_{2a}-111, an index of oxidant stress. Am J Respir Crit Care Med 1998; 158:1709–1714.

17. Finlay GA, O'Driscoll LR, Russell KJ, D'Arcy E, Materson J, Fitzgerald M, O'Connor C. Matrix-metalloproteinase expression and production by alveolar macrophages in emphysema. Am J Respir Crit Care Med 1997; 156:240–247.

18. Vignole AM, Riccobono L, Mirabella A, Profita M, Chanez P, Bellia V, Mautino G, D'Accardi P, Bousquet J, Bonsignore G. Sputum metalloproteinase-9/tissue inhibitor of metalloprotinase-1 ratio correlates with airflow obstruction in asthma and chronic bronchitis. Am J Respir Crit Care Med 1998; 158:1945–1950.

19. Nagai A, Yamawaki I, Takizawa T, Thurlbeck WM. Alveolar attachments in emphysema of human lungs. Am Rev Respir Dis 1991; 144:888–891.

20. Postma DS, Slinter HJ. Prognosis of chronic obstructive pulmonary disease: the Dutch experience. Am Rev Respir Dis 1989; 140:100–105.
21. Bates DV. Respiratory Function in Disease, 3rd ed. Philadelphia: W.B. Saunders, 1989:172–187.
22. Greaves IA, Colebatch HJ. Elastic behavior and structure of normal and emphysematous lungs postmortem. Am Rev Respir Dis 1980; 121:127–128.
23. Hogg JC, Macklem PT, Thurlbeck WA. Site and nature of airways obstruction in chronic obstructive lung disease. N Engl J Med 1968; 278:1355–1359.
24. O'Donnell SE, Sanil R, Anthonisen NR, Younis M. Effect of dynamic airway compression on breathing pattern and respiratory sensation in severe chronic obstructive pulmonary disease. Am Rev Respir Dis 1987; 135:912–918.
25. O'Donnell D, Lam M, Webb K. Measurement of symptoms, lung hyperinflation and endurance during exercise in COPD. Am J Respir Crit Care Med 1998; 158:1557–1565.
26. Javahari S, Blum J, Kazemi H. Pattern of breathing and carbon dioxide retention in chronic obstructive lung disease. Am J Med 1981; 71:228–234.
27. Rodriguez-Roisin R, Roca J. Pulmonary gas exchange. In: Calverly PM, Pride NB, eds. Chronic Obstructive Pulmonary Disease. London: Chapman & Hall, 1995:167–184.
28. Parot S, Miara B, Milic-Emili J, Gautier H. Hypoxemia, hypercapnia and breathing patterns in patients with chronic obstructive pulmonary disease. Am Rev Respir Dis 1982; 126:882–886.
29. Begin P, Grassino A. Inspiratory muscle dysfunction and chronic hypercapnia in chronic obstructive pulmonary disease. Am Rev Respir Dis 1991; 143:905–912.
30. Montes de Oca M, Celli BR. Mouth occlusion pressure, CO_2 response and hypercapnia in severe obstructive pulmonary disease. Eur Respir J 1998; 12:666–671.
31. Anthonisen NR. Prognosis in chronic obstructive pulmonary disease: results from multicenter clinical trials. Am Rev Respir Dis 1989: 133:95–99.
32. Wedzicha JA, Seemungal TAR, MacCallum PK, Paul EA, Donaldson GC, Bhowmik A, Jeffries DJ, Meade TW. Acute exacerbations of chronic obstructive pulmonary disease are accompanied by elevations of plasma fibrinogen and serum IL 6 levels. Thromb Haemost 2000; 84:210–215.
33. Niewoehner DE, Erbland ML, Deupree RH, Collins D, Gross NJ, Light RW, Anderson P, Morgan NA. Effect of systemic glucocorticoids on exacerbations of chronic obstructive pulmonary disease. N Engl J Med 1999; 340:1941–1947.
34. Thompson WH, Nielson CP, Carvalho P, Charan NB, Crowley JJ. Controlled trial of oral prednisone in outpatients with acute COPD Exacerbation. Am J Respir Crit Care Med 1996; 154:407–412.
35. Davies L, Angus RM, Caverly PM. Oral corticosteroids in patients admitted to hospital with exacerbations of chronic obstructive pulmonary disease: a prospective randomized controlled trial. Lancet 1999; 354:456–460.
36. The Lung Health Study research group. Effect of inhaled triamcinolone on the decline in pulmonary function in chronic obstructive pulmonary disease. N Engl J Med 2000; 343:1902–1909.
37. Seemungal TAR, Donaldson GC, Bhowmik A, Jeffries DJ, Wedzicha JA. Time course and recovery of exacerbations in patients with chronic obstructive pulmonary disease. Am J Respir Crit Care Med 2000; 161:1608–1613.
38. Elmaghraby Z, Hamada F, Pinto-Plata V, Livnat G, Celli B. Dyspnea during acute exacerbation (AE) of COPD is best explained by dynamic hyperinflation (DH) [abstr]. Am J Respir Crit Care Med 2001; 163:A812.

39. Livnat G, Pinto-Plata V, Girish M, Kenney L, Celli B. Clinical and physiological correlates in acute exacerbation (AE) of COPD. Am J Respir Crit Care Med 2001; 163:A769.

40. Barbera JA, Roca J, Ferrer A, Felez MA, Diaz O, Roger N, Rodriguez-Roisin R. Mechanism of worsening gas exchange during acute exacerbations of chronic obstructive pulmonary disease. Eur Respir J 1997; 10:1285–1291.

41. Brochard L, Mancebo J, Wysocki M. Noninvasive ventilation for acute exacebations of chronic obstructive pulmonary disease. N Engl J Med 1995; 333:817–822.

42. Diaz O, Iglesia R, Ferrer M, Zavala E, Santos C, Wagner PD, Roca J, Rodriguez-Roison R. Effects of noninvasive ventilation on pulmonary gas exchange and hemodynamics during acute hypercapnic exacerbations of chronic obstructive pulmonary disease. Am J Respir Crit Care Med 1997; 156:1840–1845.

43. Fuso L, Incalzi RA, Pistelli R, Muzzolon R, Valente S, Pagliari G, Gliozzi F, Ciappi G. Predicting mortality of patients hospitalized for acutely exacerbated chronic obstructive pulmonary disease. Am J Med 1995; 98:272–277.

44. Incalzi AR, Fuso L, De Rosa M, Forastiere F, Rapiti E, Nardecchia B, Pistelli R. Comorbidity contributes to predict mortality of patients with chronic obstructive pulmonary disease. Eur Respir J 1997; 10:2794–2800.

45. Seneff MG, Wagner DP, Wagner RP, Zimmerman JE, Knaus WA. Hospital and 1-year survival of patients admitted to intensive care units with acute exacerbation of chronic obstructive pulmonary disease. JAMA 1995; 274:1852–1857.

46. Nevins ML, Epstein SK. Predictors of outcome for patients with COPD requiring invasive mechanical ventilation. Chest 2001; 119:1840–1849.

19

Impact of Sleep on Acute Exacerbations of Chronic Obstructive Pulmonary Disease

WALTER T. McNICHOLAS

St. Vincent's University Hospital
University College Dublin
Dublin, Ireland

I. Introduction

Sleep is a complex process associated with recurring cycles of non–rapid eye movement and rapid eye movement (REM) sleep, each cycle lasting 90 to 120 min. Electroencephalographic (EEG) signals differ from wakefulness, particularly during non-REM sleep. The exact function of sleep is unclear, but there is no doubt that it is an essential restorative process as evidenced by experiments that have examined the physical and behavioral consequences of sleep deprivation.

Sleep has well-recognized effects on breathing, which in normal individuals have no adverse impact. These effects include a mild degree of hypoventilation with consequent hypercapnia, and a diminished responsiveness to respiratory stimuli. However, in patients with chronic lung disease such as COPD, these physiological changes during sleep may have a profound effect on gas exchange, and episodes of profound hypoxemia may develop, particularly during REM sleep (1), which may predispose to death at night, particularly during acute exacerbations (2). Exacerbations of COPD are generally accompanied by further worsening of lung mechanics and gas exchange, which adds to the detrimental effects of sleep.

II. Effects of Sleep on Respiration

The respiratory center is influenced by chemical inputs from chemoreceptors responding to changes in PaO_2, $PaCO_2$, and pH, by mechanoreceptors in the airway, lungs, and chest wall, and by behavioral inputs from higher cortical centers, transmitted via the reticular activating system (3). Removal of these inputs can markedly reduce ventilation, and in some experimental settings produces complete cessation of spontaneous breathing (4). Sleep is associated with a number of effects on respiration, including changes in central respiratory control, airways resistance, and muscular contractility.

A. Central Respiratory Effects

The onset of sleep is associated with a diminished responsiveness of the respiratory center to chemical and mechanical inputs, and to a major reduction in the stimulant effects of cortical inputs (3). These effects are more pronounced as sleep deepens, particularly during REM sleep. Ventilatory responsiveness to both hypoxia and hypercapnia are diminished. Furthermore, the respiratory muscle responsiveness to respiratory center outputs are also diminished during sleep, particularly REM sleep, although the diaphragm is less affected than the accessory muscles in this regard. There is a decrease in minute ventilation (V_E) during non-REM sleep (5), predominantly due to a reduction in tidal volume, which is associated with a rise in end-tidal PCO_2. However, part of this hypoventilation during sleep is likely a response to the lower metabolic rate during sleep, since oxygen consumption and carbon dioxide production diminishes during sleep compared to wakefulness (6). During REM sleep, both tidal volume and respiratory frequency are much more variable than in non-REM sleep, particularly during phasic REM, when there are bursts of rapid eye movement as opposed to tonic REM, where eye movements tend to be absent. Minute ventilation is lower during phasic REM than during tonic REM sleep.

These physiological changes are not associated with any clinically significant deterioration in gas exchange among normal subjects, but may produce profound hypoxemia in patients with respiratory insufficiency such as COPD. This finding is principally due to the fact that normal subjects have PaO_2 levels on the flat portion of the oxyhemoglobin dissociation curve, and thus modest falls in PaO_2 as a consequence of hypoventilation during sleep are not associated with significant falls in SaO_2 (5). However, COPD patients tend to have PaO_2 levels at or near the steep portion of the oxyhemoglobin dissociation curve, particularly during acute exacerbations. Thus, equivalent modest falls in PaO_2 during sleep may result in clinically significant falls in SaO_2. The drop in SaO_2 during sleep in COPD is further compounded by the increased work of breathing associated with chronic airflow limitation, which likely also aggravates the effects of the reduction in respiratory drive during sleep.

B. Airway Resistance

Upper airway resistance increases during sleep compared to wakefulness (7), which predisposes to upper airway occlusion and obstructive sleep apnea in susceptible individuals. In addition, lower airway patency may be compromised during sleep. The majority of normal subjects have circadian changes in airway caliber with mild nocturnal bronchoconstriction, which may be exaggerated in patients with obstructive airways disease, particularly asthma (8).

C. Rib-Cage and Abdominal Contribution to Breathing

In the supine resting state, breathing is predominantly a function of diaphragmatic contraction (9). During non-REM sleep, there is an increased rib-cage contribution to breathing and an associated increase in the respiratory EMG activity of intercostal muscles (10), with respiratory activity of the diaphragm being little increased or unchanged. The resulting expansion of the rib cage may improve mechanical efficiency of diaphragmatic contraction by optimizing the length and/or radius of curvature of the diaphragm (11). This increased efficiency of the diaphragm is reflected in an increase in the transdiaphragmatic pressure developed for a given level of diaphragmatic EMG activity.

In contrast, a reduction in rib-cage contribution to breathing has been reported during REM sleep compared to wakefulness, due to a marked reduction in intercostal muscle activity (12). Diaphragmatic EMG activity is substantially increased, while transdiaphragmatic pressure falls significantly, which implies a decrease in diaphragmatic efficiency, a pattern opposite to that seen during non-REM sleep.

D. Neuromuscular Changes During Sleep

The loss of stimulant input from the cerebral cortex is an important contributor to the hypoventilation of sleep described above, but, in addition, during REM sleep, there is a marked loss of tonic activity in the upper airway and intercostal muscles. There appears to be supraspinal inhibition of gamma motoneurons (and to a lesser extent alpha motoneurons), in addition to presynaptic inhibition of afferent terminals from muscle spindles. The diaphragm, being driven almost entirely by alpha motoneurons and with far fewer spindles than intercostal muscles, has little tonic (postural) activity and, therefore, escapes reduction of this particular drive during REM sleep (3). This helps to explain the increase in abdominal contribution to breathing in REM sleep.

The fall in intercostal muscle activity assumes particular clinical significance in patients who are particularly dependent on accessory muscle activity to maintain ventilation, such as those with COPD (13), since hyperinflation of the lungs results in flattening of the diaphragm and an associated reduction in the efficiency of diaphragmatic contraction. Diaphragmatic efficiency is further compromised by the supine posture since the pressure of abdominal contents against the diaphragm by gravitational forces contrasts with the effect of gravity in the erect posture, which tends to move abdominal contents away from the diaphragm. This pressure impairs diaphragmatic contraction during inspiration since this moves the diaphragm in a caudal direction to produce lung expansion.

E. Functional Residual Capacity

A modest, but statistically significant, fall in functional residual capacity (FRC) has been noted in healthy sleeping adults in both non-REM and REM sleep (14). This fall is not considered sufficient to cause significant ventilation to perfusion mismatching in healthy subjects, but could do so, with resulting hypoxemia, in patients with chronic lung disease. Possible mechanisms responsible for this reduction in FRC include respiratory muscle hypotonia, cephalad displacement of the diaphragm, and a decrease in lung compliance (13). This fall in FRC likely contributes to the fall in SaO_2 seen in patients with COPD through a worsening of ventilation-to-perfusion relationships, which assumes particular significance during acute exacerbations where such relationships are already compromised.

F. Overall Effects During Sleep

The above account illustrates the complex effect of sleep on respiratory function, with the overall trend being a reduction in ventilation compared to wakefulness. In normal individuals, arterial blood gases change little from wakefulness to sleep (5). However, when subjects with daytime hypoxemia, due to underlying respiratory disease, develop abnormal breathing patterns during sleep, life-threatening hypoxemia may occur (1). This partly results from the fact that a similar drop in PaO_2 will be associated with a much greater drop in SaO_2, when the subject is already hypoxemic and on the steep part of the oxyhemoglobin dissociation curve. Furthermore, the changes in rib-cage and abdominal contributions to breathing and the changes in FRC may result in worsening ventilation–perfusion relationships, which will also aggravate any tendency to hypoxemia. In addition, the reduction in ventilatory drives and changes in breathing pattern during sleep attenuate the compensatory hyperventilation seen during wakefulness in these patients. This effect on ventilation is seen particularly during periods of REM sleep. These abnormalities are most common in "blue-bloater"-type patients, who also have a greater degree of awake hypoxemia and hypercapnia than "pink-puffer"-type patients (15). However, many patients with awake arterial PO_2 (PaO_2) levels in the mildly hypoxemic range can also develop substantial nocturnal oxygen desaturation, which appears to predispose to the development of pulmonary hypertension (16). A schematic outline of the effects of sleep on respiration is given in Figure 1.

While there are few physiological studies that have examined the changes in lung mechanics during sleep in patients with exacerbations of COPD, it seems reasonable to assume that the adverse changes in lung mechanics and gas exchange that develop in association with exacerbations of COPD are even greater when asleep and likely account for the increased frequency of deaths at night in these patients (2).

III. Sleep in COPD Patients Requiring Mechanical Ventilation

There has been little research into the impact of sleep on respiratory function in patients with acute respiratory failure who are intubated and on mechanical

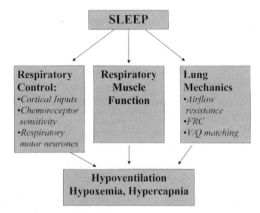

Figure 1 Schematic diagram of the effects of sleep on respiration. In each case, sleep has a negative influence that has the overall impact of producing hypoventilation and/or hypoxemia and hypercapnia. (FRC = functional residual capacity; V/Q = ventilation–perfusion.)

ventilation in the ICU setting, particularly those patients who do not have underlying chronic lung disease. Such patients would not be expected to show a significant deterioration in gas exchange during sleep, since the hypoventilation that is the principal mechanism of deteriorating gas exchange is prevented by the effects of mechanical ventilation. Changes in the rib-cage contribution and in functional residual capacity may still have some adverse effects, but these have not been well studied in mechanically ventilated patients. Most patients who are intubated and on mechanical ventilation are also paralyzed and sedated, which will further limit potential sleep-related changes in ventilation and gas exchange in such patients.

IV. Mechanisms of Nocturnal Oxygen Desaturation in COPD

Nocturnal oxygen desaturation in COPD appears to be predominantly a consequence of hypoventilation, with significant additional contributions from disturbances in ventilation–perfusion relationships.

A. Hypoventilation

Studies using noninvasive methods of quantifying respiration have shown clear evidence of hypoventilation, particularly during REM sleep, associated with periods of hypoxemia in patients with COPD (17–19), but the semiquantitative nature of these measurements makes it difficult to determine if this is the sole mechanism of oxygen desaturation, or whether other factors are involved. While there are no specific reports that have examined the mechanisms of hypoxemia during acute exacerbations of COPD, there are no specific features of such exacerbations to indicate that sleep should have any significantly different effects on gas exchange in such patients.

Numerous reports have demonstrated a close relationship between awake PaO_2 and nocturnal oxygen saturation (SaO_2) levels (18–20), and it has been proposed that nocturnal oxygen desaturation in patients with COPD is largely the consequence of the combined effects of physiological hypoventilation during sleep and the fact that hypoxemic patients show a proportionately greater fall in SaO_2 with hypoventilation than normoxemic, because of the effects of the oxyhemoglobin dissociation curve. However, it has been shown that PaO_2 falls to a greater degree during sleep among patients who show a major degree of nocturnal oxygen desaturation (19), when compared to the fall in PaO_2 during sleep among minor desaturators, which indicates that the greater fall in SaO_2 during sleep among more severely hypoxemic COPD patients is not simply a consequence of their being on the steep portion of the oxyhemoglobin dissociation curve, and that other factors must also play a part in the blood gas changes observed in these patients during sleep.

B. Altered Ventilation–Perfusion Relationships

The changes in respiratory muscle function during sleep, particularly the loss of accessory muscle contribution to breathing, also result in a decreased FRC and contribute to worsening ventilation–perfusion relationships during sleep, which further aggravates hypoxemia in COPD (13, 18–20). Given that ventilation–perfusion relationships are likely to be particularly compromised during exacerbations, particularly infective, it is likely that this mechanism assumes a particularly important role in the nocturnal hypoxemia during acute exacerbations of COPD.

Support for a role for ventilation–perfusion disturbances in the pathophysiology of nocturnal oxygen desaturation in COPD comes from the observation that PCO_2 levels rise to a similar extent in those patients who developed major nocturnal oxygen desaturation as those who developed only a minor degree of desaturation (19), which suggests a similar degree of hypoventilation in both groups, despite the different degrees of nocturnal oxygen desaturation. The much larger fall in PaO_2 among the major desaturators as compared to the minor desaturators, in conjunction with the similar rise in $PtcCO_2$ in both patient groups, suggests that in addition to a degree of hypoventilation operating in all patients, other factors such as ventilation–perfusion mismatching must also play a part in the excess desaturation of some COPD patients. Nonetheless, awake PaO_2 remains the factor that best predicts a likelihood of nocturnal oxygen desaturation.

V. Consequences of Nocturnal Hypoxemia During Acute Exacerbations of COPD

Patients with exacerbations of COPD requiring hospitalization are generally closely monitored at the time of admission, but since many such patients are admitted to general medical wards, monitoring during the night may be inadequate. This deficiency in management is unfortunate since such patients have clearly been

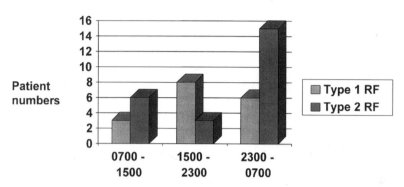

Figure 2 Time of death among patients with COPD comparing those with type 1 (nonhypercapnic) and type 2 (hypercapnic) respiratory failure (RF) and demonstrating a significant excess of death at night among those with type 2 failure. (Adapted from Ref. 2.)

shown to be at particular risk while asleep, particularly from cardiac arrhythmias and death. Ventricular arrhythmias are particularly common in exacerbations during sleep and can be prevented by the correction of hypoxemia (21, 22). Furthermore, a previous report from this department has demonstrated that patients who die in hospital with an exacerbation of COPD are significantly more likely to die at night, in contrast to patients who die from stroke or neoplasm (2). The excess nocturnal mortality is particularly seen in patients with severe hypoxemia and hypercapnia (type 2 respiratory failure) (Fig. 2).

VI. Management of Respiratory Abnormalities During Sleep in Exacerbations of COPD

The management of acute exacerbations of COPD are covered elsewhere in this book, but there are a number of aspects relevant to sleep that merit specific consideration.

A. Oxygen Therapy

The most serious consequence of hypoventilation, particularly during sleep, is hypoxemia, and appropriate oxygen therapy plays an important part in the management of any disorder associated with respiratory insufficiency during sleep. Care must be taken that correction of hypoxemia is not complicated by hypercapnia in patients with COPD, since respiratory drive in such patients may be partly dependent on the stimulant effect of hypoxemia. Therefore, the concentration of added oxygen should be carefully titrated to bring the PaO_2 up into the mildly hypoxemic range in order to minimize the tendency for carbon dioxide retention, particularly during sleep. However, the risk of CO_2 retention with supplemental oxygen therapy in such patients may have been overstated in the past, and there is evidence that CO_2 retention with oxygen supplementation during sleep is often modest, and usually nonprogressive (23). In particular, a recent report from this department has shown little risk of serious CO_2 retention with carefully controlled oxygen therapy in exacerbations of COPD, even when relatively high-flow oxygen supplementation is required to bring the SaO_2 into the region of 90 to 92% (24), a finding supported by the report of Agusti and co-authors (25).

The most common methods of low-flow oxygen therapy are nasal cannulae and Venturi facemasks. Patients requiring long-term oxygen therapy are usually given oxygen via nasal cannulae, but in patients with acute respiratory failure, face masks are often preferred (25) because of the ability to deliver higher concentrations of oxygen and to give better control of the inspired oxygen concentration (FiO_2). However, facemasks are less comfortable and are much more likely to become dislodged during sleep than nasal cannulae (26). These factors should be considered when choosing the method of oxygen delivery and the relative importance of accurate control of FiO_2 and compliance must be determined when selecting the route of oxygen delivery for each patient. Patients with hypercapnic respiratory failure benefit from the more accurate control of FiO_2 provided by facemasks, but care must be taken to ensure adequate compliance, since the abrupt withdrawal of oxygen supplementation may result in more severe hypoxemia than prior to supplementation (27). Therefore, patients in this category who tolerate facemasks poorly may be better managed by nasal cannulae.

B. Noninvasive Ventilation

Patients with COPD associated with respiratory insufficiency who fail to respond to pharmaceutical and oxygen therapy should be considered for assisted ventilation. In an acute setting, this may require intubation and ventilation, but in the past decade, increasing attention has been directed toward noninvasive methods of ventilatory support, particularly during sleep. There is growing evidence that nasal intermittent positive pressure ventilation (NIPPV) can be successfully used in the management of acute exacerbations of COPD associated with respiratory failure, and has been shown to reduce the need for intubation and mechanical ventilation in such patients (28). Since hypoxemia is most pronounced during sleep, NIPPV is particularly important at night in these patients, which requires close patient monitoring. An example of the beneficial effect of NIPPV on oxygenation during sleep in a patient with an exacerbation of COPD who also had an old thoracoplasty is given in Figure 3.

VII. Conclusion

Exacerbations of COPD represent one of the most frequent causes of in-hospital mortality in the western world and there is clear evidence that such patients are at

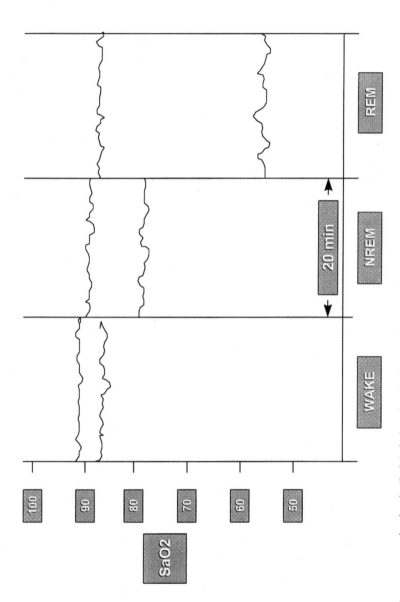

Figure 3 Oxygen saturation levels (SaO$_2$) during sleep before and after nasal intermittent positive pressure ventilation (NIPPV) in a 65-year-old male with respiratory failure due to COPD and an old thoracoplasty for tuberculosis. Each section represents 20 min of continuous record of SaO$_2$ in each of wakefulness, non-REM, and REM sleep. The lower tracings in each panel represent SaO$_2$ levels before NIPPV while the patient was receiving 28% supplemental oxygen by ventimask. The upper tracings represent the values while on NIPPV in addition to 4 L/min supplemental oxygen through the nasal mask.

particular risk while asleep. However, careful attention to preventing the adverse consequences of sleep on breathing in patients with acute exacerbations, particularly hypoxemia, can greatly improve the outcome in these patients.

References

1. Douglas NJ, Calverley PMA, Leggett RJE, Brash HM, Flenley DC, Brezinova V. Transient hypoxaemia during sleep in chronic bronchitis and emphysema. Lancet 1979; 1:1–4.
2. McNicholas WT, FitzGerald MX. Nocturnal death among patients with chronic bronchitis and emphysema. BMJ 1984; 289:878.
3. Phillipson EA. Control of breathing during sleep. Am Rev Respir Dis 1978; 118: 909–939.
4. Phillipson EA, Duffin J, Cooper JD. Critical dependence of respiratory rhythmicity on metabolic CO_2 load. J Appl Physiol 1981; 50:45–54.
5. Stradling JR, Chadwick GA, Frew AJ. Changes in ventilation and its components in normal subjects during sleep. Thorax 1985; 40:364–370.
6. White DP, Weil JV, Zwillich CW. Metabolic rate and breathing during sleep. J Appl Physiol 1985; 59:384–391.
7. Hudgel DW, Martin RJ, Johnson BJ, Hill P. Mechanics of the respiratory system and breathing pattern during sleep in normal humans. J Appl Physiol 1984; 56:133–137.
8. Hetzel MR, Clark TJH. Comparison of normal and asthmatic circadian rhythms in peak expiratory flow rate. Thorax 1980; 35:732–738.
9. Sharp JT, Goldberg NB, Druz WS, Danon J. Relative contributions of rib cage and abdomen to breathing in normal subjects. J Appl Physiol 1975; 39:608–618.
10. Tabachnik E, Muller NL, Bryan AC, Levison H. Changes in ventilation and chest wall mechanics during sleep in normal adolescents. J Appl Physiol 1981; 51:557–564.
11. Pengelly LD, Alderson AM, Milic-Emili J. Mechanics of the diaphragm. J Appl Physiol 1971; 30:797–805.
12. Tusiewicz K, Moldofsky H, Bryan AC, Bryan MH. Mechanics of the ribcage and diaphragm during sleep. J Appl Physiol 1977; 43:600–602.
13. Johnson MW, Remmers JE. Accessory muscle activity during sleep in chronic obstructive pulmonary disease. J Appl Physiol 1984; 57:1011–1017.
14. Hudgel DW, Devadetta P. Decrease in functional residual capacity during sleep in normal humans. J Appl Physiol 1984; 57:1319–1322.
15. DeMarco FJ Jr, Wynne JW, Block AJ, Boysen PG, Taasan VC. Oxygen desaturation during sleep as a determinant of the "blue and bloated" syndrome. Chest 1981; 79: 621–625.
16. Fletcher EC, Luckett RA, Miller T, et al. Pulmonary vascular hemodynamics in chronic lung disease patients with and without oxyhemoglobin desaturation during sleep. Chest 1989; 95:757–766.
17. Martin RJ. The sleep-related worsening of lower airways obstruction: understanding and intervention. Med Clin North Am 1990; 74:701–714.
18. Caterall JR, Calverley PMA, McNee W, et al. Mechanism of transient nocturnal hypoxemia in hypoxic chronic bronchitis and emphysema. J Appl Physiol 1985; 59:1698–1703.

19. Mulloy E, McNicholas WT. Ventilation and gas exchange during sleep and exercise in patients with severe COPD. Chest 1996; 109:387–394.
20. Stradling JR, Lane DJ. Nocturnal hypoxaemia in chronic obstructive pulmonary disease. Clin Sci 1983; 64:213–222.
21. Tirlapur VG, Mir MA. Nocturnal hypoxemia and associated electrocardiographic changes in patients with chronic obstructive airways disease. N Engl J Med 1982; 306(3):125–130.
22. Flick MR, Block AJ. Nocturnal vs. diurnal arrhythmias in patients with chronic obstructive pulmonary disease. Chest 1979; 75:8–11.
23. Goldstein RS, Ramcharan V, Bowes G, McNicholas WT, Bradley D, Phillipson EA. Effects of supplemental oxygen on gas exchange during sleep in patients with severe obstructive lung disease. N Engl J Med 1984; 310:425–429.
24. Moloney ED, Kiely JL, McNicholas WT. Controlled oxygen therapy and carbon dioxide retention during exacerbations of chronic obstructive pulmonary disease. Lancet 2001; 357:526–528.
25. Agusti AG, Carrera M, Barbe F, Munoz A, Togores B. Oxygen therapy during exacerbations of chronic obstructive pulmonary disease. Eur Respir J 1999; 14:934–939.
26. Costello R, Liston R, McNicholas WT. Compliance at night with low-flow oxygen therapy: a comparison of nasal cannulae and Venturi face masks. Thorax 1995; 50: 405–406.
27. West JB. Oxygen therapy. In: Pulmonary Pathophysiology. Baltimore: Williams and Wilkins, 1977:169–183.
28. Brochard L, Mancebo J, Wysocki M, et al. Noninvasive ventilation for acute exacerbations of chronic obstructive pulmonary disease. N Engl J Med 1995; 333:817–822.

20

Antibiotics

SAT SHARMA and NICHOLAS R. ANTHONISEN

University of Manitoba
Winnipeg, Manitoba, Canada

I. Introduction

In this chapter, we review the role of bacterial infections, the benefit of antibiotic therapy in AECOPD, risk stratification schemes, characteristics of an ideal antibiotic, and a brief overview of commonly prescribed antibiotics.

II. Role of Bacterial Infections and Efficacy of Antibiotic Therapy in AECOPD

The role of bacteria in causation of AECOPD has been difficult to establish, as airways of many patients with COPD are frequently colonized (1, 2). Earlier investigators focused on sputum microbiology and acute antibody response in the serum to demonstrate that infection rather than colonization led to exacerbations (3, 4). These were inconclusive and not able to substantiate the importance of bacterial infection in AECOPD.

Another way to assess the role of bacterial infection in AECOPD is to study the efficacy of antibiotic therapy. In a landmark study, Anthonisen and colleagues demonstrated that antibiotics were effective in the treatment of AECOPD (5). A cohort of 173 patients with COPD was followed for 3.5 years, 362 exacerbations

Table 1 Classification of Exacerbations

Type	Characteristics
1	Increased dyspnea, sputum volume, and sputum purulence (all three symptoms present)
2	Two of the above three symptoms present
3	One of the above symptoms present + at least one of the following: upper respiratory tract infection in the last 5 days, fever, increased wheezing, and increased cough

were treated: 180 with placebo and 182 with antibiotics. Exacerbations were classified according to three symptoms: increased dyspnea, increased sputum volume, and increased sputum purulence. Type I exacerbation was defined as the presence of all three symptoms, type II as the presence of two symptoms, and type III as the presence of only one symptom (Table 1). Therapeutic success was defined as "resolution" if all symptoms returned to baseline within 21 days, "no resolution" if all symptoms did not resolve, and "failure with deterioration" when symptoms worsened. Considering exacerbations, there was more resolution with antibiotics (68.1%) compared to placebo (55%) (Fig. 1). Deterioration occurred in 9.9% of those treated with antibiotics, compared to 18.9% with placebo (Fig. 2). The rate of peak flow recovery was faster with antibiotic treatment compared to placebo. In subgroup analysis, the success with antibiotic therapy was greatest in exacerbations classified as type 1 (62.9% vs. 43%). In type II exacerbations, antibiotics were associated with better outcome than placebo, whereas the success with antibiotic therapy was not significantly better than placebo in type III exacerbations. Similarly, deterioration occurred less frequently on antibiotic therapy in patients with type I or type II exacerbations.

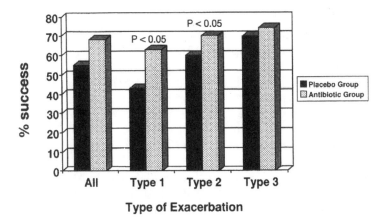

Figure 1 Rate of successful response to antibiotics or placebo in AECB, stratified according to the type of exacerbation. (Reproduced with permission from Ref. 5.)

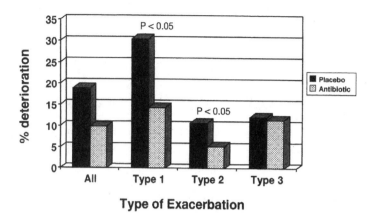

Type of Exacerbation

Figure 2 Rate of deterioration while on antibiotic or placebo in AECB, stratified according to the type of exacerbation. (Reproduced with permission from Ref. 5.)

A meta-analysis by Saint et al. reviewed randomized controlled trials published from 1955 through to 1994 (6). Nine studies met the rigorous inclusion criteria for the analysis. The outcome data were retrieved from each of the studies and transformed into units of standard deviation, and the effect size was calculated. The effect size of each study is shown in Figure 3. The overall effect size was 0.22 (95% CI, 0.10 to 0.34), indicating a benefit in antibiotic-treated patients (Fig. 3).

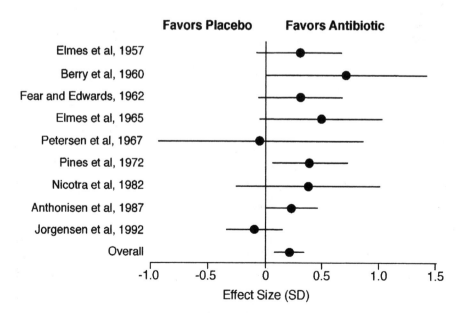

Figure 3 Overall benefit of antibiotics in the treatment of acute exacerbations of chronic bronchitis. (Reproduced with permission from Ref. 6.)

The mean change in PEFR favored the antibiotic-treated group by a difference of 10.75 L/min (95% CI, 4.96 to 16.54 L/min). The studies that included in-patients showed a greater benefit from antibiotic therapy, possibly because these exacerbations were more severe.

The three most common organisms causing AECOPD are *Hemophilus influenzae*, *Streptococcus pneumonia*, and *Moraxella catarrhalis*. In a study by Fagan and colleagues, culture of bronchial secretions obtained with bronchoscopy and protected specimen brush demonstrated that *Hemophilus parainfluenzae* was the most common pathogen (11/44), followed by *S. pneumoniae* (7/44), nontypable *H. influenzae* (6/44), and *M. catarrhalis* (3/44) (7). A variety of other gram-negative (8/44) and gram-positive (9/44) bacteria were also identified. Colonization and infection with Gram-negative organisms, including *Pseudomonas aeruginosa*, occurred in patients who had repeated courses of antibiotic therapy and, as is often the case, in bronchiectasis (8) (Table 2).

Bacterial colonization of the lower respiratory tract and recurrent infective exacerbations may play a role in progressive deterioration of lung function patients with COPD. Bacterial colonization may damage the airway epithelium, inhibit mucociliary activity, and impair local immunoglobulin and phagocytic function. The host inflammatory response of neutrophil recruitment into the bronchial mucosa could release various mediators and cytokines that enhance elastolytic activity in the lung. Products of inflammation could further impair host defense response and predispose to bacterial colonization and infections, thereby establishing a

Table 2 Pathogens Associated with Acute Exacerbations of COPD

Pathogen class	Frequency of exacerbations (%)	Specific organism	Proportion of pathogen class (%)
Viruses	30–50	Influenza A and B	30–40
		Parainfluenzae 1, 2, and 3	20–30
		Rhinovirus	15–25
		Coronavirus	10–20
		Adenovirus	5–10
		Respiratory syncytial virus	5–10
Atypical bacteria	5–10	*C. pneumoniae*	90–95
		M. pneumoniae	5–10
Bacteria	50	Nontypeable *H. influenzae*	40–60
		S. pneumoniae	15–30
		M. catarrhalis	15–30
		H. parainfluenzae	Isolated frequency but pathogenetic significance unknown
		P. aeruginosa and *Enterobacteriaceae* (*E. coli, Klebsiella*)	Isolated in severe COPD with recurrent exacerbations

self-perpetuating vicious circle of host and bacterial mediated respiratory tract damage. This process has been termed "vicious circle hypothesis" and may be responsible for progressive deterioration of lung function (9). More recently, this hypothesis was supported by Kanner et al., who demonstrated that frequent respiratory tract infections in patients with COPD led to a more rapid decline in lung function (10). Seemungal et al. contributed additional evidence to support this hypothesis demonstrating that full recovery of lung function did not occur 91 days following an acute exacerbation in approximately 7.5% of patients (11).

III. Risk Stratification and Treatment Guidelines

Patients with severe COPD have limited ventilatory reserve and acute exacerbations may cause acute respiratory failure requiring intubation and mechanical ventilation. Treatment failures in AECOPD lead to return physician visits and increase overall costs and risk of hospitalization (12). In 1995, Ball et al. found that the presence of cardiovascular comorbidity and more than four exacerbations in the previous year were associated with treatment failure (13). In a recent retrospective study, Dewan et al. reported that use of home oxygen and previous frequent exacerbations were associated with failure, while age, comorbidity, or choice of antibiotic did not affect treatment outcome (14). In other studies, advanced age, significant impairment of lung function, poor performance status, comorbid conditions, and history of previous frequent exacerbations requiring systemic corticosteroids characterized the high-risk group (15). The presence of cardiovascular comorbidity combined with greater than four exacerbations in the previous year has a sensitivity of 70% and specificity of 37% in predicting treatment failure (16). Therapy with commonly used antibiotics failed in 13 to 25% in all acute exacerbations (17). Stratification of patients into risk categories may allow physicians to select appropriate antimicrobial therapy to avoid treatment failure and improve outcome in an era of increasing antibiotic resistance.

Several risk stratification schemes have been proposed to improve initial microbial selection. In 1991, Lode (18) proposed that patients be divided into three groups based on severity of lung function, number of exacerbations each year, and presence of a comorbidity. Treatment with oral amoxicillin, doxycycline, co-trimoxazole, or a macrolide was recommended for low-risk patients (first degree). High-risk patients (second and third degree) consisted of patients with a longer history of COPD, several exacerbations each year, impaired lung function, and those hospitalized with significant comorbidity. Therapy with oral cephalosporins, amoxicillin-clavulanic acid, or quinolones was proposed for these patients (Table 3).

In 1994, Balter et al. (19) suggested that patients should be categorized into five groups: (1) patients had acute, simple bronchitis, most likely virally induced, with no previous respiratory problems; (2) patients had simple chronic bronchitis with minimal or no impairment of pulmonary function and without any risk factors; (3) patients had moderate-to-severe chronic bronchitis and other risk factors; (4) patients were similar to group 3 patients, but had other significant comorbid illnesses

Table 3 Antibiotics Used in the Treatment of Acute Exacerbations of COPD

First-line antibiotics	Second-line antibiotics
Aminopenicillins	Second-generation cephalosporins
Ampicillin	cefaclor
Amoxicillin	cefuroxime axetil
Pivampicillin	
Bacampicillin	Third-generation cephalosporins
	cefixime
Tetracylines	Amoxicillin–clavulanic acid
Tetracycline	Newer macrolides
Doxycycline	Clarithromycin
Minocycline	Azithromycin
Trimethoprim–sulfamethoxazole	Fluoroquinolones
	Ciprofloxacin
	Levofloxacin
	Moxifloxacin
	Gatifloxacin

such as congestive heart failure, diabetes mellitus, chronic renal failure, or chronic liver disease; and (5) patients were classified as having bronchiectasis. There are problems with this approach. Group 1 did not have COPD and group 5 are patients who had bronchiectasis as the predominant underlying pathology. The division between group 3 and group 4 was arbitrary and the treatment recommendations were identical.

A simpler risk stratification scheme modified from the publications of Wilson (20), Grossman (21), and others (22) is shown in Table 4. The patients could be categorized into simple and complicated AECOPD (Fig. 4). Patients with simple AECOPD have only mild-to-moderate impairment of lung function ($FEV_1 > 50\%$

Table 4 Risk Stratification of Patients with Acute Exacerbations of COPD

Classification	Characteristics
Simple chronic bronchitis	Patients with chronic bronchitis
	$FEV_1 > 50\%$ predicted
	Experience < 4 exacerbations/year
	No comorbid illness
Complicated chronic bronchitis	Patients with chronic bronchitis
	$FEV_1 < 50\%$ predicted
	Experience > 4 exacerbations/year
	Comorbid medical illness: congestive heart failure, diabetes mellitus, chronic renal failure, or chronic liver disease

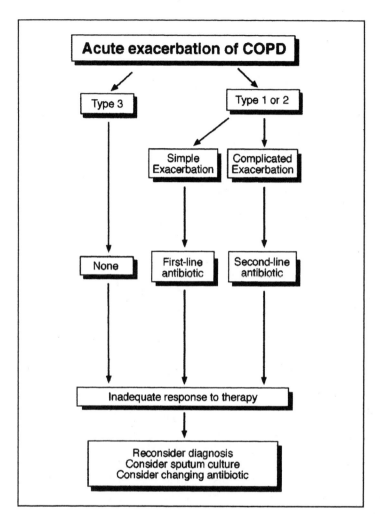

Figure 4 Proposed algorithm for choosing empirical antibiotic therapy in patients with acute exacerbation of COPD.

predicted), less than four exacerbations per year, and are colonized with *H. influenzae*, *S. pneumoniae*, and *M. catarrhalis*, although viral infections often precede bacterial superinfection. Since the consequences of treatment failure are not likely to be serious, any first-line antimicrobial agent could be used. Patients with complicated AECOPD have poorer underlying lung function (FEV$_1$ < 50% predicted) or concurrent significant medical illness (e.g., diabetes mellitus, congestive heart failure, chronic renal disease, chronic liver disease) and/or experience four or more exacerbations per year. *H. influenzae*, *S. pneumoniae*, and *M. catarrhalis* are likely to be the predominant organisms, but since treatment failure has major implications, antibiotic therapy directed toward resistant organisms is suggested. Second-line agents such as quinolones, amoxicillin-clavulanic acid, second- or third-generation cephalosporins, or the second-generation macrolides are recommended. Occasional patients with repetitive exacerbations probably have concomitant bronchiectasis and may be colonized by *P. aeruginosa*. An aggressive therapeutic approach using a quinolone with antipseudomonal activity empirically and tailoring therapy based on sputum culture is justified in these patients.

Although not prospectively tested, all the proposed classification systems emphasize identifying the high-risk population so that potentially resistant organisms can be targeted from the outset in order to reduce the risk of treatment failure.

IV. Antimicrobial Agents

In the study by Anthonisen et al. (5), antibiotics were prescribed as if they had equivalent efficacy in the treatment of AECOPD. The newer antimicrobial agents have also been studied to show equivalence with the regimens that have already been approved. Consequently, there are few data showing that one agent is superior to another because trials have not been designed with this goal in mind. Adam et al. (23) retrospectively studied the risk factors for treatment failure at 14 days after onset of AECOPD. The treatment failure was defined as return visit within 14 days with persistent or worsening symptoms. The variables associated with treatment failure were lack of antibiotic therapy and type of antibiotic used. The failure rates were 55% with amoxicillin, 8% Amox/Clavulin, 11% with TMP/SMX, and 18% with macrolides. Destache et al. (24) reported a retrospective study of 60 outpatients who developed 224 episodes of AECOPD requiring antibiotics. The antibiotics were divided into three groups: first-line (amoxicillin, co-trimoxazole, tetracycline, erythromycin), second-line (cefuroxime, cefaclor, cefprozil), and third-line (amoxicillin/clavulanate, azithromycin, ciprofloxacin). The failure rate in this study was defined as deterioration of symptoms requiring additional antibiotics within 2 weeks of initial therapy. The patients who received first-line agents had significantly higher failure rates compared to patients who received third-line agents. The patients treated with third-line agents were hospitalized less frequently and had a longer exacerbation-free interval to the next episode of AECOPD.

V. Resistance

When first described in the United States in 1974, less than 5% of isolates of *S. pneumoniae* were beta-lactamase positive. However, since the 1980s, there has been a dramatic rise in resistance to commonly used antibiotics among non-typeable *H. influenzae*, *S. pneumoniae*, and *M. catarrhalis*. In 1997, the prevalence of beta-lactamase-producing *H. influenzae* exceeded 33%, and present estimates suggest that 50% of all *H. influenzae* strains are beta-lactamase positive. Further, 35% of *H. influenzae* strains posses multiple antimicrobial mechanisms, such as beta-lactamase production and alterations in penicillin binding (25); 15% or more are cefaclor and cefprozil resistant, and 3% are azithromycin resistant (26). The prevalence of penicillin-resistant *S. pneumoniae* isolates increased from between 3 and 6% before 1991 to 43.8% in 1997 (27). Significant cross-resistance to other antibiotics has been encountered in penicillin-resistant *S. pneumoniae*. Highly resistant *S. pneumoniae* are susceptible to less than 30% of cephalosporins, and 60 to 70% are resistant to macrolides and azalides (28). However, resistance to fluoroquinolones has not been reported in *S. pneumoniae*. Similar rates of resistance have been reported in European studies (29, 30). Higher rates of resistance occur in isolates from patients who have identifiable risk factors, including age over 65 years, history of alcoholism, therapy with beta-lactam antibiotics during the past 3 months, multiple medical comorbidities, and immunosuppressive illness (31, 32).

VI. An Ideal Antibiotic

There are several theoretical characteristics that would be desirable in selecting an antibiotic for AECOPD: (1) activity against the most common and most likely etiological organisms, including *H. influenzae*, *S. pneumoniae*, and *M. catarrhalis*; (2) resistance to destruction by beta-lactamase; (3) good penetration into the sputum, bronchial mucosa, and epithelial lining fluid; (4) a mechanism of action that does not add to inflammatory events in the airway; (5) easy to take, with few side effects; (6) cost effectiveness, including the costs but also the costs of treatment failure and the duration of the exacerbation.

VII. Tetracyclines

In 1948, chlortetracycline was the first tetracycline discovered. Since then, tetracycline, demeclocycline, doxycycline, and minocycline have been synthesized for clinical use, although doxycycline and minocycline are the most frequently prescribed. The tetracyclines are broad-spectrum bacteriostatic antibiotics. They either passively diffuse or are actively transported into the bacterial cell. They inhibit ribosomal bacterial protein synthesis. The mechanism of resistance to tetracycline is to prevent accumulation of drug inside the cell by decreasing influx or increasing efflux. Many of the original trials of antibiotic therapy demonstrated that tetracycline therapy was more effective than placebo in milder infections. Tetracyclines can be used in acute exacerbations of chronic bronchitis (AECB) because they are active against *H. influenzae* and atypical pathogens, but there have been reports of increasing resistance against pneumococci (33).

VIII. Oral Penicillins and Cephalosporins

These antibiotics share a structural feature, the beta-lactam ring, and are called beta-lactam antibiotics. These antibiotics are generally bactericidal virtue of inhibition of bacterial cell wall synthesis. Beta-lactams inhibit several enzymes called penicillin-binding proteins, each involved in different aspects of cell wall synthesis. Bacterial resistance to beta-lactams may occur by either of three general mechanisms. These include (1) decreased penetration of antibiotic to the target binding protein in the bacterial plasma membrane; (2) alterations in penicillin-binding proteins; and (3) production of beta-lactamase, which may cleave the penicillins or cephalosporins. The bacteria may either synthesize beta-lactamase constitutively or initiate synthesis in the presence of antibiotics. Amoxicillin has been widely used for management of AECOPD (34). The beta-lactam antibiotics are drugs of choice in patients with mild-to-moderate exacerbations in countries where resistance among *H. influenzae* and *pneumococci* remain at low levels. Despite their relatively poor activity and suboptimal respiratory pharmacokinetics, cephalexin and cefaclor have been extensively used for the management of AECOPD. The newer cephalosporins, cefprozil and cefixime, may have some advantages such as activity against resistant pneumococci, but have not been proven to be superior to amoxicillin (35, 36) when organisms are fully sensitive to both agents.

IX. Amoxicillin–Clavulanic Acid

The combination of amoxicillin–clavulanic acid is an improvement over amoxicillin alone when prescribed for beta-lactamase-producing strains of *H. influenzae* and *M. catarrhalis.*

The addition of clavulanic acid makes the combination resistant to bacterial beta-lactamases, an important concern in patients with AECOPD. Most studies of patients with lower respiratory tract infection have shown this agent to be equivalent to standard comparators (37). Comparison with cefixime and ciprofloxacin showed better clinical success in AECOPD but no significant difference in bacterial eradication rates (38).

X. Trimethoprim–Sulfamethoxazole

Trimethoprim–sulfamethoxazole is a combination of two an antimicrobial agents that work synergistically against bacterial organisms. Both antibiotics inhibit enzyme systems involved in the bacterial synthesis of tetrahydrofolic acid. Sulfamethoxazole competes with para-aminobenzoic acid to inhibit synthesis of dihydrofolic acid. Trimethoprim binds to bacterial dihydrofolic reductase to prevent the formation of tetrahydrofolate. The combination is bactericidal, the synergism being optimal when trimethoprim and sulfamethoxazole are combined in a concentration ratio of 1:20. Resistance occurs with development of a target enzyme with decreased bacterial affinity for the drugs and via dihydrofolic reductase gene mutations. Although very popular in the 1970s and 1980s, the potential for resistance and increasing availability of safer agents has resulted in decline of the use of this antibiotic. In older studies, comparisons with oral cephalosporins have generally shown equivalent efficacy (39). Increased resistance of common respiratory pathogens to TMP-SMX in Europe and the United States is making this antibiotic less useful in the treatment of AECOPD. Penicillin-resistant pneumococci have 80 to 90% likelihood of cross-resistance to TMP-SMX (40).

XI. Newer Macrolides and Azalides

The mechanism of antibacterial action of newer macrolides is similar to that of erythromycin. These agents bind to the 50S subunit of bacterial ribosome and inhibit bacterial protein synthesis. Compared to erythromycin, these agents are more acid stable, have improved oral absorption and tolerance, and have a broader spectrum of antibacterial activity. There has been increasing resistance to macrolides among gram-positive organisms. Up to 15% of *S. pneumoniae* may have resistance to erythromycin and cross-resistance to other macrolides. Azithromycin and clarithromycin have improved pharmacokinetics and antibacterial activity against *H. influenzae* compared to erythromycin (41). The significant advantages azithromycin are enhanced potency against *H. influenzae*, once-daily administration, an abbreviated 4-day course, and perhaps a reduced frequency of relapse during extended follow-up (42, 43). Clarithromycin per se has only intermediate activity against *H. influenzae* but synergy with one of its metabolite increases its activity to satisfactory levels (44). Clinical studies of clarithromycin involving 7- to 14-day regimens in patients with mild-to-moderate infections have shown equivalence with ampicillin (45).

XII. Fluoroquinolones

Fluoroquinolones exert their antimicrobial effect by direct inhibition of bacterial DNA synthesis. DNA gyrase and topoisomerase IV are two bacterial enzymes that have essential roles in DNA replication. Fluoroquinolones bind to each of these enzymes interfering with DNA replication, leading to bacterial cell death. Resistance to fluoroquinolones occurs by mutations in the genes by encoding the subunits of DNA gyrase and topoisomerase IV. Altered permeation mechanisms may contribute to resistance by enhancing cytoplasmic membrane efflux pumps. These agents penetrate well into the respiratory secretions and bronchial mucosa, but the clinical relevance of this is uncertain. The fluoroquinolones are highly active against beta-lactamase-producing *H. influenzae* and *M. catarrhalis*. Despite a relatively high inhibitory concentration against *S. pneumoniae*, ciprofloxacin has demonstrated clinical efficacy similar to amoxicillin, clarithromycin, and cefuroxime (46). A variety of newer fluoroquinolones with longer half-lives have recently become available. The newer agents moxifloxacin and gatifloxacin have enhanced activity against pneumococci compared to ciprofloxacin, making them an effective therapy in the management of severe exacerbations (47, 48).

XIII. Summary

Antibiotics have demonstrated efficacy in the treatment of acute exacerbation of COPD. Patients with acute bronchitis without underlying lung disease or mild lung disease should not be treated with antibiotics because most likely the etiology in these patients is viral. Patients meeting Winnipeg type I or II criteria (two or three symptoms of increased dyspnea, increased sputum volume, and increased sputum purulence), who are not high risk (simple AECOPD) should be treated with traditional antibiotics termed as first-line agents, including amoxicillin, tetracycline, doxycycline, and trimethoprim–sulfamethoxazole. Cure rates with these antibiotics approach 80 to 90% in mild-to-moderate exacerbations. In patients who have more severe underlying lung disease, frequent exacerbations, and comorbid conditions, failure of initial antibiotic therapy may result in repeat visits, hospitalization, increased morbidity and mortality. In these patients (complicated AECOPD), second-line agents should be considered. Newer antimicrobial agents have largely been studied for licensing purposes, and the investigations were designed to show equivalence with regimens that have already been approved. Future studies should compare clinical efficacy of antibiotics in AECOPD using a classification system that would attempt to identify patients most likely to benefit. These studies should include well-defined prospective economic analyses with quality-of-life assessment to ascertain the cost utility of the antibiotic therapy.

References

1. Sethi S, Murphy TF. Bacterial infection in chronic obstructive pulmonary disease in 2000: a state-of-the-art review. Clin Microbiol Rev 2001; 14(2):336–363.
2. Zalacain R, Sobradillo V, Amilibia J, Barron J, Achotegui V, Pijoan JI, Llorente JL. Predisposing factors to bacterial colonization in chronic obstructive pulmonary disease. Eur Respir J 1999; 13(2):343–348.
3. Reichek N, Lewin EB, Rhoden DL, et al. Antibody responses to bacterial antigens during exacerbations of chronic bronchitis. Am Respir Dis 1970; 101:238–244.
4. Haase EM, Campagnari AA, Sarvar J, et al. Strain-specific and immunodominant surface epitopes of the P2 porin protein of non-typeable *Haemophilus influenzae*. Infect Immun 1991; 59:1278–1284.
5. Anthonisen NR, Manfreda J, Warren CPW, et al. Antibiotic therapy in exacerbations of chronic obstructive pulmonary disease. Ann Intern Med 1987; 106:196–204.
6. Saint S, Bent S. Vittinghoff E, et al. Antibiotics in chronic obstructive pulmonary disease exacerbations: a meta-analysis. JAMA 1995; 273:957–960.
7. Fagon J-Y, Chastre J, Trouillet J-L, et al. Characterization of distal bronchial microflora during acute exacerbation of chronic bronchitis. Am Rev Respir Dis 1990; 142: 1004–1008.
8. Eller J, Ede A, Schaberg T, Niederman MS, Mauch H, Lode H. Infective exacerbations of chronic bronchitis: relation between bacteriologic etiology and lung function. Chest 1998; 113(6):1542–1548.
9. Cole P, Wilson R. Host-microbial interrelationships in respiratory infection. Chest 1989; 95:217S–221S.
10. Kanner RE, Anthonisen NR, Connett JE. Lower respiratory illness promote FEV1 decline in current smokers but not ex-smokers with mild to moderate COPD: Results from lung health study. Am J Respir Crit Care Med 2001; 164:358–364.

11. Seemungal TA, Donaldson GC, Bhowmik, Jeffries DJ, Wedzicha JA. Time course and recovery of exacerbations in patients with chronic obstructive lung disease. Am J Respir Crit Med 2000; 1615:1608–1613.

12. Derenne JP, Fleury B, Pariente R. Acute respiratory failure of chronic obstructive lung disease. Am Rev Respir Dis 1988; 138:1006–1033.

13. Ball P, Harris JM, Lowson D, Tillotson G, Wilson R. Acute infective exacerbations of chronic bronchitis. Q J Med 1995; 88:61–68.

14. Dewan NA, Rafique S, Kanwar B, Satpathy H, Ryschon K, Tillotson GS, Niederman MS. Acute exacerbation of COPD: factors associated with poor treatment outcome. Chest 2000; 117(3):662–671.

15. Strom K. Survival of patients with chronic obstructive pulmonary disease receiving long-term domiciliary oxygen therapy. Am Rev Respir Dis 1993; 147:585–591.

16. Ball P, Harris JM, Lowson D, et al. Acute infective exacerbations of chronic bronchitis. Q J Med 1995; 88:61–68.

17. MacFarlane JT, Colville A, Guion A, et al. Prospective study of etiology and outcome of adult lower respiratory tract infections in the community. Lancet 1993; 341:511–514.

18. Lode H. Respiratory tract infections: when is antibiotic therapy indicated? Clin Ther 1991; 13:149–156.

19. Baiter MS, Hyland RH, Low DE, et al. Recommendations on the management of chronic bronchitis. Can Med Assoc J 1994; 151(suppl):7–23.

20. Wilson R. Outcome predictors in bronchitis. chest 1995; 108(suppl):53S–57S.

21. Grossman RF. Guidelines for the treatment of acute exacerbation of chronic bronchitis. Chest 1997; 112:310S–313S.

22. Sethi S. Etiology and management of infections in chronic obstructive pulmonary disease. Clin Pulm Med 1999; 6:327–332.

23. Adam S, Melo J, Anuzueto A. Effects of antibiotics on the recurrence rates of chronic obstructive lung disease exacerbations. Chest 1997:112, 22S.

24. Destache CJ, Dewan NA, O'Donohue, et al. Clinical and economic considerations in acute exacerbations of chromc bronchitis. J Antimicrob Chemother 1999; 43(suppl A): 107–113.

25. Doem GV, Brueggemann AB, Pierce G, Holley HP Jr, Rauch A. Antibiotic resistance among clinical isolates of *Haemophilus influenzae* in the United States in 1994 and 1995 and detection of beta-lactamase-positive strains resistant to amoxicillin-clavulanate: results of a national multicenter surveillance study. Antimicrob Agents Chemother 1997; 41(2):292–297.

26. Archibald L, Phillips L, Monnet D, McGowan JE Jr, Tenover F, Gaynes R. Antimicrobial resistance in isolates from inpatients and outpatients in the United States: increasing importance of the intensive care unit. Clin Infect Dis 1997; 24(2):211–215.

27. Doem GV, Pfaller MA, Kugler K, et al. Prevalence of antimicrobial resistance among respiratory tract isolates of *Streptococcus pneumoniae* in North America: 1997 results from SENTRY antimicrobial surveillance program. Clin Infect Dis 1999; 27:764–770.

28. Spika JS, Facklam RR, Plikaytis BD, Oxtoby MJ. Antimicrobial resistance of Streptococcus pneumoniae in the United States, 1979–1987. The Pneumococcal Surveillance Working Group. J Infect Dis 1991; 163(6):1273–1278.

29. Kayser FH, Morenzoni G, Santanam P. The second European collaborative study on the frequency of antimicrobial resistance in *H. influenzae*. Eur J Clin Microbiol Infect Dis 1990; 9:810–817.

30. Powell M, McVey D, Kassim MH, et al. Antimicrobial susceptibility of *Streptococcus pneumoniae*, *Haemophilus influenzae* and *Moraxella catarrhalis* isolated in the UK from sputa. J Antimicrob Chemother 1991; 28:249–259.

31. Kessler R, Faller M, Fourgaut G, Mennecier B, Weitzenblum E. Predictive factors of hospitalization for acute exacerbation in a series of 64 patients with chronic obstructive pulmonary disease. Am J Respir Crit Care Med 1999: 159:158–164.

32. Thornsberry C, Ogilvie, Kahn J, et al. Surveillance of antimicrobial resistance in *S. pneumonia, H. influenzae* and *M. Catarrhalis* in the United States in 1996–1997. Diagn Microbiol Infect Dis 1997; 29:249–257.

33. Mandell LA. Antibiotics for pneumonia therapy. Med Clin North Am 1994; 78: 997–1014.

34. McFarlane JT, Colville A, Guion A. Prospective study of etiology and outcome of adult lower respiratory tract infections in the community. Lancet 1993; 341:511–514.

35. Maesen FPV, Geraedts WH, Davies BI. Cefaclor in the treatment of chronic bronchitis. J Antimicrob Chemother 1990; 26:456–458.

36. Verghese A. Efficacy of cefixime in respiratory tract infections. Adv Ther 1990; 7:9–15.

37. Bernard Y, Lemenager J, Moral C. A comparative study of amoxicillin and Augmentin in the treatment of bronchopulmonary infections. In: Croydon EAP, Michel ME. Augmentin: Clavulanate-Potentiated Amoxicillin. Amsterdam: Excerpta-Medica, 1983:282–290.

38. Todd PA, Benfield P. Amoxicillin/clavulanic: an update of its antibacterial activity, pharmacokinetic properties and therapeutic use. Drugs 1990; 39:264–307.

39. Mehta S, Parr JH, Morgan DJR. A comparison of cefuroxime and co-trimoxazole in severe respiratory tract infections. J Antimicrob Chemother 1982; 9:479–484.

40. Clavo-Sanchez AJ, Giron-Gonzalez JA, Lopez-Prieto D, et al. Multivariate analysis of risk factors for infection due to penicillin resistant and multidrug resistant Streptococcus pneumonia: A multicentre study. Clin Infect Dis 1997; 24:1052–1059.

41. Ball AP. Azithromycin in the treatment of lower respiratory tract infections. Rev Contemp Pharmacother 1994; 5:351–357.

42. Hoepelma IM, Mollers MJ, vanSchie MH, et al. A short (3 day) course of azithromycin tablet versus a 10-day course of amoxicillin-clavulanic acid in the treatment of adults with lower respiratory tract infections and effects on long term outcome. Int J Antimicrob Agents 1997; 9:141–146.

43. Petrie GR, Choo Kang J, Washton H, et al. Azithromycin: an open comparison with amoxicillin in severe exacerbations of chronic bronchitis (abstr 83). Proceedings of 18th International Congress of Chemotherapy. Stockholm, June 1993.

44. Alvarez-Elcoro S, Eichel B, Ellis C, Medici TC. Erythromycin, clarithromycin, and azithromycin. Mayo Clin Proc 1999; 74:613–634.

45. Bachand RT. A comparative study of clarithromycin and ampicillin in the treatment of patients with acute bacterial exacerbation of chronic bronchitis. J Antimicrob Chemother 1991; 27(suppl A):91–100.

46. Ball AP. Evidence for the efficacy of ciprofloxacin in lower respiratory tract infections. Rev Contemp Pharmacother 1992; 3:133–142.

47. Blondeau JM. A review of the comparative in-vitro activities of 12 antimicrobial agents, with a focus on five new "respiratory quinolones." J Antimicrob Chemother 1999: 43(suppl B):1–11.

48. Chodosh S, DeAbate CA, Haverstock D, Aneiro L, Church D. Short course of moxifloxacin therapy for treatment of acute exacerbation of chronic bronchitis. Respir Med 2000; 94:18–27.

21

Bronchodilators in Acute Exacerbations of Chronic Obstructive Pulmonary Disease

CLARE D. RAMSEY and NICHOLAS R. ANTHONISEN

University of Manitoba
Winnipeg, Manitoba, Canada

I. Introduction

Acute exacerbations of chronic obstructive pulmonary disease (COPD) are attributed to a variety of triggers, most of which lead to some degree of additional airflow obstruction. The mechanisms involved probably include airway inflammation, increased mucus production, and bronchoconstriction. Obstruction to airflow leads to hyperinflation, which place the respiratory muscles at a mechanical disadvantage, increases the work of breathing, and leads to ventilation–perfusion mismatch causing hypoxemia. Although bronchoconstriction is only one contributor to airflow obstruction, it is the most rapidly reversible component and, therefore, its reversal is a major goal in the treatment of acute exacerbations of COPD. Groups of medication aimed at reversing bronchoconstriction are the inhaled bronchodilators (beta-adrenergic agonists and anticholinergics) and methylxanthines.

A. Beta-Adrenergic Agonists

Beta-adrenergic agonists, which are available in short- and long-acting formulations, are the most potent bronchodilators and have the most rapid onset of action. In the treatment of acute exacerbations of COPD, only the short-acting bronchodilators are relevant and further discussion will be limited to these preparations.

Mechanisms of Action

Beta-adrenergic agonists induce bronchodilatation by activating β_2-adrenergic receptors on the surface of airway smooth muscle cells, which in turn activate adenyl cyclase. Activation of adenyl cyclase leads to the conversion of adenosine triphosphate (ATP) to cyclic $3'5'$-adenosine monophosphate (cAMP). Increased cAMP levels cause activation of protein kinase A. This kinase, through phosphorylation of several target proteins within the cell, induces a reduction in intracellular calcium ions (Ca^{2+}), which causes relaxation of airway smooth muscle and, hence, bronchodilatation.

Smooth muscle relaxation is not limited to the airways, but includes arteries, veins, and the uterus. Other metabolic effects of β_2-adrenergic-receptor stimulation include glycogenolysis, gluconeogenesis, and insulin release.

Most beta-adrenergic bronchodilators also activate β_1- and α-receptors. Stimulation of β_1-adrenergic receptors leads to an increase in heart rate and atrial and ventricular contractility. Activation of the α-adrenergic receptors is associated with constriction of arteries and veins, contraction of the uterus, iris, urinary bladder, and stomach sphincters.

Beta-adrenergic agonists have several other effects on the airway, including inhibition of mediator release from mast and other inflammatory cells, enhancement of mucociliary clearance (1), reduction of neurotransmitter release from airway cholinergic nerves, and inhibition of bronchoconstrictor and inflammatory peptide release from sensory nerves. These effects have largely been shown in vitro and their clinical significance is not established.

Therefore, beta-agonists that are most useful for bronchodilatation are those that have mostly β_2-adrenergic activity. The basic chemical structure of these agents is a benzene ring with an ethylamine side chain. Various hydroxy side groups are added to this basic structure to form the resorcinols and saligenins, the two most commonly used groups of short-acting β_2-agonists.

Pharmacokinetics and Dosing

Short-acting β_2-agonists have an onset of action of a few minutes and peak bronchodilator effect within 10 to 30 min. The duration of action of their bronchodilator effect is up to 4 to 6 h. Different formulations have somewhat different onset and duration of action as selectivity for the β_1-receptor (Table 1).

β_2-agonists may be administered systemically or by inhalation. Systemic formulations include oral, parenteral, and subcutaneous injections. Systemic administration of β_2-agonists decreases β_2-receptor selectivity causing more side effects and, therefore, is usually reserved for situations in which administration through inhalation is not possible.

As shown in Table 1, the typical dose of albuterol/salbutamol in the acute setting is 180 µg (two puffs), by metered-dose inhaler (MDI), every 1 to 2 h. This dose can be decreased to every 4 to 6 h after initial improvement. The nebulized form can be used at a dose of 2.5 to 5.0 mg every 1 to 2 h. The continuous

Table 1 Most Commonly Used Inhaled Short-Acting β_2-Agonists

Drug	Dose	Time-to-peak effect (min)	Duration of action (h)	Beta-receptor selectivity
Salbutamol/albuterol (Ventolin, Proventil)	90 µg/dose (MDI) 2.5 mg/mL (nebulized)	30–90	3–6	$B_2 \gg B_1$
Terbutaline (Bricanyl)	500 µg/dose (turbuhaler) 5–10 mg (nebulized)	15–60	4–7	$B_2 \gg B_1$
Fenoterol (Berotec)	100–200 µg/dose (MDI) 0.5–2.5 mg (nebulized)	30–60	6–8	$B_2 > B_1$
Pirbuterol (Maxair)	200 µg/dose (MDI)	30–60	3–5	$B_2 \gg B_1$
Metaproterenol (Alupent)	650 µg/dose (MDI)	60–90	3–6	$B_2 > B_1$

MDI, metered-dose inhaler.

nebulization of β_2-agonists has not been shown to be advantageous and, hence, is not recommended in COPD (2).

Tolerance to the bronchodilator effect of β_2-agonists has been shown to occur after long-term therapy. This is likely because downregulation of β_2-receptors in the airways, which leads mainly to a decrease in the duration of bronchodilatation rather than a change in peak effect (3, 4).

Clinical Effects

In the stable COPD patient, β_2-agonists have been shown to produce bronchodilatation, improve dynamic hyperinflation, exercise capacity, and quality of life (5, 6). On the other hand, there are no randomized placebo-controlled trials examining the effects of β_2-agonist alone in acute exacerbations of COPD. Most trials have compared the effects of β_2-agonists to anticholinergics or to the combined effect of both medications. Nevertheless, β_2-agonists are considered first-line therapy as they are effective bronchodilators and have a rapid onset of action (although they produce less bronchodilatation than in patients with asthma). In patients with small improvements in spirometry (FEV_1 and FVC), symptomatic benefit is often present. Rebuck et al. (7) studied the effectiveness of the β_2-agonist, fenoterol, the anticholinergic agent, ipratropium bromide, each alone and in combination, for the management of acute exacerbations of COPD and asthma. In the COPD patients, fenoterol produced a significant increase in FEV_1 at 90 min. Karpel et al. (8) randomized 32 COPD patients with acute exacerbations to either metaproterenol sulfate or ipratropium bromide. After 90 min, patients were crossed over to receive the other medication. Metaproterenol resulted in a significant improvement in pulmonary function, with mean increases in FEV_1 and FVC of 18 and 29%, respectively. Patients who received metaproterenol were noted to have a significant initial decline in their PaO_2, which returned to baseline at 90 min.

Side Effects

As mentioned above, side effects of β_2-agonists are more common with systemic administration than with inhaled therapy, dose-related, and due to stimulation of extrapulmonary beta-receptors. Both direct stimulation of cardiac beta-receptors plus reflex cardiac stimulation secondary to peripheral vasodilatation lead to tachycardia and palpitations. Muscle tremor caused by stimulation of β_2-receptors in skeletal muscle can be quite troublesome for many patients and is the most common side effect with inhaled therapy. Hypokalemia occurs due to a shift of potassium into skeletal muscle and can be serious enough to precipitate cardiac dysrhythmias. Other metabolic effects such as increases in insulin and free fatty acids are not usually seen at therapeutic doses. β_2-agonists cause pulmonary vasodilatation in vessels previously constricted due to hypoxemia, leading to an increased ventilation–perfusion mismatch and, therefore, a fall in arterial oxygen content (8, 9). The fall in arterial oxygen content has been mostly seen with less β_2-selective agents such as metaproterenol and isoproterenol, and less with the more commonly used salbutamol/albuterol. This effect has not been documented in COPD patients as well as it has been in asthma patients.

B. Anticholinergics

Atropine is a naturally occurring tertiary ammonium compound and is the oldest known form of this class of drugs. However, its use is limited by significant side effects. The anticholinergic agents used in the management of COPD are quaternary ammonium compounds that are synthetic derivatives of atropine. The quaternary ammonium drugs have less mucosal absorption and fewer side effects. These drugs include ipratropium bromide, oxitropium bromide, and tiotropium bromide. Ipratropium bromide is the most commonly used quaternary anticholinergic agent in the treatment of COPD.

Mechanisms of Action

The parasympathetic nervous system, via the vagus nerve, plays an important role in the regulation of bronchomotor tone. Efferent preganglionic fibers of the vagus nerve travel along the airways ending in ganglia within the airways. These fibers release the neurotransmitter acetylcholine (Ach). Postganglionic muscarinic receptors, in particular subtypes M1 and M3, mediate the bronchoconstrictive effect of the vagus nerve and stimulate secretion by tracheobronchial glands. Activation of M2 receptors limits further production of Ach and protects against parasympathetic-mediated bronchoconstriction.

Anticholinergic agents inhibit the action of Ach by competing for Ach receptors. The binding of these agents to Ach receptors leads to a decrease in intracellular guanosine $3',5'$-cyclic monophosphate (cGMP) levels resulting in a decrease in bronchial smooth muscle tone. Besides their bronchodilating properties, anticholinergics reduce sputum volume without altering viscosity.

Pharmacokinetics and Dosing

The onset of action of ipratropium bromide is 60 to 90 min, which is slower than β_2-agonists, whereas its duration of action is longer (6 to 8 h). Ipratropium achieves its maximal effect in adults at a dose of 40 to 80 µg, which is the equivalent of two to four puffs by MDI (10). Higher doses may be needed during episodes of acute airflow obstruction as delivery of inhaled particles may be impaired. The optimal dose of the nebulized solution is between 50 to 125 µg (10). Both forms of medication are given at intervals of 4 to 6 h. Compared to β_2-agonist, tolerance to ipratropium has not been documented (10).

Clinical Effects

In stable COPD patients, ipratroprium bromide has been shown to alleviate dyspnea, increase exercise tolerance, and improve gas exchange (8, 11, 12). However, it has not been shown to alter the natural history of the disease (13).

In acute exacerbations of COPD, very few studies examine the us of anticholinergics alone (i.e., without β_2-agonists). The study by Rebuck et al. (7) examined the effectiveness of ipratropium in the acute setting and found a significant improvement in FEV_1 at 45 to 90 min postadministration. Karpel et al. (8), as mentioned above, also looked at the effectiveness of ipratropium bromide in the setting of acute exacerbation of COPD and found a mean increase in FEV_1 of 25% and in FVC of 22%. Ipratropium bromide is therefore considered an effective bronchodilator in the management of acute exacerbations of COPD.

Side Effects

Very few side effects occur with the inhaled anticholinergic medications because there is little systemic absorption. Despite concerns that ipratropium bromide may reduce mucociliary clearance, as seen with atropine, this effect has not been observed. Nebulized ipratropium bromide may precipitate glaucoma in elderly patients from its direct effect on the eye. This effect can be prevented by using a mouthpiece as opposed to face mask. Paradoxical bronchoconstriction with ipratropium bromide has been reported, but has been attributed mostly to additives in the nebulized solution (14). Finally, inhaled ipratropium has an unpleasant bitter taste that may affect compliance.

Comparison of β_2-Agonists and Anticholinergics

In some studies of stable COPD patients using conventional doses of both medications, the bronchodilating effects of ipratroprium bromide have been shown to be equivalent to or greater than β_2-agonists (10, 15). As we mentioned above, most trials in acute exacerbations of COPD examined the effect of β_2-agonists in comparison to anticholinergics and their combined effects. Rebuck et al. (5) compared the bronchodilator effect of fenoterol to ipratropium bromide and found that there was no difference between the two, and no further benefit from combined therapy was achieved. Karpel et al. (6), in the crossover study noted above, found that the improvement in spirometry between the two groups was similar, except that the time-to-peak effect was shorter in the metaproterenol group. No difference in hospital admission rates between the two groups was seen. A synergistic effect between metaproterenol and ipratropium was not seen, as there was no further improvement in spirometry noted during the crossover portion of the study. This study suggested that β_2-agonists and anticholinergic agents are equally effective in acute exacerbations of COPD. The ipratropium group had a small rise in PaO_2 compared to the drop in PaO_2 seen in the metaproterenol group. Therefore, in the presence of hypoxemia, ipratropium may be the better choice as it does not cause an initial decline in blood oxygenation. Several other studies have looked at combined therapy (anticholinergics and β_2-agonists) to examine whether a synergistic effect, as seen in asthma, occurs in COPD. Shrestha et al. (16) studied 76 patients with acute exacerbation of COPD. All patients were initially treated with the β_2-agonist isoetharine and then randomized to receive either ipratropium bromide or placebo in a blinded fashion. No statistical difference between the two groups was noted with regard to spirometry, adverse effects, and relapse rates. However, patients randomized to receive ipratropium bromide plus hourly β_2-agonists were discharged 91 min sooner than patients in the control group. A second study by Moayyedi et al. (17) examined 62 patients with acute exacerbation of COPD who were randomized to receive either salbutamol plus ipratropium bromide or salbutamol alone. There was no significant difference in spirometry subjective dyspnea score, or hospital stay between the two groups. O'Driscoll et al. (18) studied 125 adult patients with acute exacerbations of COPD or asthma, randomized to either nebulized salbutamol alone or in combination with ipratropium bromide. The response to treatment in the COPD patients was similar in both groups as measured by peak flows. A recent review from the Cochrane Library also concluded that both β_2-agonists and ipratropium bromide are equally effective bronchodilators in acute exacerbations of COPD (19).

There appears to be no significant difference in the bronchodilating effects between beta-agonists and anticholinergics in the setting of acute exacerbations of COPD. Beta-agonists may have a shorter time-to-peak bronchodilator effect, but the overall clinical significance of this is small.

C. Methylxanthines

The methylxanthines are a group of medications related to caffeine. They have been used for many years in the treatment of obstructive lung disease, in particular asthma and COPD. Theophylline and its intravenous formulation aminophylline, are the main methylxanthines used in the management of COPD patients. They are both 1,3-dimethylxanthines, the N-3 methyl substitution being the component that augments bronchodilator potency.

Mechanisms of Action

Despite its use for many years, the mechanism of action of theophylline at the cellular level remains unclear. Theophylline is a nonselective phosphodiesterase inhibitor causing an increase in intracellular cAMP and cGMP concentrations which, in turn, lead to bronchial smooth muscle relaxation. This bronchodilator effect is small at concentrations within the therapeutic range. Phosphodiesterase inhibition may also be responsible for the immunomodulatory and anti-inflammatory effects of this class of medications. Theophylline is also an adenosine receptor antagonist that counteracts the bronchoconstrictor effects of adenosine released from mast cells. Although this mechanism is unlikely to cause significant bronchodilatation, it may account for many of the side effects seen with theophylline such as cardiac arrhythmias, central nervous system stimulation, and diuresis. Other postulated mechanisms of action include stimulation of catecholamine release from the adrenal glands, leading to some bronchodilatation and inhibition of inflammatory mediator release from mast cells and basophils.

Several clinical observations regarding the physiological effects of methyl-xanthines, beyond bronchodilatation, have been reported. Theophylline has been shown to improve respiratory muscle function, in particular diaphragmatic contractility, and to decrease diaphragmatic fatigue, stimulate the respiratory center, and improve mucociliary clearance (20, 21, 22).

Pharmacokinetics and Dosing

While methylxanthines were used extensively in the past, their use in acute exacerbations of COPD has declined significantly over the past few years because of their relatively low potency as bronchodilators and the narrow window between the therapeutic and toxic levels. The dose–response curve of theophylline is not linear, but begins to plateau at levels of approximately 12.8 mg/dL. Therefore, the usual target range for theophylline serum concentration is 10 to 20 mg/dL. The dose required to achieve a therapeutic level is, on the other hand, quite variable due to many factors affecting theophylline clearance.

Methylxanthines are metabolized primarily by the liver. Many diseases including hepatic, cardiac (e.g., congestive heart failure), and pneumonia can alter the clearance of theophylline and, therefore, blood levels need to be monitored to avoid toxicity. The normal half-life of theophylline is 4 to 12 h but is significantly longer in congestive heart failure (up to 23 h) and liver cirrhosis (up to 26 h). In COPD patients, decreased clearance may occur due to liver congestion from cor pulmonale and due to the increased age of many of these patients. These factors must be considered when starting patients on theophylline. The loading dose, which is dependent on volume of distribution, does not require adjustment, whereas the maintenance dose must be decreased in these circumstances. Many drugs also interfere with the metabolism of theophylline and therefore a careful drug history should be taken in order to adjust the dose appropriately (see Table 2).

In severe exacerbations of COPD, intravenous aminophylline can be given at a loading dose of 5.6 mg/kg over 30 min followed by a maintenance dose of 0.5 mg/kg/h. The maintenance dose should be reduced to 0.3 mg/kg/h in the elderly and to 0.2 mg/kg/h in patients with CHF, cirrhosis, or cor pulmonale. In

Table 2   Effect of Drugs on Clearance of Theophylline

Increased clearance	Decreased clearance	
rifampin	cimetidine	
phenobarbital	erythromycin/clarithromycin	
ethanol	ciprofloxacin	
tobacco	allopurinol	methotrexate
marijuana	zileuton	propranolol
isoproterenol	estrogen	propafenone
phenytoin	fluvoxamine	ticlopidine
	verapamil	

patients already on long-acting preparations of oral theophylline, a drug level should be obtained prior to loading to avoid toxicity.

Clinical Effects

In patients with stable COPD, theophylline has been shown to improve exercise performance, reduce dyspnea, induce bronchodilatation (especially as part of a combination therapy), and perhaps improve respiratory muscle and diaphragmatic function. Other effects seen in the stable COPD patient include improved ventilation, mucociliary clearance, reduced gas trapping, and pulmonary vasodilatation (23, 24).

The role of theophylline in acute exacerbations of COPD is less clear as there are few studies addressing this issue. Rice et al. (25) randomized 28 COPD patients with acute exacerbations to receive intravenous aminophylline or placebo along with standard therapy (β_2-agonists, methylprednisolone, antibiotics, and oxygen as needed). There were no differences in spirometry (FEV_1 and FVC), dyspnea score, or arterial blood gases. The aminophylline group had an increased incidence of side effects, although this was not statistically significant. Wrenn et al. (26) randomized patients with acute exacerbations of asthma and COPD to receive either aminophylline or placebo. All patients received treatment with inhaled β_2-agonists and intravenous methylprednisolone. Spirometry (FEV_1, FVC, PEFR), incidence of side effects, patient satisfaction with treatment, and time in the emergency department was similar between the two groups. Patients who received aminophylline had a lower incidence of hospitalization, although this did not reach statistical significance when the COPD patients were analyzed separately. A third study by Seidenfeld et al. (27) involved a group of elderly men with COPD already on oral preparations of theophylline, who presented to the emergency department with an acute exacerbation. They were randomized to receive either placebo or intravenous aminophylline with inhaled bronchodilators. There was no difference between the groups with respect to spirometry, respiratory symptom scores, and number of future visits to the emergency room. Overall, theophylline has not been shown to have any additional benefit beyond that obtained from inhaled bronchodilators.

Side Effects

Significant adverse effects have occurred with the use of theophylline. The most common include, GI upset (nausea, vomiting, abdominal discomfort, and diarrhea), cardiac arrhythmias (supraventricular tachycardia and ventricular arrhythmias), central nervous system toxicity (headaches, insomnia, irritability, and seizures), and diuresis. The incidence of side effects increases at higher plasma concentrations of theophylline (greater than 20 mg/dL), although there is no predictable relationship between the serum concentration and the development of toxicity. Toxicity from theophylline can develop with both acute and chronic administration. Careful monitoring of serum levels is mandatory as clearance is variable and drug interactions are common (Table 2).

II. Method of Delivery of Bronchodilators

Historically many patients with acute exacerbations of COPD have been treated with nebulized bronchodilators, often due to patient preference and their perception that the usual therapy, the MDI, has failed. The nebulized delivery method is more labor-intensive and more expensive to administer. This has led to several studies comparing clinical and cost effectiveness of the two main methods of aerosol drug delivery, wet nebulizers and MDIs.

Turner et al. (28) performed a meta-analysis to compare the effect of bronchodilator delivery by MDI or wet nebulizer in patients with acute airflow obstruction either due to COPD or asthma. Twelve studies were included in this meta-analysis, which concluded that both delivery methods were equally effective. Spacer devices were used for MDI delivery in these studies and are therefore recommended, especially in acute exacerbations. Mandelberg et al. (29) performed a randomized, double-blind placebo-controlled trial of MDI versus nebulized salbutamol in patients with acute exacerbations of either COPD or asthma. Both methods of salbutamol delivery were equivalent with regard to improvement in FEV_1 and subjective symptom scores. In another double-blind, placebo-controlled crossover study by Berry et al. (30), 22 patients with acute exacerbations of COPD were randomized to receive albuterol either via nebulizer or MDI plus spacer. No significant difference was found in the improvement in FEV_1, FVC, and dyspnea score between the two modes of delivery. An economic evaluation of bronchodilator delivery methods in hospitalized patients, done by Turner et al. (31), found that MDIs are more cost effective than the nebulized treatments. However, effectiveness of the MDI inhalers depends on patient technique, which is likely to be worse in the acute setting. Therefore, a spacer device should be used to improve aerosol delivery and, hence, effectiveness.

III. Summary

Acute exacerbations of COPD are a common problem faced by many physicians. Bronchoconstriction plays an important role in the associated acute airflow obstruction, and therefore medications aimed at reversing this process are an important aspect of therapy.

First-line agents in acute exacerbations of COPD are the inhaled β_2-agonists and anticholinergics. Most guidelines, including the American Thoracic Society and the British Thoracic Society, suggest that either β_2-agonists or ipratropium bromide may be used as initial therapy, as there is no evidence to suggest that one agent is superior to the other. β_2-agonists have a more rapid onset of action and, hence, are often favored by many physicians in the acute setting. There is no evidence to suggest that the use of these two agents together provides any synergistic effect in COPD patients with acute exacerbations. Methylxanthines have not been shown to have any additional benefit and, therefore, their role should be limited to those patients who do not respond to inhaled bronchodilators and steroids. Methylxanthines should be used cautiously in patients at risk for toxicity. Nebulized bronchodilators should only be used when patients are too dyspneic or unable to use an MDI effectively, as they are less cost effective and provide no additional benefit. A spacer is recommended when using an MDI for bronchodilator administration.

References

1. Fazio F, Lafortuna C. Effect of inhaled salbutamol on mucociliary clearance in patients with chronic bronchitis. Chest 1981; 80:827–830.
2. Levitt MA, Gambrioli EF, Fink LB. Comparative trial of continuous nebulization versus metered-dose inhaler in the treatment of acute bronchospasm. Ann Emerg Med 1995; 26:273–277.
3. Georgopoulos D, Wong D, Anthonisen NR. Tolerance to β_2-agonists in patients with chronic obstructive pulmonary disease. Chest 1990; 97:280–284.
4. Nelson HS. β-adrenergic bronchodilators. N Engl J Med 1995; 333:499–506.
5. Guyatt GH, Townsend M, Pugsley SO, et al. Bronchodilators in chronic airflow limitation. Effects on airway function, exercise capacity and quality of life. Am Rev Respir Dis 1987; 135:1069–1074.
6. Belman MJ, Botnick, Shin JW. Inhaled bronchodilators reduce dynamic hyperinflation during exercise in patients with patients with chronic destructive pulmonary disease. Am J Respir Crit Care Med 1996; 153:967.
7. Rebuck AS Chapman KR, Abboud R, Pare PD, Kreisman H, Wolkove N, Vickerson F. Nebulized anticholinergic and sympathomimetic treatment of asthma and chronic obstructive airways disease in the emergency room. Am J Med 1987; 82:59–64.
8. Karpel JP, Pesin J, Greenberg D, Gentry E. A comparison of the effects of ipratropium bromide and metaproterenol sulfate in acute exacerbations of COPD. Chest 1990; 98:835–839.
9. Gross NJ, Bankwala Z. Effects of an anticholinergic bronchodilator on arterial blood gases of hypoxemic patients with chronic obstructive pulmonary disease. Comparison with a beta-adrenergic agent. Am Rev Respir Dis 1987; 136:1091–1094.
10. Gross NJ. Ipratropium bromide. N Engl J Med 1998; 333:499–506.
11. Mahler DA, Donohue JF, Barbee RA, et al. Efficacy of satmeterol xinafoate in the treatment of COPD. Chest 1999; 115:957–965.
12. Patakas D, Andreadis D, Mavrofridis E, Argyropoulou P. Comparison of the effects of salmeterol and ipratropium bromide on exercise performance and breathlessness in

patients with stable chronic obstructive pulmonary disease. Respir Med 1998; 92(9):1116–1121.

13. Anthonisen NR, Connett JE, Kiley JP, et al. The effects of smoking intervention and the use of an inhaled anticholinergic bronchodilator on the rate of decline of FEV_1: The Lung Health Study. JAMA 1994; 272:1497–1505.

14. Patel KR, Tullet WM. Bronchoconstriction in response to ipratropium bromide. Br Med J 1983; 286:1318.

15. Tashkin DP, Ashutosh K, Bleeker ER, et al. Comparison of the anticholinergic bronchodilator ipratropium bromide with metaproterenol in chronic obstructive pulmonary disease. Am J Med 1986; 81(suppl A):81.

16. Shrestha M, O'Brien T, Haddox R, Gourlay HS, Reed G. Decreased duration of emergency department treatment of chronic obstructive pulmonary disease exacerbations with the addition of ipratropium bromide to β-agonist therapy. Ann Emerg Med 1991; 20:1206–1209.

17. Moayyedi P, Congleton J, Page RL, Pearson SB, Muers MF. Comparison of nebulized salbutamol and ipratropium bromide with salbutamol alone in the treatment of chronic obstructive pulmonary disease. Thorax 1995; 50:834–837.

18. O'Driscoll BR, Taylor, RJ, Horsley MG, Chambers DK, Bernstein A. Nebulized salbutamol with and without ipratropium bromide in acute airflow obstruction. Lancet 1989; 1:1418–1420.

19. Brown CD, McCrory D, White J. Inhaled short-acting beta2-agonists versus ipratropium for acute exacerbations of chronic obstructive pulmonary disease (Cochrane Review). In: The Cochrane Library, Issue 4, 2001. Oxford: Update Software.

20. Murciano D, Aubier M, Lecocguic Y, Pariente R. Effects of theophylline on diaphragmatic strength and fatigue in patients with chronic obstructive pulmonary disease. N Engl J Med 1984; 311:349–353.

21. Dowell AR, Heyman A, Siecker HO, Tripathy K. Effect of aminophyhlline on respiratory-center sensitivity on Cheyne-Stokes respiration and in pulmonary emphysema. N Engl J Med 1965; 273:1447–1453.

22. Ziment I. Theophylline and mucociliary clearance. Chest 1987; 92(suppl):38S–43S.

23. Murciano D, Auclair H, Pariente R, Aubier M. A randomized controlled trial of theophylline in patients with severe chronic obstructive pulmonary disease. N Engl J Med 1989; 330:1521–1525.

24. Mahler DA, Matthay RA, Synder PE, Wells CK, Loke J. Sustained-release theophylline reduces dyspnea in nonreversible airway disease. Am Rev Respir Dis 1985; 131: 22–25.

25. Rice KL, Leatherman JW, Duane PG, Snyder LS, Harmon KR, Abel J, Niewoehner DE. Aminophylline for acute exacerbations of chronic obstructive pulmonary disease. Ann Intern Med 1987; 107:305–309.

26. Wrenn K, Slovis CM, Murphy F, Greenberg RS. Aminophylline therapy for acute bronchospastic disease in the emergency room. Ann Intern Med 1991; 115:241–247.

27. Seidenfeld JJ, Jones WN, Moss RE, Tremper J. Intravenous aminophylline in the treatment of acute bronchospastic exacerbations of chronic obstructive pulmonary disease. Ann Emerg Med 1984; 13:248–252.

28. Turner MO, Patel A, Ginsburg S, Fitzgerald JM. Bronchodilator delivery in acute airflow obstruction: A meta-analysis. Arch Intern Med 1997; 157:1736–1744.

29. Mandelberg A, Chen E, Noviski N, Priel IE. Nebulized wet aerosol treatment in emergency department—is it essential? Comparison with large spacer device for metered-dose inhaler. Chest 1997; 112:1501–1505.

30. Berry RB, Shinto RA, Wong FH, Despars JA, Light RW. Nebulizer vs spacer for bronchodilator delivery in patients hospitalized for acute exacerbations of COPD. Chest 1996; 96:1241–1246.
31. Turner MO, Gafni A, Swan D, Fitzgerald JM. A review and economic evaluation of bronchodilator delivery methods in hospitalized patients. Arch Intern Med 1996; 156:2113–2118.

22

Corticosteroids

KATHRYN L. RICE and DENNIS E. NIEWOEHNER

Minneapolis Veterans Affairs Medical Center
Minneapolis, Minnesota, U.S.A.

I. Introduction

Patients with chronic obstructive pulmonary disease (COPD) are prone to acute exacerbations that may cause a substantial decline in functional status, hospitalization, and even death. COPD exacerbations represent a major burden on health-care resources in most of the developed world (1). Viral and bacterial agents probably cause most exacerbations, and a substantial proportion can be prevented by regular immunizations (2–4). Standard treatment for established exacerbations has long included antibiotics and bronchodilators, along with oxygen and assisted ventilation in the most severely ill.

Over the past 20 years, systemic corticosteroids have assumed a more prominent role in the treatment of COPD (5). Most physicians came to regard systemic corticosteroids as a standard therapy for the in-patient and out-patient therapy of COPD exacerbations. In an effort to improve chronic symptoms and to prevent recurrent exacerbations, physicians also prescribed inhaled corticosteroids for many COPD patients and low doses of systemic corticosteroids for a selected few that were regarded as "steroid-dependent."

These practice patterns evolved without much evidence that COPD responded to corticosteroids in any clinical setting, and with the knowledge that corticosteroids have significant adverse effects. However, corticosteroids were known to be effective in asthma (6) and physicians have tended to transfer proven therapies from asthma to COPD in a somewhat uncritical manner. This phenomenon may be attributed in part to the difficulty in reliably distinguishing COPD from asthma in older patients. Patients generally regarded as suffering from COPD sometimes have selected features of asthma, such as wheezing, bronchial hyperresponsiveness, and sputum and blood eosinophilia. Other patients who suffer severe asthma from an early age may develop a clinical condition in later life that is not distinguishable from COPD. Expert panels have failed to make clear distinctions between these two conditions, and it is probably unrealistic to expect that the average practitioner could do any better.

Unanswered questions about the efficacy of corticosteroids in COPD and concern about the appropriateness of their widespread administration provided an impetus for undertaking a number of large clinical trials as well as many other investigations. Although substantive questions remain, these studies have provided much improved information about the role of corticosteroids in treating and preventing COPD exacerbations.

II. Rationale for Corticosteroid Use in COPD

A. Airway Inflammation in Stable COPD

Corticosteroids are potent anti-inflammatory agents, and the rationale for their use resides with our belief that inflammatory processes play a prominent role in the pathogenesis of COPD. Collections of macrophages and other inflammatory cells are present in the peripheral airways and alveolar spaces of healthy young smokers (7), and evidence of bronchial inflammation persists at all stages of the disease (8–12). Inflammatory cell infiltrates within airway walls consist of macrophages, neutrophils, and CD4 and CD8 T lymphocytes (13–16). The mechanisms by which these cells accumulate are poorly understood, but release of a variety of inflammatory mediators by activated macrophages, epithelial cells, and CD8+ T lymphocytes likely play a pivotal role (17). Inflammatory mediators such as tumor necrosis factor-α (TNF-α) and leukotriene B_4 (LB_4) have been detected in the sputum of stable COPD patients (17, 18).

B. Airway Inflammation in COPD Exacerbations

Inflammation is an even more prominent feature in COPD during exacerbation, purulent sputum being one of the clinical hallmarks. Some investigators reported an increase in total cell counts and in lymphocytes in sputa of patients experiencing COPD exacerbations, but considerable individual variability is apparent, perhaps due to the heterogeneous nature of the disease and to the multiple factors that may precipitate exacerbations (19). Sputum IL-6 levels are significantly increased during COPD exacerbations (19). High baseline sputum cytokine (IL-6 and IL-8) levels are also associated with more frequent exacerbations (19), and these increased cytokine concentrations are correlated with higher sputum total cell counts, particularly lymphocytes and eosinophils (19, 20). Compared to patients with infrequent exacerbations, patients who exacerbate frequently have lower levels of sputum secretory leukoproteinase, a substance with antiviral and antibacterial properties (21).

C. Corticosteroid Effects on Inflammation

The specific mechanisms by which corticosteroids suppress inflammation in stable or exacerbated COPD are very poorly understood but they appear to involve complex cellular and biochemical pathways. This has been the subject of detailed reviews (22, 23). Among many known effects, systemic corticosteroids decrease circulating lymphocytes, eosinophils, and basophils, and they deplete mucosal mast cells in asthmatic lungs. Corticosteroids suppress the expression or release of macrophage inflammatory protein 1-α (MIP-1α), monocyte chemotactic protein-1 (MCP-1), intercellular adhesion molecule-1 (ICAM-1), E-selectin, interleukins (IL) 1–6, 8, 11–13, and TNF-α. Other anti-inflammatory effects from corticosteroids may include increased gene transcriptions for the interleukin receptor antagonist and for lipocortin-1 (phospholipase A_2 inhibitor) and the suppression of platelet-activating factor activity and of nitric oxide synthase induction.

Corticosteroids may also exert beneficial effects in the airways by mechanisms that are not generally viewed as being anti-inflammatory (22). For example, corticosteroids increase transcription rates for the beta-adrenergic receptor and suppress production of the bronchoconstrictor, endothelin-1. Corticosteroids may also reduce mucus secretion in the airways and decrease microvascular leakage.

D. Clinical Studies Addressing the Mechanisms of Corticosteroid Action in COPD

Many investigators believe that eosinophils play an important role in the pathogenesis of asthma and perhaps COPD. Suppression of blood and tissue eosinophilia is a well-known effect of corticosteroids, and this has prompted clinical studies to examine the effect of systemic corticosteroids on bronchial and sputum eosinophilia. A number of small studies indicate that the presence of blood (24), sputum (25), or bronchoalveolar lavage fluid (26) eosinophilia in patients with *stable* COPD correlates with improvements in the forced expiratory volume in 1 s (FEV_1) following treatment with short-term oral corticosteroids. Similarly, a reduction in sputum eosinophil counts following a short course of prednisone is associated with improved spirometric measures, symptoms, and exercise tolerance (18, 27).

Very little is known about the molecular and cellular mechanisms by which systemic corticosteroid therapy may confer benefits in patients with *exacerbated* COPD, as there are a dearth of adequately controlled studies in this setting. Reductions in blood leukocyte counts and C-reactive protein, and increases in systemic levels of the anti-inflammatory mediator soluble interleukin 1 receptor II were reported in an uncontrolled observational study in patients with COPD exacerbations who received prednisolone in addition to bronchodilators, theophylline, and antibiotics (28).

Studies of *inhaled* corticosteroids on bronchial cell populations in COPD have yielded confusing results. In contrast to systemic corticosteroids, inhaled corticosteroids do not seem to cause a consistent decrease of bronchial eosinophilia in COPD (29, 30). Some, but not all, studies of inhaled corticosteroids in COPD patients have reported a predominant effect on airway neutrophils. Beclomethasone was found to decrease the proportion of neutrophils and increase the proportion of macrophages in induced sputum in one study of stable COPD (29). However, in another similar study, fluticasone had no effect on the numbers or proportions of sputum inflammatory cells or neutrophils (30). Other studies reported that inhaled corticosteroids increase sputum neutrophil elastase inhibitory activity, decrease sputum neutrophil chemotactic activity (31), decrease bronchoalveolar lavage myeloperoxidase activity (32), either decrease or have null effect on bronchoalveolar lavage IL-8 levels (32), and have null effects on sputum IL-8 concentrations (30).

III. Systemic Corticosteroids for COPD Exacerbations

A. Efficacy of Systemic Corticosteroids

The administration of systemic corticosteroids for COPD exacerbations became a common practice wihin the past 20 years, but it was also a contentious subject because of residual doubts concerning efficacy. Recent clinical trials have largely laid this issue to rest by showing that systemic corticosteroids do permit patients with COPD exacerbations to recover sooner.

Albert and colleagues published the first trial of systemic corticosteroids for COPD exacerbations, the results of which had a major effect on prescribing practices (33). They randomized 44 hospitalized patients to receive either intravenous methylprednisolone, 0.5 mg/kg every 6 h, or placebo for 3 days, while holding constant most other aspects of care. The FEV_1, but not the FVC or arterial blood gases, improved at a significantly faster rate in those patients who received methylprednisolone. The observation period stopped after 3 days and the investigators did not attempt to evaluate clinical endpoints.

Emerman and his associates randomized 96 patients who presented to an emergency department for COPD exacerbations to placebo or a single 100-mg dose of intravenous methylprednisolone (34). Active treatment did not improve spirometry over a 5-h observation period, nor did it reduce hospitalizations or unscheduled emergency department visits over the ensuing 48 h. The authors recognized that the duration of therapy may have been too brief to discern a beneficial effect.

Bullard and his colleagues also studied patients who presented to an emergency department (35). They randomized 113 patients to receive hydrocortisone, 100 mg I.V. every 4 h, or placebo. The patients who received active treatment did not have significantly improved peak flow rates and FEV_1 after 6 h, and they had no reduction in hospitalization, intubation, or mortality rates.

Thompson and his associated randomized 27 outpatients with COPD exacerbations to placebo or to a 9-day, tapering course of oral prednisone (36). They found that prednisone improved arterial blood gases and the FEV_1 at 3 days and at 10 days after enrollment. They also reported that prednisone-treated patients experienced significantly fewer treatment failures (0% vs. 57%, $p = 0.002$), defined as the need for open-label systemic corticosteroids or hospitalization, a conclusion that must be tempered by the small sample size.

The Cochrane Airways Group performed an interim meta-analysis on the use of corticosteroids for patients with COPD exacerbations (37). The review included the aforementioned studies along with data from several other trials that remained unpublished or had been published in abstract form only. The authors concluded that systemic corticosteroids did not significantly improve spirometry, but did significantly improve selected clinical outcomes, such as quality-of-life indices. The authors noted, however, that only a handful of the reviewed studies assessed clinical outcomes and these few studies exhibited considerable heterogeneity in their results. The authors called for further research in the form of large, multicenter trials.

The Veterans Affairs Cooperative Studies Program undertook a trial at 25 study centers to evaluate the effects of systemic corticosteroids in patients with severe COPD exacerbations. The study group, Systemic Corticosteroids in Chronic Obstructive Pulmonary Disease Exacerbations (SCCOPE), randomized 271 patients who were hospitalized with a COPD exacerbation (38). There were three treatment arms. The two active treatment arms received intravenous methylprednisolone, 125 mg every 6 h, for 3 days, followed by oral prednisone starting at 60 mg daily. One active treatment arm received a tapering dose of prednisone over 2 weeks and the second active treatment arm received a tapering dose of prednisone over 8 weeks. The placebo arm received 3 days of intravenous saline followed by inactive study capsules. Study treatments were fully blinded, and all subjects received inhaled bronchodilators and antibiotics. Follow-up continued for 6 months. The primary endpoint was treatment failure, defined as death from any cause, intubation, and mechanical ventilation, hospital readmission for COPD, or the need to intensify drug treatment. Secondary endpoints included changes in the FEV_1, hospital utilization, and all-cause mortality.

Compared to placebo, corticosteroid treatment significantly reduced the rate of treatment failure (23% vs. 33% at 30 days, $p = 0.04$; 37% vs. 48% at 90 days, $p = 0.04$) (Fig. 1).

Differences in treatment failure rates were no longer statistically significant at 6 months. Treatment with corticosteroids significantly improved the FEV_1 during the first 3 days of hospitalization by approximately 100 mL. Corticosteroids also shortened the length of initial hospital stay from 9.7 to 8.5 days ($p = 0.03$). There was no significant mortality difference between the active and the placebo treatment arms at any time. Treatment with systemic corticosteroids for 8 weeks was no more effective than treatment for 2 weeks in terms of any of the primary or secondary outcomes.

At about the same time, Davies and associates reported results from a smaller, single-center study having a design similar to that of SCCOPE (39). They

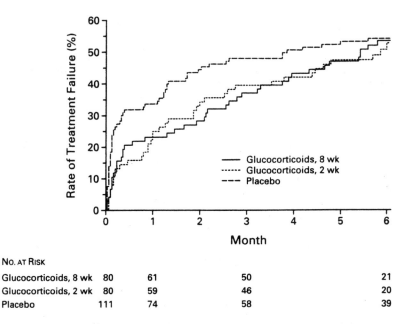

Figure 1 Rates of first treatment failure for patients hospitalized with a COPD exacerbation in the SCCOPE trial (38). Compared with the placebo arm, treatment failure rates in the combined active treatment arms are significantly ($p < 0.05$) decreased at 1 month and at 3 months, but not at 6 months. Published with permission.

randomized 56 patients who were hospitalized for COPD exacerbations to oral prednisolone, 30 mg, once daily for 2 weeks, or placebo. During the first 5 days of hospitalization, the postbronchodilator FEV_1 improved faster in the corticosteroid-treated patients by about 60 mL per day. More important, the median length of hospital stay was significantly reduced in the corticosteroid group (9 days vs. 7 days, $p = 0.027$) (Fig. 2). Corticosteroid treatment was also associated with statistically insignificant trends for improved dyspnea scores. There were no treatment-related differences in any of the efficacy outcomes after 6 weeks.

B. Adverse Effects of Short-Term Systemic Corticosteroids

Impairment of glucose tolerance is the most common adverse effect of short-term systemic corticosteroids when they are used for the treatment of COPD exacerbations. This comes as no surprise because brief exposure to systemic corticosteroids impairs glucose tolerance in normal, nondiabetic subjects (40). After 72 h of treatment, Albert and associates found that mean blood glucose levels were 25 mg/dL higher in the patients who received corticosteroids (33). Davies and colleagues reported transient glycosuria in 6 of their 29 corticosteroid-treated subjects (39). Although blood glucose was not regularly measured in the SCCOPE

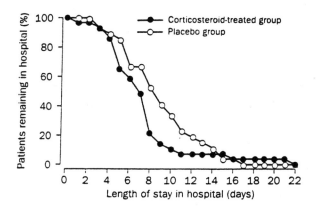

Figure 2 Proportion of patients remaining in the hospital according to treatment group after admission for a COPD exacerbation (39). Compared with placebo, the length of hospital stay was significantly reduced ($p < 0.05$) in those patients who received oral corticosteroids. (Reprinted with permission.)

trial, hyperglycemia requiring specific treatment occurred approximately four times more often in patients who received corticosteroids (38).

Systematic reviews of clinical trials indicate that brief courses of systemic corticosteroids do confer a small risk of lethal and nonlethal secondary infections (41, 42). A similarly small risk probably exists for COPD patients who receive short-term systemic corticosteroids. In the SCCOPE trial there was no statistically significant overall effect of corticosteroids on the incidence of secondary infections, although more cases of serious pneumonia were noted in patients who received 8 weeks of corticosteroids (38). Scattered cases of serious infection from *Staphylococcus aureus*, *Morganella morgagni* (42), *Legionella pneumophila*, *aspergillus* species (43–45), disseminated cytomegalovirus (43, 46), and concomitant multiple organisms (43–46) have been seen in COPD patients receiving systemic corticosteroids.

Data from a surveillance study and from a meta-analysis of clinical trials (41, 47) indicate that systemic corticosteroids may cause serious psychiatric disorders. The Boston Collaborative Drug Surveillance Program found a striking dose-dependent relationship between systemic corticosteroid administration and major psychiatric disorders (47). The incidence increased from 1.3% in patients receiving less than 40 mg of prednisone daily to 18.4% in patients receiving more than 80 mg of prednisone daily. A systematic review of many clinical trials confirmed that corticosteroid therapy is associated with a significant increase in the number of acute psychoses, but that the absolute risk may be only about 0.2% overall (41). The SCCOPE trial found no increase in the incidence of treatment-related psychiatric disorders, even though patients initially received very high doses of parenteral methylprednisolone (512 mg per day) (38). These and other trial results suggest that psychiatric complications are relatively infrequent and that most resolve quickly once the corticosteroid dose is reduced or withdrawn.

Dose-dependent reductions in inspiratory and peripheral muscle strength can occur in COPD patients who have received frequent courses of prednisone for recurrent COPD exacerbations (48). Critical illness myopathy has also been reported in patients treated for COPD or asthma with high doses of systemic corticosteroids (49, 50).

Many physicians consider bleeding from the gastrointestinal tract a complication of systemic corticosteroid therapy. However, systematic reviews on this subject have failed to find any such risk (41, 51); earlier studies suggesting such a relationship had not adjusted for concomitant use of nonsteroidal anti-inflammatory drugs. Other known complications of corticosteroids, such as cataract formation, adrenal insufficiency, and osteoporosis, are usually seen only with long-term corticosteroid use.

C. Summary

The principal lesson to be learned from these clinical trials is that systemic corticosteroids are moderately effective in hastening recovery from severe COPD exacerbations. A brief course of therapy, not to exceed 14 days, administered to patients hospitalized for COPD exacerbations, will speed recovery and shorten hospital stay by 1 or 2 days. Prednisone probably confers similar benefits when COPD exacerbations are treated in an outpatient setting. When used judiciously for short periods, the risk of a serious complication from corticosteroids appears to be acceptably low. Hyperglycemia and occasional instances of infection, myopathy, and psychosis should be anticipated in those patients who are given systemic corticosteroids.

A number of practical questions remain about the use of systemic corticosteroids for COPD exacerbations. These questions may never be answered, because huge, expensive trials would be required to provide clear answers. Neither the optimal starting dose nor the preferred route of administration is known; benefits from an small oral dose of prednisolone, 30 mg given once daily, were effective in one trial, whereas a large intravenous dose of methylprednisolone, 125 mg every 6 h, proved effective in another (38, 39). Based on the SCCOPE trial, the optimal duration of therapy is 2 weeks or less. A small, recently published trial indicated that 10 days of corticosteroid therapy were superior to 3 days in terms of spirometric changes (52). The study lacked sufficient power to draw any firm conclusions about clinical benefits. The common practice of administering tapering does of prednisone appears to be based mostly on historical precedent. Tapering seems to be unnecessary when treating asthma (53), and the same may well be true for COPD.

IV. Prevention of COPD Exacerbations

A. Efficacy of Inhaled Corticosteroids

Important long-term treatment goals in patients with COPD are to improve chronic symptoms, slow the development of the disease, decrease the number of exacerbations, and reduce mortality. Earlier trials of inhaled corticosteroids in stable COPD failed to find clear-cut benefit for any of these clinical outcomes, but most of these studies were relatively small and they may simply have lacked sufficient power to detect clinically meaningful differences (54–56). Given the increasingly widespread use of inhaled corticosteroids in COPD, there was a perceived need for better information.

Five major trials examining the effects of inhaled corticosteroids in stable COPD have now been published. The primary goal in one study was to determine if inhaled corticosteroids decreased the rate of acute exacerbations (57). The primary goal in the other four studies was to determine if inhaled corticosteroids slowed the development of COPD, as measured by age-dependent rates of decline of the FEV_1 (58–61). Additional information about clinical symptoms, health-care utilization, and exacerbation rate was collected in most of these trials.

The Copenhagen City Heart Study (CCHS) and the European Respiratory Society Study on Chronic Obstructive Pulmonary Disease (EUROSCOP) had a similar design in terms of the primary hypothesis, intervention, and patient characteristics. CCHS enrolled 290 subjects with mild COPD (mean $FEV_1 = 86\%$ of predicted) who continued to smoke cigarettes. Compared with placebo, inhaled budesonide (1200 µg per day for 6 months; 800 µg per day 30 months) had no effect on the rate of decline in FEV_1 over a 3-year period (58). There were no treatment-related differences in clinical symptoms or exacerbation rates. Failure of inhaled corticosteroids to reduce exacerbation rate might be attributed to the relatively small sample size and the mild severity of the COPD in their study population. EURO-SCOP enrolled 1277 subjects who had a mean FEV_1 that was 77% of predicted (59). Treatment with budesonide (800 µg per day) for 3 years did not significantly affect the rate of FEV_1 decline. They did not report assessments of respiratory symptoms or exacerbation rates.

The Inhaled Steroids in Obstructive Lung Disease in Europe (ISOLDE) trial enrolled 751 subjects with moderately severe COPD (mean $FEV_1 = 50\%$ of predicted) (60). The intervention was inhaled fluticasone, 1000 µg per day for 3 years, and the primary outcome was the rate of decline in the FEV_1. Fluticasone had no effect on the FEV_1 slope over time, but it did significantly improve some, but not all, secondary clinical outcomes. Of particular interest, mean exacerbation rate, as defined by worsening of respiratory symptoms treated with systemic corticosteroids or antibiotics or both, was reduced from 1.32 per year for placebo to 0.99 per year for fluticasone ($p = 0.026$).

The Lung Health Study (LHS) was also designed to detect relatively small effects of inhaled corticosteroids on the rate of decline in FEV_1 (61). LHS enrolled 1116 subjects with mild-to-moderate COPD (mean $FEV_1 = 64\%$ of predicted). Treatment with moderately high doses of triamcinolone (1200 µg per day) for an average of 40 months did not significantly alter the rate of decline in the FEV_1. Selected secondary outcomes, including respiratory symptoms, clinic visits for respiratory conditions, and hospitalization for respiratory illness, were significantly improved with triamcinolone. These results suggest that exacerbation rates may have been reduced in the active treatment group, but the investigators did not attempt to assess that outcome directly.

The International COPD Study Group trial is the only published study that was designed specifically to evaluate the efficacy of inhaled corticosteroids in preventing COPD exacerbations. This group enrolled 281 patients with moderately severe COPD (mean $FEV_1 = 57\%$ of predicted) and with a previous history of at least one exacerbation per year that required a visit to the physician or hospitalization (57). Patients were randomized to receive a relatively high dose of fluticasone (1000 μg per day) or placebo for 6 months. The study group defined an exacerbation as a worsening of COPD symptoms requiring a change in treatment. Severity of exacerbation was defined as mild (self-managed), moderate (requiring treatment by a physician or in a hospital outpatient department), or severe (resulting in hospitalization). The proportion of patients who experienced one or more COPD exacerbations over the 6-month period was designated as the primary outcome, and this proportion was not significantly changed by fluticasone (37% with placebo vs. 32% with fluticasone, $p = 0.449$) (Fig. 3). Of the patients having at least one exacerbation, fluticasone decreased the likelihood of having a moderate-to-severe exacerbation (86% with placebo vs. 60% with fluticasone, $p < 0.001$). Symptoms, including cough and daily sputum volume, but not breathlessness or the use of additional bronchodilators, were improved with fluticasone, as was exercise

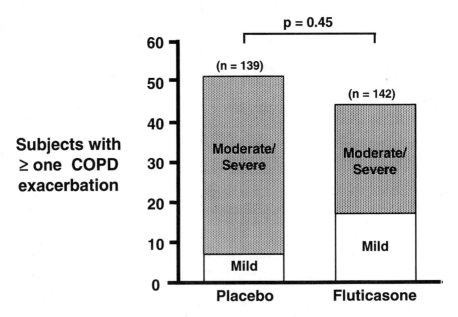

Figure 3 The proportion of COPD patients who experienced at least one exacerbation was not significantly decreased in those patients who took inhaled fluticasone, 1000 μg per day for 6 months ($p = 0.45$) (57). Of the patients experiencing an exacerbation, fluticasone decreased the likelihood of having a moderate-to-severe exacerbation (86% with placebo vs. 60% with fluticasone, $p < 0.001$). (Figure drawn from data provided in Ref. 57.)

tolerance, as assessed by the 6-min walking distance. Global efficacy ratings by both physicians and patients also favored the fluticasone-treated group.

A recent population-based, cohort study notable for its very large size ($n = 22,620$) also supports the notion that inhaled corticosteroids may prevent severe exacerbations in patients with advanced COPD (62). Using an administrative database for the Canadian province of Ontario, Sin and Tu identified all patients with a primary discharge diagnosis of COPD over a 5-year period. Over the ensuing year after discharge, the authors found that the adjusted relative risks for those patients given inhaled corticosteroids were reduced by 24% for rehospitalization and by 29% for death. The authors commented upon the inherent limitations of observational studies and called for a large randomized clinical trial to confirm these potentially important findings.

B. Efficacy of Oral Corticosteroids

Although there is little published evidence to support the practice, as many as 15% of patients with more advanced COPD may take oral corticosteroids on a regular basis (63). Patients receiving oral corticosteroids frequently have advanced COPD with a history of recurrent exacerbations or hospitalizations. It may be inferred that the goals of oral corticosteroid therapy are to prevent further exacerbations and to improve persistent daily symptoms that have responded poorly to multiple other respiratory medications.

Early randomized trials examined the effects of relatively high doses of systemic corticosteroids for relatively brief periods in patients with stable COPD. In a meta-analysis of 10 such trials, it was found that a 2-week trial of oral prednisone (30–60 mg/day), or its equivalent, resulted in a 20% or greater increase in baseline FEV_1 only 10% more frequently than did placebo (64). It was unclear whether these small, short-term spirometric changes were associated with meaningful clinical benefits, and whether the improvements were sustained.

Two relatively small trials attempted to assess the clinical benefits of oral corticosteroid therapy in stable COPD over longer periods of time. Renkema and colleagues studied 40 patients with relatively mild COPD (average baseline FEV_1 1.86 L) who did not require daily oral corticosteroids prior to entry (56). Patients received either double placebo, inhaled budesonide (1600 µg per day) plus oral placebo, or the same dose of inhaled budesonide plus low-dose daily prednisolone (5 mg) over a 2-year period. Patients in both corticosteroid treatment arms experienced improvements in respiratory symptoms, but the addition of oral corticosteroids did not confer further benefit beyond that observed with inhaled corticosteroids alone. Neither active treatment had any significant effect on the duration or frequency of COPD exacerbations. The authors hypothesized that this may have been due to the larger number of dropouts in the placebo group. Failure to see an effect could also have been due to the small sample size, the low dose of oral corticosteroid administered, or to the relatively mild severity of the disease.

Rice and associates performed a second trial involving patients with more severe disease (average baseline FEV_1 0.94 L) (65). The objective of this study was to determine whether the slow withdrawal of chronic oral corticosteroids in patients with severe, "steroid-dependent" COPD would increase the number of exacerbations over a 6-month period. The average daily dose of prednisone at the time of enrollment was 11 mg. The study was placebo-controlled such that one arm continued the same prednisone dose while the other arm decreased their prednisone dose by 5 mg per week. Patients in both treatment arms received inhaled triamcinolone (1600 µg daily). Over the 6-month study period, patients who discontinued their prednisone did not experience a significant increase in exacerbation rate, a deterioration of respiratory symptoms, or a decline in health-related quality of life. Patients who discontinued prednisone decreased their cumulative systemic corticosteroid consumption by approximately 40% and lost about 5 kg of body weight. A major limitation of this trial is, again, the small sample size (38 patients). The study does indicate that many "steroid-dependent" COPD patients can be successfully weaned from oral corticosteroid therapy. Better information about the proper role of chronic oral corticosteroid therapy in stable COPD awaits the completion of additional, larger trials.

C.   Adverse Effects from Extended Therapy with Corticosteroids

The potential benefits of long-term preventive treatment of COPD with inhaled or oral corticosteroids must be weighed against the risks of adverse side effects. This is a particularly important consideration since these patients may already be at greater risk for certain adverse corticosteroid effects due to advanced age, cigarette smoking, and sedentary lifestyle. There is considerable evidence that long-term oral corticosteroid treatment causes significant morbidity, and these adverse effects are closely related with dose and duration of treatment (41, 66–70). There is consensus that inhaled corticosteroids represent an important advance over systemic corticosteroids in terms of the benefit-to-risk ratio, at least in asthma. However, it is also recognized that inhaled corticosteroids, particularly at higher doses, are not devoid of systemic effects. Since this class of drugs is so widely used, even mild systemic effects may pose a public health problem of some magnitude, and some of these effects may not become evident for years or even decades. Due to their constrained size and length, trials have provided only limited information about long-term consequences of corticosteroid therapy, and greater reliance must be placed on various types of observational studies.

Adrenal Suppression

The suppressive effects of single or repeated doses of systemic corticosteroids are well known. Prednisone in daily doses as low as 5 mg may cause detectable decreases in the serum cortisol levels of COPD patients (56). Adrenal insufficiency and stress-induced hemodynamic instability may occur when systemic corticosteroids are withdrawn after extended therapy. This complication is much feared but probably quite rare (66, 71).

Inhaled corticosteroids are also capable of suppressing adrenal function, but generally to a lesser extent. Lipworth performed a systematic review of 27 studies, mostly of patients with asthma (68). All inhaled corticosteroid preparations suppressed adrenal function in a dose-dependent manner. At equivalent doses, fluticasone appeared to have greater effects than the other preparations tested. In terms of adrenal function, it was estimated that a fluticasone dose of 880 μg per day was equivalent to about 9 mg of oral prednisone. Among the major COPD inhaled-corticosteroid trials, only the International COPD Study Group and ISOLDE evaluated adrenal function. Both trials administered 1000 μg of fluticasone daily as the active treatment, and both found that this intervention reduced serum cortisol levels by about 10 to 15% (57, 60). Adrenal suppression to this extent probably has little clinical significance of itself, but low cortisol levels do serve as a marker of systemic absorption, and this may provoke other adverse effects of greater clinical importance.

Osteoporosis

Osteoporosis is arguably the most feared complication of extended corticosteroid therapy, and it can result in pain, increased dyspnea from thoracic vertebral compression fractures, and possibly increased mortality (72). A huge (288,470 subjects) retrospective case-control study reported that extended oral corticosteroid therapy for a variety of medical conditions confers a substantial, dose-dependent risk for fractures at multiple sites (73).

McEvoy and associates performed a cross-sectional study of 312 COPD patients that included three groups: (1) no history of inhaled or systemic corticosteroid use, (2) inhaled but no systemic corticosteroid use, and (3) systemic corticosteroid use (74). Patients with more than 6 months of lifetime exposure to prednisone had more than double the risk for having at least one vertebral fracture compared to patients with no history of corticosteroid use (adjusted OR 2.36; 95% CI 1.26 to 4.38). In addition, fractures in the oral corticosteroid group were more likely to be multiple, to be classified as severe, and to be associated with pain. Intermittent prednisone use (for more than 2 weeks but less than 6 months) or inhaled corticosteroid use was also associated with increased vertebral fracturing, but these changes were not statistically significant.

In another observational study, Iqbal and colleagues found that extended prednisone therapy had a pronounced adverse effect on bone mineral density in patients with COPD (75). They also noted a trend toward lower bone mineral densities in patients who used inhaled corticosteroids.

It has not been shown that long-term inhaled corticosteroid administration for COPD causes an increase in bone fracture rate, but numerous studies, mostly in asthmatic subjects, indicate that inhaled corticosteroids do adversely affect surrogate, biochemical markers of bone metabolism (68, 76). There is a puzzling inconsistency among these various studies, but in general, the larger the dose, the greater the effect. Two of the multicenter trials of inhaled corticosteroids in COPD measured bone mineral density in subsets of their subjects. In the EUROSCOP study, budesonide, 800 μg daily for 3 years, compared with placebo, caused a seemingly paradoxical reduction in the rate of decline in bone density in the femur

(59). This contrasts with the results from the Lung Health Study, which also measured bone mineral density in a subject subset (61). In comparison with the placebo group, they found that triamcinolone decreased bone mineral density in the femur and lumber spine by a small but statistically significant amount. EUROSCOP and ISOLDE reported no treatment-related differences in bone fracture rates, but sample sizes were not large enough and follow-ups were not long enough to detect relatively small differences (59, 61).

Ocular Effects

Chronic use of systemic corticosteroids constitutes a significant risk factor for the development of posterior subcapsular cataracts (77). Two case-controlled studies involving patients with a variety of respiratory disorders failed to discern an elevated risk for cataract development from oral corticosteroid use (67, 68). However, such a risk was identified in other studies of asthmatics that specifically focused on ocular complications (78, 79).

Inhaled corticosteroids also appear to confer a substantial risk of cataract development. Three large case-controlled studies in older adults have shown a highly significant association between the development of posterior subcapsular cataracts with the dose and duration of inhaled corticosteroid treatment (adjusted OR from 1.5 to 3.06) (80–82). High doses of inhaled corticosteroids have also been associated with an increased risk of ocular hypertension and open angle glaucoma (83).

Glucose Intolerance

Glucose intolerance is a common adverse effect of prolonged treatment with oral steroids. In a meta-analysis of 93 clinical trials involving 3335 patients who were given oral corticosteroids for a variety of conditions, treatment for longer than 3 months caused an approximately 50% increase in the occurrence of hyperglycemia and diabetes (41). Two case-controlled studies of 600 patients treated with corticosteroids for respiratory disease reported similar increases in the risk of diabetes (66, 67).

Trials and systematic reviews have not identified an increased incidence of glucose intolerance from inhaled corticosteroids (61, 68), but a few scattered case reports suggest that high doses may cause new-onset diabetes or loss of diabetic control (84, 85).

Infection

Chronic oral corticosteroids carry a small but statistically significant risk of serious infection from a variety of opportunistic and usual infections (86). A meta-analysis of 71 randomized trials that included 4198 patients with a variety of pulmonary and nonpulmonary diagnoses found a relative risk from infection of 1.6 (95% CI 1.3–1.9) in patients treated with a daily prednisone dose of >10 mg or a cumulative dose of > 700 mg (42). Serious infectious complications from inhaled corticosteroids appear to be rare, but two cases of pulmonary aspergillosis were reported in patients who were taking high doses of fluticasone (87, 88).

Skin and Cosmetic Changes

Thinning of the skin and easy bruisability occur in 50 to 80% of patients who take chronic oral corticosteroids (66, 89). Features of Cushing's syndrome, such as acne, moon facies, buffalo hump, truncal obesity, weight gain, and fluid retention, are also common and, for many patients, distressing side effects of chronic prednisone therapy (41, 66). Skin changes are not prominent with low doses of inhaled corticosteroids, but bruisability occurs in up to one-half of patients who take higher doses (89). An approximately twofold increase in the incidence of bruising was noted in several of the multicenter inhaled corticosteroid trials for COPD (59–61).

Other Effects

It has been suggested that chronic prednisone therapy causes hypertension (66, 67), but many studies are retrospective, uncontrolled, and fail to adjust for age-related changes (90). A meta-analysis of clinical trials indicated that systemic corticosteroids may confer some risk of hypertension, but details concerning case definition and descriptions of methodology were lacking in many of the trials (41). There is little information about the effects of inhaled corticosteroids on blood pressure (68). Only one of the multicenter trials of inhaled corticosteroids in COPD reported on hypertension, and in that study no effect was observed (59).

A variety of psychiatric disorders have been reported with chronic oral corticosteroid therapy, but these effects are probably rare with the low doses usually employed for COPD (47, 91). There was no increase in mental disturbances in a case-controlled series of 550 respiratory patients treated with chronic corticosteroids, only 30 of whom received more than 20 mg of prednisone per day (67). Adverse psychiatric effects from inhaled corticosteroids have been described in a few isolated case reports only (92–94).

Inhaled corticosteroids commonly cause nonspecific oral irritation, thrush, and dysphonia. This has been a consistent finding in large trials and it may affect up to 10% of patients (57, 59–61).

D. Summary

It is very clear that inhaled corticosteroids do not alter the natural history of COPD, as defined by the rate of decline in the FEV_1 over time (57, 59–61). Inhaled corticosteroids may reduce the number of exacerbations and improve selected other health outcomes in patients with severe COPD (57, 60, 61). It bears emphasizing that these health benefits were not a primary outcome in any of the trials cited, and they were achieved with relatively high doses of inhaled corticosteroids sufficient to produce discernible systemic effects. Any potential benefits of inhaled corticosteroids in COPD must be weighed against the risk of adverse drug effects. Several observational studies have implicated inhaled corticosteroids as a potent factor for the development of cataracts in elderly patients, and they may also contribute to the development of osteoporosis (68, 76, 80–82). An observational study suggesting that inhaled corticosteroids substantially reduce mortality and hospitalization rates in patients with severe COPD requires confirmation by clinical trial (62).

Available data suggest that long-term, low-dose prednisone is of limited benefit and may be safely withdrawn in many COPD patients who are using inhaled corticosteroids. However, the question of efficacy has not been assessed in a large clinical trial. Chronic prednisone is a major risk factor for the development of osteoporotic fractures, cataracts, and other adverse effects. Because of its poor risk-to-benefit ratio, an expert panel recently recommended against the use of chronic prednisone for COPD (95).

V.   Do Corticosteroid-Responsive and -Nonresponsive COPD Patients Exist?

Given the maginal benefits of corticosteroid therapy in COPD as well as their attendant side effects, it would be useful to identify those patients most likely to benefit. Current guidelines recommend a trial of inhaled or systemic corticosteroids in patients with severe COPD, using spirometry to identify those responsive patients who would presumably gain the most from long-term treatment (95). Existing clinical trials do not support this practice (60, 96), but the recommendation reflects a widespread perception that subsets of corticosteroid responders and nonresponders are to be found among COPD patients.

Responsiveness is usually defined in terms of FEV_1 improvement after a relatively short course or oral or inhaled corticosteroids. In a placebo-controlled, cross-over study, Mendella and colleagues found that stable COPD patients exhibited an apparent bimodal response to two weeks of oral methylprednisolone; 8 of 46 subjects had an average improvement of 54%, while the average response in the remainder was not significantly different from placebo (97). However, other studies of a similar design were unsuccessful in identifying such patients (98–100). Moreover, two recent multicenter trials, one in patients with stable COPD and the other in patients with exacerbated COPD, also found a relatively homogeneous response to systemic corticosteroids without evidence of a discrete responsive subset (101, 102). While these results appear to rule out a simple binary response pattern, they do not exclude other more subtle variations in corticosteroid responses.

It has been frequently suggested that certain features of asthma, such as the presence of wheezing, bronchodilator response, positive skin tests, and eosinophilia might serve as predictors of short-term steroid-responsiveness in patients with COPD (18, 24, 97, 99, 100, 103). Accumulating evidence identifies lung eosino-philia as the most promising of these predictors. Earlier studies of sputum and blood eosinophilia yielded inconsistent results (97–99). More recent single-blinded studies suggested that eosinophils in sputum, bronchoalveolar lavage, and bronchial biopsies predicted a larger FEV_1 response to oral corticosteroids (25, 26). Brightling and his associates confirmed these findings in a fully blinded, crossover trial (27). They randomized 67 patients and measured a sixfold reduction in mean sputum eosinophil count following 30 mg prednisolone daily for 2 weeks. They also found that sputum eosinophilia correlated strongly with corticosteroid responses. Those patients with the highest baseline sputum eosinophil counts had the most favorable outcomes in terms of spirometry, respiratory symptoms, and walking distance.

These provocative results suggest that a relatively simple laboratory test might permit clinicians to prescribe corticosteroids to COPD patients in a more rational manner. Confirmatory clinical studies are needed for both inhaled and systemic corticosteroid therapy in COPD.

References

1. Connors AF Jr, Dawson NV, Thomas C, Harrell FE Jr, Desbiens N, Fulkerson WJ, Kussin P, Bellamy P, Goldman L, Knaus WA. Outcomes following acute exacerbation of severe chronic obstructive lung disease. The SUPPORT investigators (Study to Understand Prognoses and Preferences for Outcomes and Risks of Treatments). Am J Respir Crit Care Med 1996; 154:959–967. [Erratum, Am J Respir Crit Care Med 1997; 155:386.]
2. Wilson R. The role of infection in COPD. Chest 1998; 115:242S–248S.
3. Nichol KL, Baken L, Nelson A. Relation between influenza vaccination and outpatient visits, hospitalization, and mortality in elderly persons with chronic lung disease. Ann Intern Med 1999; 130:397–403.
4. Nichol KL, Baken L, Wuorenma J. The health and economic benefits associated with pneumococcal vaccination of elderly persons with chronic lung disease. Arch Intern Med 1999;159: 2437–2442.
5. Jackevicius C, Joyce DP, Kesten S, Chapman KR. Prehospitalization inhaled corticosteroid use in patients with COPD or asthma. Chest 1997; 111:296–302.
6. Rowe BH, Keller JL, Oxman AD. Effectiveness of steroid therapy in acute exacerbations of asthma: a meta-analysis. Am J Emerg Med 1992; 10:301–310.
7. Niewoehner DE, Kleinerman J, Rice DB. Pathological changes in the peripheral airways of young cigarette smokers. N Engl J Med 1974; 291:755–758.
8. Martin TR, Raghu U, Maunder J, Springmeyer SC. The effects of chronic bronchitis and chronic airflow obstruction on lung cell populations recovered by broncho-alveolar lavage. Am J Respir Crit Care Med 1985; 132:254–260.
9. Thompson ABV, Daughton D, Robbins GA, Ghafouri MA, Oehklerking M, Rennard SI. Intraluminal airway inflammation in chronic bronchitis. Characterization and correlation with clinical parameters. Am J Respir Crit Care Med 1989; 140:1527–1537.
10. Lacoste JY, Bousquet J, Chanez P, Van Vyve T, Simony-Lafontaine J, Lequeu N, Vic P, Enander I, Michel FB. Eosinophilic and neutrophilic inflammation in asthma, chronic bronchitis and chronic obstructive pulmonary disease. J Allergy Clin Immunol 1993; 92:537–548.
11. Ollerenshaw SL, Woolcock AJ. Characteristics of the inflammation in biopsies from large airways of subjects with chronic airflow limitation. Am Rev Respir Dis 1992; 145:922–927.
12. Saetta M. Airway inflammation in chronic obstructive pulmonary disease. Am J Respir Crit Care Med 1999; 150(5 part 2):S17–S20.

13. Saetta M, Di Stefano A, Maestrelli P, Turato G, Ruggieri MP, Roggeri A, Calcagni P, Mapp CE, Ciaccia A, Fabbri LM. Activated T-lymphocytes and macrophages in bronchial mucosa of subjects with chronic bronchitis. Am Rev Respir Dis 1993; 147:301–306.

14. Jeffrey PK. Structural and inflammatory changes in COPD: a comparison with asthma. Thorax 1998; 53:129–136.

15. O'Shaughnessy TC, Ansari TW, Barnes NC, Jeffrey PK. Inflammation in bronchial biopsies of subjects with chronic bronchitis: inverse relationship of CD8+ T lymphocyte with FEV1. Am J Respir Crit Care Med 1997; 155:852–857.

16. Fournier M, Lebargy F, Le Roy Ladurie F, Lenormand E, Pariente R. Intraepithelial T-lymphocyte subsets in the airways of normal subjects and of patients with chronic bronchitis. Am Rev Respir Dis 1989; 140:737–742.

17. Barnes PJ. New therapies for chronic obstructive pulmonary disease. Thorax 1998; 53:137–147.

18. Keatings VM, Jatakanon A, Wordsell YM, Barnes PJ. Effects of inhaled and oral glucocorticoids on inflammatory indices in asthma and COPD. Am J Respir Crit Care Med 1997; 155:542–548.

19. Bhowmik A, Seemungal TAR, Sapsford RJ, Wedzicha JA. Relation of sputum inflammatory markers to symptoms and lung function changes in COPD exacerbations. Thorax 2000; 55:114–120.

20. Saetta M, Di Stefano A, Maestrelli P, Turato G, Ruggieri MP, Roggeri A, Calcagni P, Mapp CE, Ciaccia A, Fabbri LM. Airway eosinophilia in chronic bronchitis during exacerbations. Am J Respir Crit Care Med 1994; 150:1646–1652.

21. Gompertz S, Bayley DL, Hill SL, Stockley RA. Relationship between airway inflammation and the frequency of exacerbations in patients with smoking related COPD. Thorax 2001; 56:36–41.

22. Jantz MA, Sahn SA. Corticosteroids in acute respiratory failure. Am J Respir Crit Care Med 1999; 160:1079–1100.

23. Barnes PJ. Anti-inflammatory actions of glucocorticoids: molecular mechanisms. Clin Sci 1998; 94:557–572.

24. Harding SM, Freedman S. A comparison of oral and inhaled steroids in patients with chronic airways obstruction: features determining response. Thorax 1978; 33:214–218.

25. Pizzichini E, Pizzichini MMM, Gibson P, Parameswaran K, Gleich GJ, Berman L, Dolovich J, Hargreave FE. Sputum eosinophilia predicts benefit from prednisone in smokers with chronic obstructive bronchitis. Am J Respir Crit Care Med 1998; 158:1511–1517.

26. Chanez P, Vignola AM, O'Shaugnessy T, Enander I, Li D, Jeffery PK, Bousquet J. Corticosteroid reversibility in COPD is related to features of asthma. Am J Respir Crit Care Med 1997; 155:1529–1534.

27. Brightling CE, Monteiro W, Ward R, Parker D, Morgan MDL, Wardlaw AJ, Pavord ID. Sputum eosinophilia and short term response to prednisolone in chronic obstructive pulmonary disease: a randomised trial. Lancet 2000; 356:1480–1485.

28. Dentener MA, Creutzberg EC, Schols AMWJ, Mantovani A, van't Veer C, Buurman WA, Wouters EFM. Systemic anti-inflammatory mediators in COPD: increase in soluble interleukin 1 receptor during treatment of exacerbations. Thorax 2001; 56:721–726.

29. Confalonieri M, Mainardi E, Della porta R, Bernorio S, Gandola L, Beghe B, Spanevello A. Inhaled corticosteroids reduce neutrophilic bronchial inflammation in patients with chronic obstructive pulmonary disease. Thorax 1998; 53:583–585.

30. Culpitt SV, Maziak W, Loukdis S, Nightingale JA, Matthews JL, Barnes PJ. Effect of high dose inhaled steroid on cells, cytokines and proteases in induced sputum in chronic obstructive pulmonary disease. Am J Respir Crit Care Med 1999; 160:1635–1639:

31. Llewellyn-Jones CG, Harris TAJ, Stockley RA. Effect of fluticasone propionate on sputum of patients with chronic bronchitis and emphysema. Am J Respir Crit Care Med 1996; 153:616–621.

32. Balbi B, Majori M, Bertacco S, Convertino A, Cuomo A, Donner CF, Pesci A. Inhaled corticosteroids in COPD patients; do they have effects on cells and molecular mediators of airway inflammation? Chest 2000; 117:1633–1637.

33. Albert RK, Martin TR, Lewis SW. Controlled clinical trial of methylprednisolone in patients with chronic bronchitis and acute respiratory insufficiency. Ann Intern Med 1980; 92:753–758.

34. Emerman CL, Connors AF, Lukens TW, May ME, Effron D. A randomized controlled trial of methylprednisolone in the emergency treatment of acute exacerbations of COPD. Chest 1989; 95:563–567.

35. Bullard MJ, Liaw S-J, Tsai Y-H, Min HP. Early corticosteroid use in acute exacerbations of chronic airflow obstruction. Am J Emerg Med 1996; 14:139–143.

36. Thompson WH, Nielson CP, Carvalho P Charan NB, Crowley JJ. Controlled trial of oral prednisone in outpatients with acute COPD exacerbation. Am J Respir Crit Care Med 1996; 154:407–412.

37. Wood-Baker R, Walters EH. Corticosteroids for acute exacerbations of chronic obstructive pulmonary disease (Cochrane Review). In: The Cochrane Library, Issue 2, 2000. Oxford: Update Software.

38. Niewoehner DE, Erbland ML, Deupree RH, Collins D, Gross NJ, Light RW, Anderson P, Morgan NA. Effect of systemic glucocorticoids on exacerbations of chronic obstructive pulmonary disease. N Engl J Med 1999; 340:1941–1947.

39. Davies L, Angus RM, Calverley PMA. Oral corticosteroids in patients admitted to hospital with exacerbations of chronic obstructive pulmonary disease: a prospective randomised controlled trial. Lancet 1999; 354:456–460.

40. Pagano G, Bruno A, Cavallo-Perin P, Cesco L, Imbimbo B. Glucose intolerance after short-term administration of corticosteroids in healthy subjects. Prednisone, deflazacort, and betamethasone. Arch Intern Med 1989; 149:1098–1101.

41. Conn H, Poynard T. Corticosteroids and peptic ulcer: meta-analysis of adverse events during steroid therapy. J Intern Med 1994; 236:619–632.

42. Stuck AF, Minder CE, Frey FJ. Risk of infectious complications in patients taking glucocorticoids. Rev Infect Dis 1989; 11:954–963.

43. Weist PM, Flanigan T, Salata RA, Schleas DM, Katzman M, Lederman MM. Serious infectious complications of corticosteroid therapy for COPD. Chest 1989; 95:1180–1184.

44. Rodrigues J, Niederman MS, Fein AM, Pai PB. Nonresolving pneumonia in steroid-treated patients with obstructive lung disease. Am J Med 1992; 93:29–34.

45. Palmer LB, Greenberg HE, Schiff MJ. Corticosteroid treatment as a risk factor for invasive aspergillosis in patients with lung disease. Thorax 1991; 46:15–20.

46. Jiva TM, Kallay MC, Marin MG, Poe RH. Simultaneous legionellosis and invasive aspergillosis in immunocompetent patient newly treated with corticosteroids. Chest 1993; 104:1929–1931.

47. Boston Collaborative Drug Surveillance Program. Acute adverse reactions to prednisone in relation to dosage. Clin Pharm Ther 1972; 13:694–698.

48. Decramer M, Lacquet LM, Fagard R, Rogiers P. Corticosteroids contribute to muscle weakness in chronic airflow obstruction. Am J Respir Crit Care Med 1994; 150:11–16.

49. CPC case 11-1997. N Engl J Med 1997; 336:1079–1088.

50. Douglas JA, Tuxen DV, Home M, Scheinkestel CD, Weinmann M, Czarny D, Bowes G. Myopathy in severe asthma. Am Rev Respir Dis 1992; 146:517–519.

51. Conn HO, Blitzer BL. Nonassociation of adrenocorticosteroid therapy and peptic ulcer. N Engl J Med 1976; 294:473–479.

52. Sayner A, Aytemur ZA, Cirit M, Unsal I. Systemic glucocorticoids in severe exacerbations of COPD. Chest 2001; 119:726–730.

53. O'Driscoll BR, Kaira S, Wilson M, Pickering CAC, Carroll KB, Woodcock AA. Double-blind trial of steroid tapering in acute asthma. Lancet 1993; 341:324–327.

54. Kerstjens HAM, Brand PLP, Hughes MD, Robinson NJ, Postma DS, Sluiter HJ, Bleeker ER, Dekhuijzen PNR, de Jong PCM, Mengelers HJJ, Overbeek SE, Schoonbrood DFME, and the Dutch Chronic Non-Specific Lung Disease Study Group. New Engl J Med 1992; 327:1413–1419.

55. Dompeling E, van Schayck CP, van Grunsven PM, van Herwaarden C, Akkermans RP, Molema J, Folgering H, van Weel C. Slowing the deterioration of asthma and chronic obstructive pulmonary disease observed during bronchodilator therapy by adding inhaled corticosteroids. Ann Intern Med 1993; 118:770–778.

56. Renkema TEJ, Schouten JP, Koëter GH, Postma DS. Effects of long-term treatment with corticosteroids in COPD. Chest 1996; 109:1156–1162.

57. Paggiaro PL, Dahle R, Bakran I, Frith L, Hollingworth K, Efthimiou J, on behalf of the International COPD Study group. Multicentre randomised placebo-controlled trial of inhaled fluticasone propionate in patients with chronic obstructive pulmonary disease. Lancet 1998; 351:773–780.

58. Vestbo J, Sorensen T, Lange P, Brix A, Tone P, Viskum K. Long-term effect of inhaled budesonide in mild and moderate chronic obstructive pulmonary disease: a randomized controlled trial. Lancet 1999; 353:1819–1823.

59. Pauwels RA, Lofdahl C-G, Laitinen LA, Schouten JP, Postma DS, Pride NB, Ohlsson SV, for the European Respiratory Society Study on Chronic Obstructive Pulmonary Disease. Long-term treatment with inhaled budesonide in persons with mild chronic obstructive pulmonary disease who continue smoking. N Engl J Med 1999; 340:1948–1953.

60. Burge PS, Calverley PMA, Jones PW, Spencer S, Anderson JA, Maslen TK, on behalf of the ISOLDE study investigators. Randomised, double blind, placebo controlled study of fluticasone propionate in patients with moderate to severe chronic obstructive pulmonary disease: the ISOLDE trial. BMJ 2000; 320:1297–1303.

61. Lung Health Study Research Group. Effect of inhaled triamcinolone on the decline in pulmonary function in chronic obstructive pulmonary disease. N Engl J Med 2000; 343:1902–1909.

62. Sin DD, Tu JV. Inhaled corticosteroids and the risk of mortality and readmission in elderly patients with chronic obstructive pulmonary disease. Am J Respir Crit Care Med 2001; 164:580–584.

63. Van Andel AE, Reisner C, Menjoge SS, Witek TJ. Analysis of inhaled corticosteroid and oral theophylline use among patients with stable COPD from 1987 to 1995. Chest 1999; 115:703–707.

64. Callahan CM, Dittus RS, Katz BP. Oral corticosteroid therapy for patients with stable chronic obstructive pulmonary disease: a meta-analysis. Ann Intern Med 1991; 114:216–223.

65. Rice KL, Rubins JB, Lebahn F, et al. Withdrawal of chronic corticosteroid treatment in patients with COPD: a randomized trial. Am J Respir Crit Care Med 2000; 162:174–178.

66. Lieberman, P, Patterson R, Kunske R. Complications of long-term steroid therapy for asthma. J Allergy Clin Immunol 1972; 49:329–336.

67. Smyllie H, Connolly C. Incidence of serious complications of corticosteroid therapy in respiratory disease. Thorax 1968; 23:571–581.

68. Lipworth BJ. Systemic adverse effects of inhaled corticosteroid therapy. A systematic review and meta-analysis. Arch Intern Med 1999; 159:941–955.

69. Schlaghecke R, Kornely E, Santen R, Ridderskamp P. The effect of long-term glucocorticoid therapy on pituitary-adrenal responses to exogenous corticotropin-releasing hormone. N Engl J Med 1992; 326:226–230.

70. Walsh LJ, Wong CA, Oborne J, Cooper S, Lewis SA, Pringle M, Hubbard R, Tattersfield AE. Adverse effects of oral corticosteroids in relation to dose in patients with lung disease. Thorax 2001; 56:279–284.

71. Christy NP. Pituitary-adrenal function during corticosteroid therapy: learning to live with uncertainty. N Engl J Med 1992; 326:266–267.

72. Iqbal MM. Osteoporosis: epidemiology, diagnosis, and treatment. South Med J 2000; 93:2–18.

73. Van Staa TP, Leufkens HG, Abenhaim L, Zhang B, Cooper C. Use of oral corticosteroids and risk of fractures. J Bone Miner Res 2000; 15:993–1000.

74. McEvoy CE, Ensrud KE, Bender E, Genant HK, Yu W, Griffith JM, Niewoehner DE. Association between corticosteroid use and vertebral fractures in older men with chronic obstructive pulmonary disease. Am J Respir Crit Care Med 1998; 157:704–709.

75. Iqbal F, Michaelson J, Thaler L, Rubin J, Roman J, Nanes MS. Declining bone mass in men with chronic pulmonary disease: contribution of glucocorticoid treatment, body mass index, and gonadal function. Chest 1999; 116:1616–1624.

76. Goldstein MF, Fallon JJ Jr, Harning R. Chronic glucocorticoid therapy-induced osteoporosis in patients with obstructive lung disease. Chest 1999; 116:1733–1749.

77. Hodge WG, Whicher JP, Satariano W. Risk factors for age-related cataracts. Epidemiol Rev 1995; 17:336–346.

78. Toogood J, Markov A, Baskerville J, et al. Association of ocular cataracts with inhaled and oral steroid therapy during long-term treatment of asthma. J Allergy Clin Immunol 1993; 91:571–579.

79. Urban R Jr, Collier E. Corticosteroid-induced cataracts. Surv Ophthalmol 1986; 31:102–110.

80. Cumming RG, Mitchell P, Leeder SR. Use of inhaled corticosteroids and the risk of cataracts. N Engl J Med 1997; 337:8–14.

81. Garbe E, Suissa S, LeLorier J. Association of inhaled corticosteroid use with cataract extraction in elderly patients. JAMA 1998; 280:539–543.

82. Jick SS, Vasilakis-Scaramozza C, Maier WC. The risk of cataract among users of inhaled steroid. Epidemiology 2001; 12:229–234.

83. Garbe E, LeLorier J, Boivin JF, Suissa S. Inhaled and nasal glucocorticoids and the risks of ocular hypertension or open-angle glaucoma. JAMA 1997; 277:722–727.

84. Faul JL, Tormey W, Tormey V, Burke C. High dose inhaled corticosteroids and dose dependent loss of diabetic control. BMJ 1998; 317:1491.

85. Faul JL, Cormican U, Tormey VJ, Tormey WP, Burke CM. Deteriorating diabetic control associated with high-dose inhaled budesonide. Eur Respir 1999; 14:242–243.

86. Dale DC, Petersdorf RG. Corticosteroids and infectious diseases. Med Clin N Am 1973; 57:1277–1287.
87. Fairfax AJ, David V, Douce G. Laryngeal aspergillosis following high dose inhaled fluticasone therapy for asthma. Thorax 1999; 54:860–861.
88. Leav BA, Fanburg B, Hadley S. Invasive pulmonary aspergillosis associated with high-dose inhaled fluticasone. N Engl J Med 2000; 343:586.
89. Capewell S, Reynolds S, Shuttleworth D, Finlay AY. Purpura and dermal thinning associated with high dose inhaled corticosteroids. BMJ 1990; 300:1548–1551.
90. Jackson SW, Beevers D, Myers K. Does long-term low-dose corticosteroid therapy cause hypertension? Clin Sci 1981; 61(suppl):381–383.
91. Ling MHM, Perry PJ, Tsuang MT. Side effects of corticosteroid therapy. Arch Gen Psychiatry 1981; 38:471–477.
92. Lewis L, Cochrane G. Psychosis in child inhaling budesonide. Lancet 1983; 2:634.
93. Meysboom R. Budesonide and psychotic side effects. Ann Intern Med 1988; 109:683.
94. Connett G, Lenney W. Inhaled budesonide and behavioral disturbances. Lancet 1991; 228:634–635.
95. Pawels RA, Buist AS, Calverley PMA, Jenkins CR, Hurd SS. Global strategy for the diagnosis, management and prevention of chronic obstructive pulmonary disease: NHLBI/WHO global initiative for chronic obstructive pulmonary disease (GOLD) workshop summary. Am J Respir Crit Care Med 2001; 163:1256–1276 (www.goldcopd.com).
96. Senderovitz T, Vestbo J, Frandsen J, Maltbaek N, Norgaard M, Nielsen C, Kampmann JP. Steroid reversibility test followed by inhaled budesonide or placebo in patients with stable chronic obstructive pulmonary disease. The Danish Society of Respiratory Medicine. Respir Med 1999; 93:715–718.
97. Mendella LA, Manfreda J, Warren PW, Anthonisen NR. Steroid response in stable chronic obstructive pulmonary disease. Ann Intern Med 1982; 96:17–21.
98. Shim S, Stover DE, Williams MH Jr. Response to corticosteroids in chronic bronchitis. J Allergy Clin Immunol 1978; 62:363–367.
99. Blair GP, Light RW. Treatment of chronic obstructive pulmonary disease with corticosteroids: comparison of daily vs. alternate-day therapy. Chest 1984; 86:524–528.
100. Eliasson O, Hoffman J, Trueb D, Frederick D, McCormick JR. Corticosteroids in COPD: a clinical trial and reassessment of the literature. Chest 1986; 89:484–490.
101. Niewoehner DE, Collins D, Erbland ML. Relation of FEV_1 to clinical outcomes during exacerbations of chronic obstructive pulmonary disease. Am J Respir Crit Care Med 2000; 161:1201–1205.
102. Calverley PMA, Daniels JE. The acute effects of oral prednisolone in patients with COPD in the ISOLDE trial: responders and nonresponders. Am J Respir Crit Care Med 1996; 53(Part 2):A126.
103. Syed A, Hoeppner VH, Cockcroft DW. Prediction of nonresponse to corticosteroids in stable chronic airflow limitation. Clin Invest Med 1991; 14:28–34.

23

Oxygen Therapy During Acute Exacerbations of Chronic Obstructive Pulmonary Disease

IOANNA MITROUSKA and NIKOS M. SIAFAKAS

University Hospital of Heraklion
Heraklion, Crete, Greece

I. Introduction

Hypoxemia is frequently observed during acute exacerbation of COPD (1, 2), because of worsening of V'/Q' mismatching, and in some cases hypoventilation may also be a contributing factor. On the other hand, an increase in right-to-left shunt is not considered to be a predominant mechanism. Profound hypoxemia (PaO_2 < 60 mmHg) may lead to tissue hypoxia and cause life-threatening complications, such as myocardial, adrenal, and hepatic dysfunction as well as hypoxic encephalopathy. Obviously, treatment of this condition is oxygen therapy, the administration of increased fraction of inspired oxygen (F_IO_2). Oxygen therapy is the cornerstone of the management of severe, acute exacerbations of COPD (1–3). However, when the priority is to correct arterial hypoxemia, the other factors involved in the delivery of O_2 (hemoglobin [Hb], cardiac output) should also be taken into account (4, 5). Administration of O_2 in patients with an acute exacerbation is not without risks. Thus, as with any other drug, O_2 delivery needs proper management, having indications as well as side effects.

II. Goals of O_2 Therapy

The goal of O_2 therapy during acute exacerbations of COPD is to increase PaO_2 above 60 mmHg or to produce an arterial oxygen saturation (SaO_2) >89 to 90%.

Due to the shape of the O_2 dissociation curve, increasing the PaO_2 to values greater than 60 mmHg adds little benefit but, on the other hand, it may considerably increase the risk of CO_2 retention. It follows that O_2 therapy should be titrated to raise PaO_2 to just above 60 mmHg (6–8). Although SaO_2 can be measured noninvasively and continuously using an oximeter, it is recommended that arterial carbon dioxide tension ($PaCO_2$) and pH should be monitored, while initially titrating the O_2 flow settings and frequently thereafter until reaching a steady-state condition. It should be noted that due to lung inhomogeneity it may take 20 to 30 min to achieve a steady state after a change in F_IO_2 (1, 2, 9). Hence, measurements of arterial blood gases at shorter intervals may be misleading.

III. Physiological Effects of O_2 Therapy

Oxygen therapy provides enormous benefits in hypoxemic patients with acute exacerbations of COPD. By increasing PaO_2 pulmonary vasoconstriction, right-heart strain and global myocardial ischemia are reduced and oxygen delivery is increased (1, 2, 10, 11). Esteban et al. (12) administered controlled oxygen therapy (titrated to keep PaO_2 above 55 mmHg) in patients with acute exacerbation of COPD and severe hypoxemia ($PaO_2 < 45$ mmHg). They observed that O_2 therapy increased the O_2 delivery by approximately 74% due to an increase in arterial O_2 content. Systemic vascular resistance and cardiac output remained unchanged, while pulmonary vascular resistance decreased slightly (Fig. 1). The oxygen extraction ratio decreased by 32%. However, this pattern of hemodynamic response may not be observed in all patients (13, 14). It has been shown that some patients may respond to O_2 therapy by a decrease in cardiac output, which is associated with an unchanged O_2 delivery. The last pattern is usually observed in patients with relatively low mixed venous O_2 tension and oxygen delivery/oxygen consumption ratio (15–17).

Apart from hemodynamic effects, O_2 therapy may have other beneficial effects in hypoxemic patients with acute exacerbation of COPD. There is a substantial amount of evidence supporting the hypothesis that improving oxygen delivery to the lung enhances pulmonary defenses and augments mucociliary transport. Whether these effects are translated to better clinical outcome is not known (18). O_2 therapy may also increase cognitive function as well as function of other organs (19). It has been shown that administering O_2 in patients with COPD causes renal vasodilation, the magnitude of which is equivalent to that observed with low-dose dopamine (20). An O_2-related increase of both the urinary Na^+ excretion and the fractional excretion of filtered sodium have been also demonstrated. It appears that O_2 therapy may play a role in decreasing the edematous state, common in acute exacerbation of COPD, by interfering with renal function (21, 22).

IV. Modes of O_2 Delivery

The oldest method of O_2 delivery during acute exacerbation is via a dual-prong nasal cannulae, which has the advantages of low cost and comfort, and acceptability to

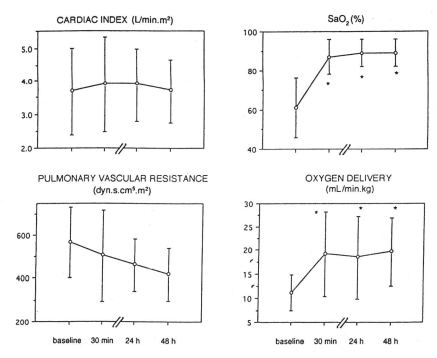

Figure 1 Changes in hemodynamic and oxgyen transport variables after administering oxygen to patients with acute exacerbation of COPD. *Indicates $p < 0.05$ for comparison with baseline. (From Ref. 12, with permission.)

most patients. The major disadvantage of this method is that the F_IO_2 cannot be precisely controlled because it is affected by the route of inhalation (mouth or nose), upper airway geometry, and breathing pattern. Therefore, by using this method of O_2 delivery, patients run the risk of under- or overtreatment. With this method, a deleterious increase of $PaCO_2$ (see below) is always a consideration. Keeping in mind that F_IO_2 may change from moment to moment, it can be estimated approximately using the following equation:

$$F_IO_2 = 20\% + (4 \times O_2 \text{ L/min})$$

Because of the above-mentioned drawbacks, delivery of O_2 by nasal prongs is not the method of choice in patients with acute exacerbation of COPD. Currently, the best method of delivering O_2 to patients during acute exacerbation is via a Venturi mask (2). These high-flow O_2 devices generally incorporate a dilution apparatus that reduces the final concentration of O_2 by entraining and adding air to the O_2 stream using the Venturi principle (23, 24). The amount of air entrained depends on the physical design of the apparatus. Use of these devices implies that the clinician wants the patient's actual F_IO_2 to be the same as the concentration delivered. This obviously requires that the volume-rate of delivery exceeds the patient's demand for inspired gas. Otherwise the O_2 mixture will be further diluted by room air inspired into the airways from around the O_2 delivery system. This becomes a major problem in tachypneic patients who have rapid inspiratory flow rates, and the problem is compounded by the rather insufficient delivery devices available. The total flow of gas through a delivery system containing an entrainment device that provides a certain flow of O_2 can be calculated as follows:

$$V'_{TOTAL}(L/min) = V'_IO_2 + V'_Iair$$

The flow of O_2 (V'_IO_2 in L/min) is set by the O_2 regulator and the final O_2 concentration delivered by the device (F_IO_2) can be easily measured with a portable O_2 analyzer or assumed to be correct as stated by the manufacturer. The flow of entrained air containing 21% O_2 can be calculated by solving for the amount of O_2 in the system:

$$F_IO_2(V'_IO_2 + V'_Iair) = (V'_IO_2 \times 1.0) + (V'_Iair \times 0.21)$$

So $V'_Iair = V'_IO_2 \times (1 - F_IO_2)/(F_IO_2 - 0.21)$
For example, a Venturi device set to deliver 31% O_2 and powered by 6 L/min O_2 would entrain:

$$V'_Iair = 6 \times (1 - 0.31)/(0.31 - 0.21) = 41.4 \text{ L/min}$$

This method has the advantage of delivering, precisely and constantly, the desired F_IO_2, provided that the F_IO_2 is $< 40\%$ (2, 9). With $F_IO_2 > 40\%$, the total flow delivered to the patient by the apparatus is reduced considerably. This under certain circumstances (high patients-inspiratory-flow demands) may decrease the actual F_IO_2 that the patient receives. It has been shown that compared with nasal prongs the Venturi mask is more efficient in achieving the target PaO_2 in patients with acute exacerbation of COPD.

The operation of a Venturi mask is based on the Bernoulli principle. One hundred percent O_2 flowing through a narrow orifice results in a high-velocity stream that entrains room air through multiple open side ports at the base of the mask. The amount of room air entrained to dilute the O_2 depends on the orifice size. A Venturi mask can provide F_IO_2 levels from 24 to 40% with great accuracy. Higher F_IO_2 is difficult to achieve because the total flow to the patient delivered by the Venturi mask may not meet the patient's flow demand, in which case room air (21% O_2) will be the additional flow and, depending on that, the final F_IO_2 will be reduced (Fig. 2).

Other systems for O_2 administration during acute exacerbation of COPD are used when very high concentrations ($F_IO_2 > 50\%$) of oxygen are needed. This, however, is uncommon in acute exacerbation of COPD and other causes for hypoxemia should be considered. A full-face mask with reservoir and one-way valve to avoid rebreathing may deliver an F_IO_2 up to 90%, provided that leaks

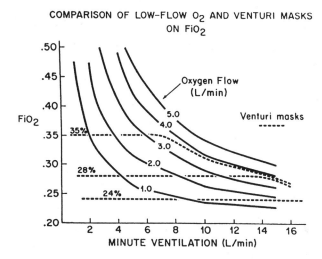

Figure 2 An approximation of the F_IO_2 of gas entering the trachea as a function of minute ventilation for patients receiving O_2 therapy in several forms. A ratio of inspiration to expiration of 1 : 2 was assumed. (From Ref. 23, with permission.)

around the face have been eliminated by tight seals. However, these masks are rarely, if ever, used during acute exacerbation of COPD because they are not easily accepted by the patients and carry significant risks of CO_2 retention. This mode of oxygen delivery should de used in the intensive care unit. Nevertheless, if the patient is still hypoxemic with an F_IO_2 of 50% delivered by a Venturi mask, noninvasive positive pressure ventilation rather than a reservoir mask should be attempted.

V. Adjusting Oxygen Delivery

As has already been stated, in acute exacerbation of COPD V'/Q' mismatching is the predominant mechanism of hypoxemia (25, 26). A true right-to-left shunt contributes very little to hypoxemia, averaging less than 5% of total blood flow (25, 26). Therefore, correction of hypoxemia in these patients usually requires small increases in F_IO_2. An F_IO_2 in the range 25 to 40% is sufficient to raise PaO_2 to > 60 mmHg in the vast majority of patients. Failure to increase PaO_2 above 60 mmHg suggests an additional process, such as atelectasis, pneumonia, pulmonary embolism, pneumothorax, right-to-left intracardiac shunt, or end-stage disease (27).

The initial setting of F_IO_2 (Venturi mask) or O_2 flow (L/min, nasal prongs) should be adjusted to bring PaO_2 to just above 60 mmHg. Table 1 shows recommended initial O_2 settings based on the value of PaO_2 breathing room air (9). However, these recommendations serve as a general guide and may not apply in an individual patient. If an oximetry is available, adjusting O_2 therapy to an SaO_2 just above 89 to 90% by titrating the F_IO_2 or O_2 flow would be helpful. Twenty to

Table 1 Recommended Initial O_2 Settings to Achieve
Arterial Oxygen Tension >7.98 kPa (60 mmHg)

Initial PaO_2 (on room air) mmHg	F_1O_2 (Venturi mask) %	O_2 flow (nasal prongs) L/min
50	24	1
45	28	2
40	32	3
35	35	4

30 min after the initiation of O_2 therapy, arterial blood gases should be obtained. PaO_2 should be in the range that has been already mentioned. At the same time, the pH and $PaCO_2$ should be observed for CO_2 retention. We should mention that many patients have chronic CO_2 elevation due to factors other than oxygen therapy (28). In this case, the pH usually is in the normal range. The goal of O_2 therapy should be to achieve a SaO_2 above 89 to 90%, without an excessive rise in $PaCO_2$ (>10 mmHg) or a decrease in pH bellow 7.25 (1, 2, 4). Thus, if hypercapnia is already present, the use of a Venturi mask for oxygen delivery is advisable. If adequate oxygenation is unachievable without progressive respiratory acidosis, then mechanical ventilatory support may be required. Figure 3 shows an algorithm for correcting hypoxemia during acute exacerbation of COPD (29).

VI. Oxygen-Induced Hypercapnia

The major concern for oxygen administration in hypoxemic patients with acute exacerbation of COPD is the risk of carbon dioxide (CO_2) retention (30, 31). The other side effects of CO_2 therapy, such as absorption atelectasis and oxygen toxicity, are not an issue in these patients. The classic explanation for CO_2 retention by O_2 therapy is that it occurs in patients with reduction or absence of sensitivity to CO_2, in which case ventilatory drive is dependent mainly on hypoxemia. CO_2 retention with O_2 therapy occurs much more often in exacerbations of COPD than in the same patients during stable conditions. It has been postulated that this is due to a difference in hypoxic ventilatory sensitivity between remissions and exacerbation (32). However, Milic-Emili and coworkers suggested that changes in the pattern of breathing may significantly contribute to CO_2 retention (33).

Approximately 25 years ago, Bone et al. (34) in a large study tried to address the issue of CO_2 retention. In 50 consecutive patients with COPD and acute respiratory failure, they administered 24 to 28% oxygen to correct the hypoxia. Twenty-six percent of these patients required mechanical ventilation because of CO_2 narcosis. These patients did not differ from the 37 patients who responded well to conventional therapy in any terms. The authors used the relationship between arterial

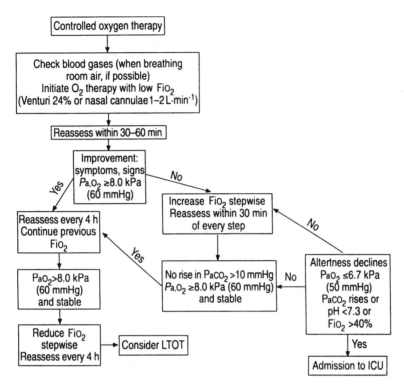

Figure 3 Algorithm for controlled oxygen therapy in acute exacerbation in COPD. F_1O_2: inspired oxygen fraction; PaO_2: arterial oxygen tension; $PaCO_2$: arterial carbon dioxide tension; LTOT: long-term oxygen therapy. (From Ref. 29, with permission.)

pH and PaO_2 at presentation to predict a respiratory failure, without taking into account the value of resting PCO_2. They concluded that hypoxemia and acidosis are more discriminatory for CO_2 retention than hypercapnia. There are some other studies indicating that oxygen administration in patients with exacerbation of COPD may result in hypercarbia but that the patients at highest risk for respiratory failure associated with oxygen administration can be identified (18, 24, 35–37).

Aubier and coworkers offered another explanation for CO_2 retention during O_2 therapy (38, 39). They studied 22 patients with chronic airways obstruction during an episode of acute exacerbation. All patients were severely hypoxic and hypercapnic and noticed that 15 min of breathing 100% oxygen resulted in an early decrease in ventilation by an average 18% of control values, followed by a slow increase to 93% of control values. At the end of a 15-min period of O_2 breathing, $PaCO_2$ had increased by an average of 23 mmHg (35%). This increase was not accompanied by an increase in expired CO_2, indicating an increase in physiological dead space. Carbon dioxide production remained stable while there was a small increase in cardiac output (7.2 to 7.5). Changes in tidal volume and breathing frequency were not statistically significant, but the calculated $V_D phys/V_T$ ratio was significantly increased (77% to 82%); however, this rise was not proportional to the $PaCO_2$ rise. The authors concluded that the rise in $PaCO_2$ was due to a deterioration in V_A/Q matching on the basis of the following statements. (1) V_E fell only 7% and thus could account only for 5 mmHg (0.66 kPa) of the $PaCO_2$ increase. (2) The Haldane effect, caused by an increase in mixed venous oxygen tension (PvO_2) contributed much less to the $PaCO_2$ rise. (3) There was a significant rise in physiological dead space while tidal volume did not change significantly. It is possible that O_2 breathing, by relieving hypoxic vasoconstriction, increased blood flow to poorly ventilated low ventilation/perfusion (V/Q) units and therefore decreased flow to high V/Q units increasing both their number and V/Q. This redistribution of blood flow would increase the physiological dead space and produce CO_2 retention. This mechanism was thought to be the most important in half of the patients studied, while in the other half hypoventilation could have explained the CO_2 retention (33, 40).

Recently the mechanism of O_2-induced hypercapnia has been reexamined in detail by Robinson et al. (Fig. 4). These authors used the multiple inert gas elimination technique to evaluate the response to 100% O_2 in patients with acute exacerbations of COPD. Two groups of patients were identified according to CO_2 response to O_2. Approximately 50% of the patients were classified as retainers ($PaCO_2$ rose by more than 3 mmHg), while the others' $PaCO_2$ remained unchanged or decreased and thus they were classified as nonretainers. The results of this study demonstrated that an overall reduction in ventilation characterizes the O_2-induced hypercapnia, as an increased dispersion of blood flow from release of hypoxic vasoconstriction occurred to a similar degree in both groups. The significant increase in wasted ventilation in the group of retainers may be a secondary effect of hypercapnia possibly related to bronchodilation (41).

In a more recent study, Moloney et al. studied 24 patients presenting to the emergency department with acute exacerbation associated with hypercapnic respiratory failure (Fig. 5). Study patients had severe airflow limitation (mean forced vital capacity 58% and mean forced expiratory volume in 1 s 37% of predicted normal values). In all patients controlled O_2 as given by Venturi mask. The oxygen concentration was adjusted every 15 to 20 min between 24% and 40% to achieve an oxygen saturation of 91 to 92%. Mean PaO_2 rose from 6.0 kPa (SD 0.8) on admission to 9.6 kPa (2.1) after 2 h of oxygen therapy; $PaCO_2$ remained unchanged (7.5 kPa vs. 7.6 kPa after oxygen therapy, mean change 0.09 kPa), and no patient developed a later rise in $PaCO_2$. Only three patients showed signs of clinically important CO_2 retention (defined as an increase in $PaCO_2 > 1$ kPa), but none of them developed CO_2 narcosis. Although there was no systematic tendency toward CO_2 retention associated with increasing $PaCO_2$ on admission, $PaCO_2$ changes with oxygen therapy were more variable in patients with a higher $PaCO_2$. Patients who had the greatest $PaCO_2$ rise with oxygen therapy were generally more hypercapnic at baseline. These findings suggest that the risk of CO_2 retention with carefully controlled oxygen therapy is very low and possible with minimal clinical significance (42).

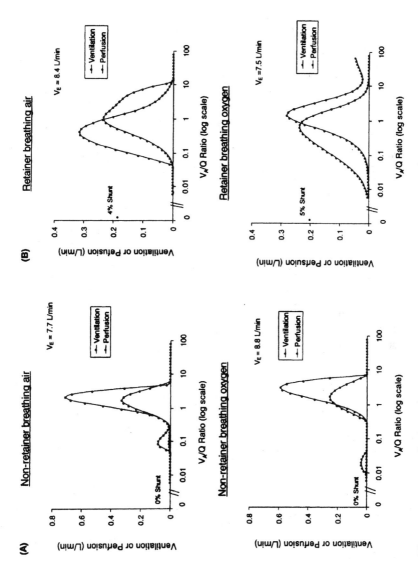

Figure 4 Typical V'/Q' distribution in two patients breathing air (upper panel) and 100% O_2 (lower panel). (A) Patient without a considerable increase in $PaCO_2$ with O_2 breathing (< 3 mmHg). (B) Patient with an increase in $PaCO_2$ with O_2 breathing (> 3 mmHg). (From Ref. 41, with permission.)

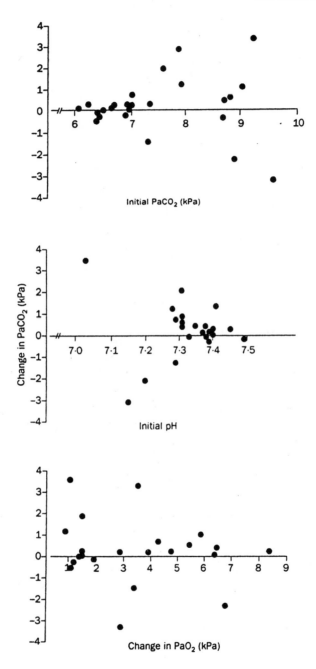

Change in PaCO₂ in first 2 h of oxygen therapy

Figure 5 Changes in $PaCO_2$ in the first 2 h of oxygen therapy in 24 hypoxemic and hypercapnic patients with exacerbations of COPD. (From Ref. 42, with permission.)

VII. Conclusion

Acute exacerbation of COPD is invariably associated with derangements of gas exchange. V'/Q' mismatching is the main pathogenetic mechanism for gas exchange abnormalities. In hypoxic patients with acute exacerbations of COPD, administration of O_2 to increase $PaO_2 > 60\,mmHg$ is a cornerstone in therapeutic interventions. A high-flow O_2 mask (Venturi mask) is the method of choice of O_2 administration because the F_1O_2 can be precisely controlled, provided that the F_1O_2 requirement is less than 40%. During O_2 therapy, the risk of CO_2 retention is always a consideration. This risk, however, is greatly minimized by carefully controlling the F_1O_2 in order to avoid excessive increase in PaO_2.

References

1. Siafakas NM, Vermeire P, Pride NB, et al. Optimal assessment and management of chronic obstructive pulmonary disease (COPD). The European Respiratory Society Task Force. Eur Respir J 1995; 8:1398–1420.
2. Pauwels RA, Buist AS, Ma P, Jenkins CR, Hurd SS. Global strategy for the diagnosis, management, and prevention of chronic obstructive pulmonary disease: National Heart, Lung, and Blood Institute and World Health Organization Global Initiative for Chronic Obstructive Lung Disease (GOLD): executive summary. Respir Care 2001; 46:798–825.
3. McCrory DC, Brown C, Gelfand SE, Bach PB. Management of acute exacerbations of COPD: a summary and appraisal of published evidence. Chest 2001; 119:1190–1209.
4. Georgopoulos D, Anthonisen NR. Continuous oxygen therapy for the chronically hypoxemic patient. Annu Rev Med 1990; 41:223–230.
5. Sherk PA, Grossman RF. The chronic obstructive pulmonary disease exacerbation. Clin Chest Med 2000; 21:705–721.
6. Fong YM, Marano MA, Moldawer LL, et al. The acute splanchnic and peripheral tissue metabolic response to endotoxin in humans. J Clin Invest 1990; 85:1896–1904.
7. Campell E. Management of respiratory failure. BMJ 1964; 2:1328–1339.
8. Spector JI, Zaroulis CG, Pivacek LE, Emerson CP, Valeri CR. Physiologic effects of normal- or low-oxygen-affinity red cells in hypoxic baboons. Am J Physiol 1977; 232:H79–H84.
9. Statement ATS. Standards for the diagnosis and care of patients with chronic obstructive pulmonary disease (COPD). Am J Respir Crit Care Med 1996; 152:S77–S120.
10. Anthonisen NR. Hypoxemia and O_2 therapy. Am Rev Respir Dis 1982; 126:729–733.
11. Fulmer JD SG. American College of Chest Physicians/National Heart, Lung, and Blood Institute National Conference on Oxygen Therapy. Heart Lung 1984: 13:550–562.
12. Esteban A, Cerda E, De La Cal MA, Lorente JA. Hemodynamic effects of oxygen therapy in patients with acute exacerbations of chronic obstructive pulmonary disease. Chest 1993; 104:471–475.
13. Ashutosh K, Mead G, Dunsky M. Early effects of oxygen administration and prognosis in chronic obstructive pulmonary disease and cor pulmonale. Am Rev Respir Dis 1983; 127:399–404.
14. Naeije R, Melot C, Mols P, Hallemans R. Effects of vasodilators on hypoxic pulmonary vasoconstriction in normal man. Chest 1982; 82:404–410.

15. DeGaute JP, Domenighetti G, Naeije R, Vincent JL, Treyvaud D, Perret C. Oxygen delivery in acute exacerbation of chronic obstructive pulmonary disease. Effects of controlled oxygen therapy. Am Rev Respir Dis 1981; 124:26–30.

16. Lejeune P, Mols P, Naeije R, Hallemans R, Melot C. Acute hemodynamic effects of controlled oxygen therapy in decompensated chronic obstructive pulmonary disease. Crit Care Med 1984; 12:1032–1035.

17. Kawakami Y, Kishi F, Yamamoto H, Miyamoto K. Relation of oxygen delivery, mixed venous oxygenation, and pulmonary hemodynamics to prognosis in chronic obstructive pulmonary disease. N Engl J Med 1983; 308:1045–1049.

18. Bach PB, Brown C, Gelfand SE, McCrory DC. Management of acute exacerbations of chronic obstructive pulmonary disease: a summary and appraisal of published evidence. Ann Intern Med 2001; 134:600–620.

19. Tarpy SP, Celli BR. Long-term oxygen therapy. N Engl J Med 1995; 333:710–714.

20. Howes TQ, Deane CR, Levin GE, Baudouin SV, Moxham J. The effects of oxygen and dopamine on renal and aortic blood flow in chronic obstructive pulmonary disease with hypoxemia and hypercapnia. Am J Respir Crit Care Med 1995; 151:378–383.

21. Sharkey RA, Mulloy EM, O'Neill SJ. The acute effects of oxygen and carbon dioxide on renal vascular resistance in patients with an acute exacerbation of COPD. Chest 1999; 115:1588–1592.

22. De Siati L, Baldoncini R, Coassin S, et al. Renal sodium excretory function during acute oxygen administration. Respiration 1993; 60:338–342.

23. Johanson J, Peters JI. Respiratory failure. In: Murray JF, Nadel JA, eds. Textbook of Respiratory Medicine. Philadelphia: W.B. Saunders Company, 1988:1973–2016.

24. Bedon GA, Block AJ, Ball WC Jr. The "28 percent" Venturi mask in obstructive airway disease. Arch Intern Med 1970; 125:106–113.

25. Rossi A, Santos C, Roca J, Torres A, Felez MA, Rodriguez-Roisin R. Effects of PEEP on VA/Q mismatching in ventilated patients with chronic airflow so obstruction. Am J Respir Crit Care Med 1994; 149:1077–1084.

26. Torres A, Reyes A, Roca J, Wagner PD, Rodriguez-Roisin R. Ventilation–perfusion mismatching in chronic obstructive pulmonary disease during ventilator weaning. Am Rev Respir Dis 1989; 140:1246–1250.

27. Rodriguez-Roisin R. Effects of mechanical ventilation on gas exchange. In: Tobin MJ, ed. Principles and Practice of Mechanical Ventilation. Vol. 1. New York: McGraw-Hill, 1994:673–693.

28. Younes M. Mechanism of respiratory failure. Curr Pulmonol 1993; 14:243–292.

29. Tzanakis IM, Siafakas NM. Oxygen therapy in chronic obstructive pulmonary disease. In: Postma DS, Siafakas NM, eds. Management of Chronic Obstructive Pulmonary Disease. Vol. 3. Sheffield, U.K.: European Respiratory Society, 1998:169–179.

30. Markello R, Winter P, Olszowka A. Assessment of ventilation–perfusion inequalities by arterial–alveolar nitrogen differences in intensive care patients. Anesthesiology 1972;37:4–15.

31. Bryan CL JS. Oxygen toxicity. Clin Chest Med 1988; 9:141–152.

32. Rudolf M, Banks RA, Semple SJ. Hypercapnia during oxygen therapy in acute exacerbations of chronic respiratory failure. Hypothesis revisited. Lancet 1977; 2:483–486.

33. Sorli J, Grassino A, Lorange G, Milic-Emili J. Control of breathing in patients with chronic obstructive lung disease. Clin Sci Mol Med 1978; 54:295–304.

34. Bone RC, Pierce AK., Johnson RL Jr. Controlled oxygen administration in acute respiratory failure in chronic obstructive pulmonary disease: a reappraisal. Am J Med 1978; 65:896–902.

35. Eldridge F, Gherman C. Studies of oxygen administration in respiratory failure. Ann Intern Med 1968; 68:569–578.
36. Warrell DA, Edwards RH, Godfrey S, Jones NL. Effect of controlled oxygen therapy on arterial blood gases in acute respiratory failure. Br Med J 1970; 1:452–455.
37. Group NOTT. Continuous or nocturnal oxygen therapy in hypoxemic chronic obstructive lung disease: a clinical trial. Ann Intern Med 1980; 93:391–398.
38. Aubier M, Murciano D, Milic-Emili J, et al. Effects of the administration of O_2 on ventilation and blood gases in patients with chronic obstructive pulmonary disease during acute respiratory failure. Am Rev Respir Dis 1980; 122:747–754.
39. Stradling JR. Hypercapnia during oxygen therapy in airways obstruction: a reappraisal. Thorax 1986; 41:897–902.
40. Hanson CW 3rd, Marshall BE, Frasch HF, Marshall C. Causes of hypercarbia with oxygen therapy in patients with chronic obstructive pulmonary disease. Crit Care Med 1996; 24:23–28.
41. Robinson TD, Freiberg DB, Regnis JA, Young IH. The role of hypoventilation and ventilation–perfusion redistribution in oxygen-induced hypercapnia during acute exacerbations of chronic obstructive pulmonary disease. Am J Respir Crit Care Med 2000; 161:1524–1529.
42. Moloney ED, Kiely JL, McNicholas WT. Controlled oxygen therapy and carbon dioxide retention during exacerbations of chronic obstructive pulmonary disease. Lancet 2001; 357:526–528.

24

Acute Exacerbations
Other Treatment

NIKOS TZANAKIS and EVA PAPADOPOULI

University of Crete Medical School
Heraklion, Crete, Greece

I. Introduction

COPD patients have one to four acute exacerbations per year on average, accounting for 16,367,000 office visits, 500,000 hospitalizations, and direct health costs of $18 billion (1, 2). During an exacerbation, there is an intensification of treatment with a hospital or intensive care unit admission often necessary. These figures demonstrate the enormous contribution of the cost of the exacerbations to the economic burden of this common disease. Thus, one of the main treatment goals for COPD patients is to reduce the number and severity of exacerbations they experience each year (3). On the other hand, reports worldwide (4) (Fig. 1) have pointed out that during exacerbations of COPD (AECOPD) the most frequent prescriptions include medication other than the conventional treatment modalities that international guidelines have recently described (3, 5, 6). This is especially true concerning AECOPD that takes place on an outpatient basis at home.

All the recently developed guideline reports have found enough evidence to make recommendations about the following therapeutic modalities in AECOPD: bronchodilators, corticosteroids, antibiotics, oxygen, and noninvasive positive-pressure ventilation (NIPPV) (3). However, difficulties exist in verifying other therapeutic practices commonly used in several clinical settings in AECOPD (7). The aim of this chapter is to evaluate and present published data on some of the

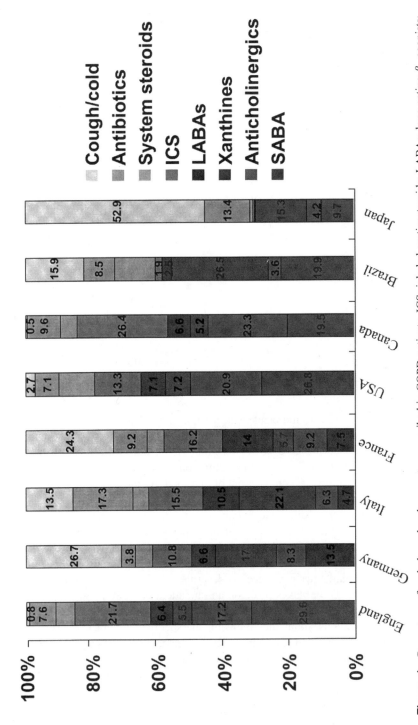

Figure 1 Percentage of each drug class by country prescribed in COPD patients. ICS: inhaled corticosteroids; LABAs: long-acting β_2-agonists; SABA: short-acting β_2-agonists. (From Ref. 4.).

Table 1 Other Therapeutic Modalities Used in Acute
Exacerbation of COPD

  I. Prevention
     A. Vaccination
     B. Immunostimulating medication
     C. Long-term antibiotic treatment
  II. Mucus clearance
     A. Expectorants, mucolytics, and mucokinetics
     B. Physical and respiratory therapies
 III. Management of pulmonary hypertension
     A. Anticoagulants
     B. Pulmonary vasodilators
     C. Phlebotomy and venesection
 IV. Respiratory stimulants
     A. Acting to respiratory drive
     B. Acting to respiratory muscles
  V. Antitussives
 VI. Nutritional support

---

current treatment practices in AECOPD that, although not generally recommended, are in use, some of them which may be beneficial in the prevention and treatment of AECOPD (Table 1).

II. Prevention

A. Vaccination

Although exacerbations may be initiated by multiple factors, the most common identifiable associations are with bacterial and viral infections. These are associated with approximately 50 to 70% and 20 to 30% of COPD exacerbations, respectively (3). Vaccination against influenza and pneumococcal infections are highly recommended in all COPD patients according to the recently reported global guidelines of management of COPD (3). Complicated influenza illness among elderly persons, including those with COPD, is responsible for hundreds of thousands of excess hospitalizations, tens of thousands of excess deaths, and billions of dollars in health-care costs (8, 9). The efficacy and cost effectiveness of influenza vaccination has been demonstrated in a large cohort study of 25,000 patients (9). In this study, it was clearly shown that vaccination was associated with a 40% reduction in the rate of hospitalization for all acute and chronic respiratory diseases including AECOPD (9). The same investigators recently reported an overwhelming reduction in the risk of death from any cause including AECOPD to be related with influenza vaccination (odds ratio—OR = 0.3; 95% CI = 0.21–0.43) (8). These studies and a recent meta-analysis concluding that influenza vaccines could reduce serious AECOPD and death by approximately 50% (8–10) clearly suggest adequate influenza vaccination of patients with COPD. Thus, vaccines containing killed or live viruses are recommended and should be given once (in autumn) or twice (autumn and winter) each year (3).

Vaccination against pneumococcal infections is recommended (3), although its value in COPD has been controversial (11). A 23-valent-pneumococcal vaccine has been used, but two randomized controlled trials evaluating its efficacy among patients with COPD failed to show a significant protective effect (12,13). In spite of these controversies, pneumococcal vaccination continues to be recommended for patients with COPD because recent randomized population-based trials (14) and meta-analysis (11) concluded that the vaccine provides partial protection against bacteremic pneumococcal pneumonia (15).

B. Immunostimulating Agents (Immunomodulators, Immunoregulators)

Immunomodulators have been used mostly in Europe for many years in an attempt to stimulate the immune system of the patients with COPD and to reduce the frequency and severity of AECOPD (5). OM-85 BV is the most important oral immunostimulating agent consisting of lyophilized fractions of the eight most common respiratory pathogens. Two studies showed that the use of an immuno-stimulator was associated with a decrease in the severity of AECOPD and shorter duration of hospitalizations (16,17). However, these studies have not been duplicated (18) and all the guideline reports are not recommending them based on the current knowledge (3, 5, 6).

C. Long-Term Antibiotic Treatment

The use of long-term antibiotic treatment of intermittent administration, intended as "prophylaxis," does not appear to be beneficial (6). As the Global Initiative for Chronic Obstructive Lung Disease (GOLD) report states; "the use of antibiotics, other than in treating infectious AECOPD is not recommended" (3).

III. Mucus Clearance

A. Expectorants, Mucolytics, and Mucokinetics

Mucus strategies, in order to facilitate the expectoration of the increased amount of sputum production during an acute exacerbation of COPD, have been cornerstones in COPD therapy for many years. Numerous medications, with supposed mucolytic properties, have been tried (19–21). Two types of drugs are used: mucolytics, which contain substances that enhance the breakdown of mucoproteins, and mucokinetics, which reduce viscosity by altering sialomucin synthesis. Both of these drugs could be given orally or parenterally (N-acetylcysteine and ambroxol can also be administered by nebulization). On the basis of our current knowledge derived from well-controlled, double-blind, randomized clinical trials (20, 22–24), pharma-cological mucus-clearance strategies have not demonstrated a reduction in the frequency, severity, and duration of AECOPD, although an improvement of the symptoms has been shown in some of them (20, 24). *N*-acetylcysteine is a mucolytic that can sever glycoprotein disulfide bonds, liquefy mucus, reduce sputum viscosity, and thin mucoid and purulent secretions of patients with COPD. In animal studies, there is evidence that *N*-acetylcysteine at high doses may also reduce the hyperplasia of bronchial mucous glands induced by smoking (25). Oral *N*-acetylcysteine has been reported to enhance the mucus clearance in patients with slow clearance (19, 26). In conclusion, mucolytics and mucokinetics have some positive short-term effects in AECOPD by improving the symptoms and may be recommended in a selected group of patients with persistent, copious, and tenacious phlegm. However, there is no evidence to indicate that these regimens affect the long-term outcome of COPD and therefore should not be prescribed routinely in AECOPD (5, 6).

B. Physical and Respiratory Therapies

Although, physiotherapy and mechanical percussion of the chest as applied by physical or respiratory therapists has been regarded as a basic therapeutic strategy in the management of AECOPD for a long time, randomized and observational studies showed no effect on several outcomes in the course of an AECOPD (27–29). In fact, the studies of Wollmer and colleagues and Campbell ct al. actually reported a harmful effect on the respiratory function of patients with AECOPD to be associated with chest physiotherapy (27, 29). The role of physiotherapy in AECOPD at home that aims to improve respiratory muscle function and to encourage sputum expectoration has not been systematically investigated, but it can be considered as part of the rehabilitation program (30). Manual or mechanical chest percussion and postural drainage could improve AECOPD outcome in patients producing more than 25 mL sputum per day or presenting with lobar atelectasis (3).

IV. Management of Pulmonary Hypertension

Oxygen therapy, careful use of diuretics, and the treatment of the underlying cause of acute exacerbation remain the mainstays of therapy of pulmonary hypertension and cor pulmonale in AECOPD (3, 5, 6). These main treatment strategies in managing pulmonary hypertension in AECOPD are discussed elsewhere. Here, the use of three other treatment strategies including anticoagulants, pulmonary vasodilators, and blood venesection in the management of pulmonary hypertension in AECOPD will be discussed (Table 1).

Patients with COPD admitted to medical wards with acute exacerbation are at moderate risk for the development of venous thromboembolism (VTE) independently of the cause of the exacerbation (31, 32). This is particularly true concerning severe AECOPD, with the patient presenting with worsening of his pulmonary hemodynamics along with an acute hemodynamic decompensation, increased hematocrit, and increased blood viscosity (5). Besides, true pulmonary embolism is one of the main causes of an acute exacerbation in COPD patients (5). Although there are no studies published with regard to the prophylactic administration of the anticoagulants in AECOPD, many clinical centers and intensive care units regularly use anticoagulants in AECOPD—if there is no major contraindication—independently of the cause of the exacerbation (31–33). Low-molecular-weight heparin in immobilized, polycythemic, or dehydrated patients with or without a history of thromboembolic disease is also recommended in the GOLD report (3). In some cases of severe AECOPD, the hematocrit is markedly elevated above 55 to 60%, while dehydration and increased blood viscosity could lead to hemodynamic decompensation and promotion of pulmonary embolism. In these cases, phlebotomy and venesection can temporarily improve patient function (5, 34–36).

The study of numerous vasodilators has been reported mainly with regard to treatment of "primary" pulmonary hypertension (37–39). Prostacyclin (37, 38) and calcium channel blockers (39) were the most promising regimens, but only those patients suffering from primary pulmonary hypertension were found to have a significant response (37–39). Ideally, a vasodilator clinically relevant to pulmonary hemodynamics should act selectively in the pulmonary rather than in the systemic circulation, with a reduction in right atrial pressure and a rise in cardiac output. Currently, inhaled nitric oxide (NO) is the only selective pulmonary vasodilator (40, 41). However, neither inhaled NO nor other vasodilators can sustain clinically relevant reductions in pulmonary vascular resistance while NO has been reported to induce hypotension and worsening of hypoxemia due to worsening of ventilation–perfusion mismatching (42). Ashutosh et al. recently reported a significant improvement of pulmonary hemodynamics in patients with COPD after inhalation of NO in combination with supplemental oxygen (43). In contrast, Baigorri et al. reported no effect of inhalation of NO in either right ventricular function or arterial oxygenation in mechanically ventilated patients with acute respiratory failure caused by acute exacerbation of COPD (44). Results of the vasodilator therapy in AECOPD with inhaled NO showed frequent side effects in some trials including a small number of COPD patients (41, 43, 45, 46). Indeed, vasodilators appear to be less effective in COPD compared to primary pulmonary hypertension. Thus, there is, at present, no justification for the use of inhaled NO in AECOPD (47, 48). The GOLD report states that in stable COPD inhaled NO is contraindicated because of alteration of the hypoxic regulation of the ventilation–perfusion balance (3).

V. Respiratory Stimulants

The imbalance between respiratory muscle function and respiratory workload is an important determinant of dyspnea and hypercapnia seen in AECOPD. Many of the respiratory, and particularly inspiratory, muscle insufficiencies are secondary to a mechanical disadvantage related to worsening of hyperinflation during AECOPD (49). Because many of the lung and airway derangements are irreversible in COPD, the respiratory drive and respiratory muscles appear to be an attractive target for therapeutic interventions (49).

Numerous respiratory stimulants aiming to enhance central respiratory drive have been investigated. Acetazolamide (50), doxapram (51, 52), almitrine (53–56), tricyclic antidepressants (57), and progestational hormones (56, 58) have been tried in the hope of improving ventilation and oxygenation, reducing hypercapnia and dyspnea either during AECOPD or in stable condition (59). Doxapram and almitrine bismesylate were the most promising central respiratory stimulants (56, 60). Although, doxapram may improve blood gas exchange in the short term, newer intervention methods such as nasal intermittent positive pressure ventilation (NIPPV) may be more effective (51). After a decade of study, almitrine still appears most promising but the controversies, side effects, and poor results observed in long-term studies limit its value in the management of COPD (59).

Stimulants of respiratory muscles have shown promise, but no evidence of improving outcome in AECOPD has emerged. However, theophylline has been shown to improve muscle function in hyperinflated severe exacerbated patients (61) and can improve nocturnal oxygen saturation (62). During the last decade methyl-xanthines have been downgraded to a minor role in AECOPD, because safer and more potent bronchodilators have been developed. Two clinical trials that were specially designed to test the role of theophylline in the treatment of AECOPD have been published (63, 64). In the study of Rice et al., no significant differences were reported between the placebo and aminophylline groups in any of the spirometric measurements or the dyspnea indexes (63). The second study—emergency depart-ment–based randomized design—investigated a mixed population of asthmatic and AECOPD patients. The authors reported a decrease in the hospital admission rate for the aminophylline group (64) for both asthma and COPD exacerbation. However, the effect of theophylline on admission rate was not statistically significant when an adjustment for multiple comparisons was performed. Moreover, no effect on spirometry was observed between aminophylline and the placebo group (64). In conclusion, the rationale for prescribing theophylline to patients with AECOPD is primarily for their bronchodilator action, and not for the stimulator effect on respiratory muscles (3). Other regimens with a probable stimulator effect on respiratory muscles include digoxin, calcium-channel blockers, anabolic steroids, and antioxidants (*N*-acetylcysteine). Their role as stimulants of the respiratory muscles on the present evidence is unclear (65). β-Agonists also have a stimulation effect on respiratory muscles, but their primary role is bronchodilation.

VI. Antitussives

Although patients with COPD on acute exacerbation experience coughing as a troublesome symptom, it has a very important protective role in airway clearance and removal of the tenacious secretions (66). The use of antitussives during AECOPD is clearly contraindicated (3, 5, 6).

VII. Nutritional Support

Malnutrition in COPD is a common finding. About 20 to 30% of COPD patients are underweight (67) and may be worse when the disease is in the advanced stage (68) or in exacerbation (69). Nutritional abnormalities can be present, even among patients with normal body mass index (BMI) (70); evidence shows, however, that patients with emphysema have poorer nutritional status than patients with features of bronchitis (71). Many causes can be associated with the poor nutritional status observed in COPD including poor dietary intake, increased satiety as a consequence of the hyperinflation, and increased energy expenditure because of the increased respiratory workload (69). Recently, investigations have focused on observations relating the weight loss and anorexia of COPD patients to elevated serum concentrations of systemic inflammatory markers such as acute-phase proteins, cytokines (TNF-α), and adhesion molecules (72). Malnourished COPD patients have a poorer prognosis after an AECOPD because of their nutritional status; decrease respiratory muscle strength alters ventilatory drive and impairs immunological defense mechanisms (69, 73). These adverse effects can be additive in AECOPD with respiratory failure and promote a more severe and prolonged course of illness. Malnutrition can also be very critical to mechanically ventilated COPD patients (69). Therefore, it is necessary to properly manage the malnutrition of patients with COPD during an acute exacerbation.

COPD patients admitted to emergency or hospital wards with acute exacerbation and respiratory failure can be candidates for nutritional support if they are already malnourished or if it is likely that malnutrition will develop because of inadequate oral intake and prolonged clinical course. Nutritional assessment is essential before an action of nutritional support takes place and can include simple and more complicated tests such as loss of weight (weight <10% of ideal weight means malnutrition), anthropometry, hepatic secretory proteins (albumin, transferring, retinol-binding protein), cellular immunity, and delayed cutaneous hypersensitivity. Finally, for a more sensitive evaluation, a multiparameter nutritional index (a combination of several single tests) can be used (69). In patients with respiratory failure, the presence or absence of invasive mechanical ventilation is the first factor in the consideration of nutritional support while the classification of the patient as hypermetabolic or simply malnourished is also an important modifier of the nutritional intervention (69). A hypermetabolic disorder is very common in AECOPD caused by infections, which can further attenuate malnutrition of the patient.

The detailed scheme of nutritional supplementation in AECOPD is beyond the scope of this review; besides, two excellent reviews have recently been published (69, 72). In general, the goals of nutritional support should focus on adequate, but not excessive, energy, nitrogen balance, preservation of lean body mass, adequate vitamins, minerals, and fat quantities. Fluids and electrolytes should be administered considering the patient's needs and hemodynamic status. Adaptation of the patient's nutritional habits should always be considered. Nutritional supplementation should be divided carefully during the day to avoid loss of appetite and adverse effects due to the worsening of hyperinflation or to the high caloric load.

References

1. Hagedorn SD. Acute exacerbations of COPD. How to evaluate severity and treat the underlying cause. Postgrad Med 1992; 91(1):105–107, 110–112.

2. Agency-for-HealthCare-Research-and-Policy. Healthcare cost and utilization project: nationwide inpatient sample for 1997. Available at: http://www.ahcpr.gov/data/hcup/hcupnet.htm.

3. Pauwels RA, Buist AS, Ma P, Jenkins CR, Hurd SS. Global strategy for the diagnosis, management, and prevention of chronic obstructive pulmonary disease: National Heart:, Lung, and Blood Institute and World Health Organization Global Initiative for Chronic Obstructive Lung Disease (GOLD): executive summary. Respir Care 2001; 46(8):798–825.

4. Rudolf M. The reality of drug use in COPD: the European perspective. Chest 2001; 117(2 suppl):29S–32S.

5. Siafakas NM, Vermeire P, Pride NB, Paoletti P, Gibson J, Howard P, Yernault JC, Decramer M, Higenbottam T, Postma DS, et al. Optimal assessment and management of chronic obstructive pulmonary disease (COPD). The European Respiratory Society Task Force. Eur Respir J 1995; 38(8):1398–1420.

6. American-Thoracic-Society-statement. American Thoracic Society statment. Standards for the diagnosis and care of patients with Chronic Obstructive Pulmonary Disease. Am J Respir Crit Care Med 1996; 152(5):S77–S120.

7. Bach PB, Brown C, Gelfand SE, McCrory DC. Management of acute exacerbations of chronic obstructive pulmonary disease: a summary and appraisal of published evidence. Ann Intern Med 2001; 134(7):600–620.

8. Nichol KL, Baken L, Nelson A. Relation between influenza vaccination and outpatient visits, hospitalization, and mortality in elderly persons with chronic lung disease. Ann Intern Med 1999; 130(5):397–403.

9. Nichol KL, Margolis KL, Wuorenma J, Von Sternberg T. The efficacy and cost effectiveness of vaccination against influenza among elderly persons living in the community. N Engl J Med 1994; 331(12):778–784.

10. Seneff MG, Wagner DP, Wagner RP, Zimmerman JE, Knaus WA. Hospital and 1-year survival of patients admitted to intensive care units with acute exacerbation of chronic obstructive pulmonary disease. JAMA 1995; 274(23):1852–1857.

11. Fine MJ, Smith MA, Carson CA, Meffe F, Sankey SS, Weissfeld LA, Detsky AS, Kapoor WN. Efficacy of pneumococcal vaccination in adults. A meta-analysis of randomized controlled trials. Arch Intern Med 1994; 154(23):2666–2677.

12. Davis AL, Aranda CP, Schiffman G, Christianson LC. Pneumococcal infection and immunologic response to pneumococcal vaccine in chronic obstructive pulmonary disease. A pilot study. Chest 1987; 92(2):204–212.

13. Leech JA, Gervais A, Ruben FL. Efficacy of pneumococcal vaccine in severe chronic obstructive pulmonary disease. CMAJ 1987; 136(4):361–365.

14. Koivula I, Sten M, Leinonen M, Makela PH. Clinical efficacy of pneumococcal vaccine in the elderly: a randomized, single-blind population-based trial. Am J Med 1997; 103(4):281–290.

15. Fein A, Fein AM. 2000. Management of acute exacerbations in chronic obstructive pulmonary disease. Curr Opin Pulm Med 2000; 6(2):122–126.

16. Collet JP, Shapiro P, Ernst P, Renzi T, Ducruet T, Robinson A. Effects of an immuno-stimulating agent on acute exacerbations and hospitalizations in patients with chronic obstructive pulmonary disease. The PARI-IS Study Steering Committee and Research Group. Prevention of Acute Respiratory Infection by an Immunostimulant. Am J Respir Crit Care Med 1997; 156(6):1719–1724.

17. Orcel B, Delclaux B, Baud M, Derenne JP. Oral immunization with bacterial extracts for protection against acute bronchitis in elderly institutionalized patients with chronic bronchitis. Eur Respir J 1994; 7(3):446–452.

18. Lusuardi M, Capelli A, Carli S, Spada EL, Spinazzi A, Donner CF. Local airways immune modifications induced by oral bacterial extracts in chronic bronchitis. Chest 103(6): 1993; 1783–1791.
19. Todisco T, Polidori R, Rossi F, Iannacci L, Bruni B, Fedeli L, Palumbo R. Effect of N-acetylcysteine in subjects with slow pulmonary mucociliary clearance. Eur J Respir Dis Suppl 1985; 139:136–141.
20. Finiguerra M, Conti P, Figura I, Legnani W, Morandini GC. Clinical study on the effects of an antibiotic and mucolytic association (amoxicillin and domiodol) in hypersecretory chronic bronchopulmonary diseases. Curr Ther Res 1982; 31:895–905.
21. Ziment I. Acetylcysteine: a drug that is much more than a mucokinetic. Biomed Pharmacother 1988; 42(8):513–519.
22. Langlands JH. Double-blind clinical trial of bromhexine as a mucolytic drug in chronic bronchitis. Lancet 1970; 1(7644):448–450.
23. Aylward M. A between-patient, double-blind comparison of S-carboxymethylcysteine and bromhexine in chronic obstructive bronchitis. Curr Med Res Opin 1973; 1(4):219–227.
24. Peralta J, Poderoso JJ, Corazza C, Fernandez M, Guerreiro RB, Wiemeyer JC. Ambroxol plus amoxicillin in the treatment of exacerbations of chronic bronchitis. Arzneimittel-forschung 1987; 37(8):969–971.
25. Jeffery PK, Rogers DF, Ayers MM. Effect of oral acetylcysteine on tobacco smoke-induced secretory cell hyperplasia. Eur J Respir Dis Suppl 1985; 139:117–122.
26. Olivieri D, Marsico SA, Illiano A, Del Donno M. In vivo measurement of drug effect on mucociliary transport. Eur J Respir Dis Suppl 1983; 128(Pt 2):551–553.
27. Wollmer P, Ursing K, Midgren B, Eriksson L. Inefficiency of chest percussion in the physical therapy of chronic bronchitis. Eur J Respir Dis 1985; 66(4):233–239.
28. Newton DA, Bevans HG. Physiotherapy and intermittent positive-pressure ventilation of chronic bronchitis. Br Med J 1978; 2(6151):1525–1528.
29. Campbell AH, O'Connell JM, Wilson F. The effect of chest physiotherapy upon the FEV_1 in chronic bronchitis. Med J Aust 1975; 1(2):33–35.
30. Donner CF, Howard P. Pulmonary rehabilitation in chronic obstructive pulmonary disease (COPD) with recommendations for its use. Report of the European Respiratory Society Rehabilitation and Chronic Care Scientific Group (S.E.P.C.R. Rehabilitation Working Group). Eur Respir J 1992; 5(2):266–275.
31. Geerts WH, Heit JA, Clagett GP, Pineo GF, Colwell CW, Anderson FA Jr, Wheeler HB. Prevention of venous thromboembolism. Chest 2001; 119(1 Suppl):132S–175S.
32. Clagett GP, Anderson FA Jr, Geerts W, Heft JA, Knudson M, Lieberman JR, Merli GJ, Wheeler HB. Prevention of venous thromboembolism. Chest 1998; 114(5 Suppl):531S–560S.
33. Fraisse F, Holzapfel L, Couland JM, Simonneau G, Bedock B, Feissel M, Herbecq P, Pordes R, Poussel JF, Roux L. Nadroparin in the prevention of deep vein thrombosis in acute decompensated COPD. The Association of Non-University Affiliated Intensive Care Specialist Physicians of France. Am J Respir Crit Care Med 2000; 161(4 Pt 1): 1109–1114.
34. Erickson AD, Golden WA, Claunch BC, Donat WE, Kaemmerlen JT. Acute effects of phlebotomy on right ventricular size and performance in polycythemic patients with chronic obstructive pulmonary disease. Am J Cardial 1983; 52(1):163–166.
35. Patakas DA, Christaki PI, Louridas GE, Sproule BJ. Control of breathing in patients with chronic obstructive lung diseases and secondary polycythemia after venesection. Respiration 1986; 49(4):257–262.

36. Klinger JR, Hill NS. Right ventricular dysfunction in chronic obstructive pulmonary disease. Evaluation and management. Chest 1991; 99(3):715–723.
37. Jones DK, Higenbottam TW, Wallwork J. Treatment of primary pulmonary hypertension intravenous epoprostenol (prostacyclin). Br Heart J 1987; 357(3):270–278.
38. Long WA, Rubin LJ. Prostacyclin and PGE1 treatment of pulmonary hypertension. Am Rev Respir Dis 1987; 136(3):773–776.
39. Rich S, Brundage BH. High-dose calcium channel-blocking therapy for primary pulmonary hypertension: evidence for long-term reduction in pulmonary arterial pressure and regression of right ventricular hypertrophy. Circulation 1987; 76(1):135–141.
40. Pepke-Zaba J, Higenbottam TW, Dinh-Xuan AT, Stone D, Wallwork J. Inhaled nitric oxide as a cause of selective pulmonary vasodilatation in pulmonary hypertension. Lancet 1991; 338(8776):1173–1174.
41. Katayama Y, Higenbottam TW, Diaz de Atauri MJ, Cremon G, Akamine S, Barbera JA, Rodriguez-Roisin R. Inhaled nitric oxide and arterial oxygen tension in patients with chronic obstructive pulmonary disease and severe pulmonary hypertension. Thorax 1997; 52(2):120–124.
42. Barbera JA, Roger N, Roca J, Rovira I, Higenbottam TW, Rodriguez-Roisin R. Worsening of pulmonary gas exchange with nitric oxide inhalation in chronic obstructive pulmonary disease. Lancet 1996; 347(8999):436–440.
43. Ashutosh K, Phadke K, Jackson JF, Steele D. Use of nitric oxide inhalation in chronic obstructive pulmonary disease. Thorax 2000; 55(2):109–113.
44. Baigorri F, Joseph D, Artigas A, Blanch L. Inhaled nitric oxide does not improve cardiac or pulmonary function in patients with an exacerbation of chronic obstructive pulmonary disease. Crit Care Med 1999; 27(10):2153–2158.
45. Dweik RA. The promise and reality of nitric oxide in the diagnosis and treatment of lung disease. Cleve Clin J Med 2001; 68(6):486, 488, 490, 493.
46. Higenbottam T, Cremona G. Acute and chronic hypoxic pulmonary hypertension. Eur Respir J 1993; 6(8):1207–1212.
47. Chiche JD, Dhainaut JF. Inhaled nitric oxide for right ventricular dysfunction in chronic obstructive pulmonary disease patients: fall or rise of an idea? Crit Care Med 1999; 27(10):2299–2301.
48. Weitzenblum E, Kessler R, Oswald M, Fraisse P. Medical treatment of pulmonary hypertension in chronic lung disease. Eur Respir J 1994; 7(1):148–152.
49. Anthonisen NR. Chronic obstructive pulmonary disease. Can Med Assoc J 1988; 138(6):503–510.
50. Teppema LJ, Dahan A. Acetazolamide and breathing. Does a clinical dose alter peripheral and central CO(2) sensitivity? Am J Respir Crit Care Med 1999; 160(5 Pt 1):1592–1597.
51. Greenstone M. Doxapram for ventilatory failure due to exacerbations of chronic obstructive pulmonary disease. Cochrane Database Syst Rev 2000; 2.
52. Whittle A. COPD guidelines. Thorax 1999; 54(4):375–376.
53. Damato S, Bellone A, Castelli T, Mendoza M, Daniele R. Breathing pattern—gas exchange relation and acute effect of almitrine in severe chronic airflow obstruction. Respiration 1988; 54(1):42–49.
54. Hawrylkiewicz I, Jedrzejewska-Makowska M, Gorecka D, Zielinski J. Effects of almitrine and oxygen on ventilation and gas exchange in patients with chronic respiratory insufficiency. Eur J Respir Dis 64(7):512–516.
55. Maxwell DL, Cover D, Hughes JM. Almitrine increases the steady-state hypoxic ventilatory response in hypoxic chronic air-flow obstruction. Am Rev Respir Dis 1985; 132(6):1233–1237.

56. Pinet C, Tessonnier F, Ravel T, Orehek J. Association of oral almitrine and medroxy-progesterone acetate: effect on arterial blood gases in chronic obstructive pulmonary disease. Respir Med 2001; 95(7):602–605.

57. Strom K, Boman G, Pehrsson K, Alton M, Singer J, Rydstrom PO, Uddenfeldt M, Ericsson CH, Ostholm B, Morlin C. Effect of protriptyline, 10 mg daily, on chronic hypoxaemia in chronic obstructive pulmonary disease. Eur Respir J 1995; 8(3):425–429.

58. Dolly FR, Block AJ. Medroxyprogesterone acetate and COPD. Effect on breathing and oxygenation in sleeping and awake patients. Chest 1983; 84(4):394–398.

59. Bardsley PA. Chronic respiratory failure in COPD: is there a place for a respiratory stimulant? Thorax 1993; 48(8):781–784.

60. Angus RM, Ahmed AA, Fenwick LJ, Peacock AJ. Comparison of the acute effects on gas exchange of nasal ventilation and doxapram in exacerbations of chronic obstructive pulmonary disease. Thorax 1996; 51(10):1048–1050.

61. Gauthier AP, Yan S, Sliwinski P, Macklem PT. Effects of fatigue, fiber length, and aminophylline on human diaphragm contractility. Am Rev Respir Dis 152(1):204–210.

62. Berry RB, Desa MM, Branum JP, Light RW. Effect of theophylline on sleep and sleep-disordered breathing in patients with chronic obstructive pulmonary disease. Am Rev Respir Dis 143(2):245–250.

63. Rice KL, Leatherman JW, Duane PG, Snyder LS, Harmon KR, Abel JR, Niewoehner DE. Aminophylline for acute exacerbations of chronic obstructive pulmonary disease. A controlled trial. Ann Intern Med 107(3):305–309.

64. Wrenn K, Slovis CM, Murphy F, Greenberg RS. Aminophylline therapy for acute bronchospastic disease in the emergency room. Ann Intern Med 1991; 115(4):241–247.

65. Ferguson GT. Update on pharmacologic therapy for chronic obstructive pulmonary disease. Clin Chest Med 2000; 21(4):723–738.

66. Irwin RS, Boulet LP, Cloutier MM, Fuller R, Gold PM, Hoffstein V, Ing AJ, McCool FD, O'Byrne P, Poe RH, Prakash UB, Pratter MR, Rubin BK. Managing cough as a defense mechanism and as a symptom. A consensus panel report of the American College of Chest Physicians. Chest 1998; 114(2 Suppl Managing):133S–181S.

67. Engelen MP, Schols AM, Baken WC, Wesseling GJ, Wouters F. Nutritional depletion in relation to respiratory and peripheral skeletal muscle function in out-patients with COPD. Eur Respir J 1994; 7(10):1793–1797.

68. Ferreira IM, Brooks D, Lacasse Y, Goldstein RS. Nutritional support for individuals with COPD: a meta-analysis. Chest 2000; 117(3):672–678.

69. Pingleton SK. Nutrition in chronic critical illness. Clin Chest Med 2001; 22(1):149–163.

70. Schols AM, Soeters PB, Dingemans AM, Mostert R, Frantzen PJ, Wouters EF. Prevalence and characteristics of nutritional depletion in patients with stable COPD eligible for pulmonary rehabilitation. Am Rev Respir Dis 147(5):1151–1156.

71. Openbrier DR, Irwin MM, Rogers RM, Gottlieb GP, Dauber JH, Van Thiel DH, Pennock BE. Nutritional status and lung function in patients with emphysema and chronic bronchitis. Chest 1983; 83(1):17–22.

72. Schols AM, Wouters EF. Nutritional abnormalities and supplementation in chronic obstructive pulmonary disease. Clin Chest Med 2000; 21(4):753–762.

73. Rochester DF, Esau SA. Malnutrition and the respiratory system. Chest 1984; 85(3):411–415.

25

Noninvasive Ventilation in Acute Exacerbations of Chronic Obstructive Pulmonary Disease

MARK W. ELLIOTT

St. James's University Hospital
Leeds, England

I. Introduction

An exacerbation of chronic obstructive pulmonary disease (COPD) of sufficient severity to necessitate hospital admission carries a poor prognosis, with a reported mortality of between 6 and 26% (1, 2). However, the outcome from invasive mechanical ventilation (IMV) in patients with COPD is disappointing, both in the short term, with reported survivals of between 20 and 50% (3), and also after hospital discharge. Studies report 1-year survivals of between 25 and 54% (4–8). Patients with COPD who require IMV may subsequently prove difficult to wean from assisted ventilation. A number of studies have shown an incidence of prolonged need for ITU ventilation in between 5 to 13% of all ventilated patients (9), and these patients have a particularly poor prognosis with a hospital mortality of 50% (10). A diagnosis of COPD has been shown to be a strong predictor of weaning difficulty (10, 11).

Therefore, there is a need for new approaches in the management of this patient group. Noninvasive positive pressure ventilation (NPPV) has a number of potential advantages compared with IMV. Physiologically, NPPV is little different from invasive mechanical ventilation; positive pressure delivered to the lungs decreases inspiratory muscle effort and respiratory rate, increases ventilation, and improves gas exchange in patients with COPD during an acute exacerbation

(12–17). For the same FiO_2, the $AaDO_2$ increases due to a rise in clearance of CO_2 and hence increased respiratory exchange ratio (14). A number of studies have evaluated the hemodynamic effects of NPPV (14, 17, 18). There is a fall in cardiac output leading to a slight decrease in systemic oxygen delivery, but this is not accompanied by a change in PvO_2 (17, 18). There appears to be no improvement in the VA/Q ratio with NPPV (14).

The obvious attraction of NPPV is the avoidance of intubation and its attendant complications, in particular, ventilator-associated pneumonia (VAP). For every day intubated, there is a 1% risk of developing VAP (19). This complication of invasive ventilation is associated with a longer ICU stay, increased costs, and a worse outcome (19, 20). With NPPV, ventilatory support can be introduced at an earlier stage in the evolution of ventilatory failure than would be usual when a patient needs to be intubated to receive ventilatory support. It is also possible to provide ventilatory support for short periods, which in some cases may be sufficient to reverse the downward spiral into life-threatening ventilatory failure. Because intermittent ventilatory support is possible, patients can cooperate with physiother-apy and eat normally (21), start mobilizing at an early stage, and communicate with medical and nursing staff and with their family; this is likely to reduce feelings of powerlessness and anxiety associated with ventilatory support (4).

However, NPPV does have limitations. Concerns have been voiced that it may delay ETI and mechanical ventilation, resulting in a worse outcome (22–24). NPPV may be time consuming for medical and nursing staff (25), although more recent data suggest that this improves with time as practitioners become more experienced (26). The nasal or face mask is uncomfortable and some patients find it claustro-phobic and unpleasant. Facial pressure sores occur in 2% of patients (15) and with NPPV the upper airway is not protected and the lower airway cannot be accessed. This therefore limits the technique's applicability to those who are unconscious or have significant secretion retention. Table 1 provides a summary of the advantages and disadvantages of NPPV.

II. NPPV in Acute Exacerbations of COPD

There have been eight prospective, randomized, controlled trials (RCT) of NPPV predominantly or exclusively in patients with an acute exacerbation of COPD,

Table 1 Advantages and Disadvantages of NPPV

Advantages	Disadvantages
Intermittent ventilation possible	Less effective?
"Early" ventilatory support an option	Mask uncomfortable/claustrophobic
Ventilation outside the ICU possible	Time-consuming
Can cooperate with physiotherapy	Facial pressure sores
Patients can eat and drink	Airway not protected
Communication easy	No direct access to bronchial tree

published both within and outside the ICU. Brochard et al. (15) showed that NPPV for patients with exacerbations of COPD in the ICU reduced the intubation ($11/43$ vs. $31/42$; $p < 0.001$) and mortality rates ($4/43$ vs. $12/42$; $p = 0.02$) compared to conventional medical therapy. NPPV also improved pH, PaO_2, respiratory rate, and encephalopathy score at 1 h and was assocatiated with a shorter hospital stay (23 days vs. 35 days; $p = 0.005$) and a lower complication rate (16% vs. 48%; $p = 0.001$). Most of the excess mortality and complications, particularly pneumonia, were attributed to ETI. These data suggest that NPPV may be superior to IMV, but importantly this was a highly selected group of patients with the majority (70%) of potentially eligible patients excluded from the study. In a smaller study ($n = 31$) in two North American ICUs, Kramer et al. (27) also showed a marked reduction in intubation rate, particularly in the subgroup with COPD ($n = 23$) (all patients 31% vs. 73%; $p < 0.05$; COPD 67% vs. 9%; $p < 0.05$). However, mortality, hospital stay, and charges were unaffected. In a further ICU study, Celikel (16) showed a more rapid improvement in various physiological parameters and a trend toward a reduction in the need for ventilatory support, but there was no difference in intubation rate or survival. However, some patients in the conventional group subsequently received NPPV; were NPPV not to have been available it is likely that a significant number of these patients would have needed to be intubated.

Martin et al. (28) reported a prospective RCT comparing NPPV with usual medical care in 61 patients, including 23 with COPD. In common with other studies, there was a significant reduction in intubation rate (6.4 vs. 21.3 intubations per 100 ICU days; $p = 0.002$), but no difference in mortality (2.4 vs. 4.3 deaths per 100 ICU days; $p = 0.21$). Although the intubation rate was lower in the COPD subgroup (5.3 vs. 15.6 intubations per 100 ICU days; $p = 0.12$), this did not reach statistical significance; this may simply reflect the small sample size. Three patients in the NPPV group and one in the control group required ETI to maximize the safety of other procedures (e.g., bronchoscopy) and two patients in the NPPV group required ETI because of hemodynamic compromise related to massive gastrointestinal bleeding. All other patients required ETI because of progressive ventilatory failure; in other words, only four of the intubations in the NPPV group were because of a failure to control respiratory failure compared with 16 in the control group.

It is important to note that to date there is no direct comparison between IMV and NPPV and the two techniques should be viewed as complementary, with NPPV considered a means of obviating the need for ETI rather than as a direct alternative. These studies, performed in ICUs (Table 2), show that NPPV is possible and that the prevention of ETI is advantageous. The mean pH in all the studies was around 7.27, indicating a severe exacerbation with a high potential mortality (2). However, the generalizability of these results into everyday clinical practice is uncertain; results achieved in enthusiastic units as part of a clinical trial may not be achievable in other units lacking the same skill levels or commitment to making NPPV work. To establish whether NPPV has a role in the "real" world, a survey was undertaken among 42 ICUs in France over a 3-week period (29), including all 689 patients who needed ventilatory support. Patients treated with NPPV represented 16% of all patients and 35% of the patients admitted without previous endotracheal intubation

Table 2 The ICU Studies

			Reduced intubation rate and survival	
Confirm the feasibility of NPPV				
Confirm the effectiveness of NPPV				
			pH	Intubation/Fails Mortality
Ref. 15	7.28	**Conv**	**74% ± 13**	**26% ± 13**
		NPPV	**26% ± 13**	**9% ± 9**
Ref. 27	7.28	**Conv**	**67% ± 26**	13% ± 17
		NPPV	**9% ± 17**	6% ± 12
Ref. 16	7.27	**Conv**	**40% ± 25**	7% ± 12
		NPPV	**7% ± 12**	0% (0/15)
Ref. 28	7.28	**Conv**	**59% ± 18**	34% ± 17
		NPPV	**28% ± 16**	16% ± 12

Were performed in selected patients (all studies excluded those needing immediate ETI)
Reduced incidence of complications, particularly infections
    16% vs. 48% (15), **18% vs. 60%** (81), **10% vs. 19%** (29)
Reduced hospital and ICU length of stay
    23 vs. 35 days (15), **9 vs. 15** days (81)

Bold indicates $p < 0.05$.

and needing ventilatory support. NPPV was employed in less than 20% of all hypoxic ARF, in half of patients with hypercapnic respiratory distress, and was never used in patients with coma. It was followed by ETI in 40% of cases. The incidence of both nosocomial pneumonia (10% vs. 19%; $p = 0.03$), and mortality (22% vs. 41%; $p < 0.001$) was lower in NPPV patients than in those with ETI (29). After adjusting for differences at baseline, Simplified Acute Physiology Score (SAPS) II (odds ratio [OR] = 1.05 per point; confidence interval [CI]: 1.04 to 1.06), McCabe/Jackson score (OR = 2.18; CI: 1.57 to 3.03), and hypoxemic ARF (OR = 2.30; CI: 1.33 to 4.01) were identified as risk factors explaining mortality; success of NPPV was associated with a lower risk of pneumonia (OR = 0.06; CI: 0.01 to 0.45) and of death (OR = 0.16; CI: 0.05 to 0.54). In NPPV patients, SAPS II and a poor clinical tolerance predicted secondary ETI. Failure of NPPV was associated with a longer length of stay.

NPPV also opens up new opportunities with regard to location and timing of intervention. With NPPV, paralysis and sedation are not needed and ventilation outside the ICU is an option; given the considerable pressure on ICU beds in some countries, the high costs, and the fact that for some patients admission to ICU is a distressing experience (30), this is an attractive option. There have been six prospective RCTs of NPPV outside the ICU, four in which NPPV was started on a general ward and two in the emergency department (Table 3). In general, these studies have shown less clear-cut results than the ICU studies. Bott et al. (31) randomized 60 patients to either conventional treatment or NPPV. NPPV was initiated by research staff who spent 15 min to 4 h initiating it (average 90 min)

Table 3 General Ward and Emergency Room Studies

	Disease (n)		Baseline pH	ETI or "surrogate"	Mortality	Mode plus settings (cmH$_2$O) and use on day 1—when stated
Bott et al.	COPD (60)	Ward	7.35	0/30 vs. 5/30	3/30 vs. 9/30	Volume cycled ventilators. Use 7.63 h on day 1
Barbe et al.	COPD (24)	ER Ward	7.33	0/12 vs. 0/12	0/12 vs. 0/12	IPAP 14.8 EPAP 5. Use 2- to 3-h sessions per day
Angus et al.	COPD (17)	Ward	7.31 vs. 7.30	0/9 vs. 5/8	0/9 vs. 3/8	IPAP 14 to 18 cmH$_2$O
Wood et al.	Mixed (27), COPD (6)	ER	7.35 vs. 7.34	7/16 vs. 5/11	4/16 vs. 0/11	—
Bardi et al.	COPD (30)	Ward	7.36 vs. 7.39	1/15 vs. 2/15	0/15 vs. 1/15	IPAP 13 EPAP 3
Plant et al.	COPD (236)	Ward	7.32 vs. 7.31	**15% vs. 27%**	**10% vs. 20%**	IPAP 10 to 20 EPAP 5 h. Use median 8 h on day 1

and led to a more rapid correction of pH and $PaCO_2$; 9 of 30 of the conventional treatment group died compared to 3 of 30 of the NPPV group. On an intention-to-treat analysis, these figures were not statistically significant, but when those unable to tolerate NPPV were excluded a significant survival benefit was seen (9/30 vs. 1/26; $p = 0.014$). Generalizability from this study, although performed on general wards, to routine practice is again difficult given that staff additional to the normal ward complement set up NPPV. The high mortality rate (30%) in the control group was surprising, considering that the mean pH was only 7.34. In addition, the low intubation rate, while reflecting U.K. practice, has been criticized.

Angus et al. (32) compared NPPV and doxapram in patients with COPD and type II respiratory failure in a small randomized trial on a general ward. NPPV resulted in a significant improvement in both PaO_2 and $PaCO_2$ at 4 h. In contrast, no fall in $PaCO_2$ occurred in those patients treated with doxapram and an initial improvement in PaO_2 was not sustained at 4 h. At both 1 and 4 h, pH was significantly better in the NPPV group as compared with the doxapram group. All the patients in the NPPV group were discharged, although one required doxapram in addition to NPPV during their acute illness; 3 of 8 patients in the doxapram group died and a further two received NPPV. This small study suggests that NPPV is more effective than doxapram in the treatment of respiratory failure associated with COPD. However, no comparisons were made of nursing workload, patient tolerance, or complication rates between the two groups. Although respiratory stimulants have been shown to improve arterial blood gas tensions, no advantage in terms of intubation rates or survival has been demonstrated (33, 34).

Barbe et al. (35) initiated NPPV in the emergency department and continued it on a general medical ward. To ease some of the problems of workload and compliance NPPV was administered for 3 h twice a day. In this small study ($n = 24$), there were no intubations nor deaths in either group and arterial blood gas tensions improved equally in both the NPPV group and in the controls. However, the mean pH at entry in each group was 7.33 and at this level of acidosis significant mortality is not expected; in other words, it was unlikely that such a small study would show an improved outcome when recovery would be expected anyway (2). In a 1-year study, Plant et al. identified all patients with an acute exacerbation of COPD admitted to two large hospitals: 953 patient episodes were identified; 20% of all patients were acidotic on arrival to the emergency department and, of these, 20% completely corrected their pH into the normal range by the time they arrived on the ward. This was independent of the severity of acidosis. There was a relationship between PaO_2 and pH suggesting that at least in some patients acidosis had been precipitated by high-flow oxygen therapy on the way to the hospital. In addition, a proportion of patients will respond to medical therapy instituted on arrival to the hospital. The message from these studies is that it is reasonable to ascertain the effect of medical therapy, particularly controlled oxygen therapy, before starting NPPV.

Wood et al. (24) randomized 27 patients with acute respiratory distress to conventional treatment or NPPV in the emergency department. Intubation rates were similar (7/16 vs. 5/11), but there was a nonsignificant trend toward increased mortality in those given NPPV (4/16 vs. 0/11; $p = 0.123$), attributed to a delay in intubation as conventional patients requiring invasive ventilation were intubated after a mean of 4.8 h compared to 26 h in those on NPPV ($p = 0.055$). It is difficult to draw many conclusions from this study since the two groups were not well matched, with more patients with pneumonia, which is associated with a reduced likelihood of success for NPPV (22), in the NPPV group and the level of ventilatory support was modest (inspiratory positive airway pressure 8 cm H_2O). The trend toward worse outcome in association with a delay in intubation reinforces the point that facilities for prompt intubation and mechanical ventilation must be in place for patients who fail NPPV.

Bardi et al. (36), in a small, prospective controlled study of 30 patients, with allocation to the control group or ventilatory support determined by availability of personnel and equipment rather than randomly, found no significant difference in in-hospital events, although there was a trend toward an advantage with NPPV.

A multicenter RCT of NPPV in acute exacerbations of COPD ($n = 236$) on general respiratory wards in 13 centers attempted to get around some of the problems of the earlier studies (37). It was designed to establish whether NPPV applied by the usual ward staff (i.e., in the "real world") for patients who remained acidotic after initial therapy was feasible and effective in the ward setting. Patients were randomized to NPPV or conventional therapy if they had a pH 7.25–7.35 inclusive, a respiratory rate > 23 breaths per minute in association with hypercapnia on arrival at the ward, after standard medical therapy had been instituted in the emergency department. The study had 80% power to detect a 50% reduction in treatment failure, a surrogate for the need for intubation, defined by a priori criteria. Ventilation was applied by the ward staff, usually nurses, but occasionally physiotherapists, using a simple S mode bilevel device according to a simple protocol. NPPV could be established (defined as > 1 h of use) in 93% of patients, similar to the 87% described by Bott et al. using research staff to initiate ventilation, and only consumed an additional 26 min of nursing time (31). In a low nurse–patient setting, subsequent compliance might be expected to deteriorate compared to studies performed in ICU or with additional staff. However, the median compliance of 8 h on day 1 and 7 h on day 2 are similar to those in the other trials [7.6 h (31) and 6 h per day (15) and 14.4 h over the first 2 days (27)]. NPPV led to a fall in respiratory rate and a more rapid improvement in pH associated with a statistically nonsignificant fall in $PaCO_2$: these changes are similar to those reported in other studies (15, 27, 31). However, by 4 h there were no physiological differences between the two groups. This may have reflected a systematic bias against finding large physiological changes in the study design. Once a patient met criteria for intubation, further gases were not included in the analysis due to the confounding effects of subsequent intervention (e.g., invasive mechanical ventilation). Hence the physiological data largely reflect the successes and excludes those that failed. Because more patients failed in the standard group, there was a bias to minimizing any difference in physiological change. The primary endpoint treatment failure was reduced from 27% to 15% by NPPV ($p < 0.05$). There was a similar reduction in ICU utilization, although this did not reach statistical significance. However, in-hospital mortality was also reduced from 20% to 10% ($p < 0.05$). Subgroup analysis suggested that the outcome in patients with pH < 7.30 after initial treatment was inferior to that in the studies performed in the ICU. Although this study attempted to be "real world," inevitably there were advantages to patients being part of a study and the ward nursing staff could receive telephone advice and support from the trial doctor and nurse. The comfort/discomfort associated with NPPV was assessed using a five-point scale and the median score on the first 3 days indicated that patients found the process "mildly uncomfortable." Relief of the unpleasant sensation of breathlessness is an important goal of therapy. NPPV was shown to be associated with a more rapid return to "normal" in this study and a greater reduction in breathlessness than conventional therapy in another study (31). Some patients do find NPPV to be unpleasant and any benefit in terms of relief of dyspnea is offset by the claustrophobia, etc., associated with the mask. If patients find NPPV unpleasant, a decision needs to be made as to how hard the patient should be encouraged to persevere. Data from this study, together with data from the ICU studies, suggest that once the pH falls below 7.30 the outcome without ventilatory support is poor, whereas above 7.30, although there is a clear advantage from NPPV, 80% of patients will get better anyway. If the pH is > 7.30 and the patient finds NPPV unpleasant, it would be reasonable to monitor carefully. Once the pH is < 7.30, however, patients should be strongly encouraged to persevere. Put another way, if the pH is between 7.30 and 7.35, NPPV is desirable whereas once the pH falls below 7.30 it can be considered necessary. Furthermore, once the pH falls below 7.30, NPPV delivered by a very simple ventilator used according to protocol on a general ward is associated with an outcome that is markedly worse than that seen when more sophisticated ventilators are used in an ICU setting.

III. Long-Term Effects of NPPV

A number of studies have looked at long-term outcome following in-hospital NPPV. Confalonieri et al. (38) compared 24 patients treated with NPPV with matched historical controls. Only two patients receiving NPPV required intubation as compared to nine controls. The in-hospital survival rates were no different, but at 12 months were significantly better in the patients receiving NPPV (71% vs. 50%). Vitacca et al. (39) also found no difference in hospital mortality in patients receiving NPPV compared to historical controls who were intubated and ventilated (20% vs. 26%); however, a survival advantage to NPPV became apparent at three (77% vs. 52%) and 12 (70% vs. 37%) months. In the study of Bardi et al. (36), patients allocated to NPPV had four exacerbations (50% received NPPV) and to the control group six exacerbations (16% received NPPV); there was a statistically significant difference in long-term survival, with a marked advantage to the NPPV group. The reasons for this were not clear, but it was postulated may have included greater improvements in pH, tidal volume, and FEV_1, compared with admission, in the NPPV group. However, the FEV_1 at discharge in the NPPV group was 50% predicted compared with 40% predicted in the control group, suggesting more severe obstructive airways disease in the controls. The fact that less patients in the control group received NPPV for subsequent exacerbations may also have been relevant. Long-term follow-up of the patients in the study by Plant et al. (40) showed median survivals of 16.8 (NPPV group) and 13.4 months (standard group) ($p = 0.12$). The trend toward improved survival with NPPV was attributable to prevention of death during the index admission.

The possible long-term survival advantage when NPPV is given during an acute exacerbation is intriguing. It has been suggested that it is due to imperfect matching of the control and patient groups (41). However, there are other possible explanations. If ICU care has been prolonged, and weaning difficult, there may be reluctance, on the part of either medical staff or the patients themselves, to consider invasive mechanical ventilation (IMV) for a subsequent exacerbation. Second, it is possible that IMV has adverse effects that may be significant later; electrophysiological and biopsy evidence of muscle dysfunction has been shown after as little as 1 week of invasive ventilation (42, 43). Such dysfunction of the respiratory muscles will reduce the capacity of the respiratory muscle pump, which may increase the risk of ventilatory failure in subsequent exacerbation. These observations, however, are speculative and need to be substantiated in further prospective, randomized studies with larger numbers of patients.

IV. Predicting the Outcome of NPPV

A number of studies have looked at predictors of outcome with NPPV (Table 4). These have been based upon information available at the time NPPV is initiated and also after a period of NPPV. Patients with high APACHE II scores, inability to minimize the amount of mouth leak (because of lack of teeth, secretions, or breathing pattern) or inability to coordinate with NPPV are less likely to improve with NPPV (44). In another study, patients who failed on NPPV had a significantly higher incidence of pneumonia (38.5% vs. 8.7%), were underweight, had a greater level of neurological deterioration, a higher APACHE II score, and a reduced compliance with ventilation as assessed by the physician in charge compared to

Table 4 Unlikely Success of NPPV

Low pH prior to starting NPPV (22, 40, 47)
pH and respiratory rate do not improve within the first few hours of NPPV (15, 22, 40, 46, 82)
High APACHE II scores (22, 44)
Poor tolerance (44)
Inability to minimize leak (44)
Excessive secretions (44)
Poor synchrony between patient and ventilator (22, 44)
Radiological consolidation (22)
Low BMI (22)
Neurological compromise (22)
Inability to perform normal activities of every day living (47)

---

those who were successfully treated (22). However, in a RCT in which NPPV was used in patients with a primary diagnosis of community-acquired pneumonia, the only advantage, compared with conventional therapy, was a better 2-month survival (88.9% vs. 37.5%; $p = 0.05$) in the subgroup who also had COPD (45). In the study of Ambrosino et al. (44), patients failing on NPPV had a significantly more abnormal $PaCO_2$ and pH before starting NPPV, although both groups had a similar PaO_2/FiO_2 ratio. Only baseline pH was found by logistic regression analysis to predict success or failure of NPPV (mean 7.28 in successful group versus 7.22 in the failure group) with a sensitivity of 97% and specificity of 71%. Plant et al. (40) confirmed that severe acidosis at baseline was associated with an increased likelihood of failure; for each nmol $[H^+]$ increase above normal, the odds ratio for failure increased by 1.22 (95% CI 1.09–1.37; $p < 0.01$). Similarly, the more severe the hypercapnia at enrollment the greater the likelihood of failure of NPPV; $PaCO_2$ (OR 1.14 per kPa 95% CI 1.14–1.81; $p < 0.01$). After 4 h of therapy, improvement in acidosis (OR 0.89 per nmol/L 95% CI 0.82–0.97; $p < 0.01$) and fall in respiratory rate (OR 0.92 per breath/min 95% CI 0.84–0.99; $p = 0.04$) were associated with success. Poponick et al. (46), however, found no relationship between baseline parameters and the likelihood of success of NPPV delivered in the emergency room with the lack of change in blood gases after a 30-min trial being the best predictor for the need for ETI. One problem with these studies is that failure criteria are likely to be something of a self-fulfilling prophecy. If it is decided that the patient will be intubated if arterial blood gas tensions do not improve after 30 min, or if there is severe acidosis so that the patient will only be given a very limited trial of NPPV, these will then become failure criteria, even though with persistence, adjustment of settings, change of interface, etc., a different outcome might have been achieved.

Patients may fail after a period of successful NPPV, with rates reported at 0 to 20% and this has been associated with a poor outcome. Moretti et al. (47) studied 137 patients admitted with COPD and acute hypercapnic respiratory failure, initially treated successfully with NPPV. Of these, 106 continued to improve and were discharged. The remaining 23% deteriorated after 48 h of NPPV. These so-called "late failures" were then assigned to either an increased number of hours of NPPV (the mean number of hours/day of NPPV at the time of late failure was 9.2) or intubation and mechanical ventilation, depending on the patients/relatives wishes. Patients assigned to increased NPPV did significantly worse—with a mortality of 92% compared with 53% in those invasively ventilated. At the time of relapse, those patients treated with increased NPPV were more acidotic than those who were intubated (pH 7.1 vs. pH 7.29) and, although this difference was not statistically significant, it is clinically significant. The lack of statistical significance probably reflects the small number of patients. The pH difference suggests that the patients who were treated with continuing NPPV were sicker than those who were intubated. There is also the possibility that patients who were not intubated were self-selected as a group with more advanced disease, since they were not offered or declined ETI. At the time of admission, late failures had significantly lower activities of daily living (ADL) scores and blood pressure, were more tachycardic, and were more likely to have associated complications, in particular hyperglycemia. pH was not different between the groups at admission, 1 h or 24 h. Using logistic regression analysis, a low pH, a low ADL score, and the presence of associated complications at admission were more likely in patients who failed after ≥ 48 h of NPPV. Interestingly, neither the APACHE II score nor age were predictive of failure.

When considering the failure of NPPV it is important to differentiate between failure of the noninvasive approach because of intolerance of the mask, etc., and failure of ventilation (i.e., patient's condition deteriorates in spite of ventilation). Invasive ventilatory support is more likely to be successful in the former situation or when intubation carries advantages over and above the provision of ventilatory support, for instance, facilitating clearance of excessive secretions.

V. Contraindications to NPPV

Coma or confusion, upper gastrointestinal bleeding, high risk of aspiration, hemodynamic instability, or uncontrolled arrhythmia have been suggested as contra-indications to NPPV (48). This is primarily for theoretical reasons and because these patients have been excluded from previous studies and not because there is any evidence that IMV is superior in these situations. A number of anecdotal reports suggest that NPPV can be used successfully. Whether NPPV should be tried in these circumstances and, if so, for how long before moving to ETI depends upon individual circumstances. If the patient has expressed a desire not to be intubated but is willing to be treated with NPPV, there are no contraindications other than conditions that make the application of a mask impossible (e.g., severe facial deformity or burns). In other situations, a short trial of NPPV with careful monitoring and ready access to intubation is unlikely to be harmful.

VI. NPPV After Invasive Ventilation

It is important to note that all the studies described above excluded patients who were deemed to require immediate intubation. In everyday practice, some patients require intubation from the outset and others after a failed trial of NPPV. Patients with COPD may be difficult to wean from invasive mechanical ventilation (49) and NPPV has been used successfully in this situation (50, 51). Nava et al. (52) performed a prospective multicenter randomized controlled trial of the use of NPPV as a means of weaning patients with COPD who had failed a T-piece weaning trial after 48 h of ETI, controlled mechanical ventilation, and aggressive suctioning to clear secretions: 56% of the patients had required ETI on presentation and 44% after a failed trial of NPPV (mean pH at presentation = 7.18). If patients failed the weaning trial, they were randomized to further intubation and mechanical ventilation or NPPV. NPPV was associated with a shorter duration of ventilatory support (10.2 days vs. 16.6 days), a shorter ITU stay (15.1 days vs. 24 days), less nosocomial pneumonia (0/25 vs. 7/25) and an improved 60-day survival (92% vs. 72%). Girault et al. (53) in a further RCT involving 33 patients showed a reduction in the duration of invasive mechanical ventilation (4.6 ± 1.9 vs. 7.7 ± 3.8 days) and a reduced mean daily ventilatory support, but an increased total duration (11.5 ± 5.2 vs. 3.5 ± 1.4 days) of ventilatory support when the noninvasive approach was used. There was no difference in percentage of patients successfully weaned or in complication rates. In patients not suitable for NPPV from the outset or those who fail, ETI for 24 to 48 h to gain control and then early extubation onto NPPV has significant advantages over prolonged ETI.

A proportion of patients weaned from invasive ventilation subsequently deteriorate and require further ventilatory support. Hilbert et al. (54) reported 30 patients with COPD who developed hypercapnic respiratory distress within 72 h of extubation. They were treated with mask bilevel pressure support ventilation. Only 6 of these 30 patients, as compared to 20 of 30 historical controls, required reintubation. Although in-hospital mortality was not significantly different, the mean duration of ventilatory assistance and length of intensive care stay related to the event were significantly shortened by noninvasive ventilation.

VII. Modes of NPPV in Acute Exacerbations of COPD

Ventilators commonly used for NPPV are either volume or pressure targeted. There are theoretical advantages to each mode, but broadly speaking they are comparable in efficacy. Volume-targeted ventilators have been shown to produce more complete off loading of the respiratory muscles, but at the expense of comfort (55). In intubated patients, however, assist-pressure-controlled ventilation has been shown to be more effective than assist-control-volume ventilation at reducing various parameters of respiratory muscle effort, although this difference was only seen at moderate tidal volumes and low flow rates (56). In stable patients, little difference in gas exchange was seen with different types of ventilators (57, 58). In terms of outcome, Vitacca et al. (59) found that there was no difference whether volume-targeted or pressure-targeted machines were used, but pressure-targeted machines were better tolerated by patients. A new mode of proportional assist ventilation (PAV) improves gas exchange and dyspnea in stable COPD (60), and has been used successfully in the treatment of acute respiratory failure of various etiologies (61). PAV delivers ventilation according to patient demand, which should theoretically be more comfortable, but makes the assumption that the patient with respiratory failure knows best what he needs in terms of ventilatory support. PAV using flow assistance and PEEP achieved greatest improvement in minute ventilation, dyspnea, and reduction in pressure-time product per breath of the respiratory muscles and diaphragm in COPD patients with acute respiratory failure (62). It has been shown to decrease patient effort and work of breathing and neuromuscular drive (P0.1) in patients with COPD being weaned off invasive mechanical ventilation (63, 64). Further data are needed comparing PAV with conventional modes of ventilation. Pressure-cycled machines are usually cheaper than volume-cycled flow generators and this, together with the fact that they tend to be better tolerated makes them the machines of first choice.

PEEP can be added during NPPV and has beneficial effects, off loading the respiratory muscles probably by counterbalancing the inspiratory threshold load imposed by intrinsic PEEP (65) and lavaging carbon dioxide from the mask (66). In a short-term study in stable patients, the addition of PEEP has been shown to reduce oxygen delivery despite an adequate SaO_2 (18). Mask continuous positive airway pressure (CPAP) has also been shown to decrease respiratory rate and the subjective sensation of dyspnea, decrease $PaCO_2$, increase PaO_2 (67), significantly improve ventilation (68), and avoid intubation and mechanical ventilation (69) in exacerbations of COPD. In stable patients, the degree of unloading with CPAP is less than with NPPV (58) and, given the lack of randomized controlled trial data on the use of CPAP in acute exacerbations of COPD (in contrast to NPPV), its use should be confined to centers in which NPPV is not available.

The use of other modes of noninvasive ventilation have been reported in patients with COPD exacerbations. In a retrospective uncontrolled study, 105 patients were successfully weaned and 93 were eventually discharged from the hospital after intermittent negative-pressure ventilation by means of an iron lung (70). Of these 105 patients, 62 were in coma and 43 had a deteriorating level of consciousness at presentation. All patients were initially ventilated continuously for 12 to 48 h and subsequently received intermittent daytime ventilation until weaned. Any subsequent exacerbation was also treated with negative-pressure ventilation. Survival was 92 and 37% at 1 and 5 years, respectively. A more recent study by the same group was carried out in 150 patients with hypoxic hypercapnic coma (including 79% patients with COPD) (71). Of the 74 patients with only COPD exacerbation as the cause of coma, treatment failed only in 19 (26%) patients including 14 (19%) who died. However, negative-pressure ventilation is only available in a few centers that have particular expertise in the technique, and in the absence of a formal controlled trial NPPV remains the noninvasive mode of choice.

Recently, the use of a helium–oxygen gas mixture in combination with noninvasive ventilation has been evaluated in 10 patients with an acute exacerbation of COPD (72). The authors found that the helium–oxygen mixture reduced patient effort and improved gas exchange at both low $(9 \pm 2\,cmH_2O)$ and high $(18 \pm 3\,cm\,H_2O)$ levels of pressure support without significantly changing breathing pattern or oxygenation. Further data, in particular on whether this approach improves outcome, are needed, but the added expense and complexity of using helium make it unlikely to be widely used.

VIII. Staffing and Economic Implications of NPPV

In an early report of the use of NPPV in six patients, Chevrolet et al. (25) found that, particularly in patients with obstructive lung disease, the technique was very time-consuming for the nurses and largely a wasted effort because eventually all patients had to be intubated. As with any new technique, there is a learning curve and the same group have subsequently published more encouraging results (26). In the ICU, where there are high nurse-to-patient ratios, any additional work associated with NPPV is unlikely to have a major effect, but the issue of medical and nursing time is very relevant if the technique is to be performed in the ward environment. Nurses and therapists will have responsibility for a much larger number of patients and any extra work associated with NPPV may mean that other tasks and patients are neglected.

In their RCT comparing standard treatment with or without NPPV in a general ward setting, Bott et al. (31) asked the senior nurse to record on a daily basis the amount of care needed using a simple visual analogue scale. They found no difference in nursing care requirements. This may have underestimated the care requirements associated with NPPV because ventilation was initiated and maintained by staff supernumerary to the normal ward complement. In another study, with more detailed analysis of nursing and therapist activity, Kramer et al. (27) found that the respiratory therapist spent more time with patients in the NPPV group compared to the standard treatment group in the first 8 h, but this difference did not reach statistical significance. The time required in the NPPV group dropped significantly in the second 8-h period. The time demands on the nurses did not differ in the two groups throughout the measurement period and neither the respiratory therapist nor the nurses considered caring for patients on NPPV as being any more difficult than the control patients. Nava et al. (73) found that in the first 48 h of assisted ventilation NPPV was no more time-consuming or demanding for staff than invasive mechanical ventilation. However, after the first few days of ventilation, NPPV was significantly less time-consuming for both medical and nursing personnel.

Since most studies report a shorter period of ventilation, ICU, and hospital stay, it has been suggested that NPPV should be cheaper than invasive mechanical ventilation (74, 75). However, patients treated with NPPV do incur substantial financial cost during their hospitalization (76). Nava et al. (73) found that the total cost per day was comparable for invasive and noninvasive ventilation when NPPV was performed on a respiratory ICU. In a study by Kramer et al. (27), the total hospital charges were 37.6 ± 7.9 (in thousands of dollars) in patients receiving NPPV versus 33.9 ± 6.9 in control patients not receiving NPPV, which was not statistically different (27). Keenan et al. performed a cost-effectiveness analysis of NPPV versus conventional therapy using base care modeled for a tertiary care, teaching hospital (77). The main outcomes modeled and calculated were costs, mortality, and intubation rates. To determine clinical effectiveness, the authors used a meta-analysis of randomized trials. Then a decision tree was constructed and probabilities were applied at each chance node using research evidence and a comprehensive regional database. They concluded that NPPV was more effective than standard treatment in reducing hospital mortality and, at the same time less expensive, with a cost saving of about $2500 per patient admission. In the multicenter study from the U.K., the incremental cost of NPPV per patient avoiding the need for intubation was £2829. However, the incremental savings per death avoided was £4114, by way of decreased ICU use, thus providing a strong economic argument for use of NPPV outside the ICU (78). The major problem with these kinds of analyses is that the different models and costs of health care in different countries, and indeed between different institutions within the same country, severely limit the generalizability. However, overall the data suggest that NPPV improves outcome at reduced cost.

IX. Conclusion

There is now robust evidence for the use of NPPV in patients with COPD. NPPV should be considered as a means of preventing, rather than a direct alternative to, ETI and mechanical ventilation. When ETI is deemed necessary, a strategy of early extubation onto NPPV should be considered. The reduction in complications, particularly pneumonia, is a consistent and important finding (15, 29, 52, 79). Because of the advantages associated with the noninvasive approach, it has become an important part of the therapeutic armamentarium of the respiratory physician and the intensivist and has recently been described as "a new standard of care" in acute exacerbations of COPD (80).

References

1. Martin TR, Lewis SW, Albert RK. The prognosis of patients with chronic obstructive pulmonary disease after hospitalization for acute respiratory failure. Chest 1982; 82(3):310–314.
2. Jeffrey AA, Warren PM, Flenley DC. Acute hypercapnic respiratory failure in patients with chronic obstructive lung disease: risk factors and use of guidelines for management. Thorax 1992; 47:34–40.
3. Hudson LD. Survival data in patients with acute and chronic lung disease requiring mechanical ventilation. Am Rev Respir Dis 1989; 140:S19–S24.
4. Seneff MG, Wagner DP, Wagner RP, Zimmerman JE, Knaus WA. Hospital and 1-year survival of patients admitted to intensive care units with acute exacerbation of chronic obstructive pulmonary disease. JAMA 1995; 274:1852–1857.
5. Anon JM, Garcia de Lorenzo A, Zarazaga A, Gomez-Tello V, Garrido G. Mechanical ventilation of patients on long-term oxygen therapy with acute exacerbation of chronic obstructive pulmonary disease: prognosis and cost-utility analysis. Intens Care Med 1999; 25:452–457.
6. Ludwigs UG, Baehrendtz S, Wanecek M, Matell G. Mechanical ventilation in medical and neurological diseases: 11 years of experience. J Intern Med 1991; 229(2):117–124.
7. Spicher JE, White DP. Outcome and function following prolonged mechanical ventilation. Arch Intern Med 1987; 147(3):421–425.
8. Sluiter HJ, Blokzijl EJ, Dijl WV, Haeringen JRV, Hilvering C, Steenhuis EJ. Conservative and respirator treatment of acute respiratory insufficiency in patients with chronic obstructive lung disease. A reappraisal. Am Rev Respir Dis 1972; 105(6):932–943.
9. Nevins ML, Epstein SK. Weaning from prolonged mechanical ventilation. Clin Chest Med 2001; 22(1):13–33.
10. Seneff MG, Zimmerman JE, Knaus WA, Wagner PD, Draper EA. Predicting the duration of mechanical ventilation—the importance of disease and patient characteristics. Chest 1996; 110:469–479.

11. Brochard L, Rauss A, Benito S, Conti G, Mancebo J, Rekik N, et al. Comparison of three methods of gradual withdrawal from ventilatory support during weaning from mechanical ventilation. Am J Respir Crit Care Med 1994; 150:896–903.

12. Girault C, Richard J, Chevron V, Tamion F, Pasquis P, Leroy J, et al. Comparative physiological effects of noninvasive assist-control and pressure support ventilation in acute hypercapnic respiratory failure. Chest 1997; 111:1639–1648.

13. Brochard L, Isabey D, Piquet J, Amaro P, Mancebo J, Messadi AA, et al. Reversal of acute exacerbations of chronic obstructive lung disease by inspiratory assistance with a face mask. N Engl J Med 1990; 323:1523–1530.

14. Diaz O, Iglesia R, Ferrer M, Zavala E, Santos C, Wagner PD, et al. Effects of noninvasive ventilation on pulmonary gas exchange and hemodynamics during acute hypercapnic exacerbations of chronic obstructive pulmonary disease. Am J Respir Crit Care Med 1997; 156:1840–1845.

15. Brochard L, Mancebo J, Wysocki M, Lofaso F, Conti G, Rauss A, et al. Noninvasive ventilation for acute exacerbations of chronic obstructive pulmonary disease. N Engl J Med 1995; 333:817–822.

16. Celikel T, Sungur M, Ceyhan B, Karakurt S. Comparison of noninvasive positive pressure ventilation with standard medical therapy in hypercapnic acute respiratory failure. Chest 1998; 114:1636–1642.

17. Confalonieri M, Gazzaniga P, Gandola L, Aiolfi S, Della Porta R, Frisinghelli A, et al. Haemodynamic response during initiation of non-invasive positive pressure ventilation in COPD patients with acute ventilatory failure. Respir Med 1998; 92:331–337.

18. Ambrosino N, Nava S, Torbicki A, Riccardi G, Fracchia C, Opasich C, et al. Hemodynamic effects of pressure support and PEEP ventilation by nasal route in patients with stable chronic obstructive pulmonary disease. Thorax 1993; 48:523–528.

19. Fagon JY, Chastre J, Hance A, Montravers P, Novara A, Gibert C. Nosocomial pneumonia in ventilated patients: a cohort study evaluating attributable mortality and hospital stay. Am J Med 1993; 94:281–287.

20. Torres A, Aznar R, Gatell JM. Incidence, risk and prognosis factors of nosocomial pneumonia in mechanically ventilated patients. Am Rev Respir Dis 1990; 142:523–528.

21. Pingleton SK. Complications of acute respiratory failure. Am Rev Respir Dis 1988; 137:1463–1493.

22. Ambrosino N, Foglio K, Rubini F, Clini E, Nava S, Vitacca M. Non-invasive mechanical ventilation in acute respiratory failure due to chronic obstructive airways disease: correlates for success. Thorax 1995; 50:755–757.

23. Ambrosino N. Noninvasive mechanical ventilation in acute respiratory failure. Eur Respir J 1996; 9:795–807.

24. Wood KA, Lewis L, Von Harz B, Kollef MH. The use of noninvasive positive pressure ventilation in the Emergency Department. Chest 1998; 113(5):1339–1346.

25. Chevrolet JC, Jolliet F, Abajo B, Toussi A, Louis M. Nasal positive pressure ventilation in patients with acute respiratory failure. Chest 1991; 100:775–782.

26. Chevrolet JC, Jolliet P. Workload on non-invasive ventilation in acute respiratory failure. In: Vincent JL, ed. Year book of Intensive and Emergency Medicine. Berlin: Springer, 1997:505–513.

27. Kramer N, Meyer TJ, Meharg J, Cece RD, Hill NS. Randomized, prospective trial of noninvasive positive pressure ventilation in acute respiratory failure. Am J Respir Crit Care Med 1995; 151:1799–1806.

28. Martin TJ, Hovis JD, Costantino JP, Bierman MI, Donahoe MP, Rogers RM, et al. A randomized, prospective evaluation of noninvasive ventilation for acute respiratory failure. Am J Respir Crit Care Med 2000; 161:807–813.

29. Carlucci A, Richard JC, Wysocki M, Lepage E, Brochard L. Noninvasive versus conventional mechanical ventilation. An epidemiologic survey. Am J Respir Crit Care Med 2001; 163(4):874–880.

30. Easton C, MacKenzie F. Sensory-perceptual alterations: delirium in the intensive care unit. Heart Lung 1988; 17:229–237.

31. Bott J, Carroll MP, Conway JH, Keilty SEJ, Ward EM, Brown AM, et al. Randomised controlled trial of nasal ventilation in acute ventilatory failure due to chronic obstructive airways disease. Lancet 1993; 341:1555–1557.

32. Angus RM, Ahmed AA, Fenwick LJ, Peacock AJ. Comparison of the acute effects on gas exchange of nasal ventilation and doxapram in exacerbations of chronic obstructive pulmonary disease. Thorax 1996; 51:1048–1050.

33. Riordan JF, Sillett RW, McNichol MW. A controlled trial of doxapram in acute respiratory failure. Br J Dis Chest 1975; 69:57–62.

34. Moser KM, Luchsinger PC, Adamson JS, McMohan SM, Schlueter DP, Spivack M, et al. Respiratory stimulation with intravenous doxapram in respiratory failure. A double-blind co-operative study. N Engl J Med 1973; 288:427–431.

35. Barbe F, Togores B, Rubi M, Pons S, Maimo A, Agusti AGN. Noninvasive ventilatory support does not facilitate recovery from acute respiratory failure in chronic obstructive pulmonary disease. Eur Respir J 1996; 9:1240–1245.

36. Bardi G, Pierotello R, Desideri M, Valdisseri L, Bottai M, Palla A. Nasal ventilation in COPD exacerbations: early and late results of a prospective, controlled study. Eur Respir J 2000; 15:98–104.

37. Plant PK, Owen JL, Elliott MW. Early use of non-invasive ventilation for acute exacerbations of chronic obstructive pulmonary disease on general respiratory wards: a multicentre randomised controlled trial. Lancet 2000; 355:1931–1935.

38. Confalonieri M, Parigi P, Scartabellati A, Aiolfi S, Scorsetti S. Nava S, et al. Noninvasive mechanical ventilation improves the immediate and long-term outcome of COPD patients with acute respiratory failure. Eur Respir J 1996; 9:422–430.

39. Vitacca M, Clini E, Rubini F, Nava S, Foglio K, Ambrosino N. Non-invasive mechanical ventilation in severe chronic obstructive lung disease and acute respiratory failure: short- and long-term prognosis. Intens Care Med 1996; 22:94–100.

40. Plant PK, Owen JL, Elliott MW. Non-invasive ventilation in acute exacerbations of chronic obstructive pulmonary disease: long term survival and predictors of in-hospital outcome. Thorax 2001; 56(9):708–712.

41. Shneerson JM. The changing role of mechanical ventilation in COPD. Eur Respir J 1996; 9:393–398.

42. Coakley JH, Nagendran K, Honavar M, Hinds CJ. Preliminary observations on the neuromuscular abnormalities in patients with organ failure and sepsis. Intens Care Med 1993; 19:323–328.

43. Coakley JH, Nagendran K, Ormerod IE, Ferguson CN, Hinds CJ. Prolonged neurogenic weakness in patients requiring mechanical ventilation for acute airflow limitation. Chest 1992; 101:1413–1416.

44. Soo Hoo GW, Santiago S, Williams AJ. Nasal mechanical ventilation for hypercapnic respiratory failure in chronic obstructive pulmonary disease: determinants of success and failure. Crit Care Med 1994; 22:1253–1261.

45. Confalonieri M, Potena A, Carbone G, Porta RD, Tolley EA, Meduri UG. Acute respiratory failure in patients with severe community-acquired pneumonia. A prospective randomized evaluation of noninvasive ventilation. Am J Respir Crit Care Med 1999; 160:1585–1591.

46. Poponick JM, Renston JP, Bennett RP, Emerman CL. Use of a ventilatory support system (BiPAP) for acute respiratory failure in the emergency department. Chest 1999; 116:166–171.

47. Moretti M, Cilione C, Tampieri A, Fracchia C, Marchioni A, Nava S. See 3288 incidence and causes of non-invasive mechanical ventilation failure after an initial (< 48 hrs) successful attempt. Thorax 2000; 55:819–825.

48. Ambrosino N. Noninvasive mechanical ventilation in acute on chronic respiratory failure: determinants of success and failure. Monald Arch Chest Dis 1997; 52:73–75.

49. Grassino A, Comtois N, Galdiz HJ, Sinderby C. The unweanable patient. Monald Arch Chest Dis 1994; 49(6):522–526.

50. Udwadia ZF, Santis OK, Steven MH, Simonds AK. Nasal ventilation to facilitate weaning in patients with chronic respiratory insufficiency. Thorax 1992; 47:715–718.

51. Restrick LJ, Scott AD, Ward EM, Feneck RO, Cornwell WE, Wedzicha JA. Nasal intermittent positive-pressure ventilation in weaning intubated patients with chronic respiratory disease from assisted positive-pressure ventilation. Respir Med 1993; 87:199–204.

52. Nava S, Ambrosino N, Clini E, Prato M, Orlando G, Vitacca M, et al. Noninvasive mechanical ventilation in the weaning of patients with respiratory failure due to chronic obstructive pulmonary disease. A randomized, controlled trial. Ann Intern Med 1998; 128:721–728.

53. Girault C, Daudenthun I, Chevron V, Tamion F, Leroy J, Bonmarchand G. Noninvasive ventilation as a systematic extubation and weaning technique in acute-on-chronic respiratory failure. A prospective, randomized controlled study. Am J Respir Crit Care Med 1999; 160:86–92.

54. Hilbert G, Gruson D, Pore L, Gbikpi-Benissan G, Cardinaud JP. Noninvasive pressure support ventilation in COPD patients with post extubation hypercapnic respiratory insufficiency. Eur Respir J 1998; 11:1349–1353.

55. Girault C, Richard JC, Chevron V, Tamion F, Pasquis P, Leroy J, et al. Comparative physiologic effects of noninvasive assist-control and pressure support ventilation in acute hypercapnic respiratory failure. Chest 1998; 111:1639–1648.

56. Cinnella G, Conti U, Lofaso F, Lorino H, Harf A, Lemaire F, et al. Effects of assisted ventilation on the work of breathing: volume-controlled versus pressure-controlled ventilation. Am J Respir Crit Care Med 1996; 153:1025–1033.

57. Meecham Jones DJ, Wedzicha JA. Comparison of pressure and volume preset nasal ventilator systems in stable chronic respiratory failure. Eur Respir J 1993; 6:1060–1064.

58. Elliott MW, Aquilina R, Green M, Moxham J, Simonds AK. A comparison of different modes of noninvasive ventilatory support: effects on ventilation and inspiratory muscle effort. Anaesthesia 1994; 49:279–283.

59. Vitacca M, Rubini F, Foglio K, Scalvini S, Nava S, Ambrosino N. Non-invasive modalities of positive pressure ventilation improve the outcome of acute exacerbations in COLD patients. Intens Care Med 1993; 19:450–455.

60. Ambrosino N, Vitacca M, Polese G, Pagani M, Foglio K, Rossi A. Short-term effects of nasal proportional assist ventilation in patients with chronic hypercapnic respiratory insufficiency. Eur Respir J 1997; 10:2829–2834.

61. Patrick W, Webster K, Ludwig L, Roberts D, Wiebe P, Younes M. Non-invasive positive-pressure ventilation in acute respiratory distress without prior respiratory failure. Am J Respir Crit Care Med 1996; 153:1005–1011.

62. Ranieri VM, Grasso S, Mascia L, Martino S, Fiore T, Brienza A, et al. Effects of proportional assist ventilation on inspiratory muscle effort in patients with chronic obstructive pulmonary disease and acute respiratory failure. Anaesthesiology 1997; 86(1):79–91.

63. Wrigge H, Golisch W, Zinserling J, Sydow M, Almeling G, Burchardi H. Proportional assist versus pressure support ventilation: effects on breathing pattern and respiratory work of patients with chronic obstructive pulmonary disease. Intens Care Med 1999; 25(8):790–798.

64. Appendini L, Purro A, Gudjonsdottir M, Baderna P, Patessio A, Zanaboni S, et al. Physiological response of ventilator-dependent patients with chronic obstructive pulmonary disease to proportional assist ventilation and continuous positive airway pressure. Am J Respir Crit Care Med 1999; 159(5 Pt 1):1510–1517.

65. Appendini L, Patessio A, Zanaboni S, Carone M, Gukov B, Donner CF, et al. Physiologic effects of positive end-expiratory pressure and mask pressure support during exacerbations of chronic obstructive pulmonary disease. Am J Respir Crit Care Med 1994; 149:1069–1076.

66. Ferguson GT, Gilmartin M. CO_2 rebreathing during BiPAP ventilatory assistance. Am J Respir Crit Care Med 1995; 151:1126–1135.

67. de Lucas P, Tarancon C, Puente L, Rodriguez C, Tatay E, Monturiol JM. Nasal continuous positive airway pressure in patients with COPD in acute respiratory failure: a study of the immediate effects. Chest 1993; 104:1694–1697.

68. Potgieter PD, Rosenthal E, Benatar SR. Immediate and long-term survival in patients admitted to a respiratory ICU. Crit Care Med 1985; 13:798–802.

69. Miro AM, Shivaram U, Hertig I. Continuous positive airway pressure in COPD patients in acute hypercapnic respiratory failure. Chest 1993; 103:266–268.

70. Corrado A, Bruscoli G, Messori A, Ghedina L, Nutini S, De Paola E, et al. Iron lung treatment of subjects with COPD in acute respiratory failure. Evaluation of short- and long-term prognosis. Chest 1992; 101:692–696.

71. Corrado A, De Paola E, Gorini M, Messori A, Bruscoli G, Nutini S, et al. Intermittent negative pressure ventilation in the treatment of hypoxic hypercapnic coma in chronic respiratory insufficiency. Thorax 1996; 51:1077–1082.

72. Jaber S, Fodil R, Carlucci A, Boussarsar M, Pigeot J, Lemaire F, et al. Noninvasive ventilation with helium–oxygen in acute exacerbations of chronic obstructive pulmonary disease. Am J Respir Crit Care Med 2000; 161:1191–1200.

73. Nava S, Evangelisti I, Rampulla C, Compagnoni ML, Fracchia C, Rubini F. Human and financial costs of noninvasive mechanical ventilation in patients affected by COPD and acute respiratory failure. Chest 1997; 111:1631–1638.

74. Vitacca M, Clini E, Porta R, Sereni D, Ambrosino N. Experience of an intermediate respiratory intensive therapy in the treatment of prolonged weaning from mechanical ventilation. Minerva Anestesiol 1996; 62:57–64.

75. Anderer W, Kunzle C, Dhein Y, Worth H. [Noninvasive ventilation in the acute care hospital—a cost factor?]. [German]. Med Klin 1997; 92(Suppl 1):119–122.

76. Criner GJ, Kreimer DT, Tomaselli M, Pierson W, Evans D. Financial implications of noninvasive positive pressure ventilation (NPPV). Chest 1995; 108:475–481.

77. Keenan SP, Gregor J, Sibbald WJ, Cook DJ, Gafni A. Noninvasive positive pressure ventilation in the setting of severe, acute exacerbations of chronic obstructive pulmonary disease: More effective and less expensive. Crit Care Med 2000; 28:2094–2102.

78. Plant PK, Owen J, Elliott MW. A cost effectiveness analysis of non-invasive ventilation (NIV) in acute exacerbations of COPD. Thorax 1999; 54(Suppl 3):A11.

79. Antonelli M, Conti G, Rocco M, Bufi M, De Blasi RA, Vivino G, et al. A comparison of noninvasive positive-pressure ventilation and conventional mechanical ventilation in patients with acute respiratory failure. N Engl J Med 1998; 339:429–435.

80. Brochard L. Non-invasive ventilation for acute exacerbations of COPD: a new standard of care. Thorax 2000; 55(10):817–818.

81. Girou E, Schortgen F, Delclaux C, Brun-Buisson C, Blot F, Lefort Y, et al. Association of noninvasive ventilation with nonsocomial infections and survival in critically ill patients. JAMA 2000; 284(18):2361–2367.

82. Meduri GU, Turner RE, Abou-Shala N, Wunderink R, Tolley E. Noninvasive positive pressure ventilation via face mask. First-line intervention in patients with acute hypercapnic and hypoxemic respiratory failure. Chest 1996; 109:179–193.

26

Invasive Mechanical Ventilation in Acute Exacerbation of Chronic Obstructive Pulmonary Disease

DIMITRIS GEORGOPOULOS

University Hospital of Heraklion
Heraklion, Crete, Greece

ANDREA ROSSI

Ospedali Riuniti di Bergamo
Bergamo, Italy

I. Introduction

Patients with acute exacerbation of chronic obstructive pulmonary disease (COPD) may need mechanical ventilatory support in order to (1) relieve excessive dyspnea; (2) improve the gas exchange; (3) sustain alveolar ventilation; and (4) unload the respiratory muscles (1, 2).

Meanwhile, there is time for other therapeutic interventions (bronchodilators, corticosteroids, antibiotics) to reverse the cause of exacerbation and to improve the functional status of the patient. During mechanical ventilatory support, the physician must aim to avoid complications related to mechanical ventilation and should initiate weaning and discontinuation of mechanical ventilation as soon as possible.

Mechanical ventilatory support can be applied in intubated and nonintubated patients with acute exacerbation of COPD (1–3). The latter is referred to as noninvasive mechanical ventilation (NIMV) (3). Because mechanical ventilation via an endotracheal tube (invasive or conventional mechanical ventilation) can be associated with a number of complications that carry their own risk of morbidity and mortality (4, 5), NIMV should be regarded as a way to avoid many of these complications and should be attempted whenever possible (see Chap. 25).

Invasive mechanical ventilation in patients with acute exacerbation of COPD is a challenge due to the complex pathophysiology of the disease (6–9) as well as the significant interaction between this pathophysiology and the process of mechanical ventilation (10, 11). Planned ventilatory strategies to achieve the goals of mechanical ventilation should take into consideration both the pathophysiology of the disease and the patient–ventilator interaction. In this review we will discuss the principles that underlie the use of conventional mechanical ventilation in patients with acute exacerbation of COPD. Weaning strategies will be reviewed separately (see Chap. 27).

II. Indications for Invasive Mechanical Ventilation

The indications for intubation and ventilatory support in patients with acute exacerbations of COPD are not clearly defined and the decision to ventilate these patients via an endotracheal tube is usually made based on the patient's condition and the physician's clinical judgment. As a general rule, conventional mechanical ventilation should be performed in the intensive care unit (ICU). Table 1 shows commonly used criteria for ICU admission, which may be modified based on local resources (2). Patients who show signs of impending acute respiratory failure and those with life-threatening acid-base status abnormalities and/or altered mental status despite aggressive therapy (including NIMV) are candidates for invasive mechanical ventilation (2) (Table 2). Although a recent uncontrolled study reported that NIMV using negative pressure ventilation was effective in patients with hypoxic–hypercapnic coma (12), this observation needs to be confirmed by randomized studies; currently coma is considered as an absolute indication for intubation. Finally, the use of invasive mechanical ventilation is also influenced by the likely reversibility of the precipitating event leading to acute exacerbation, the patient's wishes, and the availability of intensive care facilities (2).

III. Pathophysiology

Extensive review of the pathophysiology of acute exacerbation of COPD is beyond the scope of this chapter and the reader is referred to several excellent reviews (6–9).

Table 1 Indications for ICU Admission of Patients with Acute Exacerbations of COPD[a]

1. Severe dyspnea that responds inadequately to initial emergency therapy.
2. Confusion, lethargy, coma.
3. Persistent or worsening hypoxemia ($PaO_2 < 6.7$ kPa, 50 mmHg), or severe/worsening hypercapnia ($PaCO_2 > 9.3$ kPa, 70 mmHg), or severe/worsening respiratory acidosis (pH < 7.30) despite supplemental oxygen and NIPPV.

[a]Local resources need to be considered.
Source: From Ref. 2.
NIPPV: noninvasive positive pressure ventilation.

Table 2 Indications for Invasive Mechanical Ventilation

1. Severe dyspnea with use of accessory muscles and paradoxical abdominal motion.
2. Respiratory frequency > 35 breaths/min.
3. Life-threatening hypoxemia (PaO_2 < 5.3 kPa, 40 mmHg or PaO_2 < 200 mmHg).
4. Severe acidosis (pH < 7.25) and hypercapnia ($PaCO_2$ > 8.0 kPa; 60 mmHg).
5. Respiratory arrest.
6. Somnolence, impaired mental status.
7. Cardiovascular complications (hypotension, shock, heart failure).
8. Other complications (metabolic abnormalities, sepsis, pneumonia, pulmonary embolism, barotrauma, massive pleural effusion).
9. NIPPV failure (or exclusion criteria).

F_1O_2; fractional concentration of oxygen in dry inspired gas.
NIPPV: noninvasive positive pressure ventilation.
Source: From Ref. 2.

Only those aspects of the pathophysiology relevant to mechanical ventilation will be highlighted.

Multiple factors in patients with acute exacerbation of COPD cause four primary pathophysiological events (1, 2, 6–9) that should be considered when mechanical ventilation is initiated: (1) dynamic hyperinflation; (2) respiratory muscles dysfunction; (3) inefficient gas exchange; and (4) cardiovascular abnormalities. Each of these features is affected considerably by mechanical ventilation, while, on the other hand, a significant interaction between them exists.

A. Dynamic Hyperinflation

During acute exacerbations of COPD bronchoconstriction, enhanced inflammation of the airway wall, and secretions significantly worsen the abnormal resistance to airflow. The increase is much higher during expiration where the airway resistance may be severalfold higher than that during inspiration (6–9). In addition, excessive expiratory flow limitation, which is commonly present in patients with stable moderate-to-severe COPD, worsens too. The high expiratory airway resistance, combined with expiratory flow limitation, low elastic recoil, high ventilatory demands, and short expiratory time due to the high frequency of breathing (i.e., tachypnea), may not permit the respiratory system to reach the elastic equilibrium volume [i.e., passive functional residual capacity (FRC)] at end expiration. This phenomenon is commonly referred to as dynamic hyperinflation (10, 12–21) (Fig. 1). Thus, an elastic threshold load [intrinsic positive end-expiratory pressure (iPEEP)] is imposed on the inspiratory muscles at the beginning of inspiration] and increases the amount of the inspiratory effort needed to breathe (14). In addition, the respiratory system may be driven by the dynamic hyperinflation to operate near-total lung capacity (TLC) where the compliance is relatively low and the elastic work of breathing is greater than at FRC (21). Dynamic hyperinflation has several other adverse consequences (Fig. 2). First, it forces the respiratory muscles to operate at

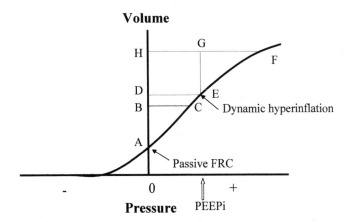

Figure 1 Static pressure–volume curve of total respiratory system. Normally the respiratory system at the end of expiration reaches passive FRC where alveolar pressure is zero (point A). Assuming that end-inspiratory lung volume is at point B the ABC area determines the inspiratory elastic work of breathing. In the dynamically hyperinflated patient, the respiratory system does not reach passive FRC and inspiration begins at higher volume where the alveolar pressure is positive (PEEPi, point E). The patient, in order to initiate flow, must first decrease the alveolar pressure to zero by contracting the inspiratory muscles (alveolar pressure must decrease from E to D). This represents an elastic threshold load, which substantially increases the work of breathing (area EDGH). The work of breathing may be further increased if the system at end inspiration approaches total lung capacity (area EFG). At presence of dynamic hyperinflation, for a given tidal volume the total work of breathing (area EDGH + EFG) is considerably higher than that without dynamic hyperinflation (area ABC).

high lung volume, which is a disadvantageous position for pressure generation (19–21). Thus, the respiratory muscles must face the increased workload while, at the same time, their capacity is reduced. Second, dynamic hyperinflation increases mean intrathoracic pressure and this may cause impaired cardiovascular function, barotrauma, patient-ventilator asynchrony, and misinterpretation of data regarding hemodynamic and respiratory system mechanics (22–26). Third, high alveolar pressure may convert more of the lung into zones 1 and 2, thereby increasing dead space and minute ventilation requirements (27). This may further worsen the gas exchange and the dynamic hyperinflation (Fig. 2).

It follows that dynamic hyperinflation plays a key role in the pathophysiology of acute exacerbations of COPD and is a fundamental mechanism leading to acute respiratory failure and the need for mechanical ventilatory support.

B. Respiratory Muscles Dysfunction

Respiratory muscles dysfunction may be the result of factors related to (1) central command; (2) neuromuscular transmission; (3) ability of the respiratory muscles to generate pressure; and (4) the translation of this pressure to flow and volume

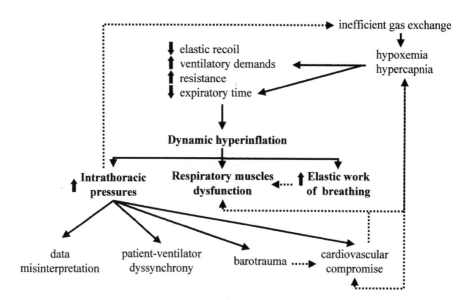

Figure 2 Determinants and consequences of dynamic hyperinflation (see text for details).

(9, 19–21). In patients with acute exacerbation of COPD, the factors that affect the ability of ventilatory muscles to generate pressure and its translation to flow and volume are most important and include dynamic hyperinflation (17, 18), excessive resistive load (28), and high ventilatory demands (29). All these pathophysiological abnormalities increase the work of breathing, a central feature of the exacerbation (14). The existence of dynamic hyperinflation is of particular concern for the function of respiratory muscles. Indeed, it has been shown that during acute exacerbation of COPD approximately half of the patient's inspiratory effort may be needed to counterbalance the elastic threshold imposed by the dynamic hyperinflation to initiate flow (30). The elastic inspiratory work of breathing would be further increased if the respiratory system, because of dynamic hyperinflation, is forced to operate at high lung volumes where compliance is relatively low (Fig. 1). At the same time, respiratory muscle dysfunction may be further aggravated by malnutrition (29), high demands for oxygen (31), cardiac output decrease (32), blood gas abnormalities (33), electrolyte disturbances (34, 35), and infections (36).

C. Inefficient Gas Exchange

Inefficient gas exchange is manifested by hypercapnia and hypoxemia and is a cardinal feature in patients with COPD needing mechanical ventilation (37, 38). Hypoxemia of variable degree, caused mainly by $\dot{V}/\dot{Q}$ mismatching, is always present (37, 38). Hypercapnia, if present, reflects both $\dot{V}/\dot{Q}$ mismatching and alveolar hypoventilation, the latter resulting from respiratory muscle dysfunction, on one hand, and increased ventilatory requirements on the other (9). Alveolar hypoventilation may also be the only pathway through which the respiratory muscles can cope with the mechanical abnormalities of the ventilatory pump (9). Finally, as a terminal event, central drive inhibition mediated through afferents from respiratory muscles may contribute to hypercapnia (39, 40).

D. Cardiovascular Abnormalities

Cardiovascular dysfunction is usually related to chronic and acute blood gas derangement, dynamic hyperinflation and increased right ventricular afterload (41–44). However, because these patients are often elderly, with several risk factors for coronary artery disease, the association with left ventricular dysfunction is potentially a frequent event (45). Although diagnosis of left heart failure may be particularly difficult in this context, its presence may considerably influence the therapeutic management as well as the prognosis.

Hypotension following intubation and passive positive pressure ventilation (controlled modes) is a common event in patients with COPD (46). The transmission of positive alveolar pressures to pleural space impedes venous return and leads to reduction in stroke volume (13, 44, 46) (Fig. 3). The situation is also aggravated when intravascular volume is reduced and by the concomitant use of sedation, circumstances associated with decreased mean systemic pressure (47). Furthermore, a greater portion of positive alveolar pressure is transmitted to pleural space if the chest wall compliance is low (obesity) and/or the lung compliance is high (emphysema) (47). Therefore, sedated and dehydrated patients with low chest wall compliance and/or high lung compliance are at high risk for cardiovascular compromise with positive pressure ventilation. All these factors may cause cardiovascular collapse, particularly if the patient is overventilated in order to correct the respiratory acidosis. Finally, dynamic hyperinflation, apart from the tendency to decrease the venous return, increases the pulmonary vascular resistance, thus raising the afterload of the right ventricle, and further compromises the right heart function (44).

Active respiratory efforts (inspiratory and expiratory) in patients breathing spontaneously or ventilated on assisted modes, may cause cardiovascular dysfunction through a number of mechanisms related to changes in preload and afterload of both ventricles (44, 48–51). Vigorous inspiratory efforts against obstructed airways increase the filling of the right heart and combined with the increased right ventricle afterload may cause a left shift in intraventricular septum, resulting in a decrease in the diastolic compliance of the left ventricle (45, 46). Meanwhile, the negative intrathoracic pressures during inspiration increase the afterload of the left ventricle and may cause a reduction of stroke volume (48, 49). These events may be associated with significant increases in end-diastolic left-ventricular pressures and may be a precipitating factor for cardiogenic pulmonary edema (45). Finally, expiratory muscle contraction, commonly observed in patients with acute exacerbations of COPD (50), increases abdominal pressure and, in the presence of

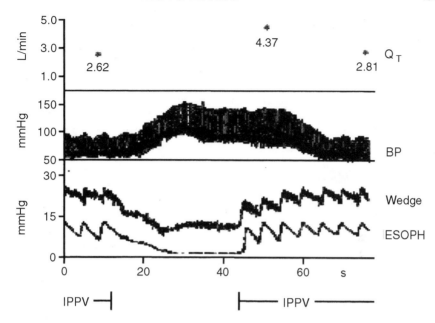

Figure 3 Effect of temporary discontinuation of intermittent positive-pressure ventilation (IPPV) on cardiac output (QT), systemic blood pressure (BP), pulmonary arterial wedge pressure, and esophageal pressure in a patient with obstructive lung disease and PEEPi. Note that IPPV is associated with a significant reduction in QT. Observe, also, that wedge pressure during IPPV is elevated by the increase in intrathoracic pressure. (From Ref. 13.)

hypovolemia, may collapse the inferior vena cava during expiration, reducing the venous return (51).

To summarize, in the passively ventilated patient, the main problem, as far as the cardiovascular system is concerned, is the decrease in venous return, while during assisted (or loaded spontaneous) breathing left ventricle afterload exposes to the risk of pulmonary edema.

IV. Evaluation of the Patient

An important step in approaching a mechanically ventilated patient with acute exacerbation of COPD is to evaluate to which extent the various aspects of the pathophysiology of the disease contribute to patient status.

Assessment of respiratory system mechanics, including dynamic hyperinflation (10), respiratory muscle function (52, 53), gas exchange properties of the lung (54), and cardiovascular functioning (41–44) should be performed rapidly. We would like to focus only on assessment of dynamic hyperinflation and respiratory system mechanics because this task plays a vital role in patient management. On the other hand, dynamic hyperinflation affects considerably the cardiovascular function, as well as that of respiratory muscles (Fig. 2).

A. Respiratory System Mechanics: Dynamic Hyperinflation

Respiratory system mechanics, including dynamic hyperinflation, can be assessed relatively easily in patients without respiratory efforts, ventilated on controlled modes, but this task is much more difficult in those with active respiratory efforts, ventilated on assisted modes.

Controlled Modes

Dynamic hyperinflation should be sought in all patients. The shape of relaxed expiratory flow-time or flow-volume curves, often depicted by the ventilator monitor, is the first clue for the presence of dynamic hyperinflation (10) (Fig. 4). The persistence of expiratory flow at the end of relaxed expiration indicates that the system is above passive functional residual capacity (FRC) and flow is driven by the positive recoil pressure of respiratory system at end expiration (PEEPi). PEEPi can be measured by comparing the end-expiratory airway occlusion pressure, easily obtained with the expiratory hold function of many ventilators, with the set level of extrinsic PEEP (occlusion method) (Fig. 4) or by measuring the amount of positive airway pressure required to initiate inspiratory flow from airway pressure and flow recordings (counterbalance method) (4, 10). Recently, Nucci and colleagues (55) developed a simple method for on-line monitoring of intrinsic PEEP in ventilator-dependent patients with relaxed respiratory muscles. This method requires neither any intervention on the patient's ventilatory pattern nor any maneuver and is reliable for a breath-by-breath monitoring of PEEPi in both patients with exacerbation of COPD or acute respiratory distress syndrome (ARDS). In relaxed patients, the magnitude of dynamic hyperinflation can be computed directly by measuring the total exhaled volume during a period of apnea (26, 56).

To access respiratory system mechanics, the technique of rapid end-inspiratory occlusion with recordings of airway pressure, airflow, and volume is commonly used and yield static end-inspiratory compliance of the respiratory system (Cst,rs) and airway resistance (Raw), as well as the additional resistance due to viscoelastic pressure dissipation and/or time-constant inequalities (ΔR) (57–59). These indices may be used to follow the effectiveness of various ventilatory strategies (60–62). However, it should be noted that expiratory resistance which is usually severalfold higher than inspiratory and largely determines the level of PEEPi, is difficult to be measured, particularly in the presence of flow limitation (26). In COPD patients, excessive expiratory flow limitation is far more relevant than any change in the so-called "ohmic" component of "resistance." The term "expiratory impedance" should include both changes in the bronchial caliber, due to inflammation of the wall, and dynamic compression of the small airways, mainly determined by the loss of alveolar attachments. However, the changes of expiratory "impedance" can be estimated indirectly by observing the indices of dynamic hyperinflation, such as the PEEPi level, which is the relevant event for clinical purposes.

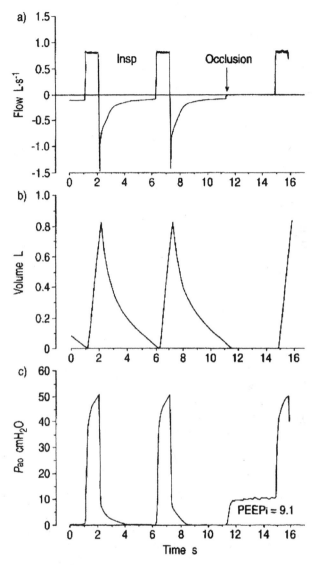

Figure 4 Flow (inspiration up), volume and airway pressure (Pao) in a patient with acute exacerbation of COPD ventilated passively on volume-controlled with constant inspiratory flow. The first mechanical inflation is regular and Pao at end expiration is apparently atmospheric. The second mechanical inflation begins when deflation is not completed as indicated by the presence of expiratory flow at that point. At the end of the second tidal expiration, the expiratory circuit is occluded (arrow) using the end-expiratory hold button of the ventilator and Pao rises to a plateau value, reflecting the end-expiratory elastic recoil of the respiratory system due to incomplete expiration (PEEPi). The value of PEEPi (9.1 cmH$_2$O) is provided by the difference between the Pao plateau pressure and Pao at the end of expiration of the breath without occlusion. (From Ref. 10.)

The shape of Paw during constant flow inflation (volume control) may also give important information regarding the severity of dynamic hyperinflation (63). For example, in the case of severe dynamic hyperinflation, the system during tidal inflation may approach volumes where compliance is reduced. This reduction will be manifested in the shape of Paw as a convexity-to-time axis (63). Ventilatory strategies planned to minimize dynamic hyperinflation may be assessed by observing the shape of Paw during constant flow inflation. This last technique is potentially very useful but has not been the object of a quantitative experiment. Finally, the rate of deflation may also be observed and quantitated using exponential analysis (64–66). Indeed, studies calculated the time constant of respiratory system during expiration in an attempt to predict the time needed to reach passive FRC (64–66). This technique, however, presents several problems and the assumptions made are not always valid (67).

Assisted Modes

Measurements of respiratory system mechanics and demonstration of dynamic hyperinflation in mechanically ventilated patients with respiratory efforts are complicated. Contrary to patients ventilated on controlled modes, there are no accepted methods of assessing the extent of dynamic hyperinflation in patients with active respiratory efforts (4). Expiratory muscle activity, common in patients with COPD, greatly influences PEEPi measurements (50, 68). Lessard et al. (68) have shown, in patients with COPD ventilated on pressure support, the persistence of expiratory muscle activity during end-expiratory occlusion despite the fact that the plateau in Paw was obtained (Fig. 5). In these patients, PEEPi should be corrected for expiratory muscle activity by concomitant inspection of gastric and esophageal pressures (10, 68). Furthermore, it has been shown that at high ventilatory demands an elastic threshold load can be present even at volumes below passive FRC, where inspiratory muscles start contracting while expiratory muscles are still active (69, 70).

With assisted modes of mechanical ventilation, the expiratory time, the real level of support, and some characteristics of the patient's respiratory efforts may vary from breath to breath. This variation may lead to breath-by-breath variability in the magnitude and consequences of dynamic hyperinflation. Because of this variability, patient data, such as hemodynamic measurements, may differ substantially between breaths, making their interpretation complicated. In addition, patient–ventilator interactions (see below) are considerably affected by the variability in dynamic hyperinflation.

Mechanisms of Dynamic Hyperinflation

Dynamic hyperinflation may exist with and without expiratory flow limitation during passive expiration (16). This difference may be important for therapeutic intervention aimed to reduce the work of breathing, for instance by application of PEEP (see below) (16, 71–73).

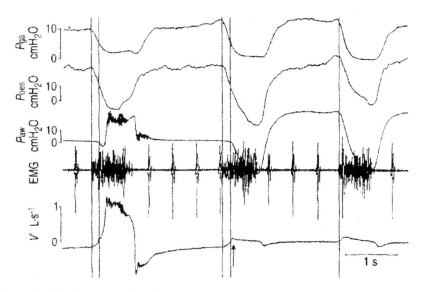

Figure 5 Gastric pressure (Pga), esophageal pressure (Peso), airway pressure (Paw), diaphragmatic electromyographic activity (EMG), and flow (V) in a patient with chronic obstructive pulmonary disease, ventilated on pressure-support mode, before and after end-expiratory occlusion (arrow). The two vertical lines traced on the inspiratory effort before occlusion are passed through the onset of inspiratory muscle activity and the point where Paw crosses baseline, respectively. Note that Pga decreased in the beginning of inspiration and increased during occlusion, indicating, respectively, relaxation and contraction of expiratory muscles. Part of the decrease in Peso in the beginning of inspiration and the increase in Paw during occlusion was due to expiratory muscles. Note, also, the plateau in Paw despite the presence of expiratory muscle activity. (From Ref. 68.)

A sharp decrease in expiratory flow after an initial spike at the beginning of expiration may be observed in patients with significant rise in expiratory impedance and usually indicates excessive flow limitation during passive expiration. The spike has been thought to represent the expulsion of air from open central airways, which is followed by dynamic compression of smaller airways causing an acute increase in expiratory impedance and a sharp decrease in expiratory flows (74). The same phenomenon may be observed during inspiration if the patient is ventilated on pressure-controlled modes [or on proportional assist ventilation (PAV)]; an early inspiratory flow spike followed by a sharp decline in inspiratory flow (75). The existence of flow limitation in patients with acute exacerbation of COPD is common and may be demonstrated by manipulating the airway opening pressure (mouth pressure) or alveolar pressure and observing the iso-volume flow. In the presence of expiratory flow limitation, changes in the difference between alveolar and mouth pressure, up to a point, have no effect on iso-volume expiratory flows and therefore do not affect the magnitude of dynamic hyperinflation (Figs. 6, 7). There are several methods of detecting expiratory flow limitation in mechanically ventilated patients

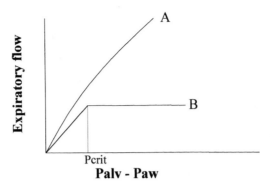

Figure 6 Iso-volume expiratory flow-pressure curves. Curve A: iso-volume flow–pressure relationship at lung volume without flow limitation. The expiratory flow is proportional to the driving pressure (alveolar pressure–mouth pressure, Palv-Paw) for expiratory flow. Curve B: iso-volume flow-pressure relationship at lung volume with flow limitation. Notice that in curve B changes of the driving pressure up to a point does not affect flow. Decreasing the driving pressures below a critical point (dashed line) causes a decrease in expiratory flow.

on controlled modes. Methods such as alteration of PEEP, external resistance, negative airway pressure during expiration and by-passing the ventilator expiratory tube have been used to manipulate the difference between alveolar and mouth pressure during expiration (26, 73, 76, 77). The demonstration of flow limitation helps the physician manage the mechanically ventilated patient more efficiently (see below).

In patients on assisted modes, demonstration of flow-limitation is complicated due to active expiratory effort that is difficult to be quantitated (4). Flow limitation should be suspected based mainly on the clinical response to graded application of PEEP (4). Increased dynamic hyperinflation due to inappropriate high level of PEEP or to the fact that the patient simply is not flow limited may be associated with increased dyspnea and cardiovascular compromise (26, 76, 78). Similar to patients on controlled modes, an initial spike in expiratory flow [and in inspiratory flow if the patient is ventilated on pressure support or proportional assist ventilation (75)] indicates severe obstruction and that flow limitation is likely present. Recently, Ninane et al. (79) applied manual compression of the abdominal wall during expiration in stable COPD patients breathing spontaneously and, by recording flow-volume curves with and without abdominal compression, were able to detect the presence of expiratory flow limitation (Fig. 8). This simple technique does not need a special device (such as the negative pressure technique) and can be applied in mechanically ventilated patients to differentiate who will benefit from PEEP application. However, similar to other methods, this technique may also be misleading if, during the procedure, the patient changes instantly the respiratory muscle activity.

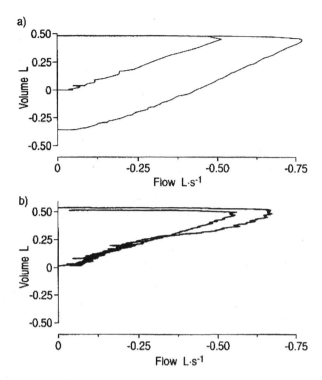

Figure 7 Expiratory flow–volume curves with and without manipulation of mouth pressure in a patient without flow limitation (a) and a patient with flow limitation (b). Mouth pressure was altered by negative expiratory pressure (NEP). At presence of flow limitation (second half of expiration) NEP does not increase expiratory flow in. (From Ref. 10.)

B. Patient–Ventilator Interactions

The patient–ventilator interaction is a key point in patient evaluation and further management. This interaction consists of two equally important aspects.

Response of Ventilator to Patient Effort

Ideally, in patients ventilated on assisted modes, all inspiratory efforts trigger the ventilator, which, depending on the mode used, supports the patient breath (4). The level of support may range from zero support, where the patient performs the total work of breathing, to near-maximum, where inspiratory muscles relax after ventilator triggering.

In assist modes, the patient must reduce airway pressure below the external PEEP level before assist begins. In some cases, the ventilator does not provide any flow until Paw decreases below a predetermined level that represents an infinity resistance (pressure triggering), while in other cases the ventilator allows air to flow

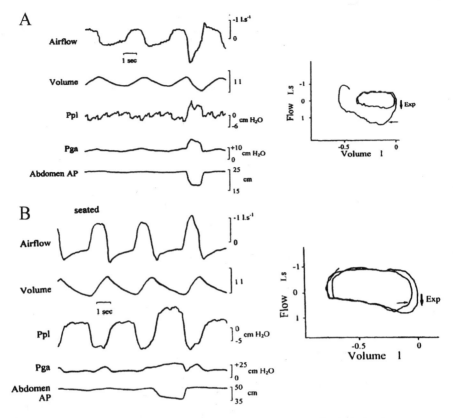

Figure 8 Left: records of airflow, volume, esophageal (Ppl), and gastric (Pga) pressure and of abdominal anterior–posterior (AP) diameter in a representative normal subject (A) and in a patient with COPD (B) breathing at rest in the seated position and then, during manual compression of the abdominal wall (MCA) during expiration. Right: corresponding records of the flow–volume curves during the MCA test (horizontal arrow) and during the preceding control breath. In the normal subject, MCA increases expiratory flow suggesting no flow limitation. On the other hand, in the patient, MCA does not increase expiratory flow despite a decrease in abdominal AP dimension, an increase in Pga and Ppl, indicating flow limitation. Exp = expiration. (From Ref. 50.)

in response to the decrease in Paw (4, 80, 81). In the last case, triggering occurs when flow from machine to patient exceeds a set level that represents a finite and often low resistance (flow triggering).

There are some important points that should be considered as far as the response of ventilator-to-patient effort concerns.

Trigger Sensitivity

In patients with COPD, considerable inspiratory effort may be needed to trigger the ventilator. This may be due to factors related both to patient and ventilator (4). An insensitive or unresponsive triggering system may impose a significant load to inspiratory muscles (80, 81). Because it is an open system, narrow endotracheal tubes, increased resistance (internal and external) to inspiratory flow, and low respiratory system compliance may significantly increase the inspiratory effort required to trigger a flow-triggering device (4). The presence of PEEPi (i.e., dynamic hyperinflation) decreases the triggering sensitivity in both pressure and flow-triggering modes of assist (4, 80). However, compared to pressure triggering, it has been shown that with flow-triggering systems the work of breathing necessary to trigger the ventilator is considerably reduced (82).

Ineffective Effort and Patient–Ventilator Dyssynchrony

In the presence of dynamic hyperinflation, there could be a situation where pressure generated by inspiratory muscles to initiate a breath is less than the positive alveolar pressure (PEEPi), due to the end-expiratory elastic recoil of the respiratory system, plus the airway pressure decrease required to trigger the ventilator, in which case inspiratory effort fails to trigger the ventilator (ineffective effort) (Fig. 9). Because lung volume continues to decline, the elastic recoil is less at the beginning of the next patient effort and the patient is in a better position to trigger the ventilator on the next spontaneous cycle. At times, more than one ineffective effort takes place before triggering occurs. In addition, in some cases ineffective efforts occur during inspiration (Fig. 10). In the presence of ineffective efforts the magnitude of dynamic hyperinflation may vary substantially from breath to breath.

Ineffective efforts may occur both with pressure- or volume-assist modes of mechanical ventilation (83–87). Causes leading to the occurrence of ineffective efforts are similar to determinants of dynamic hyperinflation (Fig. 2). Therefore, ineffective efforts occur invariably in mechanically ventilated patients with COPD (88). They have been observed even in spontaneously breathing tracheostomized COPD patients (89). The occurrence of this phenomenon is influenced by the mechanical properties of the respiratory system, the spontaneous breathing frequency, and the characteristics of the previous effective breath (11). The level of assistance, which in part drives the intensity of patient effort and determines end-inspiratory lung volume, may also be important (85–87). It is obvious that the higher the level of support (i.e., higher VT), the more frequent the occurrence of this phenomenon may be. A machine's rate may be also influenced by muscle pressure (i.e., drive) or by changing machine inspiratory time (Fig. 11). With ineffective efforts, the rate of a machine's cycle does not reflect the patient's spontaneous breathing frequency. Monitoring ventilator breathing frequency in patients with obstructive lung disease ventilated on assisted modes may thus be misleading.

With assisted ventilation, dyssynchrony between ventilator and neural timing invariably occurs in patients with COPD (83–89). With the volume-assist ventilator, inspiratory and expiratory time may bear no relationship with patient neural inspiratory and expiratory time. Ventilator inspiratory time is fixed and cannot be manipulated by the patient. With pressure support, the patient may have the ability to control inspiratory flow and, hence, inspiratory time. However, it has been shown in

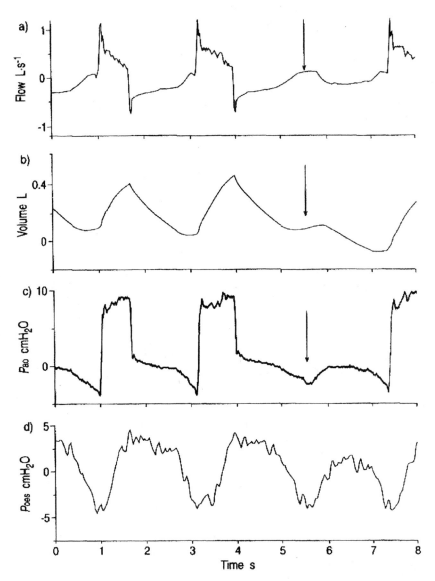

Figure 9 Flow, volume, and airway (Pao) and esophageal (Poes) pressures in a ventilator-dependent patient during pressure support. The third inspiratory effort (arrow), as indicated by the negative swings in Poes, was not able to trigger the ventilator. (From Ref. 10.)

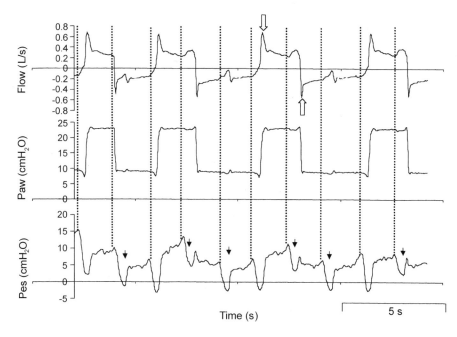

Figure 10 Flow (inspiration up), airway pressure (Paw), and esophageal pressure (Pes) in a patient with acute exacerbation of COPD ventilated on pressure support (flow triggering). Dashed vertical lines indicate the beginning of inspiratory effort. Closed arrows indicate ineffective efforts. Observe that ineffective efforts occur both during inflation and during deflation. Notice also that, at the beginning of expiration, flows after an initial increase (open arrow) decrease abruptly, a sign of severe obstruction and possibly of flow limitation. The same phenomenon, although to a lesser degree, is present at the beginning of inspiration (open arrow). Finally, notice that inspection of flow tracing is much more sensitive to detect ineffective efforts than airway pressure tracing.

patients with COPD that end-inspiratory synchrony between patient and ventilator rarely occurs (85–87, 90) (Fig. 12).

    Proportional assist ventilation (PAV), which is a new mode of mechanical ventilatory support, may partly solve the problem of patient–ventilator dyssynchrony. With PAV, pressure provided by the ventilator is proportional to instantaneous patient effort (91) and, therefore, the end of inspiratory effort should cause termination of ventilator assistance. This mode, however, is highly susceptible to PEEPi. With volume assist or pressure support, the ventilator, once triggered, delivers the set volume or pressure regardless of patient effort beyond the trigger; the patient may relax his/her respiratory muscles after triggering, leaving the ventilator to deliver the volume, which, depending on the settings, may be substantial. Contrary to other modes, with PAV the assist is linked to patient effort. If a considerable part of neural inspiration is needed to trigger the ventilator, the

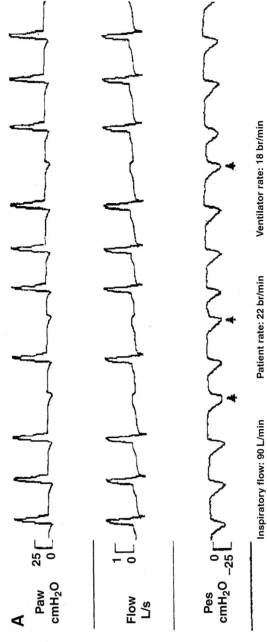

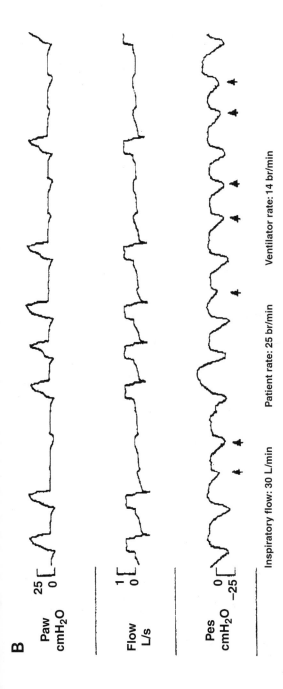

Figure 11 Airway pressure (Paw), airflow, and esophageal pressure (Pes) in a patient with chronic obstructive lung disease ventilated on assist volume–controlled mode. With this mode, every patient effort should trigger the ventilator to deliver a breath with a predetermined volume and flow-time profile. Therefore, with this mode, machine rate should be set by the patient while tidal volume (VT) and mechanical inspiratory time by the ventilator. A constant VT (0.6 L, not shown) was delivered with two different inspiratory flow rate (V_I), 90 L/min(Fig. 11A) and 30 L/min (Fig. 11B). Both at V_I of 90 and 30 L/min a significant number of ineffective efforts exist (arrows). At V_I of 90 L/min the rate of machine's cycles was 18 breaths/min, whereas patient spontaneous rate was 22 breaths/min. Minute ventilation, determined by ventilator rate and VT, was 10.8 L/min. By changing V_I to 30 L/min, we observe a decrease in machine rate and ventilation to 14 breaths/min and 8.4 L/min, respectively, despite the fact that patient breathing frequency increased from 22 to 24 breaths/min. When Pes swings are decreased, the likelihood of missing effort increases, indicating that for a given degree of PEEPi missing effort is more likely to occur when the pressure generated by inspiratory muscles is small, such as when the muscles are fatigued and/or weak or central drive is low (i.e., low PcCO$_2$). Note, also, that a considerable portion of inspiratory muscle pressure needs to trigger the ventilator and in some breaths all the muscle pressure is dissipated to trigger the ventilator and therefore neural inspiratory time ends when machine inspiratory time starts. It is obvious that machine cycles out of phase with the patient and the discrepancy vary substantially from breath to breath. Observe, finally, that at V_I of 30 L/min Paw in some breaths is convex to time axis, indicating that flow delivered by the ventilator does not meet patient instantaneous flow demands.

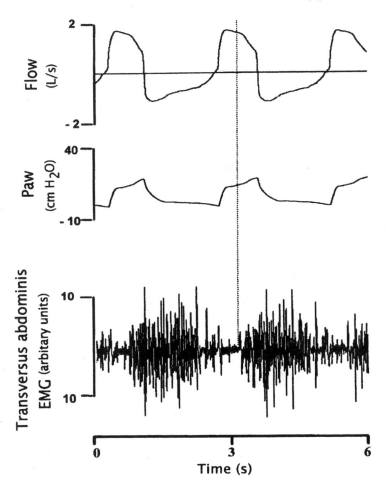

Figure 12 Recordings of flow, airway pressure (Paw), and transversus abdominis EMG in a critically ill patient with COPD receiving PS of 20 cmH$_2$O. The onset of expiratory muscle activity (vertical dotted line) occurred when mechanical inflation was only partly completed. (From Ref. 90.)

patient may terminate his or her effort soon after triggering. Thus, because the pressure provided by the ventilator is proportional to the patient effort after triggering, the delivered volume may be inadequate although the assist level is set to maximum (91). It follows that the effectiveness of PAV is highly dependent on measures aiming to decrease the dynamic hyperinflation and PEEPi. Indeed, it has been shown in difficult-to-wean COPD patients that counterbalancing PEEPi with PEEP greatly increased the efficiency of PAV to unload the respiratory muscles (Fig. 13) (92).

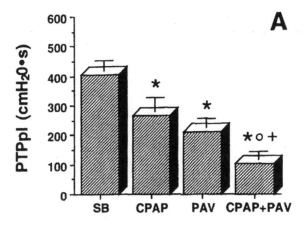

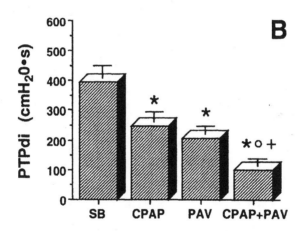

Figure 13 Changes in the pressure-time product for the inspiratory muscles (PTP$_{pl}$, A) and for the diaphragm (PTP$_{di}$, B) throughout the procedure. Bars represent means $\pm$ 1 SE. *$p < 0.05$, treatment vs. SB; °$p < 0.05$, treatment vs. CPAP; +$p < 0.05$, CPAP + PAV vs. PAV. SB: spontaneous breathing, CPAP: continuous positive airway pressure. PAV: proportional assist ventilation. Notice that the effectiveness of PAV is significantly increased by CPAP application. (From Ref. 92.)

Inspired Gas Flow

On most commercial ventilators, gas flow from the ventilator is governed by set flow or set pressure (4, 81). With set-flow modes of assist (i.e., assist-volume) any patient effort during machine-delivered breath will result in lower airway pressure provided by the ventilator in order to maintain the predetermined inspiratory flow. If gas flow from the ventilator is not sufficiently high to meet patient's flow demand, the patient will work harder than necessary to inflate the chest wall (Fig. 14). This can increase the sense of dyspnea and alter breathing pattern. It may also interfere with the weaning process. With set-pressure modes of assist (i.e., pressure support), airway pressure is fixed and the patient can increase inspiratory flow rate simply by increasing inspiratory effort (4). Nevertheless, in the face of high inspiratory drive (high inspiratory flow) many ventilators are not able to maintain Paw constant and Paw deviates from the target level (93). Therefore, the ventilatory consequences of a given increase in patient effort will be inappropriate. Furthermore, the velocity of pressurization of pressure support differs between various ventilators and this may affect the support level (94). Although a pressure-supported mode may appear more reliable to unload the respiratory muscles, for the above-mentioned reasons and because of its high initial peak flow, similar unloading can be achieved with a volume-controlled mode, provided that the peak flow rate is set properly (95). On the other hand, PAV has some theoretical advantages (91, 93) but currently this mode is under investigation and thus it is difficult to make any recommendation.

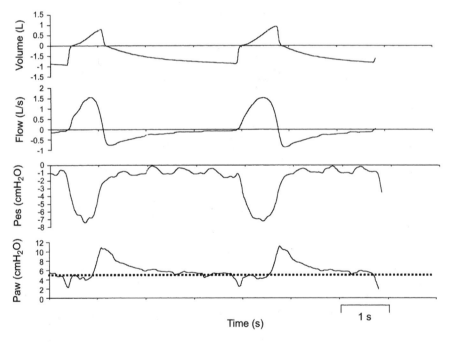

Figure 14 Flow (inspiration up), volume (volume was reset to zero at zero flow, inspiration up), esophageal and airway pressure in a patient with COPD ventilated on assist volume (inspiratory rate is predetermined). Observe that due to inadequate inspiratory flow the relatively strong inspiratory effort causes pressure provided by the ventilator (Paw) to be close to or even lower from PEEP level (dashed horizontal line) throughout inspiration, in which case the patient performs the total work of breathing while, on the other hand, the ventilator may impose a significant load by decreasing Pao below PEEP.

Response of Patient's Respiratory Effort to Ventilator-Delivered Breath

The act of breathing is not a simple mechanical event. Mechanical, chemical, reflex, and behavioral factors can affect the rate, intensity, and shape of respiratory effort (96). With assisted modalities of ventilatory support, the ventilator-delivered breath has two components, one related to machine settings and the other to patient effort (97, 98). Changes in ventilatory settings are associated with changes in flow, volume, or airway pressure delivered by the ventilator. These changes may modify the patient's respiratory effort through alterations in (1) intrinsic properties of respiratory muscles (force-length and force-velocity relationships); (2) chemical stimuli (PCO_2, PO_2); and (3) the activity of various receptors located in respiratory track, lung, and chest wall. Furthermore, changes in volume, flow, and pressure are readily perceived in awake patients and may, therefore, evoke behavioral ventilatory responses intended to enhance comfort (see Refs. 97 and 98 for review).

Some examples may be worthwhile to understand the role of ventilator-delivered breath to modify the patient's respiratory effort. It is well known that, for a given level of inspiratory muscle activation, pressure generated by the inspiratory muscles ($Pmus_i$) decreases with increasing lung volume (force-length relationship) and flow (force-velocity relationship) (99). If changes in ventilator settings result in higher inspiratory flow and inspired volume, then, for a given neural output to inspiratory muscles, $Pmus_i$ should be lower (mechanical feedback). The clinical significance of this effect is not known, but it might be of concern in patients with dynamic hyperinflation. It has been suggested that mechanical feedback, by reducing $Pmus_i$, might increase the number of ineffective efforts, particularly if impaired neuromuscular competence coexists (97). Of more importance is the role of chemical feedback. For example, changes in ventilator settings, aiming to reduce dynamic hyperinflation, may alter alveolar ventilation and, thus, PaO_2, $PaCO_2$, and pH, which, in turn, through peripheral and central chemoreceptors, affect respiratory effort, depending on chemical sensitivity and sleep/awake stage (97, 98, 100, 101). Similarly, the reflex feedback under certain circumstances may also alter, sometimes considerably, the respiratory motor output (101, 102). Thus the effect of changes in ventilator settings on dynamic hyperinflation is largely unpredictable. It follows that expected responses to change in ventilatory settings may be modified by these feedback systems, thus affecting the magnitude of pathophysiological abnormalities (97, 98). Planned ventilatory strategies should take into account the modification of patient's respiratory effort to ventilator-delivered breath (see below).

V. Ventilatory Strategies

A. Controlled Modes

With these ventilatory modes (pressure or volume controlled), the ventilator assumes the total work of breathing. Usually, controlled modes are used immediately after intubation. The duration of controlled mechanical ventilation varies between patients, depending mainly on the severity of disease. As a general rule, controlled modes should be used for a short time to avoid respiratory muscle atrophy and unnecessary prolongation of the time of mechanical ventilation (103). With these modes, patients are usually sedated and, in some cases, paralyzed, although the latter should be avoided. However, if $PaCO_2$ is well below the set point of the patient and machine rate is above the intrinsic spontaneous breathing frequency, patients may be ventilated on controlled modes being fully alert (104). This implies alveolar hyperventilation and may increase the magnitude of dynamic hyperinflation and induce alkalemia, risk factors for serious complications (5, 105). Nevertheless, this method is useful to compute respiratory system mechanics in patients ventilated on assisted modes when this is done for a brief period of time.

Oxygenation

Achievement and maintenance of an acceptable level of arterial oxygenation is the first priority (Table 3). $PaO_2 > 60$ mmHg (or $SaO_2 > 90\%$) is considered a reasonable target (106). Correction of hypoxemia in patients with obstructive lung disease usually requires small increases in the fraction of inspired O_2 (F_IO_2) and F_IO_2 in the range of 25 to 40% is sufficient to raise $PaO_2 > 60$ mmHg in the majority of patients (1, 2). Failure of this level of F_IO_2 to increase PaO_2 above 60 mmHg indicates another process, such as atelectasis, pneumonia, pulmonary embolism, pneumothorax, or intracardiac shunting (54). The other important factors of oxygen delivery to tissues, such as Hb and cardiac output, should also be taken into account (106).

Correction of Respiratory Acidosis

Correction of respiratory acidosis should be performed carefully. Patients with acute exacerbation of COPD usually have preexisting compensatory metabolic alkalosis due to chronic hypercapnia, and, thus, rapid correction of hypercapnia may cause,

---

Table 3 Targets in Controlled Modes

---

1. Acceptable PaO_2 (>60 mmHg) and adequate O_2 delivery to tissues (consider Hb, cardiac output).
2. Correction of life-threatening respiratory acidemia (pH < 7.2).
3. Relaxation of the respiratory muscles (use sedation, avoid paralysis).
4. Reduction of dynamic hyperinflation.
   a. ↓ minute ventilation (↓ VT, ↓ ventilatory demands, accept hypercapnia and mild acidemia)
   b. ↑ expiratory time (high inspiratory flow, low T_I/T_{TOT}, no end-inspiratory pause)
   c. ↓ resistance to expiratory airflow (use bronchodilators, corticosteroids, heliox, low resistance ventilator tubings and valves)
5. Switching to assisted modes whenever possible.

---

among other complications related mainly to dynamic hyperinflation, life-threatening alkalemia. The goal is to return pH toward normal, not to return the PCO_2 to normal (4, 107, 108). Nevertheless, vigorous attempts to return pH to normal by increasing minute ventilation should be avoided, because it may increase the dynamic hyperinflation. When reduction of dynamic hyperinflation is an issue (see below), and provided that intracranial hypertension and overt hemodynamic instability do not exist, acceptance of acidemia (pH > 7.2) is reasonable (109).

Relaxation of Respiratory Muscles

All patients with acute exacerbation of COPD sustain an excessive work of breathing due to multiple factors (1, 2). Furthermore, most of them are intubated and mechanically ventilated when inspiratory muscles are unable to generate sufficient alveolar ventilation, whatever the presence of peripheral or central fatigue (9). Therefore, it is usually assumed that the muscles should be put at rest for some time before switching the ventilator to assist modes. Studies have shown that more than 24 h may be needed for complete recovery of the muscles from low-frequency fatigue (28, 110). The patients, at least initially, may need sedation in order to suppress respiratory efforts. Paralysis should be avoided, because it is associated with significant side effects, such as widespread pooling of airway secretions and prolonged muscle weakness (111–115).

Minimizing the Dynamic Hyperinflation

Minimizing the magnitude of dynamic hyperinflation is a key point for the management of patients with COPD during mechanical ventilation. Dynamic hyperinflation, as discussed above, influences many aspects of the disease, as well as patient management. In patients on controlled modes, there are three strategies that can decrease dynamic hyperinflation: (1) decreased minute ventilation; (2) increased expiratory time; and (3) decreased resistance to expiratory flows (Table 1) (107, 108). If possible, all these strategies should be applied simultaneously.

Decreased Minute Ventilation

The magnitude of dynamic hyperinflation can be reduced considerably by decreasing tidal volume and breathing frequency (56). This controlled hypoventilation may cause acidemia due to respiratory acidosis. In patients with COPD, however, and contrary to asthmatics, it is often of less concern since preexisting metabolic alkalosis prevents pH from dropping to dangerous levels. Decrease of minute ventilation requirements by measures that decrease VCO_2 is also important. Fever reduction, treatment of infection, and adequate nutritional support (116, 117) may permit, by decreasing VCO_2, significant reduction of ventilation with modest increase in $PaCO_2$.

Increased Expiratory Time

At constant tidal volume and breathing frequency dynamic hyperinflation can be decreased by increasing expiratory time. This increase can be achieved by increasing

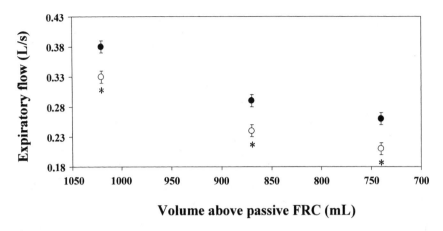

Volume above passive FRC (mL)

Figure 15   Iso-volume expiratory flows, measured at three lung volumes above passive FRC, with and without end-inspiratory pause. Closed circles: without end-inspiratory pause (EIP, 10% of T_{TOT}). Open circles: with end-inspiratory pause. For a given lung volume, EIP caused a significant decrease in iso-volume expiratory flows. (Data redrawn from Ref. 60.)

inspiratory flows at the expense of increasing peak dynamic pressures (Ppk) and by elimination of end-inspiratory pause time. This strategy, although less powerful than controlled hypoventilation, may decrease dynamic hyperinflation considerably, improving cardiovascular function and gas exchange (60). It follows that in patients with COPD, the use of Ppk to monitor complications during mechanical ventilation, such as barotrauma and hemodynamic instability, may be misleading. It is of interest to note that the use of end-inspiratory pause time increases dynamic hyperinflation not only by decreasing the time available for expiration but also by decreasing iso-volume expiratory flow because of reduction in elastic energy stored at the viscoelastic elements of the respiratory system during inspiration (60) (Fig. 15). In patients with COPD, addition of end-inspiratory pause time is not associated with improvement in gas exchange while, on the other hand, it may be detrimental causing further hyperinflation, effects that contrast with these observed in patients with severe restriction and impairment of gas exchange (ARDS) (23).

Decreased Resistance to Expiratory Flows

Obviously, in patients with COPD, the decrease of expiratory airway resistance and total impedance is of great importance (118). Bronchodilators, corticosteroids, and helium may be used for this purpose (119). In addition to bronchodilators, the decrease in the external resistance related to ventilator tubing and various devices (i.e., PEEP valves) is also a priority, although the effectiveness of these procedures may be limited by the presence of expiratory flow limitation (107, 108).

Bronchodilators. Adrenergic and anticholinergic agents and methyl-xanthines are the drugs used as bronchodilators in these patients. These agents are reviewed in detail elsewhere and only issues relevant to mechanical ventilation will be highlighted.

The anticholinergic bronchodilators are given only by inhalation because the systemic route results in nonacceptable side effects. On the other hand, adrenergic drugs might be given either systemically or by inhalation. However, contrary to general belief, intravenously or subcutaneously given adrenergic agonists, including adrenaline, do not result in greater bronchodilation than that observed with inhaled β_2-agonists, provided that the inhalation technique is proper. Indeed, studies have demonstrated that inhaled β_2-agonists are equally effective or even better than parenteral therapy (120, 121). Because parenteral therapy carries significant risks, such as hypokalemia, cardiac arrhythmias, myocardial necrosis, and lactic acidosis (122, 123), the inhaled route is preferable. Finally, methylxanthines are given only by systemic route, and a physiological study showed that IV doxophylline significantly reduces respiratory resistance in ventilator-dependent COPD patients (124). However, the narrow therapeutic range of these drugs and their significant side effects have considerably reduced their use in patients with COPD (2).

Inhaled bronchodilators in mechanically ventilated patients may be delivered either by nebulizer or by metered-dose inhaler (MDI) (119). It is generally believed that during mechanical ventilation nebulizers are superior to MDIs. However, the delivery of bronchodilators with MDI in mechanically ventilated patients has received considerable interest in recent years (125, 126). This is because the use of MDI has several advantages over the nebulizer, such as reduced cost, ease of administration, less personnel time, reliability of dosing, and a lower risk of contamination (126). Nowadays, particularly, in the era of limited financial resources, the cost of therapy is an important issue. Indeed, it has been estimated that substitution of nebulizers by MDIs in a 700-bed hospital could decrease potential patient costs of aerosol therapy by $300,000 a year (127). Moreover, the use of nebulizers under certain circumstances may lead to patient–ventilator dyssynchrony (128). Ineffective efforts have been demonstrated in patients ventilated on assisted modes of support whenever the flow rate of continuous in-line jet nebulizers exceeded the patient's inspiratory flow rate (128). This may lead to serious episodes of hypoventilation, which may not be detected by the alarm function because the bias flow introduced into the system by the continuous flow is falsely interpreted by the ventilator as representing minute ventilation. Finally, nebulizers may damage the expiratory transducer of some ventilators, making unreliable the expiratory volume measurement (129).

Although bronchodilator delivery with MDI in mechanically ventilated patients carries several advantages over the nebulizers, the use of MDIs has not gained widespread acceptance among ICU physicians. Indeed, bronchodilator delivery with MDI is considered to be relatively ineffective due to drug deposition in the ventilator circuit and endotracheal tube (130). Manthous et al. (130) reported no benefit from administration of up to 100 puffs of albuterol (9 mg) with an MDI and elbow adapter in ventilator-supported patients. This consideration, however, is not supported by recent scientific data. Studies using a spacer device instead of elbow adapter did not reconfirm these findings. Bronchodilator delivery using an MDI and a spacer device results in a significant decrease in airflow resistance (see Ref. 126 for review). Thus, a spacer device is thought to be important in order to demonstrate the efficacy of bronchodilator therapy given by MDI (Fig. 16). Provided that a proper technique of administration is used, bronchodilator therapy with MDI is clearly effective.

In patients with acute exacerbation of COPD needing ventilatory support, delivery of bronchodilators with an MDI and a spacer results in approximately 18 to 25% and 8 to 15% decrease in inspiratory airway resistance (Rmin) and total resistance of the respiratory system, respectively (125, 126). These decreases are comparable with those observed when bronchodilators were delivered with nebulizers despite the severalfold lower drug dose (131). Although expiratory resistance, a main determinant of dynamic hyperinflation, is not usually measured, indirect measurements, such as iso-volume expiratory flows or intrinsic positive-end-expiratory pressure (PEEPi), suggest an appreciable decrease in expiratory resistance (impedance) as well. Indeed, an approximately 20% reduction of PEEPi has been observed after bronchodilation therapy indicating a decrease in dynamic hyperinflation as a result of a decline in expiratory (impedance) (131-135). It is of interest to note that delivery of bronchodilators with an MDI and a spacer results in bronchodilation, which was not affected by the ventilator settings such as end-inspiratory pause, tidal volume, inspiratory flow, and ventilator mode (132-135). Thus, although aerosol deposition to target sites is influenced by several factors related to ventilator settings (136), data concerning the clinical response suggest that in everyday clinical practice, inhaled bronchodilator therapy using an MDI and a spacer is a rather simple procedure (137), and significant bronchodilation may be achieved without modification of ventilator settings.

The decrease in total resistance of the respiratory system after bronchodilator delivery with an MDI and a spacer is mainly due to Rmin decrease (i.e., airway

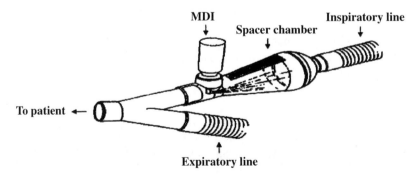

Figure 16 Schematic representation of a spacer device used to administer inhaled bronchodilator drugs with metered-dose inhalers in mechanically ventilated patients. (From Ref. 133.)

resistance), whereas the additional resistance (ΔR) due to time-constant inequalities and/or viscoelastic behavior remains unchanged (131–135). This indicates that the delivery of bronchodilators with MDI affects the smooth muscle tone of large airways. On the other hand, bronchodilators administered using nebulizers seem to elicit a parenchymal response (131). Guerin et al. (136) in a recent study administered, in mechanically ventilated COPD patients, a combination of feno-terol-ipratropium bromide either with nebulizer or MDI and found that total resistance of respiratory system, trapped end-expiratory lung volume, and PEEPi decreased similarly between the two modes of drug administration, although through different mechanisms. With a nebulizer, the reduction of total inspiratory resistance was due to a decrease in ΔR, while with MDI the decrease was due to Rmin. The authors attributed these results to the higher alveolar deposition of the total drug mass achieved with a nebulizer, although as a percent of the nominal dose the deposition was greater with MDI (136).

The optimal dose of bronchodilators delivered in mechanically ventilated patients is not clearly established. Some 10 years ago, Bernasconi and colleagues (138) showed that 1.2 mg of nebulized fenoterol did not produce any advantage over 0.4 mg in the significant improvement of respiratory mechanics. They also showed that approximately 180 min after administration respiratory resistance were essentially back to the abnormal preadministration values. Manthaus et al. (139), in patients who had Ppeak to Pp gradient of more than 15 cmH$_2$O, found that five puffs of albuterol (90 µg/puff) significantly decreased the resistive pressure. The addition of 10 more puffs further reduced, albeit slightly, the resistive pressure. Fifteen more puffs did not result in further improvement. In mechanically ventilated patients with COPD, Dhand et al. (140) have shown that the decrease in airway resistance with four puffs of albuterol was comparable to that observed with cumulative doses of 28 puffs. In a recent study, we demonstrated in patients with acute exacerbation of COPD that two puffs of salbutamol resulted in significant bronchodilation that was comparable to that observed with six puffs (134). It seems that in stable mechani-cally ventilated patients, 2 to 6 puffs of a short-acting β_2-agonist may achieve maximum or near-maximum bronchodilation with no side effects. However, some patients may require higher doses. Individual titration of the dose, such as to achieve the best bronchodilation with acceptable side effects, may be an alternative strategy as opposed to use of a standard dose (141). The optimal dose of other bronchodi-lators such as anticholinergic or long-acting β_2-agonists is not known. The optimal dose of bronchodilators administered with nebulizer is also unknown. The doses indicated in Table 4 might be used initially and then should be titrated up depending on the response and side effects (141).

The duration of the bronchodilator response in mechanically ventilated COPD patients is an important issue, which surprisingly has not been adequately studied. In a recent study, we observed that in patients with COPD six puffs of salbutamol resulted in significant bronchodilation lasting approximately 3 h (142). Duarte et al. (143) administered also in patients with COPD four and ten puffs of albuterol with MDI and a spacer and compared the duration of bronchodilation with that achieved with 2.5 mg of albuterol given with nebulizer. The authors reported that independent

Table 4 Inhaled Bronchodilator Drugs

Drug	Recommended initial dose	
Adrenergic agents (β₂-agonists)	MDI (g)	Nebulizer (mg)
Fenoterol	200–400	0.5–2.0
Salbutamol	200–400	2.5–5.0
Terbutaline	500–100	
Formoterol	24–48	
Salmeterol	100–200	
Anticholinergic agents		
Ipratropium bromide	80–160	0.25–0.5
Oxitropium bromide	400	

MDI: Metered-dose inhaler.

of the dose and mode of drug delivery the duration of bronchodilation ranged between 90 and 120 min. Bernasconi and colleagues (138) showed that 180 min after administration of nebulized fenoterol, respiratory resistance was essentially back to the abnormal preadministration values. The findings of the above studies indicate that the duration of bronchodilation in mechanically ventilated patients is decreased compared to that in ambulatory patients, in accordance with the results of Duarte et al. (144), who showed that the relative systemic bioavailability of inhaled albuterol as measured by serum level was reduced in mechanically ventilated patients. It follows that the dose interval when bronchodilator drugs are given either with MDI or with nebulizer in mechanically ventilated patients might be shorter than that in ambulatory patients.

Corticosteroids. It has been shown that, in mechanically ventilated patients with acute exacerbation of COPD, intravenous methylprednisolone acutely decreased the respiratory resistance and dynamic hyperinflation as indicated by the significant reduction of PEEPi (145). Thus, a short course of high-dose steroids may be used in these patients, but the risks of side effects should be taken into account (see Chap. 22). Among other side effects, myopathy in patients receiving neuro-blocking agents is of particular concern. Inhaled steroids might be an alternative. Nava et al. (146) have recently shown in stable COPD patients on long-term ventilatory support that inhaled fluticasone propionate for 5 days significantly decreased airway resistance and PEEPi. However, at the present stage of our knowledge, inhaled steroids do not have any role in the treatment of acute exacerbation of COPD. Extrapolation of the results by Nava and colleagues to the acute condition is not warranted.

Helium. Helium is an inert gas with unique physical properties that might be useful for various respiratory emergencies. Compared to air, helium's density is considerably lower, whereas the density of a helium–oxygen mixture (He–O_2, heliox) is directly proportional to the inspired oxygen concentration (F_1O_2) (147). At 20° C and F_1O_2 of 0.3, the density He–O_2 is approximately 40% of that of air–O_2 mixture. In mechanically ventilated patients, by substituting the air–O_2 mixture with heliox, two consequences arise. First, the lower gas density decreases the Reynold's number and thus more laminar flow conditions prevail, where the resistive pressure drop is relatively low. Second, in turbulent flow conditions, flow is inversely related to gas density, meaning that for a given driving pressure flow will be higher if gas density is lower. It follows that breathing low-density gas such as heliox is equivalent to decreasing airflow resistance (147, 148). Indeed, in mechanically ventilated patients with obstructive lung disease, heliox reduces dynamic hyperinflation and lowers peak, mean, and intrinsic positive-end-expiratory airway pressures (149). No side effects have been observed with heliox breathing. It appears that heliox is an attractive and safe treatment for dynamic hyperinflation due to high airflow resistance. Finally, the use of heliox in the ventilator circuit may improve aerosol delivery. Goode et al. (150), in an in vitro lung model of mechanical ventilation, demonstrated that heliox (80 : 20) increased significantly the albuterol delivery from both MDI and nebulizer by as much as 50%. Whether this increase is associated with better clinical outcome remains to be determined.

The use of heliox presents some problems. These are mainly related to the interference of helium with the ventilator function. Discrepancies have been found between the actual volume and O_2 delivered by the ventilator and those set by the operator (151, 152). The relationship between the actual and dialed ventilator settings depends on the type of ventilator used. This should be taken into account and, when heliox is used, correction factors should be applied in order to avoid false readings from the ventilator.

The adequacy of the above strategies to reduce the magnitude of dynamic hyperinflation might be evaluated using measurements of gas volume trapped at the end of expiration, PEEPi, and static end-inspiratory plateau pressure (Pp) (4). Parameters of hemodynamic improvement (arterial pressure, heart rate, urine output) usually follow the reduction of dynamic hyperinflation and may also be used as an index (107, 108). It is difficult, however, to establish cut-off points for dynamic hyperinflation, PEEPi, and Pp, and further studies are needed. Titration of tidal volume and breathing pattern using the static pressure–volume curve might be another approach. Keeping end-inspiratory lung volume below lung volumes at which respiratory system compliance start to diminish (upper inflection point in P–V curve), rather than aiming at specific values of dynamic hyperinflation, PEEPi and Pp may be an alternative strategy. However, at present, this technique has been applied only in patients with acute respiratory distress syndrome (153). Furthermore, the interpretation of upper inflection points is rather complicated because its occurrence may be due to diminished recruitment and not overdistention (154).

B. Assisted Modes

Compared to controlled modes, the management priorities in patients ventilated on assisted modes are somewhat different, mainly due to interaction between patient respiratory effort and ventilator function (Table 5).

As in patients on controlled modes, the achievement and maintenance of an acceptable level of arterial oxygenation and adequate oxygen delivery to tissues is,

Table 5   Targets in Assisted Modes

1. Acceptable PaO_2 (>60 mmHg) and adequate O_2 delivery to tissues (consider Hb, cardiac output).
2. Promotion of patient-ventilator synchrony.
   a. Consider the response of ventilator to patient.
      i. Maximize trigger sensitivity: (a) adjust triggering threshold; (b) reduce dynamic hyperinflation (see Table 3); (c) apply PEEP (low levels).
      ii. Consider machine inspiratory and expiratory time.
      iii. Consider inspiratory flow
   b. Consider the response of patient to ventilator.
      i. Avoid insufficient as well as excessive levels of volume and flow.
      ii. Consider the relationship between neural and ventilator breath timing.
      iii. Consider the subjective feelings of comfort and breathlessness.

apparently, the first priority and its principles will not be repeated. However, in patients ventilated on assisted modes, high levels of PaO_2 (>70 mmHg) should be avoided so as not to lead to CO_2 retention (106).

During assisted modes of ventilatory support, promotion of patient–ventilator synchrony is always a consideration. By improving patient–ventilator synchrony the main goals of ventilatory support during acute exacerbation, such as adequate oxygenation and work of breathing reduction, can be achieved. Ventilatory strategies are planned to improve both the response of ventilator-to-patient effort and the response of respiratory effort to ventilator-delivered breath.

Response of Ventilator-to-Patient Effort

Maximize Trigger Sensitivity

Manipulation of trigger sensitivity has two components, one related to the ventilator and the other to the patient. Trigger sensitivity may be altered by changing the threshold for triggering, ventilator settings, patient status, and PEEP.

The threshold for triggering (pressure or flow) should be set to possible maximum level so that auto-cycling does not occur. Decreasing the resistance of the inspiratory ventilator line and using a large-bore endotracheal tube are of particular concern in flow-triggering devices (4, 80). However, flow-triggering devices are preferable to pressure-triggering devices because with these systems the work of breathing to counterbalance PEEPi is less.

Dynamic hyperinflation significantly affects the trigger sensitivity (26). The dynamically hyperinflated patient, in order to decrease Paw and trigger the ventilator, must first generate enough pressure to counterbalance the positive-end expiratory elastic recoil. Therefore, measures that decrease the magnitude of dynamic hyperinflation increase trigger sensitivity, decrease the likelihood for ineffective efforts, and promote patient–ventilator synchrony.

In patients on assisted modes, the magnitude of dynamic hyperinflation, following a change in ventilator settings or patient status, is largely unpredictable; these changes may alter patient effort through various feedback systems (97, 98) and, therefore, modify expected responses. Keeping this consideration in mind, reduction of resistance to airflow and patient requirements for ventilation are the first measures. The use of bronchodilators and corticosteroids is well established and of great importance for dynamic hyperinflation (see above). A mixture of helium–oxygen may also be used (152). Increased metabolic rate, such as occurs during excessive nutritional support and various disease states (i.e., infection, hyperthyroidism) is likely to be detrimental for patient–ventilator synchrony (155). Panic reactions are invariably associated with increased respiratory drive. Inappropriate ventilator settings (i.e., inadequate flow rates, tidal volume, inspired oxygen percentage), machine malfunction, and patient-related acute problems (i.e., pneumothorax, deterioration of blood gases) are important causes of panic reaction (155) and should be corrected in order to abort the panic cycle. When no apparent cause is found, judicious use of sedation might be tried.

Low levels of PEEP in mechanically ventilated patients with obstructive disease and dynamic hyperinflation may increase trigger sensitivity substantially by narrowing the difference between alveolar pressure and mouth pressure at end expiration (26). Indeed, a substantial reduction of the elastic work of breathing due to PEEPi has been repeatedly demonstrated (30, 71–73) (Fig. 17). This beneficial effect of PEEP is most evident in patients exhibiting flow limitation during tidal expiration (16, 71–73). In these patients, expiratory flows are maximum and, according to the wave-speed theory of flow-limitation, wave speed has been reached and therefore pressure disturbances downstream are not able to be propagated

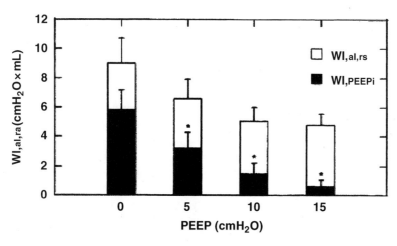

Figure 17 Average ± SE value of total static work of breathing per breath (entire bars) and work due to PEEPi (filled portion of the bars) in 10 COPD patients at four levels of external PEEP. *$p < 0.01$ relative to zero PEEP. (From Ref. 30.)

upstream (26). Thus, at presence of flow limitation, PEEP, up to a point, does not affect expiratory flow and does not cause further hyperinflation (16) (Fig. 6), in which case, after PEEP application, the difference between alveolar pressure and mouth pressure at end expiration is decreased and trigger sensitivity is increased by an amount equal to PEEP. However, expiratory flow limitation is a dynamic process and the increase in trigger sensitivity may become less than PEEP (26). On the other hand, if flow limitation does not exist, PEEP will present a back-pressure to expiratory flow and will cause further hyperinflation, thus counterbalancing the beneficial effect on trigger sensitivity. As a rule, careful reevaluation of patient status (i.e., systemic arterial pressure, comfort of the patient) should be performed after any level of applied PEEP. Airway occlusion pressure might also be used to titrate PEEP in mechanically ventilated patients with dynamic hyperinflation. Mancebo et al. (156) showed that increasing PEEP was associated with a decrease in P0.1 if dynamic hyperinflation was not affected by PEEP. On the other hand, if PEEP was excessive and thus caused further hyperinflation, P0.1 was not reduced.

Machine Inspiratory and Expiratory Time Should Correspond as Close as Possible to Patient Neural Breathing Pattern

With volume-assisted modalities of ventilatory support, machine inspiratory time is fixed and may be shorter or longer than neural inspiratory time. Changes in the latter will not result in changes in machine inspiratory time. At best, by trial and error, machine inspiratory and expiratory times may be set to correspond to neural breathing pattern in a given steady state. With pressure support, the patient has the ability to influence machine breathing pattern (4). This ability, however, may be seriously compromised by several factors related to mechanical properties of the respiratory system, characteristics of a single breath, and function of the ventilator (93). The relationship between patient and machine breathing pattern could be improved by increasing trigger sensitivity (see above), reducing the level of pressure support as much as possible, minimizing the inspiratory pressure rise time, and decreasing resistance to airflow (93).

Gas Flow from the Ventilator Should Meet Patient Flow Demands

With volume-assisted modes, inspection of airway pressure waveform may be used as a guide for setting inspiratory flow (V_I) rate. Airway pressure which is in concordance to time axis indicates insufficient inspiratory flow rates and increased patient work of breathing (Fig. 14). As a rough rule, in patients with obstructive lung disease, V_I might be set approximately to 60 to 70 L/min. Then airway pressure waveform and indices of dyspnea (Borg scale) may be used to see the appropriateness of V_I setting. It has been shown that both lower and higher than spontaneous inspiratory flow rates may increase the sense of dyspnea (157). However, because a considerable variability of V_I exists between breaths, the set V_I is likely to approach the highest flow demand and therefore exceed the average flow demand.

Theoretically, with pressure-support mode, the patient may increase V_T (tidal volume) by increasing inspiratory effort and, thus, retain considerable control over inspiratory flow pattern as well as over ventilation, key points for patient–ventilator synchrony. In addition, inspiratory flow is more likely to be adequate with the decelerating flow pattern of pressure-support ventilation than with the square-wave pattern, commonly used in assist-volume modes. For these reasons, it is generally believed that pressure support is the mode of choice in patients with COPD. However, there are no convincing data indicating that this mode is superior to other modes (4). Furthermore, it has been shown that a similar degree of unloading can be achieved with a square-wave flow pattern if inspiratory flow is sufficiently high (96). Finally, we should mention that, in the presence of high inspiratory flow demands, some old-generation ventilators, set on pressure-support mode, are not able to maintain airway pressure at a preset level (93). This may reduce inspiratory flow rates when the patient actually increases his or her flow demands. Increasing pressure support may solve this problem but, on the other hand, may increase dynamic hyperinflation and patient–ventilator dyssynchrony (93).

Response of Patient's Respiratory Effort to Ventilator-Delivered Breath

The response of patient effort to ventilator-delivered breath remains a largely unexplored issue and much work needs to be done before establishment of guidelines. Some points, however, deserve special comments.

One of the main objectives of assisted modes of mechanical ventilation in patients with acute exacerbation of COPD is to unload the respiratory muscles. This should be advantageous in terms of energy and degree of dyspnea. However, the ability of assisted modes to downregulate neural stimulation and, thus, respiratory muscle-force output has been questioned by several pieces of evidence. Data in patients with COPD during constant-flow, synchronized, intermittent mandatory ventilation (SIMV) have shown that, for a given level of assist, inspiratory effort did not differ between spontaneous and mandatory breaths (158, 159). These results indicate that inspiratory output is preprogrammed and is relatively insensitive to breath-by-breath changes in load seen during SIMV. Chemical feedback could be a critical factor for this breath programming (97). Indeed, in a series of studies in normals as well as in patients with acute lung injury, we recently demonstrated that when chemical stimulus is rigorously controlled, unloading does not result in downregulation of respiratory muscle activation; the neuromuscular output is tightly linked to CO_2 and not to load reduction (70, 100–102). Notwithstanding that the response to unloading was not examined in COPD patients, these studies emphasize the importance of chemical feedback during mechanical ventilation. It follows that mechanical ventilatory support downregulates respiratory muscle output to the extent that increases alveolar ventilation and decreases PCO_2. According to this hypothesis, baseline $PaCO_2$ plays a central role in the degree of unloading. For a given increase in alveolar ventilation, $PaCO_2$ will drop more if baseline $PaCO_2$ is high than low, due to a parabolic relation between alveolar ventilation and $PaCO_2$ (160) and, thus, the degree of unloading should be greater. This, however, should be prospectively studied.

It has been proposed, based on data from several studies, that patients with COPD should be ventilated with high inspiratory flows in order to enhance patient–ventilator interaction and by increasing the time available for expiration to reduce dynamic hyperinflation (60). However, inspiratory flow rates may affect respiratory output in a way that has been largely ignored in patient management. It has been shown in mechanically ventilated normals and critically ill patients that inspiratory flow rates exert a reflex excitatory effect on respiratory output; for a given tidal volume, increasing inspiratory flow is associated with an increase in breathing frequency (161–164). This effect persists, although to a lesser degree, during sleep (163). The strength of this reflex is not affected by breathing route (nose or mouth), temperature, and volume of inspired gas and anesthesia of upper and lower airways. It is presumed to be mediated through receptors located deep in airway mucosa or chest wall (162). Similar response was also observed with decreasing ventilator inspiratory time; for a given tidal volume and inspiratory flow, breathing frequency increased with decreasing mechanical inspiratory time brought by eliminating the end-inspiratory pause (165). The last observation indicates that the excitatory effect of high inspiratory flow might be partly mediated by the concomitant decrease in ventilator inspiratory time. Recent studies suggest that the alteration in ventilator inspiratory time affects breathing frequency via the change in the time that mechanical inflation extents into neural expiration (166).

There are at least four implications for the mechanically ventilated patient with COPD as far as this reflex response be concerned. First, an increase in level of assistance intended to decrease respiratory effort (96) is likely to be less effective than planned because of the stimulating effect of the concomitant increase in flow. Second, high inspiratory flow rates and/or short ventilator inspiratory time may cause hyperventilation with detrimental effects on dynamic hyperinflation and, under certain circumstances, respiratory alkalosis, an important cause of various arrhythmias and weaning failure (5). Third, the desired effect of manipulation of inspiratory flow and/or ventilator inspiratory time on expiratory time and thus on dynamic hyperinflation (60) may not be achieved. Fourth, the ventilatory consequences of flow or ventilator inspiratory time are likely to be different depending on sleep/awake stage (163). These findings indicate that increasing inspiratory flow rates and decreasing ventilator inspiratory time in patients with obstructive disease might not always be appropriate. It follows that the physician dealing with these patients should be aware of the function of different feedback systems when changes in ventilator settings occur. Reevaluation of the patient is mandatory.

VI. Complications

In general, complications during conventional mechanical ventilation in patients with acute exacerbation of chronic obstructive pulmonary disease are similar to those observed in other groups of patients. These complications are due to the process of intubation itself, the mechanical consequences of endotracheal tube, ventilator malfunction, infections, particularly ventilator-associated pneumonia

(VAP), the consequences of the positive-pressure breathing on the function of various organs, inappropriate ventilator management and human error (5). Extensive review of these complications is beyond the scope of this article and the reader is referred to other reviews (5). However, we think that it may be useful to address briefly the issue of barotrauma and VAP in these patients. Other complications related to the interaction of pathophysiology of the disease and the process of mechanical ventilation, such as patient-ventilator dyssynchrony, were already discussed.

Pneumothorax, pneumomediastinum, subcutaneous emphysema and other forms of extra-alveolar air detected during mechanical ventilation are collectively termed barotrauma (5). This term implies alveolar disruption from excessive alveolar distending volume. Theoretically, mechanically ventilated patients with acute exacerbation of COPD are at increased risk of barotrauma for at least three reasons: (1) the existence of dynamic hyperinflation, which leads to increased intrathoracic pressures; (2) the presence of emphysematous regions within the lungs; and (3) the significant time-constant inequalities that predispose some alveoli to high distending volumes even with low tidal volume inflation. Nevertheless, despite these theoretical considerations, recent studies have shown that patients with acute exacerbation of COPD have either no risk or an intermediate risk for barotrauma (167, 168). Perhaps, understanding the pathophysiology of the disease that led to better ventilator management may be the reason for the relatively low risk for barotrauma in these patients.

Ventilator-associated pneumonia is defined as lung infection diagnosed more than 48 h following endotracheal intubation and mechanical ventilation. VAP likely prolongs the length of ICU stay by about 4 days and is associated with a 20 to 30% increased risk of death in critically ill patients (169). Thus, VAP increases both the morbidity and mortality in these patients. The presence of COPD is an independent risk factor (among others) for developing VAP (170). Therefore, in these patients, strategies that have been shown to reduce the incidence of VAP should be employed. These include the semirecumbent position, subglottic secretion drainage, use of heat and moisture exchange filters and oral intubation, minimizing ventilator circuit manipulation and kinetic beds (171). However, the most important factor seems to be the avoidance of intubation. Indeed it has been shown mainly in patients with acute exacerbation of COPD that the use of NIMV decreased the rate of nosocomial pneumonia and nosocomial infections from 22% to 8% and from 60% to 18%, respectively (171). This decrease was associated with shorter ICU stay and lower mortality (171). It follows that the term artificial airway–associated pneumonia, rather than ventilator-associated pneumonia, advocated recently by some, may better characterize the lung infection in patients conventionally ventilated.

VII. Outcomes

Predicting the outcome of mechanically ventilated (via an artificial airway) patients with acute exacerbation of COPD is mandatory for decision making as well as information for the patient and his or her family. It is believed that invasive mechanical ventilation in this group of patients is associated generally with an uncertain prognosis (173, 174). Some investigators have also cautioned against mechanical ventilation in acute exacerbation of COPD, citing problems of prolonged weaning and ICU stay (173, 174). In addition, management of patients with acute exacerbation of COPD in a non-ICU setting has also been recommended. Recent studies, however, challenge this sentiment (175–178). Indeed it has been shown that in mechanically ventilated patients with acute exacerbation, mortality rates, lengths of ICU stay, rates of prolonged ventilation, and tracheostomy did not differ from those patients mechanically ventilated for other than COPD causes (176, 177). Furthermore, the survival rate for up to 2 years was not negatively affected by episodes of ventilation and/or tracheostomy (176). These results, however, should be interpreted with caution, especially in the face of the results of randomized studies with NIPPV showing an adverse effect of intubation and mechanical ventilation on mortality and complication rate (172).

Although mortality following an episode of acute exacerbation of COPD requiring mechanical ventilation may not be influenced by the process of mechanical ventilation, it could be affected by other factors such as premorbid conditions, functional and nutritional status at ICU entry, causes of exacerbation and comorbid illnesses (175–180). For example, it has been shown that the mortality in mechanically ventilated patients with acute exacerbation of COPD who were on long-term oxygen therapy is significantly higher than these reported by studies in unselected patients (177).

The costs of care in mechanically ventilated patients with acute exacerbation of COPD represent an outcome variable that, in the face of continuing decreasing financial resources, achieves a great deal of attention. Indeed the general cost of care for COPD is astounding. The National Lung Health Education Program Executive Committee has noted that, in 1993, the morbidity and mortality from COPD accounted for 14.7 billion dollars in U.S. medical care expenditures (181). The distribution of costs of care in mechanically ventilated patients with acute exacerbations of COPD has recently been studied by Ely et al. (177), who found that, despite similar mortality rates, lengths of ICU stay and mechanical ventilation, and rates of prolonged ventilation and tracheostomy among patients, ICU respiratory care costs were higher in patients with COPD than in patients with other causes of respiratory failure. The cost of administration of bronchodilator drugs, pulse oximetry, and CO_2 detectors was responsible for the observed difference. It seems that, as far as the cost of care is concerned, fundamental differences exist between ICU patients who are related to the nature of the disease process and physician management approaches.

Although ICU and hospital mortality is acceptable in these patients, the long-term outcome in terms of survival and functional status is questionable (Fig. 18). At 6 months, the mortality ranges between 40 to 70%, depending on the population studied, while a significant portion has poor quality of life (175, 176, 179, 180, 182). Two- and 5-year mortality rates may approach 80% and 90%, respectively (179). Age and factors related to nutritional status, such as ideal body weight and plasma

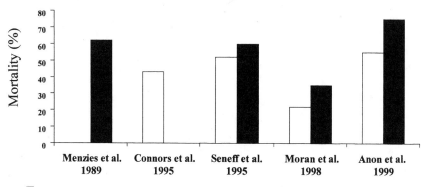

□ 6 mo ■ 1 yr

Figure 18 Six-month (open bars) and 1 year (closed bars) mortality of patients with acute exacerbation of COPD ventilated conventionally. The data of Anon et al. were from patients being on long-term home O_2 therapy. (Data based on Ref. 177.)

albumin, may be predictive of long-term outcome (176, 180). A formula for computing the probability of survival following a severe acute exacerbation of COPD has been described using readily available clinical information (170). This formula may help physicians and patients to make health-care decisions.

VIII. Conclusion

COPD is a complex disorder. The beginning of the inflammatory and destructive process affects the airways and the lungs following inhalation of noxious agents in susceptible subjects. For many years, the lungs are affected, but without symptoms. Then cough and sputum become a frequent morning event; breathing becomes difficult first during effort, then during mild-to-moderate exercise, until daily living is made miserable by unbearable dyspnea for minimal events such as slow walking, taking a shower, eating, etc. At the present time, only smoking cessation and long-term oxygen therapy are known to change the natural history of the disease. It is not known whether and how acute exacerbations affect the progression of COPD. It is, however, well established that exacerbations of COPD, particularly in patients with severe airflow limitation at rest, affect adversely both the individual patient's life and the socioeconomic variables related to COPD. Many exacerbations cause acute respiratory failure and need mechanical ventilation as a life-saving procedure. Noninvasive ventilation is effective in treating many exacerbations of COPD with mild-to-moderate respiratory acidosis, but it may fail to manage patients with severe hemodynamic instability, coma, agitation, excessive secretions, and last, but not least, severe acidosis (e.g., pH < 7.1). Therefore, though less frequent, intubation and mechanical ventilation through artificial airways remains an important procedure in the therapy of acute respiratory failure due to exacerbations of COPD. However, the physicians should be aware of the complex pathophysiology of COPD as well as of the variety of modes and patterns by which mechanical ventilation can be delivered to obtain the best possible patient–ventilation interaction. Furthermore, due to the complications related to airway intubation, the endotracheal tube should be removed as soon as possible. Mechanical ventilation could be continued by means of noninvasive ventilation until the patient can eventually be weaned from machine support and can breathe spontaneously.

References

1. Siafakas NM, Vermeire P, Pride NB, Paoletti P, Gibson J, Howard P, Yernault JC, Decramer M, Hingenbottam T, Postma DS, Rees J. Optimal assessment and management of chronic obstructive pulmonary disease. ERS—Consensus statement. Eur Respir J 1995; 8:1398–1420.
2. Pauwels RA, Buist SA, Calverely PMA, Jenkins CR, Hurd SS on behalf of the GOLD Scientific Committee. Global Strategy for the diagnosis, management and prevention of chronic obstructive pulmonary disease. NHLBI/WHO Global Initiative for chronic obstructive lung disease (GOLD)—Workshop Summary. Am J Respir Crit Care Med 2001; 163:1256–1276.
3. Evans TW. International Consensus Conferences in Intensive Care Medicine: non-invasive positive pressure ventilation in acute respiratory failure. Intens Care Med 2001; 27:166–178.
4. Slutsky AS. Mechanical ventilation. ACCP consensus conference. Chest 1993; 104:1833–1859.
5. Pingleton SK. Complications of acute respiratory failure. Am Rev Respir Dis 1988; 137:1463–1493.
6. Pride NB, Macklem PT. Lung mechanics in disease. In: Macklem PT, Mead J, eds. Handbook of Physiology. The Respiratory System. Mechanics of Breathing, Vol. 2. Bethesda, MD: American Physiological Society, 1986:659–692.
7. Hubmayr RD, Rodarte JR. Cellular effects and physiologic responses: lung mechanics. In: Cherniack NS, ed. Chronic Obstructive Pulmonary Disease. Philadelphia: Saunders, 1991:79–95.
8. Sharp J. The chest wall and respiratory muscles in airflow limitation. In: Roussos C, Macklem PT, eds. The Thorax. New York: Marcel Dekker, 1985:1155–1202.
9. Younes M. Mechanisms of ventilatory failure. Curr Pulmonol 1993; 14:243–292.
10. Rossi A, Ganassini A, Polese G, Grassi V. Pulmonary hyperinflation and ventilator-dependent patients. Eur Respir J 1997; 10:1663–1674.
11. Tobin M, Jubran A, Laghi F. Patient–ventilator interaction. Am J Respir Crit Care Med 2001; 163:1059–1063.
12. Corrado A, De Paola E, Gorini M, Messori A, Bruscoli G, Nutini S, Tozzi D, Ginanni R. Intermittent negative pressure ventilation in the treatment of hypoxic hypercapnic coma in chronic respiratory insufficiency. Thorax 1996; 51:1077–1082.
13. Pepe PE, Marini JJ. Occult positive end-expiratory pressure in mechanically ventilated patients with airflow obstruction. Am Rev Respir Dis 1982; 126:166–170.
14. Fleury B, Murciano D, Talamo C, Aubier M, Pariente R, Milic-Emili J. Work of breathing in patients with chronic obstructive pulmonary disease in acute respiratory failure. Am Rev Respir Dis 1985; 132:822–827.

15. Rossi A, Gotfried SB, Higgs BD, Zocchi L, Grasino A, Milic-Emili J. Respiratory mechanics in mechanically ventilated patients with respiratory failure. J Appl Physiol 1985; 58:1849–1858.
16. Marini JJ. Should PEEP be used in airflow obstruction? (Editorial). Am Rev Respir Dis 1989; 140:1–3.
17. Rossi A, Polese G, Brandi G, Conti G. Intrinsic positive end-expiratory pressure (PEEPi) Intens Care Med 1995; 21:522–536.
18. Younes M. Load responses, dyspnea and respiratory failure. Chest 1990; 97(Suppl): 59–68.
19. Roussos C, Macklem PT. The respiratory muscles. N Engl J Med 1982; 307:786–797.
20. Tobin MJ. Respiratory muscles in disease. Clin Chest Med 1988; 9:263–286.
21. Roussos C, Campbell EJM. Respiratory muscles energetics. In: Macklem PT, Mead J, eds. Handbook of Physiology: The Respiratory System. Mechanics of Breathing, Vol. 2. Bethesda, MD: American Physiological Society, 1986:481–509.
22. Pinsky MR. The effects of mechanical ventilation on the cardiovascular system. Crit Care Med 1990; 6:663–678.
23. Marini JJ, Ravenscraft SA. Mean airway pressure: Physiologic determinants and clinical importance–Part 2: Clinical implications. Crit Care Med 1992; 20:1604–1616.
24. Haake R, Schlichting R, Ulstad DR, Henchen R. Barotrauma. Pathophysiology, risk factors and prevention. Chest 1987; 91:608–613.
25. Rossi A, Gottfried SB, Zocchi L, Higgs BD, Lennox S, Calverley PMA, Begin P, Grassino A, Milic-Emili J. Measurement of static compliance of total respiratory system in patients with acute respiratory failure during mechanical ventilation: the effect of "intrinsic" PEEP. Am Rev Respir Dis 1985; 131:672–677.
26. Georgopoulos D, Giannouli E, Patakas D. Effect of extrinsic positive end-expiratory pressure on mechanically ventilated patients with chronic obstructive pulmonary disease and dynamic hyperinflation. Intens Care Med 1993; 19:197–203.
27. West JB, Dolley CT, Naimark A. Distribution of blood flow in isolated lung in relation to vascular and alveolar pressures. J Appl Physiol 1964; 19:713–724.
28. Roussos C, Macklem PT. Diaphragmatic fatigue in man. J Appl Physiol 1977; 43:189–197.
29. Arora NS, Rochester DF. Respiratory muscle strength and maximal voluntary ventilation in undernourished patients. Am Rev Respir Dis 1982; 126:5–8.
30. Guerin C, Milic-Emili J, Fournier G. Effect of PEEP on work of breathing in mechanically ventilated COPD patients. Intens Care Med 2000; 26(9):1207–1214.
31. Hussain SNA, Simkus G, Roussos C. Respiratory muscle fatigue, a cause of ventilatory failure in septic shock. J Appl Physiol 1985; 58:2027–2032.
32. Aubier M, Trippenbach T, Roussos C. Respiratory muscle fatigue during cardiogenic shock. J Appl Physiol 1981; 51:499–508.
33. Jardin J, Farkas G, Prefaut C, Thomas D, Macklem PT, Roussos C. The failing inspiratory muscles under normoxic and hypoxic conditions. Am Rev Respir Dis 1981; 124:274–279.
34. Aubier M, Murciano D, Lecocgnic Y, Viires N, Jacqueus Y, Squara P, Pariente R. Effect of hypophosphatemia on diaphragmatic contractility in patients with acute respiratory failure. N Engl J Med 1985; 313:420–424.
35. Malloy DW, Dhingra S, Solven FS. Hypomagnesemia and respiratory muscle power. Am Rev Respir Dis 1984; 129:497–498.
36. Rochester DF, Esau SA. Critical illness, infection and the respiratory muscles (editorial). Am Rev Respir Dis 1988; 138:258–259.

37. Rossi A, Santos C, Roca J, Torres A, Felez MA, Rodriguez-Roisin R. Effects of PEEP on VA/Q mismatching in ventilated patients with chronic airflow obstruction. Am J Respir Crit Care Med 1994; 149:1077–1084.

38. Torres A, Reyes A, Rocca J, Wagner PD, Rodriguez-Roisin R. Ventilation-perfusion mismatching in chronic obstructive pulmonary disease during ventilator weaning. Am Rev Respir Dis 1989; 140:1246–1250.

39. Cohen C, Zagelbaum G, Gross D, Roussos C, Macklem PT. Clinical manifestations of inspiratory muscle fatigue. Am J Med 1982; 73:308–316.

40. Bellemare F, Bigland-Ritchie B. Central components of diaphragmatic fatigue assessed from bilateral phrenic nerve stimulation. J Appl Physiol 1987; 62:1307–1316.

41. MacNee W. Pathophysiology of cor pulmonale in chronic obstructive pulmonary disease. Part 1. State of the art. Am J Respir Crit Care Med 1994; 150:833–852.

42. Rounds S, Hill NS. Pulmonary hypertensive diseases. Chest 1984; 85:397.

43. Walley KR, Wood LDH. Ventricular dysfunction in critical illness. In: Hall JB, Schmidt GA, Wood LDH, eds. Principles of Critical Care. New York: McGraw-Hill, 1992:1417–1436.

44. Permutt S, Wise RA. Mechanical interaction of respiration and circulation. In: Fishman A, ed. Handbook of Physiology, Vol. 3. Bethesda, MD: American Physiological Society, 1986:647–656.

45. Lemaire F, Teboul JL, Cinotti L, Giotto G, Abrouk F, Steg G, Macquin-Mavier I, Zapol WM. Acute left ventricular dysfunction during unsuccessful weaning from mechanical ventilation. Anesthesiology 1998; 69:171–179.

46. Franklin C, Samuel J, Hu TC. Life threatening hypotension associated with emergency intubation and the initiation of mechanical ventilation. Am J Emerg Med 1994; 12:425–428.

47. Cassidy SS, Schweip F. Cardiovascular effects of positive end-expiratory pressure. In: Scarf SM, Cassidy SS, eds. Heart–Lung Interaction in Health and Disease. New York: Marcel Dekker, 1989:463.

48. Scharf S, Brown R, Saunders N, Green L. Effects of normal and loaded spontaneous inspiration on cardiovascular function. J Appl Physiol 1979; 47:582–590.

49. Scharf S, Brown R, Tow D, Parisi A. Cardiac effects of increased lung volume and decreased pleural pressure. J Appl Physiol 1979; 47:257–262.

50. Ninane Y, Rypens F, Yernault JC, De Troyer A. Abdominal muscle use during breathing in patients with chronic airflow obstruction. Am Rev Respir Dis 1992; 146:16–21.

51. Takata M, Wise RA, Robotham JL. Effects of abdominal pressure on venous return: Abdominal vascular zone conditions. J Appl Physiol 1990; 69:1961–1972.

52. Rochester DF, Braun NMT. Determinants of maximal inspiratory pressure in chronic obstructive lung disease. Am Rev Respir Dis 1985; 132:42–47.

53. Moxham J. Tests of respiratory muscle function. In: Tobin MJ, ed. The Respiratory Muscles. Philadelphia: JB Lippincott, 1990:312–328.

54. Rodriguez-Roisin. Effect of mechanical ventilation on gas exchange. In: Tobin MJ, ed. Principles and Practice of Mechanical Ventilation. New York: McGraw-Hill, 1994;673–693.

55. Nucci G, Mergoni M, Bricchi C, Polese G, Cobelli C, Rossi A. On-line monitoring of intrinsic PEEP in ventilator dependent patients. J Appl Physiol 2000; 89:985–995.

56. Tuxen D, Lane S. The effects of ventilatory pattern on hyperinflation, airway pressures, and circulation in mechanical ventilation in patients with airflow obstruction. Am Rev Respir Dis 1987; 136:872–879.

57. Bates JHT, Rossi A, Milic-Emili J. Analysis of the behavior of the respiratory system with constant inspiratory flow. J Appl Physiol 1985; 58:1840–1848.

58. Gottfried SB, Rossi A, Higgs BD, Calverly PM, Zocchi L, Bozic C, Milic-Emili J. Noninvasive determination of respiratory system mechanics during mechanical ventilation for acute respiratory failure. Am Rev Respir Dis 1985; 131:414–420.

59. Guerin C, Tantucci C. Respiratory mechanics in intensive care units. Eur Respir Mon 1999; 12:255–278.

60. Georgopoulos D, Mitrouska I, Markopoulou K, Patakas D, Anthonisen NR. Effects of breathing patterns on mechanically ventilated patients with chronic obstructive pulmonary disease and dynamic hyperinflation. Intens Care Med 1995; 21:880–886.

61. Gay PC, Rodarte JC, Tayyab M, Hubmayr RD. Evaluation of bronchodilator responsiveness in mechanically ventilated patients. Am Rev Respir Dis 1987; 136:880–885.

62. Rubini F, Rampulla C, Nava S. Acute effects of corticosteroids on respiratory mechanics in mechanically ventilated patients with chronic airflow obstruction and acute respiratory failure. Am J Respir Crit Care Med 1994; 149:306–310.

63. Marini JJ. Monitoring during mechanical ventilation. Clin Chest Med 1988; 9:73–100.

64. Lourens MS, van den Berg B, Aerts JG, Verbraak AF, Hoogsteden HC, Bogaard JM. Expiratory time constants in mechanically ventilated patients with and without COPD. Intens Care Med 2000; 26:1591–1594.

65. Brunner JX, Laubscher TP, Banner MJ, Iotti G, Braschi A. Simple method to measure total expiratory time constant based on the passive expiratory flow-volume curve. Crit Care Med 1995; 23(6):1117–1122.

66. Zin WA, Pengelly LD, Milic-Emili J. Single-breath method for measurement of respiratory mechanics in anesthetized animals. J Appl Physiol 1982; 52(5):1266–1271.

67. Rossi A, Polese G. As simple as possible, but not simpler. Intens Care Med 2000; 26:1591–1594.

68. Lessard MR, Lofaso F, Bornchard L. Expiratory muscle activity increases intrinsic positive end-expiratory pressure independently of dynamic hyperinflation in mechanically ventilated patients. Am J Respir Crit Care Med 1995; 151:562–569.

69. Gallagher CG, Younes M. Effect of pressure assist on ventilation and respiratory mechanics in heavy exercise. J Appl Physiol 1989; 66:1824–1837.

70. Georgopoulos D, Mitrouska I, Webster K, Bshouty Z, Younes M. Effects of inspiratory muscle unloading on the response of respiratory output to CO_2. Am J Respir Crit Care Med 1995; 151:A639.

71. Petrof BJ, Legare M, Goldberg P, Milic-Emili J, Gottfried SB. Continuous positive airway pressure reduces work of breathing and dyspnea during weaning from mechanical ventilation. Am Rev Respir Dis 1990; 141:281–289.

72. Rossi A, Brandolese R, Milic-Emili J, Gottfried SB. The role of PEEP in patients with chronic obstructive pulmonary disease during assisted ventilation. Eur Respir J 1990; 3:818–822.

73. Gay PC, Rodarte JR, Hubmayr RD. The effects of positive end-expiratory pressure on inso-volume flow and dynamic hyperinflation in patients receiving mechanical ventilation. Am Rev Respir Dis 1989; 139:621–626.

74. Knudson RJ, Mead J, Knudson DE. Contribution of airway collapse to supramaximal expiratory flows. J Appl Physiol 1974; 36:653–657.

75. Younes M, Kun J, Masiowski B, Webster K, Roberts D. A method for noninvasive determination of inspiratory resistance during proportional assist ventilation. Am J Respir Crit Care Med 2001; 163:50–60.

76. Ranieri MV, Giuliani R, Cinnella G, Peske C, Brienza N, Ippolito EL, Pomo V, Fiore T, Gottfried SB, Brienza A. Physiologic effects of positive end-expiratory pressure in patients with chronic obstructive pulmonary disease during acute ventilatory failure and controlled mechanical ventilation. Am Rev Respir Dis 1993; 147:5–13.

77. Valta P, Corbeil C, Lavoie A, Campodonico R, Koulouris N, Chasse M, Braidy J, Milic-Emili J. Detection of expiratory flow limitation during mechanical ventilation. Am J Respir Crit Care Med 1994; 150:1311–1317.

78. O'Donnell DE. Breathlessness in patients with chronic airflow limitation: mechanisms and management. Chest 1994; 106:904–912.

79. Ninane V, Leduc D, Kafi SA, Nasser M, Houa M, Sergysels R. Detection of expiratory flow limitation by manual compression of the abdominal wall. Am J Respir Crit Care Med 2001; 163(6):1326–1330.

80. Sassoon CSH. Mechanical ventilation design and function: the trigger variable. Respir Care 1992; 36:815–828.

81. American Association for Respiratory Care. Consensus statement on the essentials of mechanical ventilation. Respir Care 1992; 37:1000–1008.

82. Ranieri VM, Mascia L, Petruzzelli V, Bruno F, Brienza A, Giuliani R. Inspiratory effort and measurement of dynamic intrinsic PEEP in COPD patients: effects of ventilator triggering systems. Intens Care Med 1995; 21(11):896–903.

83. Braschi A, Iotti G, Rodi G, Emmi V, Salagallini G. Dynamic pulmonary hyperinflation (DPH) during intermittent mandatory ventilation (IMV). Intens Care Med 1988; 14:89.

84. Fernandez R, Benito S, Blanch LL, Net A. Intrinsic PEEP: a cause of inspiratory muscle ineffectivity. Intens Care Med 1988; 15:51–52.

85. Fabry B, Guttmann J, Eberhard L, Bauer T, Haberthur C, Wolff G. An analysis of desynchronization between the spontaneous breathing patient and ventilator during inspiratory pressure support. Chest 1995; 107:1387–1394.

86. Nava S, Bruschi C, Rubini F, Palo A, Iotti G, Brashi A. Respiratory response and inspiratory effort during pressure support ventilation in COPD. Intens Care Med 1995; 21:871–879.

87. Jubran A, Van De Graaf WB, Tobin M. Variability of patient-ventilator interaction with pressure support ventilation in patients with chronic obstructive pulmonary disease. Am J Respir Crit Care Med 1995; 152:129–136.

88. Rossi A, Appendini L. Wasted efforts and dyssynchrony: is the patient-ventilator battle back? (Editorial). Intens Care Med 1995; 21:867–870.

89. Purro A, Appendini L, De Gaetano A, Gudjonsdottir M, Donner CF, Rossi A. Physiologic determinants of ventilator dependence in long-term mechanically ventilated patients. Am J Respir Crit Care Med 2000; 161(4 pt 1):1115–1123.

90. Parthasarathy S, Jubran A, Tobin MJ. Cycling of inspiratory and expiratory muscle groups with the ventilator in airflow limitation. Am J Respir Crit Care Med 1998; 158(5 Pt 1):1471–1478.

91. Younes M. Patient-ventilator interaction with pressure-assisted modalities of ventilatory support. Sem Respir Med 1993; 14:299–322.

92. Appendini L, Purro A, Gudjonsdottir M, Baderna P, Patessio A, Zanaboni S, Donner CF, Rossi A. Physiologic response of ventilator-dependent patients with chronic obstructive pulmonary disease to proportional assist ventilation and continuous positive airway pressure. Am J Respir Crit Care Med 1999; 159(5 Pt 1):1510–1517.

93. Mancebo J, Amaro P, Mollo JL, Lorino H, Lemaire F, Brochard L. Comparison of the effects of pressure support ventilation delivered by three different ventilators during weaning from mechanical ventilation. Intens Care Med 1995; 21:913–919.

94. Cinnella G, Conti G, Lofaso F, Lorino H, Harf A, Lemaire F, Brochard L. Effects of assisted ventilation on the work of breathing: volume-controlled versus pressure-controlled ventilation. Am J Respir Crit Care Med 1996; 153:1025–1033.
95. Younes M, Remmers J. Control of tidal volume and respiratory frequency. In: Hornbein TF, ed. Regulation of Breathing. New York: Marcel Dekker, 1981:621–671.
96. Georgopoulos D, Roussos C. Control of breathing in mechanically ventilated patient. Eur Respir J 1996; 9:2151–2160.
97. Younes M, Georgopoulos D. Control of breathing relevant to mechanical ventilation. In: Marini J, Slutsky A, eds. Physiological Basis of Ventilatory Support. New York: Marcel Dekker, 1998:1–74.
98. Younes M. A model for the relation between respiratory neural and mechanical outputs. I Theory. J Appl Physiol 1981; 51:963–978.
99. Mitrouska I, Xirouchaki N, Patakas D, Siafakas N, Georgopoulos D. Effects of chemical feedback on respiratory motor and ventilatory output during different modes of assisted mechanical ventilation. Eur Respir J 1999; 13:873–882.
100. Xirouchaki N, Kondili E, Mitrouska I, Siafakas N, Georgopoulos D. Early and late response of respiratory motor output to varying pressure support level in mechanically ventilated patients. Eur Respir J 1999; 14:508–516.
101. Kondili E, Prinianakis G, Anastasaki M, Georgopoulos D. Acute effects of ventilator settings on respiratory motor output in patients with acute lung injury. Intens Care Med 2001; 27:1147–1157.
102. Le Bourdelles G, Viires N, Boczkowsi J, Setar N, Pavlovic D, Aubier M. Effects of mechanical ventilation on diaphragmatic contractile properties in rats. Am J Respir Crit Care Med 1994; 149:1539–1544.
103. Simon PM, Skatrud JB, Badr MS, Griffin DM, Iber C, Dempsey JA. Role of airway mechanoreceptors in the inhibition of inspiration during mechanical ventilation in humans. Am Rev Respir Dis 1991; 144:1033–1041.
104. Ayres SM, Crace WJ. Inappropriate ventilation and hypoxemia as causes of cardiac arrhythmias. The control of arrhythmias without antiarrhythmic drugs. Am J Med 1969; 46:495–505.
105. Georgopoulos D, Anthonisen NR. Oxygen therapy. Curr Pulmonol 1990; 11:221–246.
106. Georgopoulos D, Rossi A, Moxham J. Ventilatory support in COPD. Eur Respir Monogr 1998; 7:189–208.
107. Georgopoulos D, Brochard L. Ventilatory strategies in acute exacerbations of COPD. Eur Respir Monogr 1998; 8:12–44.
108. Feihl F, Perret C. Permissive hypercapnia: how permissive should we be? Am J Respir Crit Care Med 1994; 150:1722–1737.
109. Laghi F, D'Alfonso N, Tobin MJ. Pattern of recovery from diaphragmatic fatigue over 24 hours. J Appl Physiol 1995; 79:539–546.
110. Hansen-Flaschen J, Cowen J, Raps EC. Neuromuscular blockade in the Intensive Care Unit. More than we bargained for. Am Rev Respir Dis 1993; 147:234–236.
111. Shapiro JM, Condos R, Cole RP. Myopathy of status asthmaticus: relation to neuromuscular blockade and corticosteroid administration. J Intens Care Med 1993; 8:144–152.
112. Douglas JA, Tuxen DV, Horne M, Scheinkestel CD, Weinmann M, Czarnyu D, Bowes G. Myopathy in severe asthma. Am Rev Respir Dis 1992; 146:517–519.
113. Griffin D, Fairman N, Coursin D, Rawsthorne L, Grossman JE. Acute myopathy during treatment of status asthmaticus with corticosteroids and steroidal muscle relaxants. Chest 1992; 102:510–514.

114. Manthous CA, Chatila W. Prolonged weakness after withdrawal of atracurium. Am J Respir Crit Care Med 1994; 150:1441–3.
115. Dark DS, Pingleton SK, Kerby GR. Hypercapnia during weaning: A complication of nutritional support. Chest 1985; 88:141–143.
116. Al-Saady NM, Blackmore CM, Bennett ED. High fat, low carbohydrate, enteral feeding lowers $PaCO_2$ and reduces the period of ventilation in artificially ventilated patients. Intens Care Med 1989; 15:290–295.
117. Mancebo J, Amaro P, Lorino H, Lemaire F, Harf A, Brochard L. Effects of albuterol inhalation on the work of breathing during weaning from mechanical ventilation. Am Rev Respir Dis 1991; 144:95–100.
118. Kondili E, Georgopoulos D. Aerosol medications. Respir Clin North Am 2002; 8:309–334.
119. Salmeron S, Brochard L, Mal H, et al. Nebulized versus intravenous albuterol in hypercapnic acute asthma: multicenter, double blind, randomised study. Am J Respir Crit Med 1994; 149:1466–1470.
120. Williams SJ, Winner SJ, Clark TJH. Comparison of inhaled and intravenous terboutaline in acute severe asthma. Thorax 1981; 36:629–631.
121. Kurland G, Williams Lewiston NJ. Fatal myocardial infarction during continuous infusion of intravenous isoproterenol during therapy of asthma. J Allergy Clin Immunol 1979; 63:407–411.
122. O'Connel MB, Iber C. Continuous intravenous terbutaline infusions for adult patients with status asthmaticus. Ann Allergy 1990; 64:213–218.
123. Dhand R, Tobin M. Bronchodilator delivery with metered-dose inhalers in mechanically ventilated patients. Eur Respir J 1996; 9:585–595.
124. Poggi R, Brandolese R, Bernasconi M, Manzin E, Rossi A. Doxophylline and Respiratory Mechanics: short term effects in mechanically ventilated patients with airflow obstruction and respiratory failure. Chest 1989; 96:772–778.
125. Georgopoulos D, Mouloudi E, Kondili E, Klimathianaki M. Bronchodilator delivery with metered-dose inhaler during mechanical ventilation. Crit Care 2000; 4:227–234.
126. Bowton DL, Goldsmith WM, Haponic EF. Substitution of metered-dose inhalers for hand nebulizers: success and cost-saving in a large acute care hospital. Chest 1992; 101(2):305–308.
127. Beaty CD, Ritz RH, Benson MS. Continuous in-line nebulizers complicate pressure support ventilation. Chest 1989; 96(6):1360–1363.
128. Hess D. Aerosol bronchodilator delivery during mechanical ventilation nebulizer or inhaler? Chest 1991; 100:1103–1104.
129. Manthous CA, Hall JB, Schmidt GA, Wood LD. Metered-dose inhaler versus nebulized albuterol in mechanically ventilated patients. Am Rev Respir Dis 1993; 148:1567–1570.
130. Guerin G, Chevre A, Dessirier P, Poucet T, Becquemin MH, Dequiu PF, Le Guellec C, Jacques D, Fournier G. Inhaled fenoterol-ipratropium bromide in mechanically ventilated patients with chronic obstructive pulmonary disease. Am J Respir Crit Care Med 1999; 159:1036–1042.
131. Mouloudid L, Katsanoulas K, Anastasaki M, Askitopoulou E, Georgopoulos D. Bronchodilator delivery by metered-dose inhaler in mechanically ventilated patients with chronic obstructive pulmonary disease—Influence of end-inspiratory pause. Eur Respir J 1998; 12:165–169.
132. Mouloudi L, Katsanoulas K, Anastasaki M, Xoing S, Georgopoulos D. Bronchodilator delivery by metered-dose inhaler in mechanically ventilated patients with chronic

obstructive pulmonary disease—Influence of tidal volume. Intens Care Med 1999; 25:1215–1221.

133. Mouloudi L, Prinianakis G, Kondili E, Georgopoulos D. Bronchodilator delivery by metered-dose inhaler in mechanically ventilated patients with chronic obstructive pulmonary disease—Influence of flow pattern. Eur Respir J 2000; 16:263–268.

134. Mouloudi L, Prinianakis G, Kondili E, Georgopoulos D. Bronchodilator delivery by metered-dose inhaler in mechanically ventilated patients with chronic obstructive pulmonary disease—Influence of flow rate. Intens Care Med 2001; 27:42–46.

135. Fink JB, Dhand R, Duarte AG, Jenne JW, Tobin MJ. Deposition of aerosol from metered-dose inhaler during mechanical ventilation: an in vitro model. Am J Respir Crit Care Med 1996; 154(2 pt 1):382–387.

136. Bauer TT, Torres A. Aerosolized beta2-agonists in the intensive care unit: just do it. Intensive Care Med 2001; 27(1):3–5.

137. Manthous CA, Chatila W, Schmitdt GA, et al. Treatment of bronchospasm by meter-dose inhaler albuterol in mechanically ventilated patients. Chest 1995; 107:210–213.

138. Bernasconi M, Brandolese R, Poggi R, Manzin E, Rossi A. Dose-response effects and time-course of inhaled fenoterol on respiratory mechanics and arterial oxygen tension in mechanically ventilated patients with chronic airflow obstruction. Intens Care Med 1990; 16:108–114.

139. Dhand R, Duarte AG, Jubray A, Jenne JW, Fink JB, Fahey PJ, Tobin MJ. Dose-response to bronchodilator delivered by metered dose inhaler in ventilator-support patients. Am J Respir Crit Care Med 1996; 154(2 pt 1):388–393.

140. Georgopoulos D, Bruchardi H. Ventilatory strategies in status asthmaticus. Eur Respir Monogr 1998; 8:45–83.

141. Mouloudi L, Maliotakis Ch, Kodili E, Kafetzakis A, Georgopoulos D. Duration of salbutamol induced bronchodilation delivered by metered dose inhaler in mechanically ventilated COPD patients. Mon Arch Chest Dis 2001; 56:189–194.

142. Duarte AG, Momii K, Bidani A. Bronchodilator therapy with metered-dose inhaler and spacer versus nebulizer in mechanically ventilated patients: comparison of magnitude and duration of response. Respir Care 2000; 45(7):817–823.

143. Duarte AG, Dhand R, Reid R, Fink JB, Fahey PJ, Tobin MJ, Jenne JW. Serum albuterol levels in mechanically ventilated patients and healthy subjects after metered-dose inhaler administration. Am J Respir Crit Care Med 1996; 154(6 pt 1):1658–1663.

144. Nava S, Compagnoni ML. Controlled short-term trial of fluticasone propionate in ventilator-dependent patients with COPD. Chest 2000; 118(4):990–999.

145. Papamoscou D. Theoretical validation of the respiratory benefits of helium-oxygen mixtures. Respir Physiol 1995; 99:(1)183–190.

146. Murray JF. Ventilation. In: Murray JF, ed. The Normal Lung. 83–107, 1986.

147. Tassaux D, Jolliet P, Roeseler J, Chevrolet JC. Effects of helium-oxygen on intrinsic positive end-expiratory pressure in intubated and mechanically ventilated patients with severe chronic obstructive pulmonary disease. Crit Care Med 2000; 28(8):2721–2728.

148. Goode ML, Fink JB, Dhand R, Tobin MJ. Improvement in aerosol delivery with helium-oxygen mixtures during mechanical ventilation. Am J Respir Crit Care Med 2001; 163(1):109–114.

149. Devabhaktuni VG, Torres A Jr, Wilson S, Yeh MP. Effect of nitric oxide, perfluorocarbon, and heliox on minute volume measurement and ventilator volumes delivered. Crit Care Med 1999; 27(8):1603–1607.

150. Tassaux D, Jolliet P, Thouret JM, Roeseler J, Dorne R, Chevrolet JC. Calibration of seven ICU ventilators for mechanical ventilation with helium-oxygen mixtures. Crit Care Med 1998; 26(2):290–295.

151. Roupie E, Dambrossion M, Servillo G, Mentec H, El Atrous S, Beydon L, Brun-Bruisson C, Lemaire F, Brochard L. Titration of tidal volume and induced hypercapnia in acute respiratory distress syndrome. Am J Respir Crit Care Med 1995; 152:121–128.

152. Hickling KG. The pressure-volume curve is greatly modified by recruitment. A mathematical model of ARDS lungs. Am J Respir Crit Care Med 1998; 158:194–202.

153. Marcy TW, Marini JJ. Respiratory distress in the ventilated patient. Clin Chest Med 1994; 15:55–73.

154. Mancebo J, Albaladejo P, Touchard D, Bak E, Subirana M, Lemaire F, Harf A, Brochard L. Airway occlusion pressure to titrate positive end-expiratory pressure in patients with dynamic hyperinflation. Anesthesiology 2000; 93(1):81–90.

155. Manning HL, Molinary EJ, Leiter JC. Effect of inspiratory flow rate on respiratory sensation and pattern of breathing. Am J Respir Crit Care Med 1995; 151:751–757.

156. Marini JJ, Smith TC, Lamb VJ. External work output and force generation during synchronized intermittent mechanical ventilation. Effects of machine assistance on breathing effort. Am Rev Respir Dis 1988; 138:1169–1179.

157. Imsand C, Feihl F, Perret C, Fitting JW. Regulation of inspiratory neuromuscular output during synchronized intermittent mechanical ventilation. Anesthesiology 1994; 80:13–22.

158. Kryger MH. Respiratory failure: Carbon dioxide. In: Kryger MH, ed. Introduction to Respiratory Medicine. New York: Churchill Livingstone, 1990:211–226.

159. Puddy A, Younes M. Effect of inspiratory flow rate on respiratory output in normal subjects. Am Rev Respir Dis 1992; 146:787–789.

160. Georgopoulos D, Mitrouska I, Bshouty Z, Webster K, Anthonisen NR, Younes M. Effects of breathing route and airway anesthesia on the response of respiratory output to inspiratory flow rates. Am J Respir Crit Care Med 1996; 153:168–175.

161. Georgopoulos D, Mitrouska I, Bshouty Z, Anthonisen NR, Younes M. Effects of NREM sleep on the response of respiratory output to inspiratory flow. Am J Respir Crit Care Med 1996; 153:1624–1630.

162. Corne S, Webster K, Younes M. Effects of inspiratory flow on diaphragmatic motor output in normal subjects. J Appl Physiol 2000; 89(2):481–492.

163. Corne S, Gillespie D, Roberts D, Younes M. Effect of inspiratory flow rate on respiratory rate in intubated ventilated patients. Am J Respir Crit Care Med 1997; 156(1):304–308.

164. Laghi F, Segal J, Choe WK, Tobin MJ. Effect of imposed inflation time on respiratory frequency and hyperinflation in patients with chronic obstructive pulmonary disease. Am J Respir Crit Care Med 2001; 163(6):1365–1370.

165. Gammon RB, Shin MS, Buchalter SE. Pulmonary barotrauma in mechanical ventilation. Patterns and risk factors. Chest 1993; 104(3):971.

166. Gammon RB, Shin MS, Groves RH Jr, Hardin JM, Hsu C, Buchalter SE. Clinical risk factors for pulmonary barotrauma: a multivariate analysis. Am J Respir Crit Care Med 1995; 152(4 Pt 1):1235–1240.

167. Cook D. Ventilator associated pneumonia: perspective on the burden of illness. Intens Care Med 2000; 26:S31–S37.

168. Cook DJ, Walter SD, Cook RJ, Griffith LE, Gyatt GH, Leasa D, Jaeschke RZ, Brun-Buisson C. Incidence of and risk factors for ventilator-associated pneumonia in critically ill patients. Ann Intern Med 1999; 130(12):1027–1028.

169. Morehead RS, Pinto SJ. Ventilator-associated pneumonia. Arch Intern Med 2000; 160(13):1926–1936.
170. Girou E, Schortgen F, Delclaux C, Brun-Buisson C, Blot F, Lefort Y, Lemaire F, Brochard L. Association of noninvasive ventilation with nosocomial infections and survival in critically ill patients. JAMA 2000; 284(18):2361–2367.
171. Muir JF, Levi-Valenci P. When should patient with COPD be ventilated? Eur J Respir Dis 1987; 70:135–139.
172. Editorial. To ventilate or not. Lancet 1991; 337:463–464.
173. Seneff MG, Wagner DP, Wagner RP, Zimmerman J, Knaus WA. Hospital and 1-year survival of patients admitted to intensive care units with acute exacerbations of chronic obstructive pulmonary disease. JAMA 1995; 274:1852–1857.
174. Moran J, Green J, Homan S, Leeson J, Leppard P. Acute exacerbation of COPD and mechanical ventilation: a reevaluation. Crit Care Med 1998; 26:71–78.
175. Ely EW, Baker AM, Evans GW, Haponik EF. The distribution of cost of care in mechanically ventilated patients with obstructive pulmonary disease. Crit Care Med 2000; 28:408–413.
176. Nevins ML, Epstein SK. Predictors of outcome for patients with COPD requiring invasive mechanical ventilation. Chest 2001; 119(6):1840–1849.
177. Anon JM, Lorenzo AG, Zanazaga A, Gomez-Tello V, Garrido G. Mechanical ventilation of patients on long term oxygen therapy with chronic obstructive pulmonary disease: prognosis and cost-analysis. Intens Care Med 1999; 25:452–457.
178. Connors AF, Dawson NV, Thomas C, Harrell FE, Desbiens N, Fulkerson WJ, Kussin P, Bellamy P, Goldman L, Knaus W. Outcome following acute exacerbations of severe chronic obstructive lung disease. Am J Respir Crit Care Med 1996; 154:959–967.
179. The National Lung Health Education Program Executive Committee: Strategies in preserving lung health and preventing COPD and associated diseases. Chest 1998; 113:123S–163S.
180. Menzies R, Gibbons W, Goldberg P. Determinants of weaning and survival among patients with COPD who require mechanical ventilation for acute respiratory failure. Chest 1989; 95(2):398–405.

27

Weaning from the Ventilator

AMAL JUBRAN

Edward Hines, Jr., Veterans Affairs Hospital
and Loyola University of Chicago
  Stritch School of Medicine
Hines, Illinois, U.S.A.

AIMAN TULAIMAT

Loyola University of Chicago
  Stritch School of Medicine
Hines, Illinois, U.S.A.

Patients with COPD account for 13% of all patients receiving mechanical ventilation; COPD is the most common indication for mechanical ventilation in North America (1). Although often life saving, mechanical ventilation is associated with several major complications. Accordingly, it is important to discontinue mechanical ventilation and extubate the patient at the earliest possible time. While it is possible to wean the majority of patients from mechanical ventilation without much difficulty, 25 to 30% of patients repeatedly fail weaning trials (2, 3). These difficult-to-wean patients account for a considerable proportion of the workload in an intensive care unit (ICU) (1). In a survey of ventilator-supported patients, over 40% of total ventilator time was consumed by weaning the patient from the ventilator (4) and, in patients with COPD, weaning constituted 59% of the total ventilator time.

I. Pathophysiological Determinants of Weaning Outcome

The pathophysiological factors that determine a patient's ability to tolerate discontinuation of ventilator support are adequacy of pulmonary gas exchange and performance of the respiratory muscle pump. In addition, psychological factors play an important role in determining weaning outcome (5).

A. Adequacy of Pulmonary Gas Exchange

Some patients with COPD who fail a trial of spontaneous breathing develop an increase in arterial carbon dioxide tension ($PaCO_2$) (6). The term hypoventilation is used synonymously with hypercapnia. But a reduction in alveolar ventilation could be due to either a decrease in overall minute ventilation or in ratio of V_T to physiological deadspace (7, 8). In patients failing a weaning trial, the minute ventilation in itself is not a significant determinant of CO_2 retention, as it is similar in weaning failure and weaning success patients (9). Instead the increase in $PaCO_2$ is due to rapid, shallow breathing, with consequent increase in physiological dead space (Fig. 1).

Attempts to resume spontaneous respiration following a period of mechanical ventilation may result in hypoxemia. Employing the multiple inert gas to study gas exchange, investigators (10) reported that discontinuation of mechanical ventilation and resumption of spontaneous breathing were associated with further worsening of ventilation perfusion (V/Q) mismatching. Despite the deterioration in V/Q relationship, arterial O_2 tension (PaO_2) did not decrease because there was a simultaneous increase in cardiac output. Unfortunately, comparable detailed investigations of gas exchange in patients failing a weaning trial have not been conducted.

A. Respiratory Muscle Performance

Impairment of the respiratory muscle pump is probably the most common cause of failure to wean from mechanical ventilation. Such impairment may result from an

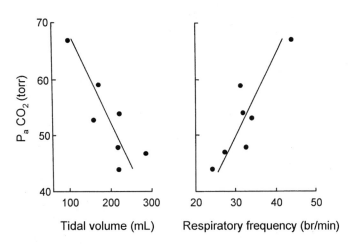

Figure 1   Relationship between tidal volume (V_T) and respiratory frequency with carbon dioxide tension ($PaCO_2$) in seven patients who failed a spontaneous breathing trial. $PaCO_2$ was significantly correlated with V_T ($r = 0.84$; $p < 0.025$) and frequency ($r = 0.87$; $p < 0.025$); 81% of the variance in $PaCO_2$ could be explained by the changes in these two variables. (From Ref. 9, with permission.)

Table 1 Respiratory Muscle Pump Failure

Decreased respiratory neuromuscular capacity
Decreased respiratory center output
Phrenic nerve dysfunction
Respiratory muscle pump dysfunction
  Hyperinflation
  Decreased oxygen delivery
  Respiratory acidosis
  Mineral and electrolyte abnormalities
  Malnutrition
  Respiratory muscle fatigue

Increased respiratory muscle pump load
Increased ventilatory requirements
  Increased CO_2 production
  Increased deadspace ventilation
Increased mechanical loads
  Increased airway resistance
  Increased dynamic lung elastance
  Increased intrinsic PEEP

---

imbalance between respiratory neuromuscular capacity and respiratory load (Table 1) (11).

B. Decreased Respiratory Neuromuscular Capacity

Respiratory Center Output

Patients who fail a trial of weaning from mechanical ventilation commonly develop respiratory acidosis, which naturally raises the suspicion of respiratory center depression. However, indices of drive, such as airway occlusion pressure at 0.1 s ($P_{0.1}$) or mean inspiratory flow (V_T/T_I), are usually above the normal range in such patients (12–15). Furthermore, an increase in V_T/T_I has been observed in patients who developed severe alveolar hypoventilation during an unsuccessful weaning trial (9). In most patients, however, the level of drive is not appropriately increased for the level of chemical stimulation (9, 16). It has been suggested that during weaning failure, it would be clever for the respiratory control system to decrease its output as a way of avoiding contractile fatigue of the respiratory muscles; such a strategy has been termed central fatigue (17). On the contrary, patients with COPD who failed a weaning trial developed >40% increase in total pressure generated by the respiratory muscles between the beginning and end of the trial (6). These data indicate that downregulation of the respiratory motor output is not common in patients who fail a weaning trial.

    Dunn and colleagues (15) assessed respiratory control during weaning by measuring the inspiratory on-switch threshold to CO_2 (18). Ventilator settings were initially altered to achieve suppression of phasic inspiratory activity. Carbon dioxide was then added to the inspired gas, and the lowest alveolar PCO_2 that produced the reappearance of inspiratory efforts was defined as the CO_2 recruitment threshold. Seven patients who failed a weaning trial developed a 3 mmHg increase in $PaCO_2$ relative to their recruitment threshold (mean increase, 5 ± 5 mmHg). In contrast, five patients who sustained spontaneous breathing for 60 min without distress maintained their spontaneous $PaCO_2$ close to their recruitment threshold (mean difference, 1.2 mmHg). These findings suggest that even mild elevations in $PaCO_2$ above the recruitment threshold produce respiratory distress during the weaning process.

Phrenic Nerve Function

Approximately 25 to 75% of patients undergoing coronary artery bypass surgery develop a raised left hemidiaphragm that is associated with decreases in lung volume and maximal inspiratory pressure (19, 20). Electrophysiological studies indicate that about 10% of these patients have evidence of phrenic nerve injury (20–22), and thus abnormalities in phrenic nerve function should be suspected if weaning proves difficult in the postoperative period.

Respiratory Muscle Dysfunction

Respiratory muscle dysfunction is believed to be a major mechanism of weaning failure in patients with COPD (23). Several factors that affect the geometrical arrangement of the respiratory muscles can result in ineffective force generation. Patients who fail weaning commonly develop tachypnea, and the resulting decrease in expiratory time becomes insufficient for lung emptying leading to dynamic hyperinflation (9). Hyperinflation has a number of adverse effects: respiratory muscles operate at an unfavorable position of their length–tension curve; flattening of the diaphragm increases the radius of curvature, and, thus, according to Laplace's law, tension within the muscle is less effectively translated into transdiaphragmatic pressure; the "bucket handle" movement of the lower rib cage is decreased as a result of a decrease in the zone of apposition and by the switch from an axial to a medial orientation of the muscle fibers; and the inwardly directed elastic recoil of the chest wall poses an added elastic load (11).

Respiratory muscle performance can also be impaired as a result of asynchronous and paradoxic motion of the rib cage and abdomen. In a study employing quantitative assessment of asynchrony and paradox, patients who failed a weaning trial displayed significantly greater asynchrony and paradox of the rib cage and abdomen than patients with a successful outcome (24). Such a manner of breathing is extremely inefficient and it poses a marked increase in the energy costs for a given level of ventilation.

The O_2 supply to a muscle is decreased secondary to decreases in cardiac output (25), O_2 content of arterial blood (hypoxemia, anemia) (26), or O_2 extraction (sepsis) (27). In a study in patients with COPD who failed a trial of weaning from mechanical ventilation, Lemaire et al. (28) observed an increase in transmural pulmonary artery occlusion pressure, which was attributed to an increase in left ventricular afterload as a result of markedly negative pleural pressure swings. More recently, Jubran et al. (29) investigated the importance of hemodynamic performance in determining weaning outcome in eight ventilator-supported patients who failed a trial of spontaneous breathing and 11 patients who tolerated a trial and were successfully extubated. Immediately before the trial, mixed venous oxygen saturation (SvO_2) was no different between the two groups. Mixed venous oxygen saturation progressively decreased over the course of the trial in the failure group, whereas it remained unchanged in the success group (Fig. 2). Although oxygen consumption was similar in the two groups, the manner in which these demands were met differed between the groups. In the success group, oxygen transport increased, mainly due to an increase in cardiac index; in the failure group, the increase in demand was met by an increase in oxygen extraction, resulting in a decrease in SvO_2. The inability of the failure group to increase oxygen transport was partly due to the increase in right- and left-ventricular afterload (Fig. 3). The low SvO_2 in the failure group combined with greater venous admixture led to rapid arterial desaturation. These data indicate that an inability to increase oxygen delivery to the tissues, including the respiratory muscles, during a period of increased O_2 demand can contribute to the development of acute respiratory failure.

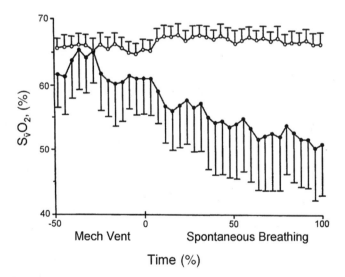

Figure 2 Ensemble averages of the interpolated values of mixed venous oxygen saturation (S_vO_2) during mechanical ventilation and a trial of spontaneous breathing in the success group (open symbols) and failure group (closed symbols). During mechanical ventilation, S_vO_2 was similar in the two groups. Between the onset and the end of the trial, S_vO_2 decreased in the failure group ($p < 0.01$), whereas it remained unchanged in the success group. Over the course of the trial, S_vO_2 was lower in the failure group than in the success group ($p < 0.02$). (Bars represent SE.) (From Ref. 29, with permission.)

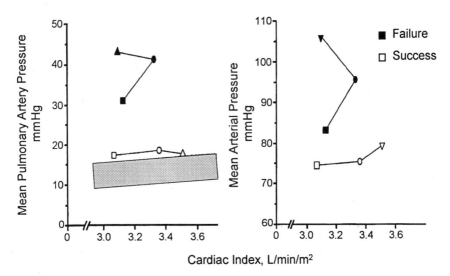

Figure 3 Mean pulmonary artery pressure and mean arterial pressure versus cardiac index during mechanical ventilation (squares) and at the onset (circles) and end (triangles) of a spontaneous breathing trial in the success (open symbols) and failure group (closed symbols). The shaded area represents the normal range of increase in pulmonary artery pressure with cardiac index. In the success group, cardiac index increased between mechanical ventilation and the end of the trial, mean pulmonary artery pressure remained slightly above the normal range, and mean arterial pressure remained unchanged. In contrast, in the failure group, cardiac index was similar during mechanical ventilation and at the end of the weaning trial, but mean pulmonary artery pressure and mean arterial pressure were higher by the end of the trial ($p < 0.025$ and $p < 0.05$, respectively). The increases in mean pulmonary artery pressure and mean arterial pressure, together with the lack of change in cardiac index, strongly suggest increases in right- and left-ventricular afterload in the failure group. (From Ref. 29, with permission.)

Acute respiratory acidosis, equivalent to a $PaCO_2$ of approximately 56 torr—a common occurrence in weaning failure patients—has been shown to cause a decrease in the contractility and endurance time of the diaphragm in healthy subjects (30). Metabolic abnormalities such as hypophosphatemia, hypokalemia, hypocalcemia, or hypomagnesemia may adversely affect respiratory muscle function. Endocrine disturbances such as hyperthyroidism or hypothyroidism may impair respiratory muscle function, as may corticosteroid therapy. Drug-induced disorders need to be considered, such as the occurrence of prolonged respiratory muscle weakness after discontinuation of neuromuscular blocking agents (31). Malnutrition is particularly common in critically ill patients and is associated with decreases in the ventilatory response to hypoxia, diaphragmatic mass and thickness, and respiratory muscle strength and endurance.

Respiratory muscle fatigue has been considered a major cause of weaning failure (32), although definite proof of its role is not available (9). In one of the first studies to use weaning failure as a model of acute ventilatory failure, Cohen et al.

(32) observed a shift in the power spectrum of the diaphragmatic electromyogram (EMG), which they considered to signify fatigue. Initially, this interpretation was readily and widely accepted because it is hard to conceive of a group of patients who are at greater risk of respiratory muscle fatigue than patients who fail a weaning trial. It is now recognized that the EMG power spectrum is influenced by several factors and does not necessarily signify impaired muscle contractility (33).

The question of whether or not weaning failure in an individual patient is due to respiratory muscle fatigue, which in part is due to structural damage in the muscles, is of vital importance for several reasons. Rest is the only means of reversing fatigue, and for the respiratory muscles this means mechanical ventilation. If a patient develops respiratory muscle fatigue during the course of an unsuccessful weaning attempt, it is likely that the new structural injury to the muscles will impair the patient's performance and represent an additional medical complication for this patient. Trying to minimize the risk of fatigue by postponing attempts at weaning places the patient at risk for the many complications associated with mechanical ventilation. Moreover, excessive muscle rest can cause muscle atrophy, thus initiating a vicious cycle (34, 35). These issues are compounded by the lack of simple, reliable means of detecting respiratory muscle fatigue in critically ill patients.

Tension–time index (TTI), which quantifies the magnitude and duration of inspiratory muscle contraction, appears to be the best available framework for considering the risk of respiratory muscle fatigue (36). In a recent study, TTI was measured in 17 patients with COPD who failed a trial of weaning from mechanical ventilation and 14 patients who tolerated such a trial and were extubated (6). At the onset of the trial, TTI was no different in the two groups. TTI, however, increased over the course of the trial whereas it remained unchanged in the success group (Fig. 4). Five of the failure patients developed a TTI greater than 0.15—a value that has been shown to be associated with respiratory muscle fatigue. These results suggest that respiratory muscle fatigue may be responsible for some instances of weaning failure in patients with COPD.

Vassilakopoulos et al. (37) measured TTI during passive ventilation after a patient failed a weaning trial and repeated these measurements later on when the patient tolerated the weaning trial and was subsequently extubated successfully. They found that TTI was higher when patients were failing a weaning trial than when they were successfully extubated. These findings provide further support for the importance of respiratory muscle dysfunction as a determinant of weaning failure.

C. Increased Respiratory Muscle Pump Load

An increase in the load on the respiratory muscle pump may result from increased ventilatory requirements or increased mechanical loads (Table 1).

D. Increased Ventilatory Requirements

Increased ventilatory requirements may result from increased CO_2 production and increased deadspace ventilation. An increase in CO_2 production predisposes to the

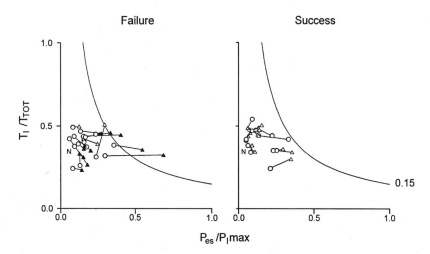

Figure 4 The relationship between mean esophageal pressure/maximum inspiratory pressure ratio (P_{es}/P_I max) and duty cycle (T_I/T_{TOT}) in ventilator-supported patients with COPD who failed a trial of spontaneous breathing and patients who tolerated the trial. Circles and triangles represent values at the start and end of the trial, respectively; closed symbols indicate patients who developed an increase in P_aCO_2 during the trial. Five of the 17 patients in the failure group developed a tension time index of >0.15 (indicated by the isopleth), suggesting respiratory muscle fatigue. N represents value in a normal subject. (From Ref. 6, with permission.)

development of CO_2 retention, but it is never the sole cause of hypercapnia. An important cause of increased CO_2 production can be administration of excessive carbohydrate calories during enteral or parenteral nutrition. Administration of carbohydrates in excess of metabolic needs results in a marked increase in CO_2 production (38). In normal subjects, the increase in alveolar ventilation prevents the development of hypercapnia. This is not possible in patients with respiratory compromise, and several patients have been reported to develop hypercapnia when given excessive nutritional support at the time of being weaned from mechanical ventilation.

Deadspace Ventilation

Physiological dead space is usually related to tidal volume (i.e., V_D/V_T) and in healthy subjects the V_D/V_T ratio is between 0.33 and 0.45. Dead space is increased in a number of disease states and requires an increase in minute ventilation if hypercapnia is to be prevented. If CO_2 production is high, an increase in V_D/V_T to 0.6 or above is generally considered to predict an unsuccessful weaning outcome because the associated increase in minute ventilation necessary for satisfactory gas exchange causes marked encroachment on ventilatory reserve; however, exceptions do exist (39). In addition, patients with increased deadspace frequently have decreased lung compliance and increased airway resistance which cause further increases in the work of breathing. However, the importance of V_D/V_T as a determinant of weaning outcome has not been systematically studied in a large group of patients.

E. Increased Mechanical Load

Patients with COPD who fail a trial of spontaneous breathing develop a substantial increase in respiratory effort, reaching more than four times the normal value at the end of the trial (Fig. 5) (6). To determine the factors responsible for the increased effort, measurements of respiratory mechanics were obtained in patients with COPD during a trial of weaning from mechanical ventilation (6). At the onset of the trial of spontaneous breathing, inspiratory resistance was similar in those patients who failed

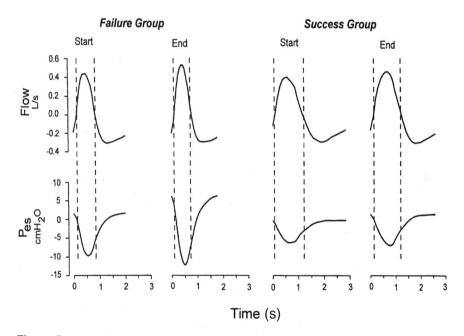

Figure 5 Ensemble average plots of flow and esophageal pressure (Pes) at the start and end of a trial of spontaneous breathing in 17 ventilator-dependent patients who failed the trial and 14 patients who tolerated the trial and were successfully extubated. At the start of the trial, the inspiratory excursions in Pes was greater in the failure group, and it showed a further increase by the end of the trial. To generate these plots, flow and Pes tracings were divided into 25 equal time intervals over a single respiratory cycle for each of the five breaths for each patient in the two groups. For a given patient, the five breaths from the start of the trial were then superimposed and aligned with respect to time, and the average at each time point was calculated. The group mean tracings were then generated by ensemble averaging of the individual mean from each patient. The same procedure was performed for breaths at the end of the trial. (From Ref. 6, with permission.)

the trial as well as in those who were successfully extubated; at the end of the trial, resistance increased in the failure group, whereas it remained unchanged from the start of the trial in the failure group (Fig. 6). The increase in resistance in the failure group could have resulted from several mechanisms: (1) an increase in flow, but this is unlikely since flow increased by the same extent over the course of the trial in the success group; (2) a decrease in lung volume, but this is unlikely since the failure group also developed an increase in intrinsic positive end-expiratory pressure (PEEPi); (3) accumulation of secretions, but the airway of all the patients were suctioned before the trial; and/or (4) development of bronchoconstriction, since patients with COPD are known to exhibit heightened airway reactivity (40).

At the start of the spontaneous breathing trial, dynamic lung elastance was higher in the failure group than in the success group; at the end of the trial, elastance was more than twofold higher in the failure group than in the success group (Fig. 6). The mechanism of the increase in dynamic elastance in the failure group is unknown and it may reflect dynamic hyperinflation (6).

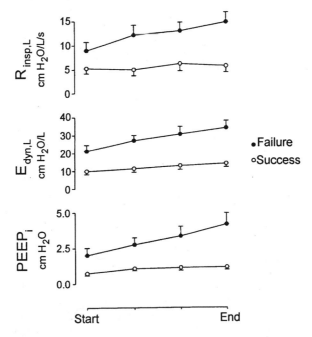

Figure 6 Inspiratory resistance of the lung ($R_{insp,L}$), dynamic lung elastance ($E_{dyn,L}$), and intrinsic positive end-expiratory pressure ($PEEP_i$) during a trial of spontaneous breathing in weaning success and weaning failure patients. Data displayed were obtained during the second and last minute of the trial, and at one-third and two-thirds of the trial duration. Between the onset and the end of the trial, increases in $R_{insp,L}$ ($p < 0.009$), $E_{dyn,L}$ ($p < 0.0001$), and $PEEP_i$ ($p < 0.0001$) occurred in the failure group, and increases in $E_{dyn,L}$ ($p < 0.0006$) and $PEEP_i$ ($p < 0.02$) occurred in the success group. Over the course of the trial, the failure group had higher values of $R_{insp,L}$ ($p < 0.003$), $E_{dyn,L}$ ($p < 0.0006$), and $PEEP_i$ ($p < 0.0009$) than the success group. (From Ref. 6, with permission.)

PEEPi was higher in the failure group than in the success group at the onset of spontaneous breathing trial. At the end of the trial, PEEPi increased in the failure group and it increased slightly in the success group (Fig. 6). The progressive increase in PEEPi in the failure group may be due to dynamic hyperinflation, and this possibility is supported by the fact that 85% of the variance in PEEPi was accounted for by inspiratory resistance, respiratory frequency, and tidal volume (V_T) (6).

Respiratory muscle energy expenditure, quantitated in terms of pressure–time produce (PTP), was not different between the failure and success groups at the onset of the trial (6). Throughout the course of the trial, PTP was higher in the failure group than in the success group. Partitioning of upper bound PTP into its resistive, $PEEP_i$ and non-$PEEP_i$ elastic components revealed that, by the end of the trial, all three components increased in the failure group whereas only the resistive and non-$PEEP_i$ elastic components increased in the success group.

To determine if the derangements in pulmonary mechanics in the weaning failure patients were evident even before undertaking a trial of spontaneous breathing, passive mechanics were measured in weaning failure and weaning success patients right before they were taken off the ventilator before the weaning trial (41). Respiratory system resistance was no different between the two group of patients. When resistance was partitioned into the ohmic component, reflecting airway resistance, and the component arising from stress inhomogeneities in the system secondary to pendelluft and viscoelastic properties, no differences were observed between the two groups. Likewise, dynamic elastance of the respiratory system ($E_{dyn,rs}$) was found to be similar between the groups before the trial. Dynamic elastance ($E_{dyn,L}$) was significantly higher in the failure group than in the success group (Fig. 7), but the individual values showed a considerable overlap among the patients in the two groups so limiting its usefulness in signaling a patient's ability to sustain spontaneous ventilation. That the respiratory mechanics were similar in the two groups before the start of the weaning trial suggests that an unknown mechanism associated with the act of spontaneous breathing caused the worsening of respiratory mechanics in patients with COPD who cannot be weaned from mechanical ventilation.

The imbalance between respiratory neuromuscular capacity and respiratory load as a mechanism of long-term ventilator dependency was recently investigated by Purro et al. (42). Patients who were chronically dependent on mechanical ventilation had decreases in V_T and respiratory muscle strength, high respiratory drive, and abnormal lung mechanics. As a result, the authors concluded that respiratory distress and CO_2 retention were due to an imbalance between workload and inspiratory muscle strength.

II. Predicting Weaning Outcome

It is desirable to have objective measurements, viz., predictive indices, that decrease dependence on the wisdom and skill of an individual physician (43). By identifying the earliest time that a patient is able to resume and sustain spontaneous ventilation,

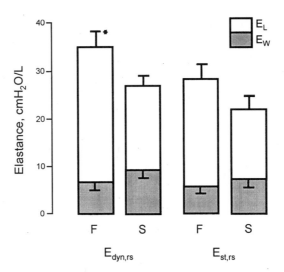

Figure 7 Dynamic ($E_{dyn,rs}$, overall column height) and static ($E_{st,rs}$, overall column height) elastances of the respiratory system in the weaning failure (F) and weaning success (S) groups during passive ventilation; the clear portions of the columns represent lung elastance while the shaded portions represent chest wall elastance. $E_{dyn,L}$ was higher in the failure group than in the success group ($p < 0.01$), and $E_{dyn,rs}$ tended to be higher in the failure group ($p = 0.07$); $E_{dyn,w}$ was not different between the two groups. $E_{st,L}$ tended to be higher in the failure group than in the success group ($p = 0.07$), while $E_{st,rs}$ and $E_{st,w}$ were not significantly different between the two groups. Upward directed bars represent $\pm$ SE of lung elastance (E_L), while downward directed bars represent $\pm$ SE of chest wall elastance (E_W). (From Ref. 41, with permission.)

such indices help to avoid unnecessary prolongation of the period of ventilator support. In addition, by identifying patients who are likely to fail a trial of spontaneous breathing, such indices can prevent a premature weaning attempt and the development of severe cardiorespiratory and/or psychological decompensation. Finally, these indices assess many different physiological functions and thus they may provide insight into the reasons for ventilator dependency in an individual patient and suggest alterations in management (43). Stroetz and Hubmayr (44) showed that clinicians were commonly inaccurate in predicting weaning outcome— positive predictive value of 0.67, negative predictive value of 0.50—emphasizing the need for predictive indices. More recently, Ely et al. (45) reported that the systematic use of weaning predictors resulted in better patient outcome than reliance on clinical judgment of the attending physician.

A. Arterial Oxygenation

Discontinuation of ventilator support is generally not contemplated in a patient with persistent hypoxemia [e.g., PaO_2 of <55 mmHg with an inspired oxygen concentration (F_IO_2) of ≥ 0.40]. Of the indices of gas exchange that can be calculated from conventional arterial blood gases, the arterial/alveolar O_2 tension ratio (PaO_2/P_AO_2) is preferred, as it is more stable with changing levels of F_IO_2 than the alveolar–arterial PO_2 gradient. However, when a PaO_2/P_AO_2 ratio of 0.35 was prospectively evaluated, it had a positive predictive value of only 0.59 and a negative predictive value of only 0.53 (46).

B. Maximal Inspiratory Pressure

Maximal inspiratory pressure ($P_I max$), a global assessment of the strength of all the respiratory muscles, is one of the classic indices used to predict weaning outcome (47). Values more negative than $-30\,cmH_2O$ are thought to predict weaning success, while values less negative than $-20\,cmH_2O$ predicted weaning failure (48). However, these criteria are frequently falsely positive and negative (49, 50).

Since published reports vary in design (retrospective, prospective), method of determining $P_I max$ (20-s occlusion, best of three attempts), weaning techniques (trials of spontaneous breathing, intermittent mandatory ventilation, pressure support), and definitions of weaning success and weaning failure, it is not surprising that the accuracy of $P_I max$ determination varies noticeably between reports. In general, the sensitivity of $P_I max$ is about 0.80, meaning that about 80% of patients who succeed in a weaning trial have a $P_I max$ value that predicts success (i.e., $<-30\,cmH_2O$). However, the specificity was generally 0.25, meaning that only a minority (25%) of patients who fail a weaning trial have a $P_I max$ value that predicts weaning failure (i.e., $>-30\,cmH_2O$). $P_I max$ measurements are more helpful in understanding the reason why a particular patient has failed a weaning trial, rather than in deciding when to attempt a weaning trial (33).

The poor predictive power of $P_I max$ may be due to the difficulty in making the measurement in uncooperative patients. In an attempt to obtain more reproducible recordings, a two-step modification was introduced consisting of a one-way valve to ensure that inspiration begins at a low lung volume and maintaining the period of occlusion for 20 s (51, 52). However, when the predictive power of $P_I max$ measurements using this technique was evaluated prospectively (46), a value of $-30\,cmH_2O$ remained a poor predictor of weaning outcome: positive predictive value of 0.58 and negative predictive value of 0.55. Thus, standardizing the method of measurement did not improve its usefulness as a predictor of weaning outcome.

C. Minute Ventilation

A minute ventilation of less than $10\,L/min$ has been suggested as another index to predict weaning (48). However, in most studies, minute ventilation has been shown to be little better than guesswork in predicting outcome (46, 49, 53).

D. Airway Occlusion Pressure

The airway pressure measured at 0.1 s after commencing an inspiratory effort against an occluded airway ($P_{0.1}$) has been evaluated as a predictor of weaning outcome by a number of investigators (12–14, 16, 54–57). Patients failing a weaning trial were found to have higher values of $P_{0.1}$ than successfully weaned patients. At first glance, it might seem surprising that a supranormal respiratory drive predisposes toward ventilatory failure. In reality, however, the increased $P_{0.1}$ values reflect respiratory distress and signify the response of the respiratory centers to respiratory compromise.

Most of these studies were based on a relatively small patient population, and the threshold value of $P_{0.1}$ was selected in a post hoc manner—a step known to overestimate the accuracy of a predictive index (58). To date, Sassoon and Mahutte (59) conducted the only prospective study examining the accuracy of $P_{0.1}$ as a weaning predictor. A $P_{0.1}$ of $\leq 5.5 \, cmH_2O$ had a sensitivity of 0.95 for predicting weaning success, but specificity was only 0.40. The investigators combined $P_{0.1}$ with an index of rapid shallow breathing, the frequency-to-tidal volume ratio (f/V_T), and found that product ($P_{0.1} \times f/V_T$) increased the specificity to 0.64, but the sensitivity remained the same as for $P_{0.1}$ alone. However, when the data were examined using receiver-operating curve analysis, the area under the curve for $P_{0.1} \times f/V_T$ product was not statistically different than that for f/V_T alone.

The only study that could not document an elevated respiratory center drive in weaning failure patients was the study by Pourriat et al. (60). This group of investigators obtained measurements of the $P_{0.1}$ and ventilatory responses to hypercapnia in 13 patients with COPD who were being weaned from mechanical ventilation. The responses were lower in six patients who failed the weaning trial, but the differences between the failure and success groups did not reach significance. They also administered doxapram, a respiratory analeptic agent, as a means of evaluating respiratory center reserve. Doxapram had no significant effect on the $P_{0.1}$ or ventilatory responses to hypercapnia in either patient group. Interestingly, doxapram produced an increase in end-expiratory lung volume (as detected by inductive plethysmography), which was significantly greater in patients who failed the weaning trial than in the success group.

E. Rapid Shallow Breathing

Patients who failed a weaning trial developed an immediate increase in respiratory frequency (f) upon discontinuation of ventilator support (9). Measurements of f and V_T can be obtained using a simple hand-held spirometer attached to the endotracheal tube while the patient breathes room air spontaneously for 1 min (46). In 100 patients in a medical intensive care unit, measurements of f and V_T were combined into an index of rapid shallow breathing—the f/V_T ratio. In the original study by Yang and Tobin (46), an f/V_T value of 105 breaths/min/L best differentiated patients who were successfully weaned from those in whom weaning failed in an initial "training data set" obtained in 36 patients. The predictive power of this value was then assessed in 64 patients who constituted the "prospective-validation data set." The positive and negative predictive values were 0.78 and 0.95, respectively. Analyzing the data with receiver-operating characteristic (ROC) curves, the area under the curve for the f/V_T was the highest of 10 weaning predictors evaluated in that study (Fig. 8). It is of note that the areas under the curves for conventional weaning

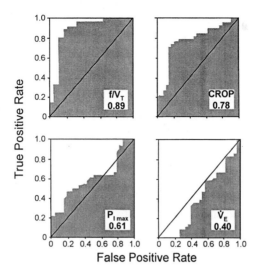

Figure 8 Receiving-operative-characteristic (ROC) curves for frequency/tidal volume (f/V_T) ratio, CROP index (an index that integrates measurements of dynamic compliance, respiratory rate, arterial blood oxygenation, and maximal inspiratory pressure $(P_I max)$, $P_I max$ and minute ventilation (V_E) in 36 patients who were successfully weaned and 28 patients who failed a weaning trial. A ROC curve is generated by plotting the proportion of true positive results against the proportion of false positive results for each value of a test. The curve for an arbitrary test that is expected a priori to have a discriminatory value appears as a diagonal line, whereas a useful test has an ROC curve that rises rapidly and reaches a plateau. The area under the curve (shaded) is expressed (in box) as a proportion of the total area. (From Ref. 62, with permission.)

indices, such as minute ventilation (0.40) and $P_I max$ (0.61) were not significantly greater than that of an arbitrary test that is expected a priori to have no discriminatory value.

The data of Yang and Tobin (46) were reanalyzed in terms of likelihood ratio (61). The likelihood ratio for $f/V_T < 80$ breaths/min/L is 7.53 times more likely to occur in a patient who is subsequently successfully weaned than in a patient who will fail a weaning trial; a likelihood ratio of 5 to 10 is considered to produce moderate and useful shifts in pretest to post-test probability. On the other hand, an f/V_T ratio greater than 100 breaths/min/L is only 0.04 as likely to occur in a patient who will be successfully weaned as in a patient who subsequently fails a weaning trial; a likelihood ratio of < 0.10 is considered to produce large and often convincing changes in the probability of a given diagnosis (in this case weaning failure) (62).

Since the original description of the f/V_T ratio (46), several investigators have examined its accuracy as a predictor of weaning outcome (59, 63–69). Many of the studies, however, did not follow closely the methodology of the original report. For example, Lee et al. (63) reported that eight of nine patients who failed a weaning trial had a f/V_T ratio of 105 breaths/min/L; they concluded that the f/V_T ratio was not helpful. However, the f/V_T measurements were performed during pressure support (level not stated), which is known to decrease f and increase V_T; it is hardly surprising that the f/V_T threshold value developed during unassisted breathing will not apply during pressure support. In contrast to the study of Lee et al. (63), Epstein (64) followed the original methodology and measured f/V_T with a bedside spirometer during spontaneous breathing. Of 84 patients with $f/V_T < 100$ breaths/ min/L who were extubated, 14 patients required reintubation within 72 h, yielding a positive predictive value of 0.83—equivalent to that originally reported, 0.78.

In a subsequent study of 218 patients in a medical intensive care unit who were extubated, Epstein and Ciubotaru (65) found that the negative predictive value for f/V_T was only 0.28, in contrast to the value of 0.95 reported by Yang and Tobin (46). In a study in 183 postoperative patients being weaned from mechanical ventilation, Jacob et al. (66) found that f/V_T had a relatively low negative predictive value, 0.50, while its positive predictive value was 0.94. These latter two studies (65, 66) demonstrate the importance of a factor often ignored when comparing negative predictive values in different studies of any index used in monitoring and decision making (i.e., the influence of pretest probability on the relevant outcome, in this instance, weaning failure) (62).

According to Bayes' theorem, the negative predictive value (also referred to as post-test probability of failure) of f/V_T is highly dependent on the pretest probability of failure (PPF) (i.e., the prevalence of failure in that study) (59):

Post-test probability of failure for $f/V_T > 100 =$

$$\frac{PPF \times TNR}{(PPF \times TNR) + (PPS \times FNR)}$$

where TNR is true negative rate, PPS is pretest probability of success, and FNR is false negative rate.

Epstein and Ciubotaru (65) examined the accuracy of f/V_T in predicting the patient's ability to tolerate extubation, and thus, they selected patients who had already tolerated a weaning trial. The pretest probability of failure was very low in their study, 0.16, compared to the value of 0.44 obtained in the study by Yang and Tobin (46); likewise, the pretest probability of weaning failure was only 0.08 in the study by Jacob et al. (66). The influence of the pretest probability of failure on the negative predictive value of f/V_T is shown in Figure 9. For certain true and false negative rates (46), the negative predictive value of f/V_T is fairly high when the pretest probability of failure is in question (i.e., ~ 0.50), as in the study of Yang and Tobin (46), and it drops sharply when the pretest probability of failure is less than 0.20, as in the studies of Epstein and Ciubotaru (65) and Jacob et al. (66).

In a randomized trial, Ely et al. (45) examined whether a two-stage approach to weaning—systematic measurement of predictors, including f/V_T, followed by a single daily trial of spontaneous breathing—would expedite the pace of weaning. Over a 9-month period, ventilator-supported patients were screened each morning for five factors: arterial blood oxygenation of a $PaO_2/F_IO_2 > 200$; PEEP $\leq$

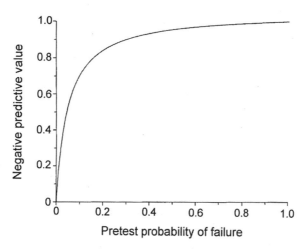

Figure 9 Negative predictive value (i.e., post-test probability of weaning failure) for a respiratory frequency/tidal volume $\geq$ 105 breaths/min/L. Calculations are based on a true negative rate of 0.64 and false negative rate of 0.03, and are performed using Bayes' formula (see text). The negative predictive value remains above 0.87 until a pretest probability of failure of 0.25 is reached, after which it falls precipitously. (From Ref. 62, with permission.)

$5\,cmH_2O$; $f/V_T \leq 105$ breaths/min/L; intact cough on suctioning; and absence of infusions of sedative or vasopressor agents. Patients who met all five criteria underwent a 2-h trial of spontaneous breathing the same morning. If the patient did not develop clinical signs of distress (2, 3), the trial was considered successful, and the patient's physician was notified of this result. The control group was screened daily but did not undergo the spontaneous breathing trial. Although the patients assigned to the two-stage approach had more severe disease, they were weaned twice as fast as those assigned to the control group. The rate of complications, reintubation, and ICU costs was also lower with the two-stage approach than with the conventional approach (45). An improved outcome, however, was not observed when the two-stage approach was applied in neurosurgical patients (69).

III. Methods of Discontinuing Mechanical Ventilation

Several methods for discontinuing ventilator support exist (70). The oldest approach is the use of intermittent trials of spontaneous breathing using a T-tube circuit. Intermittent mandatory ventilation (IMV) and, later, pressure-support ventilation (PSV) were introduced, wherein weaning is accomplished by a gradual reduction in the level of ventilator assistance and a progressive increase in the amount of respiratory work performed by the patient. In an international prevalence study in 412 medical–surgical intensive care units and 1600 patients aimed at defining the characteristics of conventional mechanical ventilation, the overall methods for weaning patients from mechanical ventilation varied considerably among countries (1) (Table 2). The most common method of weaning was PSV; the combination of PSV and IMV was the second most frequently used method in the United States despite its being the only technique of weaning whose efficacy has not been adequately examined.

A. Intermittent Mandatory Ventilation

With IMV, the patient receives periodic positive pressure breaths from the ventilator at a preset volume and rate, and spontaneous breathing between the mandatory breaths is also allowed. When this mode was first introduced, it was thought to represent a major advance in that it combined volume assistance with spontaneous breathing, and thus it was hoped that it would provide respiratory muscle rest and also protect against muscle deconditioning. However, patients have difficulty in adapting to the intermittent nature of ventilator assistance, and studies have demonstrated that inspiratory muscle effort is equivalent for the spontaneous and assisted breaths (71, 72). At a moderate level of machine assistance (i.e., where the ventilator accounted for 20 to 50% of the total ventilation), electromyographic activity of the diaphragm and the sternomastoid muscles was equivalent for assisted and spontaneous breaths (72). These findings suggest that the respiratory center output is preprogrammed and that it does not adjust to breath-to-breath changes in load as occur during IMV. Accordingly, IMV may contribute to the development of respiratory muscle fatigue or prevent recovery from it, which could adversely delay the weaning process. In a group of healthy subjects in whom diaphragmatic fatigue was induced, diaphragmatic contractility remained significantly depressed for at least 24 h (73). In difficult-to-wean patients, recovery from fatigue may be even slower. Thus, a mode of ventilation that provides inadequate respiratory muscle rest, such as IMV, is likely to delay rather than facilitate weaning. Indeed, a number of randomized controlled trials have shown that IMV was the least effective technique for weaning patients from mechanical ventilation (2, 3).

B. Pressure Support Ventilation

Pressure support ventilation (PSV) augments every spontaneous effort with a fixed amount of positive pressure (70, 74, 75). With this mode, the patient has control over the respiratory frequency (f), inspiratory time, and V_T (76, 77). Although there is no flow setting with PSV, the initial peak flow rate determines the speed of pressurization and the initial pressure ramp profile (78–80). Pressure support is very effective in decreasing patient effort (Fig. 10), although the degree of inspiratory muscle unloading is variable among patients, with a coefficient of variation of up to 96% among patients (75).

There is no consensus as to the appropriate level of PSV for an individual patient. Breathing pattern is commonly employed in tailoring the settings on a mechanical ventilator to a patient's needs. In particular, f and V_T are routinely used to select an optimal level of pressure support ventilation (75, 81, 82). In patients with

Table 2 Methods of Weaning According to Country[a]

	USA/Canada	Spain	Argentina	Brazil	Chile	Portugal	Uruguay	Total
	(n = 274)	(n = 108)	(n = 39)	(n = 39)	(n = 9)	(n = 32)	(n = 19)	(n = 520)
Weaning								
PS	45	23	28	28	33	31	21	36
SIMV	5	1	13	3	—	6	16	5
SIMV + PS	32	25	3	36	44	6	47	28
Intermittent SB trials	6	39	33	8	22	37	10	17
Daily SB trial	3	6	10	8	—	—	—	4
Others[b]	9	5	13	18	—	19	5	9

[a]Results are shown as percentage of ventilated patients.
[b]Other methods of weaning were: BIPAP or the combination of two or more methods.
PS = pressure support; SIMV = synchronized intermittent mandatory ventilation; SB = spontaneous breathing.
Source: From Ref. 1.

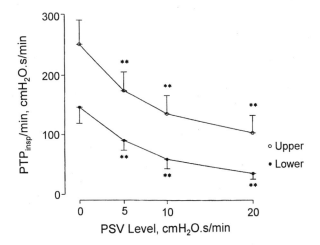

Figure 10 Upper and lower bound inspiratory pressure-time product (PTP_{insp}) per minute during unassisted breathing (i.e., pressure support ventilation (PSV) level of $0 \, cmH_2O$) and at PSV levels of 5, 10, and $20 \, cmH_2O$. Upper and lower bound PTP_{insp} decreased with increasing levels of PSV ($p < 0.001$ in each instance). The distance between the two lines reflects the amount of PTP_{insp}/min resulting from $PEEP_i$. Bars, $\pm$ SE. ** signifies $p < 0.01$ for comparison of a level of PSV with unassisted breathing. (From Ref. 75, with permission.)

COPD during PSV, $f = 30$ breaths/min was more accurate than $V_T > 0.6 \, L$ in predicting a level of inspiratory effort that is unlikely to induce respiratory muscle fatigue (75). More recently, an algorithm for adjustment of PSV using measurements of f, V_T, heart rate, and oxygen saturation and based on a fuzzy logic algorithm was introduced (83). The attractiveness of using fuzzy logic is that it naturally allows for control algorithms to be based on human experience rather than on deterministic mathematical models. The fuzzy logic algorithm did not behave erratically and provided stable recommendations. The authors conclude that fuzzy logic appears promising as a means of automating the weaning process using PSV.

PSV is commonly used to counteract the resistance imposed by the endo-tracheal tubes and ventilator circuits (84). Theoretically, this should help with weaning because a patient who is comfortable at the level of PSV that compensates for imposed work should be able to sustain ventilation following extubation. However, the level of PSV necessary to abolish imposed work varied considerably ($3–14 \, cmH_2O$) from patient to patient (84). Moreover, the notion that a patient who can breathe comfortably at a PSV of 6 to $8 \, cmH_2O$ should be able to tolerate extubation has been challenged by recent reports demonstrating that work generated by breathing through swollen airways following extubation was identical to that generated by breathing through an endotracheal tube (85). As a result, any information about the likelihood that a patient can tolerate extubation will be underestimated if PSV is employed as the weaning technique.

Termination of the inspiratory phase of PSV is based on a fall in the inspiratory flow rate to some predesignated value, such as 25% of the peak. Patients with COPD who commonly have an increased time constant, more time is required for inspiratory flow to fall to the threshold value required for termination of inspiratory assistance by the ventilator. As a result, mechanical inflation will persist in neural expiration. In a study of 12 patients with COPD during PSV, five recruited their expiratory muscles while the machine was still inflating, indicating that the patient was "fighting the ventilator" (Fig. 11) (75, 86). This patient–ventilator asynchrony may have detrimental effects on the weaning process in some patients. Algorithms that achieve better coordination between the end of mechanical inflation and the onset of a patient's expiration should lessen this form of patient–ventilator asynchrony, although such algorithms have yet to be evaluated in patients (87, 88).

When patients fail a weaning trial, mechanical ventilation is reinstituted until the next weaning attempt. During this interval, it is essential that the ventilator provide satisfactory respiratory muscle rest. Clinicians assume that the mere act of connecting a patient to a ventilator will rest his muscles. In fact, patients can have difficulty even in triggering the machine (89) (Fig. 12). When receiving high levels of PSV or assist-control ventilation, about 30% of a patient's inspiratory efforts may fail to trigger the ventilator (74). These ineffective efforts increased with increasing levels of assistance as a result of the accompanying decrease in drive and increase in volume (Fig. 13). Moreover, the breaths preceding nontriggering efforts had shorter

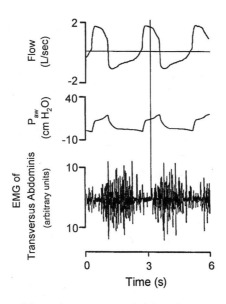

Figure 11 Recordings of flow, airway pressure (Paw), and transverses abdominis EMG in a critically ill patient with COPD receiving PS of 20 cmH$_2$O. The onset of expiratory muscle activity (vertical line) occurred when mechanical inflation was only partly completed. (From Ref. 86, with permission.)

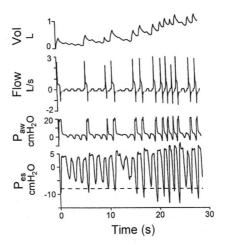

Figure 12 Recordings of tidal volume, flow, airway pressure (Paw), and esophageal pressure (Pes) in a patient with chronic obstructive pulmonary disease receiving pressure support ventilation. Approximately half of the patient's inspiratory efforts do not succeed in triggering the ventilator. Triggering occurred only when the patient generated a Pes more negative than $-8\,cmH_2O$ (indicated by the dashed horizontal line), which was equal in magnitude to the opposing elastic recoil pressure. (From Ref. 89, with permission.)

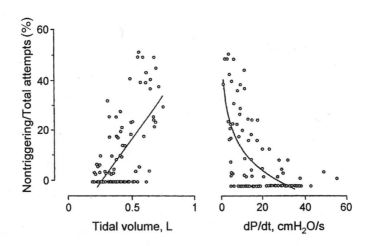

Figure 13 Relationship between the number of nontriggering attempts as a percentage of total inspiratory attempts versus tidal volume (V_T) and respiratory drive (dP/dt) in 11 ventilator-dependent patients. The number of unsuccessful attempts was significantly correlated with tidal volume ($r = 0.66$; $p < 0.0001$) and dP/dt ($r = -0.63$; $p < 0.0001$). (Based on data from Ref. 74.)

respiratory cycle times and expiratory time and higher static PEEPi than breaths preceding triggered efforts. These findings suggest that ineffective triggering did not result from a decrease in the magnitude of effort, but rather from inspiratory efforts that were premature and insufficient to overcome the elevated elastic recoil pressure associated with dynamic hyperinflation. An elevated PEEPi may result from an increase in elastic recoil pressure or expiratory muscle activity. The relative contribution of these two factors to ineffective triggering was examined in healthy subjects receiving PSV and in whom airflow limitation and hence PEEPi was induced with a Starling resistor (86). The magnitude of expiratory effort did not differ before triggering and nontriggering attempts; in contrast, elastic recoil was higher before nontriggering attempts than triggering attempts. These data indicate that nontriggering was caused by the elastic recoil fraction of PEEPi rather than that resulting from expiratory effort.

C. Spontaneous Breathing Trials

With this approach, physicians typically begin with brief trials of spontaneous breathing through a T-tube system (approximately 5 min) and then the patient is reconnected to the ventilator. The duration of the trials is gradually increased according to the patient's performance. The optimal duration of rest between the trials has never been defined, but commonly is as little as 1 to 3 h. Likewise, the optimal duration of such trials of spontaneous breathing has not been determined. Some physicians limit the trial to 1 h or less, while others extend a trial to as long as 24 h. The decision to extubate is based on clinical assessment during the course of the trial, usually supplemented by measurement of arterial blood gases. A problem with this approach is that performance of several T-tube trials in a day can be quite labor intensive for the ICU staff. Alternatively, spontaneous breathing trials can be performed once a day, lasting for up to 2 h. If this trial is successful, the patient is extubated. If the patient fails the trial, then mechanical ventilation is reinstituted for 24 h to allow the respiratory muscles to rest before another trial is performed (73). Esteban et al. (3) showed that performing a trial of spontaneous breathing once a day was as effective as multiple trials. Indeed, 76% (416 of 546) of patients were extubated after tolerating a spontaneous breathing trial for 2 h without clinical distress. In a recent study (90), spontaneous trials lasting for a half hour were as effective as those trials lasting 2 h. However, this study was not limited to difficult-to-wean patients.

D. Efficacy of Weaning Techniques

Two rigorously controlled multicenter studies compared the efficacy of IMV, PSV, and trials of spontaneous breathing (2, 3). Both studies reported that IMV delayed the weaning process. Brochard et al. (2) found that weaning time was significantly shorter with PSV than the combination of IMV and trials of spontaneous breathing. In contrast, using a similar experimental design, Esteban et al. (3) found that a once-daily trial of spontaneous breathing led to extubation about three times more quickly than did IMV, and about twice as quickly as PSV. There was no difference in the rate of successful weaning between a once-daily trial of spontaneous breathing and intermittent trials of spontaneous breathing (attempted at least twice a day), nor between IMV and PSV. The findings in these two studies are complementary; both demonstrate that the pace of weaning depends on the manner in which the technique is applied. When IMV and trials of spontaneous breathing are employed in a constrained way, weaning is delayed compared with PSV. When a spontaneous breathing trial is employed once a day, weaning is expedited.

In a recent randomized trial in long-term weaning units, Vitacca et al. (91) compared the efficiency of two weaning techniques, twice-daily T-piece trials or PSV with twice-daily decrements in inspiratory pressure, in 54 patients with COPD requiring mechanical ventilation for more than 15 days. Weaning success rates were virtually identical between the two groups (73 vs. 77%), and mortality rates and length of stay in the weaning unit and hospital did not differ significantly. Although not statistically significant, weaning time appeared to be shorter for T-piece trials than for PSV. Unfortunately, the study was not sufficiently powered to detect a difference between the two groups; therefore, the likelihood that T-piece trials are more efficient than PSV in weaning patients requiring prolonged mechanical ventilation cannot be excluded (92).

An implied goal of the various weaning techniques is to recondition respiratory muscles that may have been weakened during the period of mechanical ventilation. Theoretically, a once-daily trial of spontaneous breathing alternating with a prolonged period of rest may be the most effective method of eliciting adaptive changes. This approach meets the three principal requirements of a condition program: overload, specificity, and reversibility (23). During the trial, patients breathe against an elevated intrinsic load, thus satisfying the overload requirement. Specificity is also satisfied in that the trial is an endurance stimulus and the desired objective is enhanced endurance. Finally, the use of a daily trial prevents regression of the adaptive stages. It must be emphasized that this reasoning is based on indirect evidence and the effect of different weaning techniques on respiratory muscle reconditioning has not been investigated.

IV. Extubation

In contrast to the discontinuation of mechanical ventilation, indices that reliably predict the development of complications following extubation have not been developed. The risk of an unsuccessful extubation increases in patients with upper airway obstruction and in those patients who are unable to clear their secretions (93). Although absence of a gag reflex is commonly considered a contraindication to extubation, $\sim 20\%$ of healthy subjects may not have a gag reflex, and aspiration pneumonia may still occur in those who do (94). An indirect measurement of upper airway patency is the documentation of the absence of an audible air leak after deflation of the endotracheal tube balloon—so-called cuff leak test (95). Using the difference between inspiratory tidal volume and the averaged expiratory tidal volume after balloon deflation as a measure of the cuff leak volume, Miller and

Cole (96) found that a cuff leak less than 110 mL was a good predictor of postextubation stridor in a general medicine ICU population. However, the cuff leak test was found to be inaccurate when used in postoperative cardiothoracic surgery patients (97). Particular caution is required when planning extubation in a patient with copious airway secretions. In a recent study, Khamiees et al. (98) reported that patients with moderate or abundant secretions were more than eight times as likely to have unsuccessful extubation as those with little or no secretions. Patients with weak cough were four times as likely to have unsuccessful extubation as those with stronger cough. Moreover, the inability of the patient to propel secretion onto a white card held 1 to 2 cm from the endotracheal tube predicted unsuccessful extubation.

Extubation failure, or the need for reintubation, occurs in about 10 to 20% of patients (2, 3, 67, 90, 99). Mortality among patients who require reintubation is higher than those who can tolerate extubation (90, 99). In a recent study, Esteban et al. (90) reported that mortality was 5% in patients who succeeded in a trial of spontaneous breathing and did not require reintubation. In contrast, patients who succeeded in the trial and were extubated but then required reintubation had a mortality rate of 33%. The reason for the higher mortality in patients who require reintubation is not known; it does not appear to be related to the development of new problems unrelated to the disease that initially precipitated the need for mechanical ventilation, nor to complications related to the reinsertion of the tube (90, 100). Instead, the need for reintubation may be a marker of a more severe underlying disease.

In the Esteban study (90), respiratory frequency measured during the trial of spontaneous breathing was high in the patients who failed the spontaneous breathing trial, but the values were similar in the patients who were successfully extubated and in those requiring reintubation (90) (Fig. 14). These data may lead to the conclusion that breathing pattern does not predict the need for reintubation. The study, however, was not designed to determine if breathing pattern can predict the need for reintubation. Patients who failed the weaning trial had a much higher frequency and, if extubated, it is likely that many of them would require reintubation.

Studies of self-extubation can also provide useful information concerning the complications of inappropriate extubation. The incidence of self-extubation can vary from 4 to 11% (101–103). In a prospective study, Tindol et al. (102) reported that 6 of 13 (46%) episodes of self-extubation required reintubation within 24 h; no deaths were associated with these unplanned extubations. In a recent case-control study of 75 patients who self-extubated, 42 (56%) required reintubation. Self-extubation did not influence mortality, but patients who required reintubation had prolonged mechanical ventilation, longer ICU stay, and increased need for chronic care compared with a matched control group (104). In contrast, Coplin et al. (105) recently reported that brain-injured patients whose extubation was delayed developed pneumonia twice as often and had longer ICU and hospital stays than patients who were extubated within 48 h of meeting weaning criteria.

Laryngeal incompetence and aspiration are significant potential problems following extubation. In a study addressing the incidence of aspiration in 64 patients

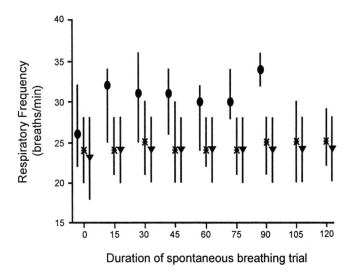

Figure 14 Respiratory frequency in successfully extubated patients (triangles), reintubated patients (stars), and patients who failed the trial of spontaneous breathing (circles) according to the time elapsed from the onset of the trial. In the group that failed the trial, the incremental areas under the curves for respiratory frequency were greater for both trial times. (From Ref. 90, with permission.)

who had been intubated for 8 to 28 h during and after elective cardiac bypass surgery, aspiration was detected in 33% of those challenged immediately following extubation, and in 20 and 5% of those who were challenged at 4 and 8 h after extubation, respectively (106). Laryngeal edema is an uncommon but potentially serious complication following extubation. In a study of 700 critically ill, intubated patients, the overall incidence of laryngeal edema following extubation was 4.2%, and it occurred more commonly in patients who had been intubated for >36 h than in those who had been intubated for a shorter period; administration of dexamethasone 1 h before extubation did not prove useful in preventing laryngeal edema, regardless of intubation duration (107). More recently, studies have indicated that breathing a helium–oxygen mixture may be beneficial in decreasing airway resistance and the effort to breathe in certain patients who are at risk for postextubation obstruction (108, 109).

V. Summary

Discontinuation of mechanical ventilation in patients with COPD is easy in the majority of patients, but a substantial proportion develop difficulties. These patients account for a disproportionate amount of health-care costs, and they pose enormous clinical, economical, and ethical problems. The major pathophysiological mechanism responsible for the failure to wean from mechanical ventilation is the inability of the respiratory muscles to cope with the abnormal pulmonary mechanics. To decide whether a patient can tolerate the discontinuation of mechanical ventilation, it is necessary to perform simple objective physiological measurements; bedside clinical examination is not sufficient to guide this decision. An index of rapid shallow breathing, the frequency-to-tidal-volume ratio, appears to be a much more accurate predictor than traditional indices such as maximum inspiratory pressure or minute ventilation. A number of different weaning techniques are available, and of these a once-daily trial of spontaneous breathing appears to be more expeditious.

References

1. Esteban A, Anzueto A, Alia I, Gordo F, Apezteguia C, Palizas F, Cide D, Goldwaser R, Soto L, Bugedo G, Rodrigo C, Pimentel J, Raimondi G, Tobin MJ. How is mechanical ventilation employed in the intensive care unit? An international utilization review. Am J Respir Crit Care Med 2000; 161:1450–1458.
2. Brochard L, Rauss A, Benito S, Conti G, Mancebo J, Rekik N, Gasparetto A, Lemaire F. Comparison of three methods of gradual withdrawing from ventilatory support during weaning from mechanical ventilation. Am J Respir Crit Care Med 1994; 150:896–903.
3. Esteban A, Frutos F, Tobin MJ, Alia I, Solsona JF, Valverdu I, Fernandez R, de la Cal MA, Benito S, Tomas R, Carriedo D, Macias S, Blanco J. A comparison of four methods of weaning patients from mechanical ventilation. N Engl J Med 1995; 332:345–350.
4. Esteban A, Alia I, Ibanez J, Benito S, Tobin MJ. Modes of mechanical ventilation and weaning. A national survey of Spanish hospitals. The Spanish Lung Failure Collaborative Group. Chest 1994; 106:1188–1193.
5. Criner G, Isaac L. Psychological problems in the ventilator-dependent patient. In: Tobin MJ. Principles and Practice of Mechanical Ventilation. New York: McGraw-Hill, Inc., 1994:1163–1175.
6. Jubran A, Tobin MJ. Pathophysiological basis of acute respiratory distress in patients who fail a trial of weaning from mechanical ventilation. Am J Respir Crit Care Med 1997; 155:906–915.
7. Sorli J, Grassino A, Lorange G, Milic-Emili J. Control of breathing in patients with chronic obstructive pulmonary disease. Clin Sci Mol Med 1978; 54:295–304.
8. Jubran A. Rapid shallow breathing: causes and consequences. In: Mancebo J, Net A, Brochard L, eds. Mechanical Ventilation and Weaning. Berlin: Springer-Verlag, 2002: 161–168.
9. Tobin MJ, Guenther SM, Perez W, Mador MJ, Semmens BJ, Allen SJ, Lodato RF, Dantzker DR. The pattern of breathing during successful and unsuccessful trials of weaning from mechanical ventilation. Am Rev Respir Dis 1986; 134:1111–1118.
10. Torres A, Reyes A, Roca J, Wagner PD, Rodriguez-Roisin R. Ventilation-perfusion mismatching in chronic obstructive pulmonary disease during ventilator weaning. Am Rev Respir Dis 1989; 140:1246–1250.
11. Jubran A, Parthasarathy S, Hypercapnic respiratory failure during weaning: neuromuscular capacity versus muscle loads. Respir Care Clin N Am 2000; 6:385–405.
12. Herrera M, Blasco J, Venegas J, Barba R, Dublas A, Marquez E. Mouth occlusion pressure ($P_{0.1}$) in acute respiratory failure. Intens Care Med 1985; 11:134–139.
13. Sassoon CSH, Te TT, Mahutte CK, Light RW. Airway occlusion pressure: an important indicator for successful weaning in patients with chronic obstructive pulmonary disease. Am Rev Respir Dis 1987; 135:107–113.

14. Murciano D, Boczkowski J, Lecocguic Y, Milic-Emili J, Pariente R, Aubier M. Tracheal occlusion pressure: a simple index to monitor respiratory muscle fatigue during acute respiratory failure in patients with chronic obstructive pulmonary disease. Ann Intern Med 1988; 108:800–805.

15. Dunn WF, Nelson SB, Hubmayr RD. The control of breathing during weaning from mechanical ventilation. Chest 1991; 100:754–761.

16. Montgomery AB, Holle RHO, Neagley SR, Pierson DJ, Schoene RB. Prediction of successful ventilator weaning using airway occlusion pressure and hypercapnic challenge. Chest 1987; 91:496–499.

17. Bellemare F, Bigland-Ritchie B. Central components of diaphragmatic fatigue assessed by phrenic nerve stimulation. J Appl Physiol 1987; 62:1307–1316.

18. Prechter GC, Nelson SB, Hubmayr RD. The ventilatory recruitment threshold for carbon dioxide. Am Rev Respir Dis 1990; 141:758–764.

19. DeVita MA, Robinson LR, Rehder J, Hattler B, Cohen C. Incidence and natural history of phrenic neuropathy occurring during open heart surgery [see comments]. Chest 1993; 103:850–856.

20. Estenne M, Yernault JC, DeSmet JM, DeTroyer A. Phrenic and diaphragm function after coronary artery bypass grafting. Thorax 1985; 40:293–299.

21. Markand ON, Moorthy SS, Mahomed Y, King RD, Brown JW. Postoperative phrenic nerve palsy in patients with open-heart surgery. Ann Thorac Surg 1985; 39:68–73.

22. Wilcox P, Baile EM, Hards J, Muller NL, Dunn L, Pardy RL, Pare PD. Phrenic nerve function and its relationship to atelectasis after coronary artery bypass surgery. Chest 1988; 93:693–698.

23. Tobin MJ, Laghi F, Jubran A. Respiratory muscle dysfunction in mechanically ventilated patients. Mol Cell Biochem 1998; 179:87–98.

24. Tobin MJ, Guenther SM, Perez W, Lodato RF, Mador MJ, Allen SJ, Dantzker DR. Konno-Mead analysis of ribcage-abdominal motion during successful and unsuccessful trials of weaning from mechanical ventilation. Am Rev Respir Dis 1987; 135:1320–1328.

25. Aubier M, Viires N, Syllie G, Mozes R, Roussos C. Respiratory muscle fatigue during cardiogenic shock. J Appl Physiol 1981; 51:499–508.

26. Jardim J, Farkas G, Prefaut C, Thomas D, Macklem PT, Roussos C. The failing inspiratory muscles under normoxic and hypoxic conditions. Am Rev Respir Dis 1981; 124:274–279.

27. Hussain SN, Simkus G, Roussos C. Respiratory muscle fatigue: a cause of ventilatory failure in septic shock. J Appl Physiol 1985; 58:2033–2040.

28. Lemaire F, Teboul JL, Cinotti L, Giotto G, Abrouk F, Steg G, Macquin-Mavier I, Zapol WM. Acute left ventricular dysfunction during unsuccessful weaning from mechanical ventilation. Anesthesiology 1988; 69:171–179.

29. Jubran A, Mathru M, Dries D, Tobin MJ. Continuous recordings of mixed venous oxygen saturation during weaning from mechanical ventilation and the ramifications thereof. Am J Respir Crit Care Med 1998; 158:1763–1769.

30. Juan G, Calverley PM, Talamo C, Schnader J, Roussos C. Effect of carbon dioxide on diaphragmatic function in human beings. N Engl J Med 1984; 310:874–879.

31. Hansen-Flaschen J, Cowen J, Raps EC. Neuromuscular blockade in the intensive care unit: more than we bargained for. Am Rev Respir Dis 1993; 147:234–236.

32. Cohen C, Zagelbaum G, Gross D, Roussos C, Macklem PT. Clinical manifestations of inspiratory muscle fatigue. Am J Med 1982; 73:308–316.

33. Tobin MJ, Laghi F. Monitoring of respiratory muscle function. In: Tobin M, ed. Principles and Practice of Intensive Care Monitoring. New York: McGraw-Hill, 1998:497–544.

34. Le Bourdelles G, Viires N, Boczkowski J, Seta N, Pavlovic D, Aubier M. Effects of mechanical ventilation on diaphragmatic contractile properties in rats. Am J Respir Crit Care Med 1994; 149:1539–1544.

35. Anzueto A, Peters JI, Tobin MJ, de los Santos R, Seidenfeld JJ, Moore G, Cox WJ, Coalson JJ. Effects of prolonged controlled mechanical ventilation on diaphragmatic function in healthy adult baboons. Crit Care Med 1997; 25:1187–1190.

36. Bellemare F, Grassino A. Effect of pressure and timing of contraction on human diaphragm fatigue. J Appl Physiol 1982; 53:1190–1195.

37. Vassilakopoulos T, Zakynthinos S, Roussos C. The tension-time index and the frequency/tidal volume ratio are the major pathophysiologic determinants of weaning failure and success. Am J Respir Crit Care Med 1998; 158:378–385.

38. Silberman H, Silberman AW. Parenteral nutrition, biochemistry, and respiratory gas exchange. J Parenter Enteral Nutr 1986; 10:151–154.

39. Teres D, Roizen MF, Bushnell LS. Successful weaning from controlled ventilation despite high deadspace-to-tidal volume ratio. Anesthesiology 1973; 39:656–659.

40. Ramsdell JW, Nachtway FS, Moser KM. Bronchial hyperactivity in chronic obstructive bronchitis. Am Rev Respir Dis 1982; 126:829–832.

41. Jubran A, Tobin MJ. Passive mechanics of lung and chest wall in patients who failed and succeeded in trials of weaning. Am J Respir Crit Care Med 1997; 155:916–921.

42. Purro A, Appendini L, De Gaetano A, Gudjonsdottir M, Donner CF, Rossi A. Physiologic determinants of ventilator dependence in long-term mechanically ventilated patients. Am J Respir Crit Care Med 2000; 161:1115–1123.

43. Tobin MJ, Alex CG. Discontinuation of mechanical ventilation. In: Tobin MJ, ed. Principles and Practice of Mechanical Ventilation. New York: McGraw-Hill, Inc., 1994:1177–1206.

44. Stroetz RW, Hubmayr RD. Tidal volume maintenance during weaning with pressure support. Am J Respir Crit Care Med 1995; 152:1034–1040.

45. Ely EW, Baker AM, Dunagan DP, Burke HL, Smith AC, Kelly PT, Johnson MM, Browder RW, Bowton DL, Haponik EF. Effect on the duration of mechanical ventilation of identifying patients capable of breathing spontaneously. N Engl J Med 1996; 335:1864–1869.

46. Yang K, Tobin MJ. A prospective study of indexes predicting outcome of trials of weaning from mechanical ventilation. N Engl J Med 1991; 324:1445–1450.

47. Jubran A. Advances in respiratory monitoring during mechanical ventilation. Chest 1999; 116:1416–1425.

48. Sahn SA, Lakshminarayan S. Bedside criteria for discontinuation of mechanical ventilation. Chest 1973; 63:1002–1005.

49. Tahvanainen J, Salenpera M, Nikki P. Extubation criteria after weaning from intermittent mandatory ventilation and continuous positive airway pressure. Crit Care Med 1983; 11:702–707.

50. Chatilla W, Jacob B, Guaglionone D, Mantous CA. The unassisted respiratory rate-to-tidal volume ratio accurately predicts weaning outcome. Am J Med 1996; 101:61–67.

51. Marini JJ, Smith TC, Lamb V. Estimation of inspiratory muscle strength in mechanically ventilated patients: the measurement of maximal inspiratory pressure. J Crit Care 1986; 1:32–38.

52. Multz AS, Aldrich TK, Prezant DJ, Karpel JP, Hendler JM. Maximal inspiratory pressure is not a reliable test of inspiratory muscle strength in mechanically ventilated patients. Am Rev Respir Dis 1990; 142:529–532.

53. Alvisi R, Volta CA, Righini ER, Capuzzo M, Ragazzi R, Verri M, Candini G, Gritti G, Milic-Emili J. Predictors of weaning outcome in chronic obstructive pulmonary disease. Eur Respir J 2000; 15:656–662.

54. Fernandez R, Cabrera J, Calaf N, Benito S. $P_{0.1}/P_I$max: an index for assessing respiratory capacity in acute respiratory failure. Intens Care Med 1990; 16:175–179.

55. Gandia F, Blanco J. Evaluation of indexes predicting the outcome of ventilator weaning and value of adding supplemental inspiratory load. Intens Care Med 1992; 18:327–333.

56. Conti G, De Blasi R, Pelaia P, Benito S, Rocco M, Antonelli M, Bufi M, Mattia C, Gasparetto A. Early prediction of successful weaning during pressure support ventilation in chronic obstructive pulmonary disease patients. Crit Care Med 1992; 20:366–371.

57. Capdevila XJ, Perrigault PF, Perey PJ, Roustan JPA, d'Athis F. Occlusion pressure and its ratio to maximum inspiratory pressure are useful predictors for successful extubation following T-piece weaning trial. Chest 1995; 108:482–489.

58. Tobin MJ, Gardner WN. Monitoring of the control of breathing. In: Tobin MJ, ed. Principles and Practice of Intensive Care Monitoring. New York: McGraw-Hill, 1998; 415–464.

59. Sassoon CSH, Mahautte CK. Airway occlusion pressure and breathing pattern as predictors of weaning outcome. Am Rev Respir Dis 1993; 148:860–866.

60. Pourriat JL, Baud M, Lamberto C, Fosse JP, Cupa M. Effects of doxapram on hypercapnia response during weaning from mechanical ventilation in COPD patients. Chest 1992; 101:1639–1643.

61. Jaechke RZ, Meade MO, Guyatt GH, Keenan SP, Cook DJ. How to use diagnostic test articles in the ICU: diagnosing wean ability using f/V_T. Crit Care Med 1997; 25:514–521.

62. Tobin MJ. Noninvasive monitoring of ventilation. In: Tobin MJ, ed. Principles and Practice of Intensive Care Monitoring. New York: McGraw-Hill, 1998; 465–495.

63. Lee KH, Hui KP, Chan TB, Tan WC, Lim TK. Rapid shallow breathing (frequency-tidal volume ratio) did not predict extubation outcome. Chest 1994; 105:540–543.

64. Epstein SK. Etiology of extubation failure and the predictive value of the rapid shallow breathing index. Am J Respir Crit Care Med 1995; 152:545–549.

65. Epstein SK, Ciubotaru RL. Influence of gender and endotracheal tube size on pre-extubation breathing pattern. Am J Respir Crit Care Med 1996; 154:1647–1652.

66. Jacob B, Chatila W, Manthous CA. The unassisted respiratory rate/tidal volume ratio accurately predicts weaning outcome in postoperative patients. Crit Care Med 1997; 25:253–257.

67. Vallverdu I, Calaf N, Subirana M, Net A, Benito S, Mancebo J. Clinical characteristics, respiratory functional parameters, and outcome of a two-hour T-piece trial in patients weaning from mechanical ventilation. Am J Respir Crit Care Med 1998; 158:1855–1862.

68. Maldonado A, Bauer TT, Ferrer M, Hernandez C, Arancibia F, Rodriguez-Roisin R, Torres A. Capnometric recirculation gas tonometry and weaning from mechanical ventilation. Am J Respir Crit Care Med 2000; 161:171–176.

69. Namen AM, Ely EW, Tatter SB, Case LD, Lucia MA, Smith A, Landry S, Wilson JA, Glazier SS, Branch CL, Kelly DL, Bowton DL, Haponik EF. Predictors of successful extubation in neurosurgical patients. Am J Respir Crit Care Med 2001; 163:658–664.

70. Tobin MJ. Advances in mechanical ventilation. N Engl J Med 2001; 344:1986–1996.

71. Marini JJ, Smith TC, Lamb VJ. External work output and force generation during synchronized intermittent mechanical ventilation: effect of machine assistance on breathing effort. Am Rev Respir Dis 1988; 138:1169–1179.

72. Imsand C, Feihl F, Perret MD, Fitting JW. Regulation of inspiratory neuromuscular output during synchronized intermittent mandatory ventilation. Anesthesiology 1994; 80:13–22.

73. Laghi F, D'Alfonso N, Tobin MJ. Pattern of recovery from diaphragmatic fatigue over 24 hours. J Appl Physiol 1995; 79:539–546.

74. Leung P, Jubran A, Tobin MJ. Comparison of assisted ventilator modes on triggering, patient effort, and dyspnea. Am J Respir Crit Care Med 1997; 155:1940–1948.

75. Jubran A, Van de Graaff WB, Tobin MJ. Variability of patient-ventilator interaction with pressure-support ventilation in patients with COPD. Am J Respir Crit Care Med 1995; 152:129–136.

76. Brochard L. Pressure support ventilation. In: Tobin MJ, ed. Principles and Practice of Mechanical Ventilation. New York: McGraw-Hill, 1994; 239–257.

77. MacIntyre NR. Respiratory function during pressure support ventilation. Chest 1986; 89:677–683.

78. Jubran A. Inspiratory flow rate: more may not be better [editorial; comment]. Crit Care Med 1999; 27:670–671.

79. Bonmarchand G, Chevron V, Menard JF, Girault C, Moritz-Berthelot F, Pasquis P, Leroy J. Effects of pressure ramp slope values on the work of breathing during pressure support ventilation in restrictive patients. Crit Care Med 1999; 27:715–722.

80. Bonmarchand G, Chevron V, Chopin C, Jusserand D, Girault C, Moritz F, Leroy J, Pasquis P. Increased initial flow rate reduces inspiratory work of breathing during pressure support ventilation in patients with exacerbation of chronic obstructive pulmonary disease. Intens Care Med 1996; 22:1147–1154.

81. Brochard L, Harf A, Lorino H, Lemaire F. Inspiratory pressure support prevents diaphragmatic fatigue during weaning from mechanical ventilation. Am Rev Respir Dis 1989; 139:513–521.

82. MacIntyre NR, Ho L. Effects of initial flow rate and breath termination criteria on pressure support ventilation. Chest 1991; 99:134–138.

83. Nemoto T, Hatzakis GE, Thorpe CW, Olivenstein R, Dial S, Bates JH. Automatic control of pressure support mechanical ventilation using fuzzy logic. Am J Respir Crit Care Med 1999; 160:550–556.

84. Brochard L, Rua F, Lorino H, Lemaire F, Harf A. Inspiratory pressure support compensates for the additional work of breathing caused by the endotracheal tube. Anesthesiology 1991; 75:739–745.

85. Straus C, Louis B, Isabey D, Lemaire F, Harf A, Brochard L. Contribution of the endotracheal tube and the upper airway to breathing workload. Am J Respir Crit Care Med 1998; 157:23–30.

86. Parthasarathy S, Jubran A, Tobin MJ. Cycling of inspiratory and expiratory muscle groups with the ventilator in airflow limitation. Am J Respir Crit Care Med 1998; 158:1471–1478.

87. Parthasarathy S, Jubran A, Tobin MJ. Assessment of neural inspiratory time in ventilator-supported patients. Am J Respir Crit Care Med 2000; 162:546–552.

88. Yamada Y, Du HL. Analysis of the mechanisms of expiratory asynchrony in pressure support ventilation: a mathematical approach. J Appl Physiol 2000; 88:2143–2150.

89. Tobin MJ, Jubran A. Pathophysiology of failure to wean from mechanical ventilation. Schweiz Med Wochenschr 1994; 124:2139–2145.

90. Esteban A, Alia I, Tobin MJ, Gil A, Gordo F, Vallverdu I, Blanch L, Bonet A, Vazquez A, de Pablo R, Torres A, de la Cal MA, Macias S. Effect of spontaneous breathing trial

duration on outcome of attempts to discontinue mechanical ventilation. Am J Respir Crit Care Med 1999; 159:512–518.

91. Vitacca M, Vianello A, Colombo D, Clini E, Porta R, Bianchi L, Arcaro G, Vitale G. Guffanti E, Lo CA, Ambrosino N. Comparison of two methods for weaning patients with chronic obstructive pulmonary disease requiring mechanical ventilation for more than 15 days. Am J Respir Crit Care Med 2001; 164:225–230.

92. Hill NS. Following protocol: weaning difficult-to-wean patients with chronic obstructive pulmonary disease. Am J Respir Crit Care Med 2001; 164:186–187.

93. Epstein SK. Predicting extubation failure: is it in (on) the cards? Chest 2001; 120:1061–1063.

94. Kulig K, Rumack BH, Rosen P. Gag reflex in assessing level of consciousness [letter]. Lancet 1982; 1:565.

95. Fisher MM, Raper RF. The 'cuff-leak' test for extubation. Anaesthesia 1992; 47:10–12.

96. Miller RL, Cole RP. Association between reduced cuff leak volume and postextubation stridor. Chest 1996; 110:1035–1040.

97. Engoren M. Evaluation of the cuff-leak test in a cardiac surgery population. Chest 1999; 116:1029–1031.

98. Khamiees M, Raju P, DeGirolamo A, Amoateng-Adjepong Y, Manthous CA. Predictors of extubation outcome in patients who have successfully completed a spontaneous breathing trial. Chest 2001; 120:1262–1270.

99. Epstein SK, Ciubotaru RL, Wong JB. Effect of failed extubation on the outcome of mechanical ventilation. Chest 1997; 112:186–192.

100. Epstein SK, Ciubotaru RL. Independent effects of etiology of failure and time to reintubation on outcome for patients failing extubation. Am J Respir Crit Care Med 1998; 158:489–493.

101. Coppolo DP, May JJ. Self-extubations. A 12-month experience. Chest 1990; 98:165–169.

102. Tindol GA, Jr., DiBenedetto RJ, Kosciuk L. Unplanned extubations. Chest 1994; 105:1804–1807.

103. Whelan J, Simpson SQ, Levy H. Unplanned extubation. Predictors of successful termination of mechanical ventilatory support. Chest 1994; 105:1808–1812.

104. Epstein SK, Nevins ML, Chung J. Effect of unplanned extubation on outcome of mechanical ventilation. Am J Respir Crit Care Med 2000; 161:1912–1916.

105. Coplin WM, Pierson DJ, Cooley KD, Newell DW, Rubenfeld GD. Implications of extubation delay in brain-injured patients meeting standard weaning criteria. Am J Respir Crit Care Med 2000; 161:1530–1536.

106. Burgess GE, III, Cooper JR, Jr., Marino RJ, Peuler MJ, Warriner RA, III. Laryngeal competence after tracheal extubation. Anesthesiology 1979; 51:73–77.

107. Darmon JY, Rauss A, Dreyfuss D, Bleichner G, Elkharrat D, Schlemmer B, Tenaillon A, Brun-Buisson C, Huet Y. Evaluation of risk factors for laryngeal edema after tracheal extubation in adults and its prevention by dexamethasone. A placebo-controlled, double-blind, multicenter study. Anesthesiology 1992; 77:245–251.

108. Jaber S, Fodil R, Carlucci A, Boussarsar M, Pigeot J, Lemaire F, Harf A, Lofaso F, Isabey D, Brochard L. Noninvasive ventilation with helium-oxygen in acute exacerbations of chronic obstructive pulmonary disease. Am J Respir Crit Care Med 2000; 161:1191–1200.

109. Jaber S, Carlucci A, Boussarsar M, Fodil R, Pigeot J, Maggiore S, Harf A, Isabey D, Brochard L. Helium-oxygen in the postextubation period decreases inspiratory effort. Am J Respir Crit Care Med 2001; 164:633–637.

28

Rehabilitation and Acute Exacerbations of Chronic Obstructive Pulmonary Disease

NICOLINO AMBROSINO

University Hospital
Cisanello-Pisa, Italy

ROBERTO PORTA

Scientific Institute of Gussago
Gussago, Italy

I. Aims of Pulmonary Rehabilitation

Only long-term oxygen therapy (LTOT) and smoking cessation improve survival in patients with chronic obstructive pulmonary disease (COPD) (1, 2). Although the primary pathological changes are confined to the lungs, the consequent physical deconditioning and emotional responses contribute importantly to morbidity. Increased breathlessness leads to inactivity and consequent peripheral muscle deconditioning, resulting in a vicious cycle that leads to further inactivity, social isolation, fear of dyspnea, and depression. Patients with severe COPD become less mobile and reduce their activities of daily living (ADL). In a survey of patients with severe COPD treated with LTOT, 50% of patients with Medical Research Council (MRC) dyspnea grade 5 did not leave the house and up to 78% were breathless walking around at home and performing ADL (3). Pulmonary rehabilitation programs (PRP) break this downward cycle (4). Furthermore, the utilization of health-care services by COPD patients is related more to respiratory and peripheral muscle force than to airway obstruction (5) and in patients hospitalized due to AECOPD, 1-year survival was reported to be independently related, among other factors, to body mass index (BMI) and prior functional status (6). Peripheral and respiratory muscle function, nutritional status, and ADL are all conditions that can be positively influenced by multidisciplinary rehabilitation.

Once recognized as an art of medical practice (7), pulmonary rehabilitation has been defined as "a multidimensional continuum of services directed toward persons with pulmonary disease and their families, usually by an interdisciplinary team of specialists, with the goal of achieving and maintaining the individual's maximum level of independence and functioning in the community" (8). Pulmonary rehabilitation reduces symptoms, increases functional ability, and improves Health-Related Quality of Life (HRQL) in individuals with chronic respiratory diseases even in the face of irreversible abnormalities of lung architecture. These benefits are possible since often much of the disability (the inability to perform an activity within the normally expected range because of lung disease) and *handicap* (the disadvantage resulting from an impairment or disability within the context of the patient's ability to perform in society or fill expected roles) result not from the functional respiratory disorder (the *impairment*) per se but from secondary morbidity that is often treatable if recognized. For example, although the severity of neither airway obstruction nor hyperinflation in COPD do change appreciably with rehabilitation, it results in reversal of muscle deconditioning and better pacing, enabling these patients to walk further with less breathlessness (9).

Although *any patient* with symptomatic COPD or other chronic respiratory disease should be considered for PRP, the key to success is the individual tailoring of the program. The improvement attributable to individual elements of a program are difficult to assess because of the multidisciplinary nature of pulmonary rehabilitation and the wide range of therapeutic modalities (Table 1).

A clear distinction must be made between pulmonary rehabilitation and chest physiotherapy (CP) which are not synonyms. Chest physiotherapy is a component of pulmonary rehabilitation, often but not always included in PRP, with specific indications. In this chapter we will examine the role of PRP, if any, in reducing incidence of AECOPD and their consequences in terms of consumption of health

Table 1 Components of Pulmonary
Rehabilitation Programs

Optimization of pharmacological therapy
Smoking cessation
Education
Breathing exercises
Chest physiotherapy
Exercise training
Respiratory muscle training
Peripheral muscle training
Occupational therapy
Long-term oxygen therapy
Respiratory muscle rest (mechanical ventilation)
Psychosocial support
Nutrition

---

resources. The role of CP and other PRP components during AECOPD, if any, will be also described.

II. Results of Rehabilitation

The benefits of pulmonary rehabilitation in stable COPD patients include improved exercise tolerance and symptoms and decreased health-care expenditure, in particular, reduced use of expensive medical resources. Published results provide a scientific basis for the overall intervention as well as for its specific components (10–14). After rehabilitation, patients report improved HRQL with a reduction in respiratory symptoms, increase in exercise tolerance, and ability to perform ADL, more independence, and improvement in psychological function with less anxiety and depression and increased feelings of hope, control, and self-esteem (15). Studies that have examined the individual components of rehabilitation have shown that even patients with severe disease can learn to understand their disease better, increase their ADL, and improve their exercise tolerance (10, 16, 17). Pulmonary rehabilitation for patients with COPD does not result in significant changes in lung function (15).

III. Effects of Rehabilitation on AECOPD

Several reports (12–14, 18, 19) confirm that a PRP for COPD patients, including lower and upper limb exercise training, and education can achieve benefits that persist up to 2 years. Troosters et al. (18) in a randomized controlled study of a 6-month outpatient PRP including cycling, walking, and strength training versus usual medical care, evaluated patients at the end and after 18 months of follow-up. Among the patients who completed the 6-month PRP, outpatient training resulted in significant and clinically relevant changes in 6-min walking distance, maximal exercise performance, peripheral and respiratory muscle strength, and HRQL. Most of these effects persisted 18 months after starting the program. No information on the long-term effects on AECOPD was given. Griffiths et al. (13), in a randomized controlled study versus standard medical management, evaluated the effect of outpatient rehabilitation on the use of health care and patients' well being over 1 year. Compared with the control group, the rehabilitation group showed greater improvements in walking ability and in general and disease-specific health status. Although there was no difference between the rehabilitation and control groups in the number of patients admitted to the hospital, the number of days these patients spent in the hospital differed. The rehabilitation group had more primary care consultations at the general practitioner's office than the control group, but fewer primary care home visits (13). In another randomized, controlled study versus standard care, Guell et al. (14) examined the short- and long-term effects of an outpatient PRP for COPD patients. These authors found significant differences between groups in dyspnea, walking test, and in day-to-day dyspnea, fatigue and emotional function measured by the Chronic Respiratory Disease Questionnaire.

The improvements were evident at the third month and continued with somewhat diminished magnitude in the second year of follow-up. Moreover, the rehabilitation group experienced a significant reduction in AECOPD but not in the number of hospitalizations. In another randomized, controlled study (20), COPD patients were evaluated 1 year after completing an 8-week outpatient PRP. Patients were randomly divided into two groups. One group repeated the PRP 1 year later, the other did not. Both groups were evaluated 2 years after the first PRP. Among other results, these authors (20) found that the hospitalizations per year (Fig. 1) and AECOPD (Fig. 2) per patient significantly decreased in both groups in the 2 years following the first PRP, when compared to the 2 years prior. Nevertheless, in comparison to the 12-month follow-up, at 24 months a further reduction in AECOPD per year was observed only in patients performing both PRPs but not in the other group (20). Therefore, it seems that an additional yearly PRP may be useful in further reducing the number of AECOPD not requiring hospitalization. Which component of the program most influenced this result is still unclear. Most COPD patients in both groups had quit smoking in the last 2 years prior to the first PRP, and this may have influenced the AECOPD in the following years. The educational program performed may have resulted in better self-management of the disease (12).

Although we can only speculate on the causes of reduced hospitalizations and AECOPD, a direct effect of exercise conditioning cannot be ruled out. Indeed, it has been demonstrated that in COPD patients the utilization of health-care services is related to ventilatory and peripheral muscle force (5), and that ability to perform ADL is associated with a better survival after an exacerbation requiring ICU ad-mission (6). Furthermore, it has recently been observed that PRP-induced improve-ments in exercise tolerance are associated with increases in exhaled nitric oxide (eNO) (21). This may suggest an association between physical fitness and eNO with resulting beneficial effects of training on the respiratory and cardiovascular systems. Although it has been shown that hospitalizations and AECOPD are important determinants of health status in COPD patients (22, 23), whether the maintenance of good HRQL observed in patients undergoing PRP (13, 14, 20) is related to reduced hospitalizations and AECOPD is still speculative.

In conclusion, there is evidence that PRP may be useful in reducing AECOPD and related hospitalizations. Which component is most responsible for this effect needs further clarification.

IV. Pulmonary Rehabilitation During AECOPD

A. Chest Physiotherapy Techniques

During AECOPD, many factors, such as viral and bacterial airway infections, stimulate increased mucus production, alter its viscoelastic properties, and impair airway mucociliary clearance mechanisms. Mucus hypersecretion and impaired tracheobronchial clearance are frequent in patients with COPD. Although increased airway secretions may correlate weakly with airflow obstruction, chronic mucus hypersecretion does correlate with hospital admissions for AECOPD (24) and may

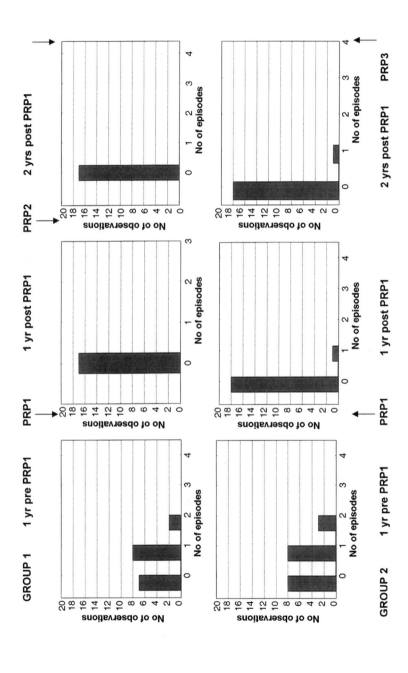

Figure 1 Frequency distribution of hospitalizations during 1 year prior to and the 2 years following the PRP1 in patients completing two PRP (upper panel) and patients performing one PRP (lower panels). Compared with before the PRP, both groups of patients showed a significant reduction in hospitalizations, without any differences between groups. (From Ref. 20, with permission.)

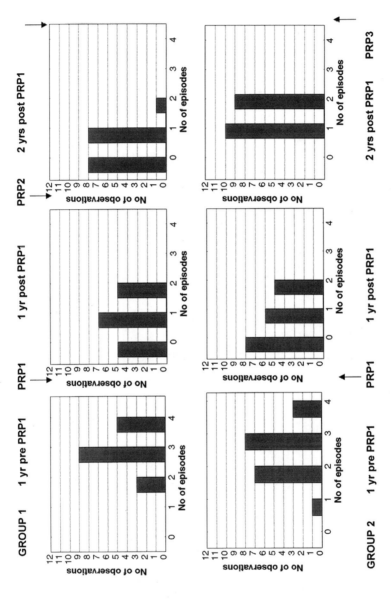

Figure 2 Frequency distribution of AECOPD during 1 year prior to and the 2 years following the PRP1 in patients completing two PRP (upper panel) and patients performing one PRP (lower panels). Compared with before the PRP, both groups of patients showed a significant reduction in AECOPD; nevertheless, in comparison to 12 month, at the 24-month follow-up, a further reduction in year AECOPD was observed only in patients performing both PRPs but not in the other group.

Table 2 Techniques to Mobilize
Airway Secretions

Directed coughing
Manual or mechanical percussion
Postural drainage
Intermittent positive pressure breathing
Positive expiratory pressure (PEP)
Bland aerosol therapy
Systemic hydration
Nasotracheal suctioning
Minitracheotomy

contribute to the risk of death in patients with severe ventilatory impairment (25). Chest physiotherapy is a cornerstone of PRP (7–9) and is commonly aimed at enhancing airway secretion clearance. The efficacy of CP techniques in patients with chronic bronchitis and emphysema has often been inferred from investigations of patients with cystic fibrosis and bronchiectasis. The role of CP during AECOPD is unclear. Several measures have been proposed to mobilize airway secretions (Table 2) and several excellent reviews have focused on them (26–28).

Postural Drainage

"Conventional" postural drainage (PD) is usually defined as the use of gravity-assisted positions, deep breathing exercises with or without chest clapping, chest shaking, or chest vibrations and coughing when secretions reach the upper airways. Gravity-assisted positioning has been shown to be more effective than cough alone (29) and more effective than the use of either coughing or breathing exercises in the sitting position (30). A similar technique is a maneuver of slow expiration with the glottis open in the lateral posture (ELTGOL, from the French) (31). This is an airway clearance treatment that uses lateral posture and lung volumes from functional residual capacity (FRC) to residual volume (RV). The theoretical aim of this technique is to control expiratory flow rate to avoid airway compression and paroxysmal cough (31).

Forced Exhalations

Chest physiotherapy, used when there is mucus stasis or difficulty in expectorating mucus, is focused on increasing mucus transport by using an external force. The most important mucus transport mechanism in COPD patients is expiratory flow. Several studies have shown that forced exhalations are the most effective airway clearance techniques used by physiotherapists (32, 33). Forced exhalations are even effective in patients who rarely expectorate sputum (34).

Using forced exhalations with open glottis, so called "huffing," instead of coughing, lung volume and expiratory force can more easily be varied than with coughing because coughing is more reflex in nature and under less voluntary control. Forced exhalation from mid-lung volume, combined with breathing exercises and coughing, is known as the forced expiratory technique (FET) or active cycle of breathing training (ACBT). A technique known as autogenic drainage (AD) uses very gentle exhalations from low lung volumes (28).

Repetitive Coughing

Based on experimental data (35) it could be argued that repetitive coughing with short intervals is more effective than single coughs; however, the clinical effectiveness of this approach remains to be proven. Some patients use this technique spontaneously.

Manual Compression

A forced expiratory flow can also be induced by the application of a force on the thorax. This is especially relevant in case of severely reduced expiratory muscle force. A full expiratory maneuver can be induced by manual compression on the thorax. In this technique, the compression direction follows the bucket handle and pump handle movement of the ribs, and on the abdomen, pushing the diaphragm into the thorax. In this case, the mechanisms involved in mucus transport are essentially the same as during a voluntary forced expiratory maneuver.

Vibration of the Thorax

Vibration or oscillations of the thorax may also produce small coughs superimposed on tidal breathing. The airflow of these induced coughs appears to be dependent on the frequency of the applied vibration/oscillation (36). The optimal frequency may vary between subjects, but usually is around 15 Hz. Conventional manual chest clapping is usually performed with a frequency of about 5 Hz and has little or no effect (32). Vibration/oscillation with higher frequencies seems to be promising, but further studies are needed to validate these techniques. In patients who cannot sufficiently clear their lungs by means of forced exhalations, vibration or oscillation can be applied under careful clinical monitoring in order to evaluate effectiveness. Nevertheless, revisions of literature on manual chest percussion (37) or mechanical percussors (38) concluded that there is a physiological rationale and a place for the use of percussion, but that the clinical evidence is inconclusive.

Positive Expiratory Pressure Breathing

When there is severe mucus plugging completely obstructing the airways there is no local air flow and thus no mucus transport by expiratory flow. It has been proposed that PEP breathing may help to bring in air behind the mucus plugs. Positive expiratory pressure (PEP) is usually applied by breathing through a face mask or a mouth piece with an inspiratory tube containing a one-way valve, and an expiratory tube containing an expiratory resistance. It results in a positive expiratory mouth pressure throughout exhalation. Usually mouth pressures of 10 to 20 cmH$_2$O are recommended, although pressures of 5 cmH$_2$O can also have a significant effect on lung volumes (39).

Increasing the volume of air in obstructed airways could potentially be achieved by several mechanisms. It is possible that PEP breathing results in a pressure difference between open and obstructed airways, increasing airflow through collateral pathways from open to obstructed parts of the lungs (40). PEP breathing may also lead to a temporary increase in FRC (39) decreasing the airway resistance and thereby possibly opening closed airways (41). In patients with COPD, forced expirations showed better mucociliary clearance after PD, including deep breathing, than after PEP (42). Therefore, PEP breathing should only be used in special individual cases under close evaluation of benefit.

High-Frequency Chest Wall Oscillations and Intrapulmonary Percussive Ventilation

During high-frequency chest wall oscillations (HFCWO), positive pressure air pulses are applied to the chest wall. It is hypothesized that increases in mucus clearance may be due to an increase in mucus/airflow interaction and/or a shearing mechanism leading to a decrease in the viscoelastic properties of mucus (43). Arens et al. (44) compared HFCWO with conventional CP. Both regimens were equally safe and effective and it was suggested that the self-applied HFCWO would provide an adequate alternative to conventional therapy. This was in agreement with a review of literature (45).

Another form of HFCWO applies external high frequency oscillations by means of a cuirass, and it has been proposed as a means to enhance expectoration (46).

A self-administered device to deliver a PEP and oscillatory vibration of the air within the airways has been proposed (Flutter VRP1). This device was found to be as effective as conventional CP in stable COPD patients (47).

B. Chest Physiotherapy During AECOPD

In the "Exacerbation Management" section of the European Respiratory Society Consensus Statement on COPD (48), it is suggested to "encourage sputum clearance by coughing" and "consider home physiotherapy." The recent NHLBI/WHO global initiative for chronic obstructive lung disease (GOLD) workshop summary (49), in the section: "Other measures" of the chapter on the treatment of AECOPD, stated that " ... Further treatment measures that can be used in the hospital include: fluid administration...; nutrition...; *sputum clearance (by stimulating coughing and low volume forced expirations). Manual or mechanical chest percussion and postural drainage may be beneficial in patients producing > 25 mL sputum per day or with lobar atelectasis.*" Nevertheless, no reference is given to support these statements. Indeed, a previous ATS statement on COPD (50) had reported that scant scientific evidence supported the application of CP techniques in hospitalized patients with AECOPD uncomplicated by bronchiectasis. Despite this declared lack of evidence, the clinical guidelines of the same ATS Statement (50) rather surprisingly suggested that PD, chest percussion, and chest vibration may be used—

with careful monitoring—after pretreatment with inhaled bronchodilators in patients with more than 25 mL of expectorated sputum a day.

On the contrary, on the basis of randomized controlled trials of CP and one observational study, a recent position paper (51) concluded that mechanical percussion of the chest as applied by physical and respiratory therapists was ineffective and perhaps even detrimental in the treatment of patients with AECOPD. In a comparative physiological study, Bellone et al. (52) found that PD, flutter, and ELTGOL were safe and effective in removing secretions without causing undesirable effects on oxygen saturation, but flutter and ELTGOL were more effective in prolonging secretion removal in AECOPD than PD. Nevertheless, previous studies by Anthonisen et al. (53) showed that CP applied to patients with AECOPD, by means of expansion exercises, PD, and vibrations, had no effect on temperature curves, sputum volume, or blood gases as compared to patients treated with conventional therapy. None of the randomized trials (54–56) reported any improvement in dynamic lung volumes, either FEV_1 or FVC. Newton and Bevans (54) reported no differences in lung function, blood gases, and hospital stay when compared with conventional treatment alone. Campbell et al. (55) showed that PD, percussion, cough, and vibrations induced a significant fall in FEV_1 not observed with PD and cough alone. Wollmer published similar results (56).

C. Breathing Control Techniques

The technique of coordinating the breathing process was previously widely used in rehabilitation but now receives less emphasis. When the term "breathing retraining" is used, it is usually referred to these techniques, including pursed-lip and diaphragmatic breathing.

Pursed-Lip Breathing

Pursed-lip breathing (PLB) is often used unconsciously by patients with COPD to enhance exercise tolerance during dyspnea and increased ventilatory demand. They inhale through the nose and then exhale slowly through pursed lips (57). Pursed-lip breathing results in slower and deeper breaths with significant increase in oxygenation and in a shift in ventilatory muscle recruitment from the diaphragm to the accessory muscles of ventilation (58, 59). During exercise, the shift to PLB results in decreased dyspnea (60).

Diaphragmatic Breathing

The description of "diaphragmatic" (DB) or "abdominal" breathing is not identical in every publication. Usually the patient is told to move the abdominal wall exclusively during inspiration and to reduce upper rib cage motion (61, 62). Theoretically, DB aims to improve chest wall motion and ventilation distribution, decrease energy cost of breathing, decrease the contribution of rib cage muscles, decrease dyspnea, and improve exercise performance. All studies show that patients are able to voluntarily change the breathing pattern to more abdominal movement and less thoracic excursion (61, 63). However, some studies observed that DB was accompanied by increased asynchronous and paradoxical breathing movements (63, 64).

Few studies addressed the effects of DB on work of breathing (WOB), oxygen cost, and mechanical efficiency of breathing. McKinley et al. (65) found a tendency of an increased WOB during DB by measurement of the pressure-volume curve before and after the exercises in six patients with COPD. Increased oxygen cost of breathing during DB was also reported in a time series experiment. This was associated with increased asynchronous breathing and reduction of mechanical efficiency during DB compared to natural breathing (63).

Slow and Deep Breathing

Several authors observed a significant drop of respiratory rate (RR), and significant rises of tidal volume (VT) and PaO_2 during imposed low-frequency breathing at rest in patients with COPD (66–68). Unfortunately, these improvements were counterbalanced by an increased WOB. Slow breathing caused a 15% increase of oxygen consumption (68). Contrary, Paul et al. (69) reported a significant fall in minute ventilation (V'_E) and dead space ventilation, while alveolar ventilation was unchanged. In addition, Bellemare and Grassino (70) demonstrated that fatigue of the diaphragm developed earlier during slow and deep breathing (increased inspiratory to total respiratory time ratio (T_I/T_{TOT}) with the same V'_E. This resulted in a significant increase of the relative force of contraction of the diaphragm, as assessed by the transdiaphragmatic to maximal transdiaphragmatic pressure ratio (Pdi/Pdi_{max}), forcing it into the critical zone of muscle fatigue.

D. Breathing Exercises During AECOPD

Slow and deep breathing improves breathing efficiency and SaO_2 at rest. A similar tendency was observed during exercise, but this needs further research. However, this type of breathing is associated with breathing pattern prone to induce respiratory muscle fatigue (70). This may be even worse during AECOPD. Vitacca et al. (71) investigated the impact of deep DB on blood gases, breathing pattern, pulmonary mechanics and dyspnea in severe hypercapnic COPD patients *recovering from an* AECOPD. Transcutaneous partial pressure of CO_2 ($PtcCO_2$) and O_2 ($PtcO_2$) and SaO_2, breathing pattern, V'_E and mechanics were continuously monitored during natural breathing and DB, respectively. Subjective rating of dyspnea was performed by means of a visual analog scale. In comparison to natural breathing, deep DB was associated to to a significant increase in V_T and a significant reduction in RR resulting in increased V'_E, significant increase in $PtcO_2$, and significant decrease in $PtcCO_2$. During DB, dyspnea significantly worsened and inspiratory muscle effort did increase as demonstrated by an increase in esophageal pressure swings, pressure-time product, and WOB (71).

Therefore, there is no evidence of any role of "breathing exercises" during AECOPD.

V. Pulmonary Rehabilitation in the Intensive Care Unit

Endotracheal intubation and mechanical ventilation are often needed in patients with AECOPD who may undergo difficulties in the weaning process and related need of tracheostomy. AECOPD represent 13% of indications to mechanical ventilation (72). These patients are considered to be the most difficult to wean from the ventilator (73). The major mechanism underlying the need of prolonged mechanical ventilation in AECOPD patients has been reported as the association between abnormal lung mechanics, in particular intrinsic positive end expiratory pressure (PEEPi), lung resistances, and reduced pressure-generating capacity of the inspiratory muscles because of pulmonary hyperinflation (74). Respiratory and skeletal muscle weakness and prolonged inactivity lead to severe curtailment of even the simplest ADL (75, 76).

In most hospitals in developed countries, physiotherapy is seen as an integral part of the management of patients in the intensive care unit (ICU). The precise role that physiotherapists play in the ICU varies considerably from one unit to the next depending on factors such as country, local tradition, staffing levels, training, and expertise (77). Furthermore, the recent development of the respiratory intensive care units (RICU) enables medical staff to work in a specialized environment in which medical and paramedical teams are familiar with and well trained in the care and management of severely ill respiratory patients, including treatment of AECOPD with invasive and noninvasive mechanical ventilation (78).

A recent European survey (79) reported that 38% of the hospitals had more than 30 physiotherapists working in the hospital, but 25% had no exclusive ICU physiotherapist. Thirty-four percent had a physiotherapist available during the night, and 85% during the weekend. In almost 100% of ICUs, the physiotherapist performed respiratory therapy, mobilization, and positioning. The physiotherapist played an active role in the adjustment of mechanical ventilation in 12% of the respondent units, in weaning from mechanical ventilation in 22% of units, in extubation in 25%, and in the implementation of noninvasive mechanical ventilation in 46%. Differences in the role of the physiotherapist were apparent between countries (79) and a growing need of a more specialized "respiratory therapist" like in the United States was claimed (80).

The definition of the components of PRP in ICU/RICU is difficult, as it is sometimes hard to distinguish between the role of nurses and physiotherapists. For example, a major goal of the rehabilitation process is early mobilization. The initial step before ambulation is sitting up in bed, followed by sitting in a chair. In addition to avoiding the adverse effects of prolonged inactivity, there are several advantages to early get out of bed to chair activity (e.g., fewer difficulties with fluid shifts from the periphery to the lungs and improvements in ventilation, mobilization of secretions, and well being) (81, 82). Clearly, this activity is on the borderline between nurses' and physiotherapists' duties.

Make et al. (83) found that only 5 of 16 ventilator-dependent patients did not benefit from a PRP started after their admission to an ICU, while Foster et al. (84), in an uncontrolled study, found improvement in exercise tolerance, pulmonary function, and arterial blood gases in a subset of COPD patients with severe hyper-capnia, some of whom had been transferred directly from an ICU. These data suggest that, for patients recovering from AECOPD, early institution of a PRP may be useful in improving the outcome. Nevertheless, despite the fact that several reviews (77), book chapters (79, 81, 82, 85), and position papers (9) have pointed out the importance of physiotherapy in an ICU for severely ill patients suffering from different pathologies, only three investigations have commented on the possible utility of a rehabilitation program in the outcome of their patients (86–88). Unfortunately, no data were reported for these studies (86–88). In the only prospective, controlled, and randomized study, Nava et al. (89) compared the effects of early stepwise comprehensive rehabilitation plus standard therapy with the effects of standard therapy and progressive ambulation only, on exercise tolerance and dyspnea in patients recovering from AECOPD, which in most cases had required mechanical ventilation. Patients in the study received pulmonary rehabilitation that consisted of tasks of increasing difficulty such as passive mobilization, early ambulation, respiratory and lower skeletal muscle training and, if patients were able, complete lower extremity training on a treadmill. Control patients received standard medical therapy plus a basic deambulation program. Sixty-one out of 80 patients were mechanically ventilated at admission and most of them were bedridden. Twelve of the 60 patients of the study group and 4 out of the 20 control patients died during their RICU stay and 9 patients required invasive mechanical ventilation at home after discharge. The mean total length of stay was 38 days in study group and 33 days in controls. Most patients of both groups regained the ability to walk. At discharge, 6-min walking distance test and inspiratory muscle strength improved only in study group, whereas dyspnea improved in both groups but the improvement was more marked in the study group (89). What are the clinical correlates in term of HRQL and outcome of these physiological results are still to be defined.

VI. Pulmonary Rehabilitation During Mechanical Ventilation

A. Difficult-to-Wean Patients

Hospitalization for AECOPD is associated to in-hospital mortality of 6 to 26% (90). Furthermore, it is estimated that 1 to 5% of mechanically ventilated patients repeatedly fail attempts at weaning from mechanical ventilation and face a substantial risk of becoming chronic ventilator-dependent patients who cannot sustain spontaneous breathing for more than a few hours (91). This proportion increases to as much as 31 to 56% in some RICU where difficult-to-wean patients are located (91, 92). Studies of predictors, protocols, and specific weaning strategies have been largely confined to patients intubated for short periods of time (73, 93–95). A recent review of literature (96) on weaning techniques used in intubated patients with different etiologies (a minority with COPD) admitted to general ICUs was unable to identify a superior weaning technique between the two most widely used modalities (namely, spontaneous breathing trials and reducing levels of inspiratory pressure support) (73, 93). Furthermore, recent trials have demonstrated that simply introducing a protocol or guideline to the weaning process leads to a decrease in weaning time independent of the mode used (94, 97). These results have been confirmed also in difficult-to-wean patients (98).

Remarkably, little literature exists regarding the ICU/RICU physiotherapist, especially in the treatment of AECOPD. Ciesla (99) noted that the efficacy of CP has been well demonstrated, resulting in a reduced incidence of pulmonary infection and improved pulmonary function. Others have emphasized the important role of the physiotherapist in ICU (100). Some studies have been conducted on the role of the physiotherapist in weaning patients from mechanical ventilation. Cohen et al. (101) suggested that "a team approach" to weaning, with the team composed of a physician, a respiratory therapist, and the bedside nurse, reduced the duration and cost of mechanical ventilation and improved the weaning success rate. Ely et al. (94) suggested that daily screening of respiratory function by the respiratory therapist, with trials of spontaneous breathing in appropriate patients, could reduce the duration of mechanical ventilation and the cost of intensive care and was associated with fewer complications than standard care. More recently, Horst et al. (102) reported that protocol-based weaning by respiratory therapists leads to more rapid extubation and reduced hospital stays than physician-directed weaning. Hall et al. (103) suggested that the presence of a physiotherapist in the weaning team is associated with reduced patient anxiety. Other groups have also documented the benefits of including a physiotherapist in the weaning team (97, 104).

B. Noninvasive Mechanical Ventilation

Physiotherapists may also be involved in the monitoring and adjustment of noninvasive positive pressure ventilation (nPPV), a process requiring considerable time (105) and constant availability, particularly at initiation (106). Indeed, the effectiveness of nPPV with all modalities depends on strict staff supervision by nurses and physiotherapists. Chevrolet et al. (107) found that acute nPPV was very time consuming in COPD patients for the nursing staff. However, in that study, no comparison with the time consumed to deliver standard therapy was reported, and Bott et al. (108) found that the amount for nursing care required to treat AECOPD with nPPV was not different in comparison to patients undergoing standard medical therapy. In a study by Kramer et al. (109), respiratory therapists tended to spend more time at the bedside of patients receiving nPPV than in control patients but the difference was not statistically significant. Furthermore, there was a significant drop in the amount of time therapists spent at the bedside of nPPV patients during the second 8-h period. In addition, therapists and nurses rated the difficulty of caring for patients receiving nPPV as no greater than for control patients. Nava et al. (105) have shown that in an experienced unit, nPPV is neither more time consuming nor more costly than endotracheal intubation. Nevertheless, in a prospective, randomized controlled study of nPPV versus standard medical therapy in community-acquired pneumonia (CAP) (110), COPD patients randomized to nPPV had a lower intensity of nursing care workload. In acute respiratory failure due to severe CAP, also Jolliet et al. (111) showed that no increase in nursing time consumption may be attributable to the use of nPPV. In a study by Plant et al. (112) performed in the ward, in comparison to standard medical therapy, nPPV led to a modest 26-min increase in nursing workload in the first 8 h of the admission. No difference was identified after 8 h. Hilbert et al. (113) evaluated prospectively the assistance time spent by nurses in relation to ventilatory time when nPPV was used in a sequential mode, in COPD patients with either AECOPD or postextubation hypercapnic respiratory insufficiency in a medical ICU. The nurse time was not different between the two populations in the study; the nurse time consumption per session was 25% of the ventilatory time during the first 24 h after enrollment and dropped significantly to 15% of the ventilatory time after the first 24 h. There are, however, no data on the effect of nPPV on the care of other patients, nor whether the outcome would have been better if the nurses had spent more time with the patients receiving nPPV. In other words, good results with nPPV might be obtained at the expense of the care of other patients. Nurses are responsible for clinical care during nPPV. They monitor clinical parameters such as patient comfort, use of accessory muscles, cyanosis, vigilance, and vital signs.

C. Nursing Workload in a RICU

Assistance to patients by nursing staff may differ according to the time spent in assistance to mechanical ventilation (either invasive or noninvasive) (114), the severity of symptoms, the neurological condition, the kind of pharmacological therapies, the patient's self-care or the ability to perform a specific function. Nursing workload devoted to noninvasive mechanical ventilation, a modality specifically performed in the RICUs (i.e., mask preparation, education, assistance procedures during pauses of noninvasive ventilation) has been shown not to be more time consuming than standard medical therapy (109). It needs no more than 20% of the total shift time and does not differ from nursing workload within the first 48 h of invasive mechanical ventilation (105).

Evaluating patients' level of dependency by scoring nursing activities through a new scale (Dependence Nursing Scale: DNS) (115) we studied 111 patients consecutively admitted to our RICU over 1 year needing nPPV for acute on chronic respiratory failure (33 patients), prolonged weaning from mechanical ventilation (33 patients), or cardiopulmonary monitoring (45 patients). DNS describes patients' dependency needing increasing levels of nursing commitment according to 13 tasks. Each task scores from 0 (no dependency) to a variable maximum increasing by 1. DNS total score ranges 0 to 45 (115). At admission (T0), demographic, anthropometric data, severity of disease (APACHE II score), nursing workload by the nine equivalents of nursing manpower use score (NEMS) (116), and inspiratory muscle strength (maximal respiratory pressure, MIP) were recorded. DNS was computed both at T0 and at discharge (T1). Mortality rate and days spent in the RICU were also recorded. DNS and NEMS at T0 were significantly higher in diffult-to-wean patients than in other groups. All the tasks except tracheotomy care significantly improved resulting in significant decrease of DNS for all patients respectively. At T0,

DNS was significantly better correlated to NEMS ($r = 0.70$) than to Apache II, MIP, and days of hospitalization. Therefore, in patients admitted to a RICU for different causes, the nurse workload in patients with AECOPD requiring RICU admission is greater in difficult-to-wean patients than due to nPPV, giving a further justification to the use of this technique in AECOPD. DNS is able to describe the dependency level of different kinds of patients and better reflects the global nursing workload than illness clinical severity and inspiratory muscle function (115).

Prevention of Pulmonary Complications

There are theoretical reasons why physiotherapy may be routinely required in intubated patients receiving mechanical ventilation with the intention of preventing complications. Many factors may adversely affect airway clearance, including the presence of an artificial airway, inadequate humidification, medications, underlying pulmonary disease, and mucosal damage as a result of suction (117). Furthermore, an effective CP, successful in enhancing airway clearance, might enable patients to undergo nPPV. Nevertheless, the expectation that physiotherapy provided a few times a day (in addition to routine nursing care) will decrease the incidence of pulmonary complications may be realistic, provided that many of the major causative factors responsible for the high incidence of complications are addressed (e.g., prolonged immobility, microaspiration, reduced host defenses, poor nutritional status, colonization of ventilator circuits, and antibiotic treatment leading to lower airway colonization and superinfection) (118–120).

Given the overall limited evidence regarding the effectiveness of physiotherapy in the ICU (Table 3) and the results of one study in which twice-daily physiotherapy did not reduce the incidence of nosocomial pneumonia (121), it could be argued that the routine use of respiratory physiotherapy for all patients is not evidence-based and therefore unsupportable (77). In this framework, the role of physiotherapy in prevention of nosocomial pneumonia in patients with AECOPD undergoing mechanical ventilation is even more obscure.

VII. Summary

Pulmonary rehabilitation reduces symptoms, increases functional ability, and improves health-related quality of life (HRQL) in individuals with chronic respiratory diseases, even in the face of irreversible abnormalities of lung architecture. Although *any patient* with symptomatic COPD or other chronic respiratory disease should be considered for pulmonary rehabilitation programs (PRP), the key to success is the individual tailoring of the program. The improvement attributable to individual elements of a program are difficult to assess, due to the multidisciplinary nature of pulmonary rehabilitation and the wide range of therapeutic modalities. There is evidence that PRP may be useful in reducing AECOPD and related hospitalizations. What component is most responsible for this effect needs further clarification.

Table 3 Evidence-Based Recommendations for Physiotherapy in the ICU with Permission

Strong evidence that:

Physiotherapy is the treatment of choice in patients with acute lobar atelectasis

Prone positioning improves oxygenation for patients with severe ARF or ARDS

Positioning in side lying improves oxygenation for patients with unilateral lung disease

Hemodynamic status should be monitored during physiotherapy to detect side effects of treatment

Sedation before physiotherapy will decrease or prevent adverse hemodynamic or metabolic responses

Preoxygenation, sedation, reassurance are necessary before suction to avoid suction-induced hypoxemia

Continuous rotational therapy decreases the incidence of pulmonary complications

Moderate evidence that:

Multimodality physiotherapy has a short-lived beneficial effect on respiratory function

Manual hyperinflation may have a short beneficial effect on respiratory function, but hemodynamic status, airway pressure, or VT should be monitored to detect any deleterious side effects of treatment

Increased intracranial pressure and cerebral perfusion pressure should be monitored on appropriate patients during physiotherapy to detect any deleterious side effects of treatment

Limited or no evidence that:

Routine physiotherapy in addition to nursing care prevents pulmonary complications commonly found in ICU patients

Physiotherapy is effective in the treatment of pulmonary conditions commonly found in ICU patients (with the exception for acute lobar atelectasis)

Physiotherapy facilitated weaning, decreases length of stay in the ICU or hospital, and reduces mortality and morbidity

Positioning (with exception for acute lobar atelectasis), percussion, vibrations, suction, or mobilization are effective components of physiotherapy for ICU patients

Limb exercises prevent loss of joint range or soft-tissue length, or improve muscle strength and function, for ICU patients.

Source: Ref. 77.

Although recommended by some guidelines, on the basis of randomized controlled trials, chest physiotherapy, as applied by physical and respiratory therapists, was ineffective and perhaps even detrimental in the treatment of patients with AECOPD. Breathing exercises, applied during AECOPD or during the recovery phase, may be useless if not detrimental.

In most hospitals in developed countries physiotherapy is seen as an integral part of the management of patients in ICU. The precise role that physiotherapists play in the ICU varies considerably from one unit to the next depending on factors such as country, local tradition, staffing levels, training and expertise. Furthermore, the recent development of the respiratory intensive care units enables medical staff to work in a specialized environment in which medical and paramedical teams are familiar with and well trained in the care and management of severely ill respiratory patients, including treatment with invasive and noninvasive mechanical ventilation.

References

1. Report of British Research Medical Council Working Party. Long-term domiciliary oxygen therapy in chronic hypoxic cor pulmonale complication in chronic bronchitis and emphysema. Lancet 1981; 1:681–686.
2. Anthonisen NR, Connett JE, Kiley JP, Altose MD, Bailey WC, Buist AS, Conway WA Jr, Enright PL, Kanner RE, O'Hara P. Effects of smoking intervention and the use of an inhaled anticholinergic bronchodilator on the rate of decline of FEV_1. JAMA 1994; 272(19):1497–1505.
3. Restrick LJ, Paul EA, Braid GM, Cullinan P, Moore-Gillon J, Wedzicha JA. Assessment and follow up of patients prescribed long term oxygen therapy. Thorax 1993; 48:708–713.
4. Donner CF, Decramer M. Pulmonary Rehabilitation. Eur Respir Monogr 2000; 5:1–199.
5. Decramer M, Gosselink R, Trooster T, Verschueren M, Evers G. Muscle weakness is related to utilization of health care resources in COPD patients. Eur Respir J 1997; 10:417–423.
6. Connors AF Jr, Dawson NV, Thomas C, Harrel FE Jr, Desbiens N, Fulkerson WJ, Kussin P, Bellamy P, Goldman L, Knaus WA. Outcomes following acute exacerbation of severe chronic obstructive lung disease. Am J Respir Crit Care Med 1996; 154:959–967.
7. Donner CF, Howard P. Pulmonary rehabilitation in chronic obstructive pulmonary disease (COPD) with recommendations for its use. Eur Respir J 1992; 5:266–275.
8. NIH Workshop Summary: Pulmonary Rehabilitation Research. Am J Respir Crit Care Med; 1994; 149:825–833.
9. American Thoracic Society. Pulmonary Rehabilitation 1999. Am J Respir Crit Care Med 1999; 159:166–168.
10. Berry MJ, Rejeski WJ, Adair NE, Zaccaro D. Exercise rehabilitation and chronic obstructive pulmonary disease stage. Am J Respir Crit Care Med 1999; 160:1248–1253.
11. Goldstein RS, Gort EH, Stubbing D, Avendano MA, Guyatt GH. Randomised controlled trial of respiratory rehabilitation. Lancet 1994; 344:1394–1397.
12. Ries AI, Kaplan RM, Limberg TM, Prewitt LM. Effects of pulmonary rehabilitation on physiologic and psychosocial outcomes in patients with chronic obstructive pulmonary disease. Ann Intern Med 1995; 122:823–832.
13. Griffiths TL, Burr ML, Campbell IA, Lewis-Jenkins V, Mullins J, Shiels K, Turner-Lawor PJ, Payne N, Newcombe RG, Ionescu AA, Thomas J, Tunbridge J. Results at 1 year of outpatient multidisciplinary pulmonary rehabilitation: a randomized controlled trial. Lancet 2000; 355:362–368.
14. Guell R, Casan P, Belda J, Sangenis M, Morante F, Guyat GH, Sanchis J. Long-term effects of outpatient rehabilitation of COPD. A randomized trial. Chest 2000; 117:976–983.
15. ACCP/AACVPR. Pulmonary rehabilitation. Joint ACCP/AACVPR evidence-based guidelines. Chest 1997; 112:1363–1396.
16. Stiebellehner L, Quittan M, End A, Wieselthaler C, Kleptko W, Haber P, Burghuber OC. Aerobic endurance training programme improves exercise performance in lung transplant recipients. Chest 1998; 113:906–912.

17. Criner GJ, Cordova FC, Furukawa S, Kuzma AM, Travaline JM, Leyenson V, O'Brien GM. Prospective randomized trial comparing bilateral lung volume reduction surgery to pulmonary rehabilitation in severe chronic obstructive pulmonary disease. Am J Respir Crit Care Med 1999; 160:2018–2027.

18. Troosters T, Gosselink R, Decramer M. Short- and long-term effects of outpatient rehabilitation in patients with chronic obstructive pulmonary disease: a randomized trial. Am J Med 2000; 109:207–212.

19. Foglio K, Bianchi L, Bruletti G, Battista L, Pagani M, Ambrosino N. Long-term effectiveness of pulmonary rehabilitation in patients with chronic airway obstruction (CAO). Eur Respir J 1999; 11:125–132.

20. Foglio K, Bianchi L, Ambrosino N. Is it really useful to repeat outpatient pulmonary rehabilitation programs in patients with chronic airway obstruction? A 2-year controlled study. Chest 2001; 119:1696–1704.

21. Clini E, Bianchi L, Foglio K, Porta R, Vitacca M, Ambrosino N. Effect of pulmonary rehabilitation on exhaled nitric oxide in patients with chronic obstructive pulmonary disease. Thorax 2001; 56:519–523.

22. Osman IM, Godden DJ, Friend JA, Legge JS, Douglas JG. Quality of life and hospital re-admission in patients with chronic obstructive pulmonary disease. Thorax 1997; 52:67–71.

23. Seemungal TA, Donaldson GC, Paul EA, Bestall JC, Jeffries DJ, Wedzicha JA. Effect of exacerbation on quality of life in patients with chronic obstructive pulmonary disease. Am J Respir Crit Care Med 1998; 157:1418–1422.

24. Vestbo J, Knudsen KM, Rasmussen FV. The value of mucus hypersecretion as a predictor of mortality and hospitalization: an 11-year register-based follow-up study of a random population sample of 876 men. Respir Med 1988; 83:207–211.

25. Speizer FE, Fay ME, Dockery DW, Ferris BG Jr. Chronic obstructive pulmonary disease mortality in six U.S. cities. Am Rev Respir Dis 1989; 140(suppl):S49–S55.

26. Pryor JA. Physiotherapy for airway clearance in adults. Eur Respir J 1999; 14:1418–1424.

27. Langenderfer B. Alternatives to percussion and postural drainage. J Cardiopulmonary Rehabil 1998; 18:283–289.

28. Van der Schans CP, Rubin BK, Olseni L, Postma DS. Airway clearance techniques. In: Ambrosino N, Donner CF, Rampulla C, eds. Topics in pulmonary rehabilitation. Pi-Me press, Pavia, 1999, pp. 229–242.

29. Loring MI, Denning CR. Evaluation of postural drainage by measurement of sputum volume and consistency. Am J Phys Med 1971; 50:215–219.

30. Steven MH, Pryor JA, Webber BA, Hodson ME. Physiotherapy versus cough alone in the treatment of cystic fibrosis. NZ J Physiother 1992; 20:31–37.

31. Postiaux G, Lens E, Alsteewns C. L'expiration lente totale glotte ouverte en decubitus lateral (ELTGOL): nouvelle manouvre pour la toilette bronchique objectivee par videobronchographie. Ann Kinesither 1987; 14:341–350.

32. van der Schans CP, Piers DA, Postma DS. Effect of manual percussion on tracheobronchial clearance in patients with chronic airflow obstruction and excessive tracheobronchial secretion. Thorax 1986; 41:448–452.

33. van Hengstum M, Festen J, Beurskens C, Hankel M, Beekman F, Corstens F. Conventional physiotherapy and forced exhalation manoeuvres have similar effects on tracheobronchial clearance. Eur J Respir Dis 1988; 1:758–761.

34. Hasani A, Pavia D, Agnew JE, Clarke SW. Regional mucus transport following unproductive cough and forced exhalation technique in patients with airways obstruction. Chest 1994; 105:1420–1425.

35. Zahm JM, King M, Duvivier C, Pierrot D, Girod S, Puchelle E. Role of simulated repetitive coughing in mucus clearance. Eur Respir J 1991; 4:311–315.
36. Hansen LG, Warwick WJ. High-frequency chest compression system to aid in clearance of mucus from the lung. Biomed Instrum Technol 1990; 24:289–294.
37. Gallon A. The use of percussion. Physiotherapy 1992; 78:85–89.
38. Thomas J, DeHueck A, Kleiner M, Newton J, Crowe J, Mahier S. To vibrate or not to vibrate: usefulness of the mechanical vibrator for clearing bronchial secretions. Physiother Can 1995; 47:120–125.
39. van der Schans CP, van der Mark ThW, de Vries G, Piers DA, Beekhuis H, Dankert-Roelse JE, Postma DS, Koëter GH. Effect of positive expiratory pressure breathing in patients with cystic fibrosis. Thorax 1991; 46:252–256.
40. Menkes HA, Traystman RJ. State of the art. Collateral ventilation. Am Rev Respir Dis 1977; 116:287–309.
41. Peters RM. Pulmonary physiologic studies of the perioperative period. Chest 1976; 76:576–584.
42. Olséni L, Midgren B, Hörnblad Y, Wollmer P. Chest physiotherapy in chronic obstructive pulmonary disease: forced expiratory technique combined with either postural drainage or positive expiratory pressure breathing. Respir Med 1994; 88:435–440.
43. Tomkiewicz RP, Biviji A, King M. Effects of oscillating air flow on the rheological properties and clearability of mucous gel simulants. Biorheology 1994; 31:511–520.
44. Arens R, Gozal D, Omlin KJ, Vega J, Boyd KP, Keens TG, Woo MS. Comparison of high-frequency chest compression and conventional chest physiotherapy in hospitalized patients with cystic fibrosis. Am J Respir Crit Care Med 1994; 150:1154–1157.
45. Hansen LG, Warwick WJ, Hansen KL. Mucus transport mechanisms in relation to the effect of high frequency chest compression (HFCC) on mucus clearance. Pediatr Pulmonol 1994; 17:113–118.
46. Scherer TA, Barandun J, Martinez E, Wanner A, Rubin EM. Effect of high-frequency oral airway and chest wall oscillation and conventional chest physical therapy on expectoration in patients with stable cystic fibrosis. Chest 1998; 113:1019–1027.
47. Ambrosino N, Callegari G, Galloni C, Brega S, Pinna G. Clinical evaluation of oscillating positive expiratory pressure for enhancing expectoration in diseases other than cystic fibrosis. Monaldi Arch Chest Dis 1995; 50:269–275.
48. Siafakas NM, Vermeire P, Pride NB, Paoletti P, Gibson J, Howard P, Yernault JC, Decramer M, Higenbottam T, Postma DS, Rees J. ERS Consensus Statement. Optimal assessment and management of chronic obstructive pulmonary disease (COPD). Eur Respir J 1995; 8:1398–1420.
49. Pauwels RA, Buist AS, Calverley PMA, Jenkins CR, Hurd SS on behalf of the GOLD Scientific Committee Global strategy for the diagnosis, management and prevention of chronic obstructive lung disease. NHLBI/WHO global initiative for chronic obstructive lung disease (GOLD) workshop summary. Am J Respir Crit Care Med 2001; 163:1256–1276.
50. American Thoracic Society. Standards for the diagnosis and care of patients with chronic obstructive pulmonary disease. Am J Respir Crit Care Med 1995; 152:S77–S120.
51. Bach PB, Brown C, Gelfand SE, McCrory DC. Management of acute exacerbations of chronic obstructive pulmonary disease: a summary and appraisal of published evidence. Ann Intern Med 2001; 134:600–620.
52. Bellone A, Lascioli R, Raschi S, Guzzi L, Adone R. Chest physical therapy in patients with acute exacerbation of chronic bronchitis: effectiveness of three methods. Arch Phys Med Rehabil 2000; 81:558–560.

53. Anthonisen F, Riis F, Sogaard-Andersen T. The value of lung physiotherapy in the treatment of acute exacerbations in chronic bronchitis. Acta Med Scand 1964; 175:715–719.

54. Newton DA, Bevans HG. Physiotherapy and intermittent positive-pressure ventilation of chronic bronchitis. Br Med J 1978; 2:1525–1528.

55. Campbell AH, O'Connell JM, Wilson F. The effect of chest physiotherapy upon the FEV$_1$ in chronic bronchitis. Med J Aust 1975; 1:33–35.

56. Wollmer P, Ursing K, Midgren B, Eriksson L. Inefficiency of chest percussion in the physical therapy of chronic bronchitis. Eur J Respir Dis 1985; 66:233–239.

57. Rodenstein DO, Stanescu DC. Absence of nasal airflow during pursed lips breathing. The soft palate mechanism. Am Rev Respir Dis 1983; 128:716–718.

58. Tiep BL, Burns M, Kao D, Madison R, Herrera J. Pursed lips breathing training using ear oximetry. Chest 1986; 90:218–221.

59. Breslin EH. The pattern of respiratory muscle recruitment during pursed-lips breathing. Chest 1992; 101:75–78.

60. Gosselink R, Foglio K, Ambrosino N. Breathing exercises. In: Ambrosi N, Donner CF, Rampulla C, eds. Topics in Pulmonary Rehabilitation. Pavia: Pi-Me Press, 1999: 209–228.

61. Sackner MA, Gonzalez HF, Jenouri G, Rodriguez M. Effects of abdominal and thoracic breathing on breathing pattern components in normal subjects and in patients with COPD. Am Rev Respir Dis 1984; 130:584–587.

62. Sharp JT, Danon J, Druz WS, Goldberg NB, Fishman H, Machnach W. Respiratory muscle function in patients with chronic obstructive pulmonary disease: its relationship to disability and to respiratory therapy. Am Rev Respir Dis 1974; 110:154–168.

63. Gosselink RAAM, Wagenaar RC, Sargeant AJ, Rijswijk H, Decramer MLA. Diaphragmatic breathing reduces efficiency of breathing in chronic obstructive pulmonary disease. Am J Respir Crit Care Med 1995; 151:1136–1142.

64. Willeput R, Vachaudez JP, Lenders D, Nys A, Knoops T, Sergysels R. Thoracoabdominal motion during chest physiotherapy in patients affected by chronic obstructive lung disease. Respiration 1983; 44:204–214.

65. McKinley H, Gersten JW, Speck L. Pressure-volume relationships in emphysema patients before and after breathing exercises. Arch Phys Med Rehabil 1961; 42:513–517.

66. Sergysels R, Willeput R, Lenders D, Vachaudez JP, Schandevyl W, Hennebert A. Low frequency breathing at rest and during exercise in severe chronic obstructive bronchitis. Thorax 1979; 34:536–539.

67. Motley HL. The effects of slow deep breathing on the blood gas exchange in emphysema. Am Rev Respir Dis 1963; 88:484–492.

68. Weitzenblum E, Moyes B, Vandevenne A, Hirth C, Methlin G. Regional ventilation and perfusion during diaphragmatic breathing in patients with severe chronic bronchitis. Clin Respir Physiol 1980; 16:263.

69. Paul G, Eldridge F, Mitchell J, Fiene T. Some effects of slowing respiration rate in chronic emphysema and bronchitis. J Appl Physiol 1966; 21:877–882.

70. Bellemare F, Grassino A. Force reserve of the diaphragm in patients with chronic obstructive pulmonary disease. J Appl Physiol 1983; 55:8–15.

71. Vitacca M, Clini E, Bianchi L, Ambrosino N. Acute effects of deep diaphragmatic breathing in COPD patients with chronic respiratory insufficiency. Eur Respir J 1998; 11:408–415.

72. Esteban A, Anzueto A, Alia I, Gordo F, Apezteguia C, Palizas F, Cide D, Goldwaser R, Soto L, Bugedo Rodrigo C, Pimentel J, Raimondi G, Tobin MJ. How is mechanical

ventilation employed in the intensive care unit? An international utilization review. Am J Respir Crit Care Med 2000; 161:1450–1458.

73. Brochard L, Rauss A, Benito S, Conti G, Mancebo J, Rekik N, Gasparetto A, Lemaire F. Comparison of three methods of gradual withdrawal from ventilatory support during weaning from mechanical ventilation. Am J Respir Crit Care Med 1994; 150:896–903.

74. Purro A, Appendini L, De Gaetano A, Gudjonsdottir M, Donner CE, Rossi A. Physiologic determinants of ventilator dependence in long-term mechanically ventilated patients. Am J Respir Crit Care Med 2000; 161:1115–1123.

75. Wiles CM. Neurological complications of severe illness and prolonged mechanical ventilation. Thorax 1996; 512:540–544.

76. Latronico N, Fenzi F, Recupero D, Guarneri B, Tomelleri G, Tonin P, De Maria G, Antonini L, Rizzuto N, Candiani A. Critical illness myopathy and neuropathy. Lancet 1996; 347:1579–1582.

77. Stiller K. Physiotherapy in intensive care. Towards an evidence-based practice. Chest 2000; 118:1801–1813.

78. Confalonieri M, Gorini M, Ambrosino N, Mollica C, Corrado A. Respiratory intensive care units in Italy: a national census and prospective cohort study. Thorax 2001; 56:373–378.

79. Norrenberg M, Vincent JL. A profile of European intensive care unit physiotherapists. Intens Care Med 2000; 26:988–994.

80. Nava S, Ambrosino N. Rehabilitation in the ICU: the European phoenix. Intens Care Med 2000; 26:841–844.

81. Bishop KL. Pulmonary rehabilitation in the intensive care unit. In: Fishman P, ed. Pulmonary Rehabilitation. New York: Marcel Dekker Inc, 1996:725–738.

82. Vitacca M. Pulmonary rehabilitation in the intensive care unit. In: Ambrosino N, Donner CF, Rampulla C, eds. Topics in Pulmonary Rehabilitation. Pavia: Pi-Me, 1999:417–431.

83. Make B, Gilmartin M, Brody JS, Snider CL. Rehabilitation of ventilator-dependent subjects with lung disease. The concept and initial experience. Chest 1984; 138:1519–1523.

84. Foster S, Lopez D, Thomas HM III. Pulmonary rehabilitation in COPD patients with elevated PaCO$_2$. Am Rev Respir Dis 1988; 138:1519–1523.

85. Sergysels R. Chest physiotherapy from chronic to acute respiratory failure in chronic obstructive lung disease. In: Derenne JP, Whitelaw WA, Similowski T, eds. Acute Respiratory Failure in Chronic Obstructive Pulmonary Disease. New York: Marcel Dekker Inc, 1996:615–634.

86. Nava S, Rubini F, Zanotti E, Ambrosino N, Bruschi C, Vitacca M, Fracchia C, Rampulla C. Survival and prediction of successful ventilator weaning in COPD patients requiring mechanical ventilation for more than 21 days. Eur Respir J 1994; 7:1645–1652.

87. Spicher JE, White DP. Outcome and function following prolonged mechanical ventilation. Arch Intern Med 1987; 147:421–425.

88. Gracey DR, Naessens JM, Krishan I, Marsh HM. Hospital and post-hospital survival in patients mechanically ventilated for more than 29 days. Chest 1992; 101:211–214.

89. Nava S. Rehabilitation of patients admitted to a Respiratory Intensive Care Unit. Arch Phys Med Rehabil 1998; 79:849–854.

90. Nevins ML, Epstein SK. Predictors of outcome for patients with COPD requiring invasive mechanical ventilation. Chest 2001; 119:1840–1849.

91. Celli BR. Home mechanical ventilation. In: Tobin MJ, ed. Principles and Practice of Mechanical Ventilation. New York: McGraw-Hill Inc, 1994:619–629.

92. Scheinhorn D, Chao DC, Stearn-Hassenpflug M, La Bree LD, Heltsley D. Post-ICU mechanical ventilation. Treatment of 1123 patients at a regional weaning center. Chest 1997; 111:1654–1659.

93. Esteban A, Frutos F, Tobin M, Alia I, Solsona J, Valverdu I, Fernandez R, De La Cal MA, Benito S, Tomas R, Carriedo D, Macias S, Blanco J. A comparison of four methods of weaning from mechanical ventilation. N Engl J Med 1995; 332:345–350.

94. Ely EW, Baker AM, Dunagan DP, Burke HR, Smith AC, Kelly PT, Johnson MM, Browder RW, Bowton DL, and Haponik EF. Effect of the duration of mechanical ventilation of identifying patients capable of breathing spontaneously. N Engl J Med 1996; 335:1864–1869.

95. Vallverdù I, Calaf M, Subirana M, Net A, Benito S, Mancebo J. Clinical characteristics, respiratory functional parameters and outcome of a two-hour T-piece-trial in patients weaning from mechanical ventilation. Am J Respir Crit Care Med 1998; 158:1855–1862.

96. Butler R, Keenan SP, Inman KJ, Sibbald WJ, Block G. Is there a preferred technique for weaning the difficult-to-wean patient? A systematic review of the literature. Crit Care Med 1999; 27:2331–2336.

97. Kollef MH, Shapiro SD, Silver P, St John RE, Printice D, Sauer S, Ahrens TS, Shannon W, Baker-Clinkscale D. A randomized controlled trial of protocol-directed versus physician-directed weaning from mechanical ventilation. Crit Care Med 1997; 25:567–574.

98. Vitacca M, Vianello A, Colombo D, Clini E, Porta R, Bianchi L, Arcaro G, Vitale G, Guffanti E, Lo Coco A, Ambrosino N. Comparison of two methods for weaning COPD patients requiring mechanical ventilation for more than 15 days. Am J Respir Crit Care Med 2001; 164:225–230.

99. Ciesla ND. Chest physical therapy for patients in the intensive care unit. Phys Ther 1996; 76:609–625.

100. Kida K, Jinno S, Nomura K, Yamada K, Katsura H, Kudoh S. Pulmonary rehabilitation program survey in North America, Europe and Tokyo. J Cardiopulm Rehabil 1998; 18:301–308.

101. Cohen IL, Ban N, Strosberg MA, Weinberg PF, Wacksman RM, Milistein BH, Fein IA. Reduction of duration and cost of mechanical ventilation in an intensive care unit by use of ventilatory management team. Crit Care Med 1991; 19:1278–1284.

102. Horst HM, Mouro D, Hall-Jenssens RA, Pamukov N. Decrease in ventilation time with a standardized weaning process. Arch Surg 1998; 133:483–488.

103. Hall JB, Wood LD. Liberation of the patient from mechanical ventilation. JAMA 1987; 257:1621–1628.

104. Wood G, MacLeod B, Moffatt S. Weaning from mechanical ventilation: physician-directed vs a respiratory-therapist-directed protocol. Respir Care 1995; 40:219–224.

105. Nava S, Evangelisti I, Rampulla C, Compagnoni ML, Fracchia C, Rubini F. Human and financial costs of non-invasive mechanical ventilation in patients affected by chronic obstructive pulmonary disease and acute respiratory failure. Chest 1997; 111:1631–1638.

106. Ambrosino N, Corrado A. Chronic obstructive pulmonary disease with acute respiratory failure. In: Muir JF, Simonds AK, Ambrosino N. Non-invasive Mechanical Ventilation. Eur Respir Mon 2001; 6(16):11–32.

107. Chevrolet JC, Jolliet P, Abajo B, Toussi A, Louis M. Nasal positive pressure ventilation in patients with acute respiratory failure. Difficult and time-consuming procedure for nurses. Chest 1991; 100:775–782.

Ambrosino and Porta

108. Bott J, Carroll MP, Conway JH, Keilty SE, Ward EM, Brown AM, Paul EA, Elliott MW, Godfrey RC, Wedzicha JA. Randomized controlled trial of nasal ventilation in acute ventilatory failure due to chronic obstructive airways disease. Lancet 1993; 341:1555–1557.

109. Kramer N, Meyer TJ, Meharg J, Cece RD, Hill NS. Randomized, prospective trial of noninvasive positive pressure ventilation in acute respiratory failure. Am J Respir Crit Care Med 1995; 151:1799–1806.

110. Confalonieri M, Potena A, Carbone G, Della Porta R, Tolley EA, Meduri GU. Acute respiratory failure in patients with severe community-acquired pneumonia. A prospective randomised evaluation of noninvasive ventilation. Am J Respir Crit Care Med 1999; 160:1585–1591.

111. Jolliet P, Abajo B, Pasquina P, Chevrolet JC. Non-invasive pressure support ventilation in severe community-acquired pneumonia. Intens Care Med 2001; 27:812–821.

112. Plant PK, Owen JL, Elliott MW. Early use of non-invasive ventilation for acute exacerbations of chronic obstructive pulmonary disease on general respiratory wards: a multicentre randomised controlled trial. Lancet 2000; 355:1931–1935.

113. Hilbert G, Gruson D, Vargas F, Valentino R, Portel L, Gbikpi-Benissan G, Dupon M, Reiffers J, Cardinaud JP. Noninvasive ventilation for acute respiratory failure. Quite low time consumption for nurses. Eur Respir J 2000; 16:710–716.

114. Ambrosino N, Vitacca M, Rampulla C. Standards for rehabilitative strategies in respiratory diseases. Monaldi Arch Chest Dis 1995; 50:293–318.

115. Clini E, Vitacca M, Ambrosino N. Dependence Nursing Scale (DNS): a new method to assess the effect of nursing workload in a respiratory intermediate intensive care unit. Respir Care 1999; 44:29–37.

116. Reis-Miranda D, Moreno R, Iapichino G. Nine equivalents of nursing manpower use score (NEMS). Intens Care Med 1997; 23:760–765.

117. Pingleton SK, Rossi A. Respiratory and non respiratory complications of critical illness. In: Parrillo JE, Bone RC. Critical Care Medicine. Principles of Diagnosis and Management. St Louis: Mosby, 1995:755–780.

118. Bowton DL. Nosocomial pneumonia in the ICU: year 2000 and beyond. Chest 1999; 115(suppl):28S–33S.

119. Kolleff MH. The prevention of ventilator-associated pneumonia. N Engl J Med 1999; 340:627–634.

120. Vincent JL. Prevention of nosocomial bacterial pneumonia. Thorax 1999; 54:544–549.

121. Ntoumenopoulos G, Gild A, Cooper DJ. The effect of manual lung hyperinflation and postural drainage on pulmonary complications in mechanically ventilated trauma patients. Anaesth Intens Care 1998; 26:492–496.

29

Home Management of Exacerbations of Chronic Obstructive Pulmonary Disease

JOSEP ROCA,
ALBERT ALONSO,
and MANEL BORRELL

University of Barcelona–
Corporació Sanitària Clínic (CSC)
Barcelona, Spain

CARME HERNÁNDEZ

Hospital Clinic
Barcelona, Spain

PAULA de TOLEDO

Polytechnic University of Madrid
Madrid, Spain

I. Lessons from Observational Studies

Patients with chronic obstructive pulmonary disease (COPD) who show repeated emergency room (ER) consultations and/or hospital admissions due to exacerbations present a rapid progress of the disease severity with deterioration of health-related quality of life (HRQL) and poor survival (1–5). Consequently, prevention of exacerbations constitutes an important endpoint in COPD management (6–8).

The lack of an operational definition of exacerbation (6–10) constrains the design of efficient prevention strategies and constitutes a limitation for a proper evaluation of the literature on the issue. Studies using an operational definition of exacerbation based on ER admissions/hospitalizations likely introduce a bias leading to an emphasis on severe episodes, together with a significant under-estimation of the prevalence of acute episodes (11, 12).

Exacerbations leading to ER admissions are responsible, however, for the important dysfunctions observed in the delivery of health-care services, particularly during winter outbreaks of COPD exacerbations. Moreover, most of our current knowledge in this area comes from the analysis of acute episodes that require ER consultations/in-hospital admissions (2–3, 13–16), as summarized in Table 1.

Table 1   Observational Studies on COPD Exacerbations

Key Remarks

COPD exacerbations represent an increasing burden on health-care systems worldwide (57).

Hospitalizations due to exacerbations generate a major portion (>70%) of the overall expenses of the disease (58).

Conventional medical care fails to further reduce hospitalization rates substantially.

Exacerbations requiring hospitalization show high rates of early readmissions after discharge (25–35% within 2 months) (30–34).

Predictors of unexpected hospitalizations (2, 3, 13–15)

History of repeated hospitalizations (three or more per year)[a]

Low FEV_1

Pulmonary and systemic effects of hypoxemia

Hypercapnia

Low daily physical activity

Endpoints

Prevention of exacerbations in frail patients

Optimal medical care of COPD patients with exacerbation

Prevention of hospitalizations triggered by exacerbations

Prevention of early readmissions after discharge.

[a]The following variables have been suggested to increase patient's frailty: (1) poor management of comorbid conditions; (2) lack of appropriate social support; (3) poor knowledge of the disease and inappropriate skills for self-management of the disease; and (4) high level of anxiety-depression, but further studies are needed to validate the role of these factors on exacerbations.

Current clinical guidelines for COPD (6–8, 17) provide recommendations to modulate some of the predictors of unexpected hospitalizations. Moreover, significant advances have recently occurred in the field of rehabilitation. Physical deconditioning has been identified as a relevant predictor of hospital admissions (2, 3, 16) and awareness on the positive effects of skeletal muscle training (18–20) is steadily growing among professionals. However, despite this undeniable progress in the management of COPD, we are still confronted with a poor understanding of the underlying factors favoring "frequent hospitalizations" in frail patients (21).

Available data strongly indicate that interventions on the determinants of frailty in COPD patients require a global approach that conventional health-care delivery does not foresee. An extraordinary effort must be devoted to introduce flexibility into health-care systems. This, in turn, would facilitate the implementation of innovative ways of chronic care management based on integrative patient-centered care, as discussed extensively below.

The first part of the present chapter reviews previous experiences and trends on homecare services for COPD patients: home hospitalization/early discharge programs and home support services. The main focus of the chapter, however, is dedicated to new developments in COPD management based on the conceptual framework of the chronic care model (22–25). Because information sharing is a pivotal aspect of this model of care, we hypothesize that information technologies

(IT) will become an essential component for a successful deployment of the new modalities of health care. In this regard, the chapter describes the basic features of the CHRONIC project*, as one of the ongoing experiences on IT that shows the potential in this field. The analysis of the clinical aspects of CHRONIC is followed by a brief description of the technological platform that supports the project.

A first feasibility analysis of home management of acute exacerbations as an alternative to hospital admission in exacerbated COPD patients was reported in 1999 in a noncontrolled study using a hospital-based team (26). The rationale for this approach was that a significant portion of these patients, especially those without severe comorbidities, do not require intensive investigations, complex therapy, or continuous monitoring. Moreover, it has been shown that prolonged hospitalizations in advanced COPD patients can be harmful because of increased associated risks such as nosocomial infections and the deleterious effects of high doses of systemic steroids on skeletal muscle (6–8).

In the initial experience by Gravil et al. (26), as well as in subsequent studies indicated below, specialized respiratory nurses played a pivotal role in the programs. It is shown that nurse-based assessment in the ER helps to identify the cohort of patients who can be treated in the community with adequate support. These nurses can also manage the home-care program under remote medical supervision. There has been controversy regarding the effects of home hospitalization schemes on costs. Two randomized controlled trials (27–29) reported that home hospitalization significantly increased health-care costs for COPD patients. These two trials, however, analyzed a very small sample of patients whose severity of illness was not delineated.

A. Feasibility of Home Hospitalization and Early Discharge

Three controlled trials (30–32) conducted in the United Kingdom and a more recent study from Spain (33) have shown both safety and cost reduction when these type of services, either home hospitalization directly from the ER or early discharge from the hospital, are applied to properly selected COPD patients with a well-defined intervention at home.

These results provide ground to consider home hospitalization a practical alternative to in-patient hospitalization in cohorts of selected individuals that could encompass up to 30 to 40% of the patients admitted in the ER because of an exacerbation. Similarly, early discharge from the hospital seems to be an adequate option to prevent unnecessarily prolonged hospitalizations in severe exacerbations. In summary, home hospitalization and early discharge should be looked at as

---

*CHRONIC, an Information Capture and Processing Environment for Chronic Patients in the Information Society, is a project funded by the European Union (1999-IST-12158) running from January 2000 to December 2002. Controlled clinical pilots on chronic respiratory diseases are conducted in Barcelona (Spain) and Leuven (Belgium); patients with chronic heart failure are studied in Leuven and neurological disorders in Milan (Italy). The Barcelona team is the Project coordinator.

potential alternatives to be indicated on an individual basis by the hospital-based home-care team. Besides, the results of these studies seem to support the notion that the efficacy of these home-care services is not dependent on the specificities of the health-care system if the logistics are managed by the hospital. Thus, while the National Health Service in the United Kingdom has a consolidated network of primary-care physicians playing as "gate keepers" who are responsible for a rather low percentage of patient's self-referrals to hospital ER (on average 20–30% countrywide, and as low as 1% in 30, the figure in Spain can be as high as 70% (13, 15, 16).

B. Limitations of the Current Home Hospitalization/Early Discharge Programs

According to the above-mentioned studies, the efficacy of home-care programs to prevent short-term relapses was not higher than in the conventional model of treatment. Despite noticeable differences in the health-care systems between UK and Spain mentioned above, the two countries showed unacceptably high rates of early relapses—between 25 to 35% of the patients required readmission within 2 months (30–34). These figures are similar in other European countries. High rates of relapses were reported in a recent study done in five main city hospitals in Barcelona (13, 15, 16). Also, a 50% hospital readmission rate within 6 months after discharge has been reported in the USA (2).

Failure of home hospitalization and/or early discharge programs to prevent early relapses might be due to fragmentation of care in the current health-care systems. All these studies were conducted by hospital-based teams that provided information to primary care on a regular basis, but without establishing real interactions among the different levels of care. In other words, though these programs implied quite a substantial redefinition of the roles of doctors and specialized nurses such changes took place only at the hospital. It can be hypothesized that similar programs carried out in the context of a regional health-care network aiming at continuum of care, as described in Figures 1 and 2, can successfully prevent relapses. A distributed model of care based on a close collaboration between health-care levels (22–25) is strongly suggested for further developments of home hospitalization/early discharge programs.

A proper design of these interventions in a regional health-care network requires better knowledge of the clinical and social factors predicting likelihood of success of home hospitalization programs. Information provided by multivariate analysis of existing data (26, 30–34) might help to decide on the distribution of responsibilities across the system aiming at collaborative work between health-care levels. Recommendations on curricula requirements for the specialized respiratory nurses and other allied health-care professionals devoted to home care, as well as appropriate clinical guidelines in this field, are urgently needed.

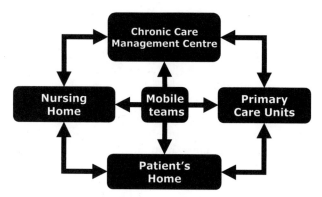

Figure 1 Scheme of a regional health-care network for care of chronic respiratory patients. The health-care sector in Barcelona includes a population of 400,000 inhabitants covered by public and private providers.

II. Home Support Services

In spite of the existing gray areas, the positive results of home-care programs are sufficiently encouraging to explore an extended application of home services. Main targets of home support services are indicated in Table 2. They should be the basis for the definition of patterns of care to be shared by professionals working at different levels of the system. As indicated above, distribution of specific tasks between primary-care teams and specialized teams is clearly beyond the scope of the current chapter.

A. Prevention of Unplanned Hospitalizations

While positive effects of a nurse-directed, multidisciplinary intervention have shown (35–38) to improve HRQL, decrease frequency of unplanned hospitalizations, reduce costs, and improve survival in elderly patients with chronic heart failure,

Table 2 Patterns of Care for Home-Based Services

Home Hospitalization and Early Discharge Programs
Home Support Services
   Prevention of hospitalizations in frail patients
   Programs targeting specific aspects:
      Oxygen therapy
      Home rehabilitation
      Noninvasive home ventilation
      Home monitoring (frail patients, tests)
   End-stage disease:
      Palliative care
      End-of-life programs

there is no information in the respiratory field. There are few small studies (39–44) on the impact of a multidisciplinary program on clinically stable but frail patients. None of them, however, provided strong conclusions on the efficacy of such programs in COPD patients, nor the clues to organize a proper cost-efficacy trial. Because of the clinical differences between COPD and chronic heart failure, the design of cardiac protocols can not be extrapolated to respiratory patients.

As indicated in the section on early relapses, excessive fragmentation of services between primary care and specialists, as well as the need for a proper identification of variables determining frailty in COPD patients (Table 1) are likely the most important factors explaining the lack of data in the respiratory field. Controlled pilot studies examining the predictive value of frailty factors on unexpected hospitalizations are needed to design multidisciplinary preventive strategies of hospitalizations in COPD patients that should be evaluated in terms of cost-efficacy analysis.

B. Programs Targeting Specific Aspects

We will only pinpoint the trends observed in three areas that are showing novel developments. First, the entire rationale for oxygen therapy is based on keeping diurnal blood levels of arterial blood oxygenation in the flat portion of the oxy-hemoglobin dissociation curve. Without disputing the physiological basis for this approach, it is increasingly accepted that both pulmonary and systemic effects of cell hypoxia are more reliable predictors of the disease severity than the diurnal PaO_2 measured at rest (3, 45). Moreover, it is acknowledged that polyglobulia is a specific but poorly sensitive biomarker of cell hypoxia. Further knowledge on the molecular consequences of cell hypoxia will likely trigger substantial changes in the clinical monitoring and management of chronic respiratory failure in COPD patients.

Second, skeletal muscle training is becoming a relevant part of the non-pharmacological treatment of the disease no longer constrained to advanced COPD patients. The predictive value of physical activity on hospitalizations (2, 3, 16), together with recent data on the molecular basis of physiological training effects (19, 20) open new avenues in the treatment of both normal and low fat free mass COPD patients. Cost-efficient strategies for rehabilitation, including remotely controlled home programs (46, 47), should be designed and the results properly assessed. Finally, despite the rather negative reports on noninvasive home ventilation of COPD patients (48), there is convincing evidence that appropriate identification of candidates and adequate delivery of ventilation are key aspects to achieve successful outcomes in this therapy, which should be analyzed in an extensive multicenter approach.

C. Palliative Care and End-of-Life Programs

The palliative care and end-of-life needs for COPD patients have been properly identified and consensus on the protocols can be achieved rather easily, based on published reports (49–52). But identification of the transition from active care to palliative care in COPD patients remains a pending issue. A similar problem occurs for end-of-life programs. Our hypothesis is that these programs cannot be successfully approached in the present model of acute care. Again, fragmentation of healthcare services and poor involvement of the patient (and caregiver) in the management of the disease preclude the progress in this area. Decisions in this field should be taken on an individual basis with a multidisciplinary approach because of both technical and ethical reasons. An active patient's partnership with professionals that have been involved in the patient's care at different levels of the system is required.

III. The Chronic Care Model

This section describes the main features of a novel approach for the management of chronic disorders (Fig. 2) (22–25). The underlying hypothesis is that the relevant limitations of the ongoing home-care programs for chronic respiratory patients described in the previous sections can be properly addressed within the frame of the new model of care.

Current health-care systems are essentially oriented to acute illnesses with special focus on symptoms and laboratory results thus favoring an expeditious resolution of immediate problems. However, this acute-care paradigm is no longer adequate for the current changes in health-care problems, because it focuses more on physician's treatment rather than in patient's active role in the self-management of his or her disease. As a result, the interactions between patient and doctor are often

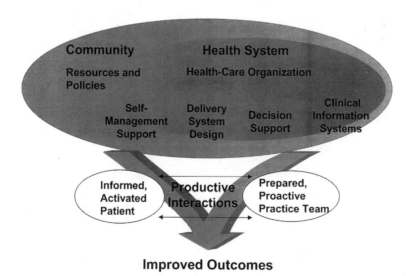

Improved Outcomes

Figure 2   The chronic care model proposes a patient-centered approach with special emphasis on shared-care arrangements across the health-care system. Key features of the model are the development of innovative home-based services with involvement of patients (and caregivers) as partners in the management of the disease.

frustrating for both of them. Unfortunately, the acute-care model is perpetuated by out-dated health-care training curricula.

Health-care systems will evolve by moving toward a model of care that can better address chronic conditions. The chronic care model defines new relationships between patients and professionals, and promotes reengineering of the roles of health-care professionals within and between levels of care. As indicated in the introduction, extensive use of user-friendly internet-based technologies seems to be an essential component of the model to support its progressive implementation.

The new model (22–25) proposes a patient-centered approach with an emphasis on shared-care arrangements across the health-care system (between specialized care at the hospital and primary care) and within the multidisciplinary primary-care team. Key features (22–25) are the development of innovative home-based services with involvement of patients (and caregivers) as partners in the management of the disease. The primary health-care center organizes and coordinates the care of the chronically ill person through a team composed of physicians, nurses, and/or community health/social workers. This team aims at optimizing patient outcomes through ongoing interactions during which they (1) collect and review patient's registries and take appropriate action; (2) help patients (and caregivers) to set goals and solve problems for improved self-management; (3) apply or reinforce proven clinical and behavioral interventions; and (4) assure a continuous follow-up of the disease. The link between the primary-care team and the hospital is often led by a nurse who plays a bridging role with the specialist. This prompts a redefinition of the roles and skills of the specialized nurses and other allied health-care professionals in this model, which in turn makes it necessary to reexamine the interactions of these professionals with physicians. The model also strengthens the role of the caregiver. In this scenario (Fig. 2), adequate standardization of procedures and fluent communication across the system becomes mandatory. This is the role that information technologies are to play in this new setting, facilitating information sharing and collaboration among different actors and health-care levels (53). Moreover, novel educational tools and continuous professional development can be integrated into practice and thus become relevant building blocks in the implementation of the chronic care model.

IV. CHRONIC Project: Innovative Home-Based Services

One of the pivotal aspects of the CHRONIC project (see footnote, p. 533) is to perform controlled clinical trials addressed to evaluate efficacy and associated costs of innovative home-based services. An important goal of the project is to assess the added value of internet-based technologies to facilitate a progressive deployment of the chronic care model. The characteristics of the technology used are described below in the section devoted to the technological platform. The CHRONIC platform integrates the use of traditional communication tools such as the phone with up-to-date technologies described below. Essential aims are to facilitate information sharing within the regional health-care network and use of user-friendly interfaces.

Home care in this model aims at a comprehensive approach of the management of target elderly chronic respiratory patients often showing several co-morbid conditions*. Home-based services are not conceived as an alternative to in-patient hospitalization, but as part of a continuum of care within a regional health-care network (Fig. 1). With special emphasis on the interactions among different public and private providers playing at different levels of the system (primary-care teams, convalescence centers, and the tertiary hospital). The system must avoid fragmentation of services by ensuring effective functional relationships across health-care levels. A well-defined distribution of responsibilities within the primary-care team and with the specialized team should be properly settled. The design of evidence-based patterns of care aiming to achieve preestablished endpoints for the management of the disease constitutes a pivotal aspect for the success. A continuous follow-up shall be established to facilitate validation of the patterns of care, as described in Table 2. In this context, timely information about patients, and populations of patients, is a critical feature to achieve effective care. A disease registry for individual practices that includes tracking of clinical information and outcomes should be mandatory. Health-care providers that have access to the registry can plan and deliver care in a timely and appropriate manner. Empowerment of patients and caregivers to ensure effective self-management helps patients and families to adhere to regimens in ways to minimize complications, symptoms, and disability. Patients and their caregivers need to be informed about self-management strategies and be appropriately motivated to adopt healthy lifestyles.

A. Home Hospitalization/Early Discharge

In the pilot phase, the approach described above has shown to be particularly successful for home hospitalization and early discharge in a group of 222 patients admitted in the emergency room of two main city hospitals because of an exacerbation, as reported in detail in (34). The intervention carried out in the home hospitalization group, described in Table 3, generated better outcomes than conventional care (Fig. 3), which included: (1) lower in-patient hospitalization rates; (2) lower rate of short-term relapses requiring ER admissions; (3) clinically relevant improvement in health-related quality of life, as assessed by the Saint George Respiratory Questionnaire (SGRQ); (4) higher degree of patient satisfaction; and (5) an important positive impact on knowledge of the disease and on patient self-management of the chronic condition, as described in Figure 4. The results were obtained with a rather modest use of the resources allocated to home support. Only a small portion of the five potential nurse visits was used (on average 1.7 nurse visits at home) during the 2-month follow-up period. Despite a free-phone access ensured to all patients, the average number of patient phone calls to the nurse was only 0.76.

---

*In a representative group of 222 COPD patients (73 ± 8.5 years) admitted at the ER of two tertiary hospitals (52) because of an exacerbation of the disease, 95% of them presented one or more comorbid conditions (on average 3.1 concomitant disorders), chronic heart disease being one of the most common problems, present in approximately 35% of the COPD patients.

Table 3 Description of the Nurse-Driven Intervention in the Home Hospitalization Group

---

1. Assessment on ER Admission by the Specialized Team
   Characteristics of the exacerbation, comorbidities, and response to treatment at the
     emergency room (ER)
   Baseline conditions of the patient (*duration 1.5 h*): (1) health-related quality of life; (2)
     health-care resources in the previous year; (3) fragility risk factors; and (4) knowledge
     of the disease and compliance to therapy
   Decision on discharge from the ER or after a short period of in-patient hospitalization
     based on 1 and 2.
2. Treatment at Discharge
   Pharmacological therapy of COPD and comorbidities
   Nonpharmacological treatment (*duration 2 h*)[a]
3. Home Hospitalization (HH) and 8-Week Follow-Up
   First nurse visit at home at 24 h (*duration 1 h*)
     Assessment of the response to pharmacological treatment
     Introduction of changes under remote physician's supervision
     On-site assessment of fragility factors
     Action plan revisited and education reinforced
   Eight-week follow-up
     Number of home visits and duration of HH were decided by the nurse
     Patient free-phone access to the nurse was ensured
     Nurse phone calls to patient to reinforce the action plan
   Failure of the program
     >5 nurse home visits during the 8-weeks follow-up
     New problem requiring ER admission
4. Assessment After 2 Months Follow-Up

Source: Ref. 34.

[a]The nonpharmacological therapy included: (a) education on knowledge of the disease; adherence to treatment; and recognition/prevention of triggers of exacerbation; (b) selection of appropriate equipment at home; training on administration of pharmacological treatment; (c) smoking cessation; (d) patient empowerment on daily life activities: hygiene, dressing, household tasks; leisure activities; breathing exercises; and, skeletal muscle activity; (e) nutrition recommendations; and (f) socialization and changes in lifestyle.

The average overall costs per home hospitalization patient were substantially lower than in conventional care essentially due to less days of in-patient hospitalization. While all previous studies assessing either home hospitalization or early discharge (26, 30–33) have shown that the approach is safe, this was the first report that clearly demonstrated beneficial effects of the intervention compared with conventional care of COPD exacerbations. The study also indicates that improvement of outcomes was associated with a reduction of direct costs. Like other reports (26, 30–33), it was demonstrated that home hospitalization was suitable only in a subset of exacerbations that must be selected at the hospital after proper assessment by a specialized team. It is of note that patients with baseline low mobility and those unable to improve their daily physical activity after the intervention (Table 1, Fig. 4) showed

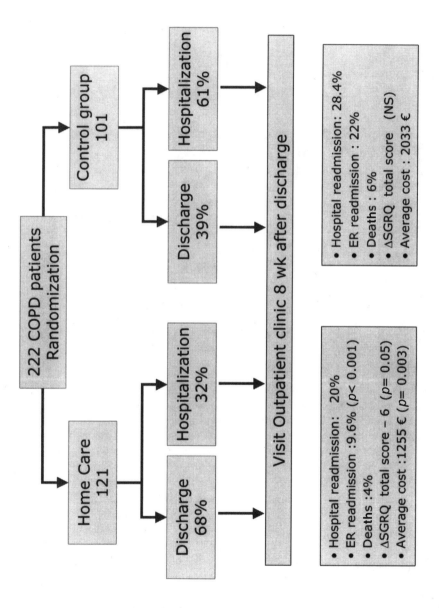

Figure 3 Barcelona home hospitalization study: profile of patient recruitment and summary of the main outcomes. (From Ref. 34.)

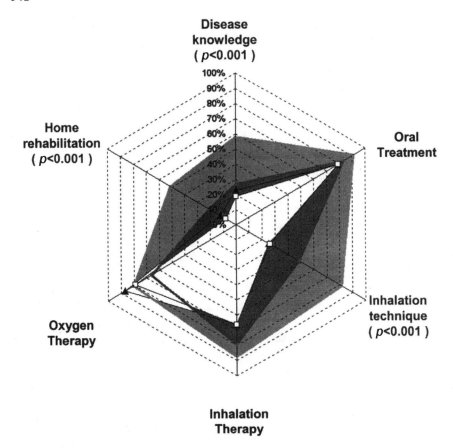

Figure 4   Knowledge of the disease and self-management of the chronic condition in the home hospitalization study (34). Results are expressed as percent of patients. On admission (inner limits: HH, triangles; and, controls, squares), no differences were seen in any of the six dimensions of the graph. No changes in the control group (dark gray area) were observed during the 8-week follow-up period, but marked beneficial effects were detected in the HH group (light gray area). It is of note that both baseline results and changes in home rehabilitation were associated with the success of the intervention measured by lack of early readmissions (and survival) after discharge.

lower health-related quality of life and higher risk of relapse after discharge from the hospital.

The positive effects of the educational intervention on patient's behavior are indicated in Figure 4. It is acknowledged, however, that the relatively short-term follow-up (2 months) might limit the generalization of the results. The pivotal effects of education on self-management of asthma have been widely demonstrated over the last years (54–56), but evidence in this regard is just being collected for COPD patients. We identify this area as a key field for the development of future guidelines for chronic respiratory diseases linking the different levels of the healthcare system.

B. Characterization of Target Subsets of Patients

An important step in the process of setting home-based health-care services is a proper characterization of the target population of candidates for the different patterns of care. This aspect is particularly important in chronic respiratory patients because of the limitations of operational criteria for diagnosis for different disease categories at primary-care level (COPD, chronic asthma, bronchiectasis, etc.). Moreover, specific endpoints for each pattern of care have not been established yet.

C. Prevention of Unplanned Hospitalizations

The analysis carried out above highlights the need for a comprehensive design of community-based multidisciplinary services to prevent unexpected hospitalizations in elderly chronic respiratory patients ensuring an appropriate cost-efficacy ratio of the setting. Preliminary results of a pilot carried out, as part of the chronic project seems to generate positive results in terms of effective prevention of both unexpected hospitalizations and ER admissions after 1-year follow-up. Moreover, the pilot is facilitating the identification of frailty criteria to predict high risk of relapse after discharge.

D. Programs Targeting Specific Aspects

Specific programs for control of oxygen therapy, noninvasive home ventilation, home rehabilitation, transient or long-term home monitoring of target groups of patients shall be included as part of the spectrum of home-based services. Also, specific offers oriented to social support or remote alarms for elderly patients should be considered in a comprehensive program. Distribution of responsibilities and particulars of the interactions between primary-care teams and specialized teams must be defined for each specific pattern of care (Table 2).

Palliative care and end-of-life programs deserve particular attention in this setting. The chronic care setting should provide continuous follow-up of target populations with availability of the patient's registries. This setting, together with patient empowerment for self-management of the disease, should generate an adequate scenario for the deployment of end-of-life programs.

V. CHRONIC Project: The Technological Platform

The CHRONIC project integrates both traditional and innovative technologies to support new models of health-care provision by developing an information environment for the care of target chronic patients (Figs. 5, 6). The principal elements of the CHRONIC technological platform are the following:

1. *The chronic care management center* (CCMC) is the core of the system. It is the single entry point for the patient to access health-care services, regardless of the provider. From the CCMC, patient's request is handled by allocating the most suitable resource (hospital and ER departments, primary-care centers, or any other related providers). At the same time, in the CCMC, information on patient status, actions taken and consumption of resources is collected. From the technical point of view, the CCMC uses advanced call center technologies coupled to a patient management module (PMM). The call center supports different modes of operation. In normal mode, incoming calls are attended by a tele-operator whereas in automatic mode a virtual response unit (VRU) takes control over them thus assuring round the clock coverage.

2. *The patient management module* is a web-based application that provides access and facilitates the management of the records of the patients

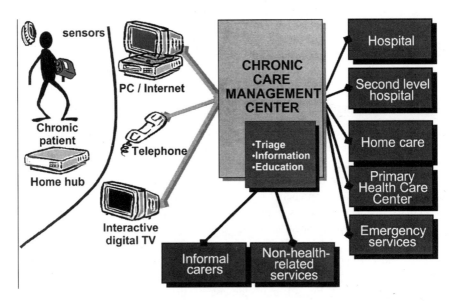

Figure 5 The CHRONIC project (1999-IST-12158) evaluates a new model of integrated healthcare services addressed to target populations of patients with chronic disorders. The core of the system is the chronic care management center (CCMC) that channels patient's requests to the appropriate health-care level through nurse-driven programs aiming to provide a continuum of care. The technological platform based on internet technologies facilitates the interactions among professionals and the management of patient registries, including monitoring of biological signals. The CCMC is also a vehicle for continuous education of patients and professionals.

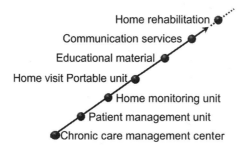

Figure 6 List of services either available or planned during the lifespan of the CHRONIC project. The system facilitates access to information for case management, teleconsultation, telemonitoring and advising, as well as rehabilitation sessions for patient empowerment and care optimization.

included in a home-care program. The information managed by the module is encoded and accessibility relies on the use of digital certificates. The module accesses information on: (1) interactions of the patient with the call center (calls made, answers to triage questionnaires, etc.); (2) monitoring data and results of the automated data analysis; (3) patient's clinical record and follow-up (frailty score, treatment plan, and follow-up reports made by health-care professionals at any level of the system); and (4) professional utilities such as home-visit agenda, list of pending problems, etc. The module is designed in such a way that the different sections can be accessed and updated from any point of care, including the patient's home. In the latter, the module is accessed through the home visit mobile unit.

3. *The home visit mobile unit* is a small size laptop computer running an application similar to the PMM that supports communication with the CCMC. This means that patient information can be accessed and updated remotely. It is also possible to manage the agenda of the health professional, to consult educational material or to perform on-site measurements such as forced spirometry. The communication is based on standard GSM and GPRS cards.

4. *The patient home unit* consists of a central device (namely a home hub) and a set of sensors (wireless ECG and pulse oximetry; spirometry; and, blood pressure). The system is designed to provide a user-friendly interface for patients that are not familiar with computers. It uses the standard TV set as a display and navigation through menus is managed by means of a remote control. The functionalities of the unit include: monitoring of biomedical signals, video conferencing, access to web based educational multimedia material and exchange of messages with the CCMC. The system is connected to the CCMC using internet protocols through private providers and public networks. Security of data transmission relies on the https protocol and digital certificates.

VI. Summary

Health-care systems in developed countries are facing a period of profound changes resulting from a variety of factors, including demography and advances in technology. Aging of the population together with a high prevalence of concurrent chronic disorders generate an extensive use of health-care and social services. Recent projections (57) indicate boosting of these two factors at least up to the year 2020. Moreover, because of specific characteristics of patients with chronic comorbid conditions, a substantial degree of flexibility of health-care services is increasingly required. Overall, these phenomena are the main cause of dysfunction in the traditional health-care models that are essentially focused on acute care. Integration of health-care delivery across systems aiming to provide a continuum of care to target populations of patients with severe chronic diseases seems to be the emerging model most suitable to provide effective and efficient health care services. In this context, managerial aspects of exacerbated COPD patients must be revisited and innovative home-based services, in conjunction with in-patient hospitalization, will be addressed. They must be understood as part of the continuum of care for chronically ill patients. Despite the promising results of these new approaches in the treatment of COPD exacerbations, prevention of early relapses after discharge is still an important challenge. Progressive deployment of these new patient-centered services should be done under the frame of a properly designed cost-effectiveness analysis.

The results of the CHRONIC project, described in the chapter, should enable health-care organizations to take advantage of information technologies, to achieve a better use of the available resources to provide citizens with a more usable and high-quality service, creating added value. The chronic care platform derived from the project will favor new organizational schemes facilitating the deployment of the chronic care model. The platform can be also used in other scenarios: acute patients after surgery or any other reasons; patients requiring regular monitoring of treatment, etc. The system can also evolve as a platform to support knowledge management tools useful for the development of new methods for continuous professional development required to face rapidly evolving requirements of health care.

Acknowledgments

We are grateful to all the partners of the CHRONIC project: CSC, Barcelona (E), Marta Serdà, Felip Burgos, Jose Luís Valera, Conchi Gistau, José A. Montero, Xavier Pastor and Bernat Sifre; UPM, Madrid (E), Francisco del Pozo, Paula de Toledo, Silvia Jiménez; CESTEL, Madrid (E), Fernando Ortiz, Luis Mena, Max Godoy, José Luís Sirera; CSIC-CNM, Barcelona (E), Jordi Aguiló, Luís Sanchez, Antón Guimerà; SMS, Milano (I), Alessandro Falco, Daniela Balconi; SMS, Madrid (E), Begoña Andrés, José J. Moratillas; ICP, Milano (I), Andrea Mattiussi, Angelo Antonini (Parkinson Center); MC, Milano (I), Carlo Castiglioni, Elvia Battaglia; TILAB, Turín (I), Fabrizio Moggio, Marco Mercinelli; KUL, Leuven (B), Marc

Decramer, Thierry Troosters, Walter Droogne, F. Van de Werf; EW, Paris (F), Peter Sylvester, Nicolas Pougetoux; ALAMO, Madrid (E), Miguel Angel García Matatoros, Alberto Marcos; UB, Barcelona (E), Ramon Farré; ECOMIT, Barcelona (E), Carmen Céinos.

Supported by Grants AATM 8/02/99 from the Agencia d'Avaluació de Tecnología Mèdica; FIS 98/0052-01 from the Fondo de Investigaciones Sanitarias; SEPAR 1998; CHRONIC project (IST-1999/12158) from the European Union (DG XIII); and, Comissionat per a Universitats i Recerca de la Generalitat de Catalunya (1999-SGR-00228).

References

1. Jones PW. Issues concerning health-related quality of life in COPD. Chest 1995; 107 (5 Suppl):187S–193S.
2. Connors AF, Dawson NV, Thomas C, Harrell FE, Desbiens N, Fulkerson WJ, Kussin P, Bellamy P, Goldman L, Knaus WA. Outcomes following acute exacerbation of severe chronic obstructive lung disease. Am J Respir Crit Care Med 1996; 154:959–967.
3. Kessler R, Faller M, Fourgaut G, Mennecier B, Weitzenblum E. Predictive factors of hospitalization for acute exacerbation in a series of 64 patients with chronic obstructive pulmonary disease. Am J Respir Crit Care Med 1999; 159:158–164.
4. Jones PW. Health status measurement in chronic obstructive pulmonary disease. Thorax 2001; 56:880–887.
5. Stoller JK. Acute exacerbations of chronic obstructive pulmonary disease. N Engl J Med 2002; 346(13):988–994.
6. Pauwels RA, Buist AS, Calverley PM, Jenkins CR, Hurd SS. Global strategy for the diagnosis, management, and prevention of chronic obstructive pulmonary disease. NHLBI/WHO Global Initiative for Chronic Obstructive Lung Disease (GOLD) Workshop summary. Am J Respir Crit Care Med 2001; 163(5):1256–1276.
7. Siafakas NM, Vermeire P, Pride NB, Paoletti P, Gibson J, Howard P, Yernault JC, Decramer M, Higenbottam T, Postma DS, Rees J. Optimal assessment and management of chronic obstructive pulmonary disease (COPD). The European Respiratory Society Task Force. Eur Respir J 1995; 8(8):1398–1420.
8. American Thoracic Society. Standards for the diagnosis and care of patients with chronic obstructive pulmonary disease. Am J Respir Crit Care Med 1995; 152:S77–S120.
9. Anthonisen NR, Manfreda J, Warren CP, Herschfield ES, Harding GKM, Nelson NA. Antibiotic therapy in exacerbations of chronic obstructive pulmonary disease. Ann Intern Med 1987; 106:196–204.
10. Rodríguez-Roisin R. Toward a consensus definition for COPD exacerbations. Chest 2000; 117:398S–401S.
11. Seemungal TA, Donaldson GC, Bhowmik A, Jeffries DJ, Wedzicha JA. Time course and recovery of exacerbations in patients with chronic obstructive pulmonary disease. Am J Respir Crit Care Med 2000; 161(5):1608–1613.
12. Seemungal TA, Donaldson GC, Paul EA, Bestall JC, Jeffries DJ, Wedzicha JA. Effects of exacerbation on quality of life in patients with COPD. Am J Respir Crit Care Med 1998; 157:1418–1422.
13. Garcia-Aymerich J, Barreiro E, Farrero E, Marrades RM, Morera J, Anto JM. Patients hospitalized for COPD have a high prevalence of modifiable risk factors for exacerbation (EFRAM study). Eur Respir J 2000; 16(6):1037–1042.

14. Antó JM, Vermeire P, Vestbo J, Sunyer J. Epidemiology of chronic obstructive pulmonary disease. Eur Respir J 2001; 17:982–994.

15. García-Aymerich J, Monso E, Marrades RM, Escarrabill J, Félez MA, Sunyer J, Antó JM. Risk factors for hospitalization for a chronic obstructive pulmonary disease exacerbation. Efram study. Am J Respir Crit Care Med 2001; 164:1002–1007.

16. García-Aymerich J, Farrero E, Felez MA, Izquierdo J, Marrades RM, Escarrabill J, Antó JM and the EFRAM investigators. Risk factors for hospitalization for a COPD: a propsective study. Thorax 2003; 58:100–105.

17. Barberà JA, Peces-Barba G, Agusti AG, Izquierdo JL, Monso E, Montemayor T et al. Clinical guidelines for the diagnosis and treatment of chronic obstructive pulmonary disease. Arch Bronconeumol 2001; 37(6):297–316.

18. Maltais F, Leblanc P, Simard C et al. Skeletal muscle adaptation to endurance training in patients with Chronic Obstructive Pulmonary Disease. Am J Respir Crit Care Med 1996; 154:442–447.

19. Sala E, Roca J, Marrades RM, Alonso J, Gonzalez de Suso JM, Moreno A, Barbera JA, Nadal J, Jover L, Rodriguez-Roisin R. Effects of endurance training on skeletal muscle bioenergetics in chronic obstructive pulmonary disease. Am J Respir Crit Care Med 1999; 159:1726–1734.

20. Rabinovich RA, Ardite E, Troosters T, Carbo N, Alonso J, Gonzalez de Suso JM, Vilaro J, Barbera JA, Figueras M, Argiles J, Fernandez-Checa JC, Roca J. Reduced Muscle Redox Capacity after Endurance Training in Patients with Chronic Obstructive Pulmonary Disease. Am J Respir Crit Care Med 2001; 164:1114–1118.

21. Nichol KL, Baken L, Nelson A. Relation between influenza vaccination and outpatient visits, hospitalization, and mortality in elderly persons with chronic lung disease. Ann Intern Med 1999; 130:397–403.

22. Wagner EH. The role of patient care teams in chronic disease management. BMJ 2000; 320(7234):569–572.

23. Wagner EH. Meeting the needs of chronically ill people. BMJ 2001; 323(7319):945–946.

24. Wagner EH, Glasgow RE, Davis C, Bonomi AE, Provost L, McCulloch D, Carver P, Sixta C. Quality improvement in chronic illness care: a collaborative approach. J Comm J Qual Improv 2001; 27(2):63–80.

25. Innovative care for chronic conditions. Meeting report 30–31 May 2001. WHO/MNC/CCH/01.01.

26. Gravil JH, Al Rawas OA, Cotton MM, Flanigan U, Irwin A, Stevenson RD. Home treatment of exacerbations of chronic obstructive pulmonary disease by an acute respiratory assessment service. Lancet 1998; 351(9119):1853–1855.

27. Shepperd S, Harwood D, Gray A, Vessey M, Morgan P. Randomized controlled trial comparing hospital at home care with inpatient hospital care. II: cost minimization analysis. BMJ 1998; 316(7147):1791–1796.

28. Ruchlin HS, Dasbach EJ. An economic overview of chronic obstructive pulmonary disease. Pharmacoeconomics 2001; 19(6):623–642.

29. Coast J, Richards SH, Peters TJ, Gunnell DJ, Darlow MA, Pounsford J. Hospital at home or acute hospital care? A cost minimization analysis. BMJ 1998; 316(7147):1802–1806.

30. Skwarska E, Cohen G, Skwarski KM, Lamb C, Bushell D, Parker S et al. Randomized controlled trial of supported discharge in patients with exacerbations of chronic obstructive pulmonary disease. Thorax 2000; 55(11):907–912.

31. Cotton MM, Bucknall CE, Dagg KD, Johnson MK, MacGregor G, Stewart C, Stevenson RD. Early discharge for patients with exacerbations of chronic obstructive pulmonary disease: a randomized controlled trial. Thorax 2000; 55(11):902–906.

32. Davies L, Wilkinson M, Bonner S, Calverley PM, Angus RM. "Hospital at home" versus hospital care in patients with exacerbations of chronic obstructive pulmonary disease: prospective randomized controlled trial. BMJ 2000; 321(7271):1265–1268.

33. Sala E, Alegre L, Carrera M, Ibars M, Orriols FJ, Blanco ML, Carceles F, Bertran S, Mata F, Font I, Agusti AG. Supported discharge shortens hospital stay in patients hospitalized because of an exacerbation of COPD. Eur Respir J 2001; 17(6):1138–1142.

34. Hernandez C, Casas A, Escarrabill J, Alonso J, Puig-Junoy J, Farrero E, Vilagut G, Collivinent B, Rodriguez-Roisin R, Roca J and partners of the CHRONIC project. Home hospitalization of exacerbated COPD patients. Eur Respir J 2002; 21:58–67.

35. Stewart S, Marley JE, Horowitz JD. Effects of a multidisciplinary, home-based intervention on unplanned readmissions and survival among patients with chronic congestive heart failure: a randomised controlled study. Lancet 1999; 354:1077–1083.

36. Stewart S, Vandenbroek AJ, Pearson S, Horowith JD. Prolonged beneficial effects of a home-based intervention on unplanned readmissions and mortality among patients with congestive heart failure. Arch Intern Med 1999; 159(3):257–261.

37. Stewart S, Pearson S, Horowitz JD. Effects of a home-based intervention among patients with congestive heart failure discharged from acute hospital care. Arch Intern Med 1998; 158(10):1067–1072.

38. Rich MW, Beckham V, Wittenberg C, Leven CL, Freedland KE, Carney RM. A multidisciplinary intervention to prevent the readmission of elderly patients with congestive heart failure. N England J Med 1995; 333:1190–1195.

39. Mundinger MO, Kane RL, Lenz ER, Totten AM, Tsai WY, Cleary PD, Friedewald WT, Siu AL, Shelanski ML. Primary care outcomes in patients treated by nurse practitioners or physicians: a randomized trial. JAMA 2000; 283(1):59–68.

40. Littlejohns P, Baveystock CM, Parnell H, Jones PW. Randomised controlled trial of the effectiveness of a respiratory health worker in reducing impairment, disability, and handicap due to chronic airflow limitation. Thorax 1991; 46:559–564.

41. Campbell M, Stockdale-Woolley R, Nair S. Respi-care. An innovative home care program for the patient with chronic obstructive pulmonary disease. Chest 1991; 100:607–612.

42. Farrero E, Escarrabill J, Prats E, Maderal M, Manresa F. Impact of a hospital-based home-care program on the management of COPD patients receiving long-term oxygen therapy. Chest 2001; 119:364–369.

43. Güell R, González A, Morante F, Sangnenís C, Sotomayor C, Caballero C, Sanchís J. Mejor en casa: un programa de asistencia continuada para los pacientes con enfermedad respiratoria crónica avanzada. Arch Bronconeumol 1998; 34:541–546.

44. Smith BJ, Appleton SL, Bennett PW, Roberts GC, Del Fante P, Adams R, Trott CM, Allan DP, Southcott AM, Ruffin RE. The effect of a respiratory home nurse intervention in patients with chronic obstructive pulmonary disease (COPD). Aust NZ J Med 1999; 29:718–725.

45. Prabhakar NR. Sleep apneas. An oxidative stress? Am J Respir Crit Care Med 2002; 165:859–860.

46. Morgan MDL (chairman). BTS standards of care subcommittee on pulmonary rehabilitation. Thorax 2001; 56:827–883.

47. Giffiths T, Burr ML, Campbell IA, Lewis-Jenkins V, Mullins J, Shiels K, Turner-Lawlor PJ, Payne N, Newcombe RG, Ionescu AA, Thomas J, Tunbridge J. Results of 1 year of outpatient multidisciplinary pulmonary rehabilitation: a randomized controlled trial. Lancet 2000; 355:362–368.

48. Casanova C, Celli BR, Tost L, Soriano E, Abreu J, Velasco V, Santolaria F. Long-term controlled trial of nocturnal nasal positive pressure ventilation in patients with severe COPD. Chest 2000; 118:1582–1590.

49. Rahow MW, McPhee SJ. End-of-life literature. Chest 2001; 120:1426–1427.
50. Rahow MW, Hardie GE, Fair JM, McPhee SJ. End-of-life care content in 50 textbooks from multiple specilities. JAMA 2000; 283:771–778.
51. Billing JA. Palliative care. BMJ 2000; 321:555–558.
52. Luce JM, Luce JA. Management of dypsnea in patients with far-advanced lung disease. JAMA 2001; 285:1331–1337.
53. Petty TL. Technology transfer and continuity of care by a "consultant." Ann Intern Med 2000; 132:587–588.
54. Brooks CM, Richards JM, Kohler CL, Soong SJ, Martin B, Windsor RA, Bailey WC. Assessing adherence to asthma medication and inhaler regimens: a psychometric analysis of adult self-report scales. Med Care 1994; 32(3):298–307.
55. Gallefoss F, Bakke PS. How does patient education and self-management among asthmatics and patients with chronic obstructive pulmonary disease affect medication? Am J Respir Crit Care Med 1999; 160(6):2000–2005.
56. Watson PB, Town GI, Holbrook N, Dwan C, Toop LJ, Drennan CJ. Evaluation of a self-management plan for chronic obstructive pulmonary disease. Eur Respir J 1997; 10(6):1267–1271.
57. Murray CJ, Lopez AD. Global mortality, disability, and the contribution of risk factors: Global Burden of Disease Study. Lancet 1997; 349(9063):1436–1442.
58. Strassels SA, Smith DH, Sullivan SD, Mahajan PS. The costs of treating COPD in the United States. Chest 2001; 119(2):344 352.

30

Hospital Management of Acute Exacerbations of Chronic Obstructive Pulmonary Disease

ALVAR G.N. AGUSTÍ, MIGUEL CARRERA, and ERNEST SALA

Son Dureta Hospital
Palma de Mallorca, Spain

I. Introduction

This chapter presents an integrated view of the management of patients hospitalized because of an acute exacerbation of COPD (AECOPD) (1–5). It does not address the management of AECOPD in the community, nor does it discuss in depth the individual aspects of each of the different therapeutic options available (Table 1, Evidence A–D), because both are covered at length in other chapters of this book.

The management of AECOPD in hospital can pursue several goals, including (2, 5) (1) the stabilization of the respiratory and hemodynamic situation of the patient; (2) the recovery or improvement (if possible) of the baseline clinical condition of the patient; (3) the correct diagnosis of the causes of the AECOPD; (4) the assessment of the severity of the baseline disease (COPD) as well as the identification of any potential comorbid condition present; (5) the education of the patient on the proper use of medications and therapeutic devices, as well as on an adequate, health-promoting lifestyle to engage with after discharge; and, finally (6) the assessment of the need of additional treatment at home, such as pulmonary rehabilitation and/or domiciliary oxygen therapy. The achievement of these different goals requires the management of the patient in different areas/settings of the hospital [emergency room, hospitalization ward, intensive care unit (ICU)]. The text that follows discusses (1) the initial management of the patient with AECOPD in the

Table 1 Description of Levels of Evidence

Evidence category	Sources of evidence	Definition
A	RCTs; rich body of data	Evidence is from endpoints of well-designed RCTs that provide a consistent pattern of findings in the population for which the recommendation is made. Category A requires substantial numbers of studies involving substantial numbers of participants.
B	RCTs; limited body of data	Evidence is from endpoints of intervention studies that include only a limited number of patients, posthoc or subgroup analysis of RCTs, or meta-analysis of RCTs. In general, Category B pertains when few randomized trials exist, they are small in size, or they were undertaken in a population that differs from the target population of the recommendation, or the results are somewhat inconsistent.
C	Nonrandomized trials; observational studies	Evidence is from outcomes of uncontrolled or nonrandomized trials or from observational studies.
D	Panel consensus judgment	This category is used only in cases where the provision of some guidance was deemed valuable but the clinical literature addressing the subject was deemed insufficient to justify placement in one of the other categories. The Panel Consensus is based on clinical experience or knowledge that does not meet the above-listed criteria.

RCTs, randomized controlled trials.

emergency room; (2) the criteria for hospitalization; (3) the management of AECOPD in the ward; (4) the management of AECOPD in the ICU; and (5) the criteria for discharge from each of these different care levels (ICU, ward); and (6) identification of unresolved issues that need more research and speculates on potential future alternatives.

II. Initial Management in the Emergency Room

A. Assessment of Severity

Table 2 presents the main components of the initial evaluation of a patient with suspected AECOPD in the emergency room. The information provided by the clinical history, physical examination, chest x-ray, and arterial blood gas values allows to (1) establish the diagnosis of AECOPD; (2) grade its severity; (3) identify

Table 2 Initial Components of Emergency Room Evaluation of Patients with AECOPD

Clinical history
    Baseline respiratory status
    Smoking history
    Previous exacerbations and whether they require hospitalization
    Sputum volume and color
    Baseline resting dyspnea
    Prior measurements of lung function and arterial blood gases
    Length and rate of onset of symptoms
    Level of activity
    Home therapeutic regimen and compliance
    Social circumstances
    Comorbid conditions
    Severity of symptoms
    Cor pulmonale
    Bronchospasm
    Pneumonia
    Hemodynamic instability
    Level of consciousness
    Paraxodical abdominal retractions
    Use of accessory respiratory muscles
    Acute comorbid conditions
Laboratory
    Blood gases
    ECG
    Chest radiograph
    Whole blood count and biochemical test
    Sputum culture

---

its causes; and (4) decide the need for hospitalization, oxygen therapy and/or ventilatory support (6, 7) (evidence D). In contrast, the severity of airflow obstruction present when the patient was clinically stable (before AECOPD) is useless to assess the severity of the current episode of AECOPD, the need for hospitalization and/or the time for discharge (6–8). Finally, it is necessary to rule out (and treat, if necessary) other morbid conditions that can contribute to worsen the clinical situation of the patient, such as heart failure, pulmonary emboli, pneumonia, and/or intake of sedatives, among others. These, however, should not be conceptually considered *causes* of AECOPD (9). This consideration is important in order to dissect clearly the mechanisms of AECOPD (and, therefore, its appropriate management) from that of other disease states that may impact on the patient with COPD, independently of his (her) basic disease process.

B. Initial Therapeutic Measures

Oxygen Therapy

If the clinical condition of the patient allows it, arterial blood gases should be measured before starting oxygen therapy. The goal of oxygen therapy is to achieve an arterial partial pressure of O_2 (PaO_2) greater than 60 mmHg (8.0 kPa) or an arterial oxyhemoglobin saturation value (SaO_2) higher than 90%. To avoid a simultaneous rise in arterial PCO_2 and a fall in arterial pH, the lowest inspiratory fraction of oxygen (FiO_2) should be used (evidence A) (2–5, 10).

Bronchodilators

The administration of aerosolized, short-acting β_2-agonists (Table 3) is the bronchodilator treatment of choice in the initial management of AECOPD (evidence A) (2, 3, 10). If this does not result in a rapid clinical improvement, the combination with anticholinergic bronchodilators is recommended (evidence B) (2, 5, 8, 10). The use of subcutaneous or intravenous β_2-agonists is not recommended for routine use. It can be considered in life-threatening conditions and when the inhaled route is not available.

Steroids

Oral or intravenous steroids are efficacious in the treatment of AECOPD (evidence A) and should therefore be used routinely (6, 7, 10). An initial dose of 0.5 mg/kg of 6–8 h of prednisolone has been empirically recommended (evidence D) (3, 4, 10). Given that undesirable side effects (mostly hyperglycemia) are not rare (11), whether smaller doses may be equally effective needs to be tested prospectively.

Antibiotics

The use of antibiotics in the management of AECOPD is controversial. When invasive and sophisticated research techniques (such as the endoscopic sampling of

Table 3   Bronchodilator Dosages in AECOPD

	MDI (µg)	Nebulizer (mg)	Endovenous (mg/min)	Time to onset (min)	Time to peak (min)	Duration (h)
Fenoterol	100–200	0.5–	—			4–6
Salbutamol	100–200	2.5–5	4	3–5	60–90	4–6
Terbutaline	250–500	5–10	0.005	3–5	60–90	3–6
Formoterol	12–24	—	—	5	60–90	11–12
Salmeterol	50–100	—	—	45–60	120–240	11–12
Ipratropium Br.	40–80	0.25–0.5	—	5–15	60–120	6–8

the tracheo-bronchial secretions with a protected brush) are used in patients with AECOPD, only in about 65% of all episodes can bacteria be identified (12–16). It would be then in these cases (but not in the 35% remaining) where antibiotics may play a role in the management of AECOPD. However, these research techniques can not be used routinely in practice and the identification of this particular subset of AECOPD episodes just on clinical grounds is difficult. Because of these difficulties, therefore, and following Anthonisen pioneering work (17), antibiotics are recommended for the management of AECOPD in those episodes that fulfill at least two of the following criteria: increased breathlessness, increased volume of expectoration or increased sputum purulence. These criteria have been later extended to all those AECOPD episodes accompanied by acute (or acute on chronic) respiratory failure (evidence B) (3–5, 7, 10).

Other Measures

A proper assessment of the clinical condition of the patient in the emergency room may advocate the need of other therapeutic measures, including the administration of fluids and electrolytes and the use of diuretics, anticoagulants and any other drug deemed necessary for the treatment of the individual patient under examination.

III. Criteria for Hospitalization

After the assessment in the emergency room and the initiation of the treatment measures discussed above, a decision on the need for hospitalization or discharge, as well as on the precise care level needed in the former case (ward, ICU), has to be taken. However, there is no single clinical or biological marker useful for this purpose. This decision has to be based upon the global interpretation (necessarily of subjective nature) of the clinical condition of the patient, the response to the therapeutic measures instituted and the severity of any comorbid condition present. Table presents a summary of the criteria generally recommended for such decision (evidence D) (2–5, 10). Although, individually, none of these criteria constitutes an absolute indication for hospitalization, the greater the number present the more likely is the need for hospital care.

IV. Management in the Ward

A. Pharmacological Measures

Bronchodilators

Short-acting β_2-agonists and anticholinergic drugs constitute the cornerstone of bronchodilator treatment of AECOPD during hospitalization (evidence A) (7, 15).

Despite the fact that both have similar bronchodilator potency (6, 7, 18), the former is normally recommended for its faster onset of action (evidence A) (2, 10). When the clinical response to high doses of inhaled short-acting β_2-agonists is unsatisfactory, anticholinergics are also recommended (2–5, 10). Whether the

Table 4   Indications for Hospitalization in AECOPD

Failure to respond to initial medical management
Increased dyspnea plus inability to eat, sleep and/or walk between rooms
Insufficient home support
Altered mental status
Cyanosis
Rapid onset of symptoms
Prolonged and progressive symptoms before emergency visit
Severe comorbidities or poor general condition
Worsening peripheral edema
Changes on the chest radiograph
Arterial pH < 7.35
Temperature $> 38.5°C$
Respiratory frequency > 25 breaths/min
Heart rate > 110 beats/min
Acute respiratory failure
Diagnostic uncertainty

combination of both (short-acting β_2-agonists and anticholinergics) is better than the use of high doses of any one of them alone is controversial (10, 18).

In the management of hospitalized patients with AECOPD, short-acting β_2-agonists and anticholinergics are normally given every 4 to 6 h (Table 3). This period of time can be shortened if required by the clinical condition of the patient (2). The inhaled route is recommended for their administration because of its high efficacy and low rate of side effects (evidence A) (6, 7). In hospitalized patients, nebulizers are commonly used for this purpose but metered-dose inhaler devices (MDI) are equally effective if the patient is able to coordinate and perform the inhalatory maneuver correctly (evidence A) (2, 7).

When the response to inhaled treatment with short-acting β_2-agonists and anticholinergics is unsatisfactory, intravenous treatment with methylxanthines can also be considered (bolus of aminophylline of 2.5–5 mg/kg over 30 min, followed by a maintenance perfusion of 0.5 mg/kg/h) (evidence B) (2, 3, 10, 19, 20). If used, monitoring of theophylline plasma levels is mandatory (2–4, 10, 19).

To date, there is no evidence to recommend the use of long-acting β_2-agonists in the management of AECOPD. This is, however, an area that clearly needs research, particularly in those patients who were already being treated with such drugs when clinically stable (21).

Steroids

The systemic administration of glucocorticoids is efficacious in the hospital management of AECOPD (evidence A) (6, 7, 10). Its use enhances the recovery of airflow obstruction (as assessed by FEV_1), shortens hospital stay, and reduces the number of readmissions due to AECOPD (7, 11, 22, 23). However, their optimal dose (and timing for tapering) has not been determined precisely. Normally, prednisolone is recommended (empirically) at a dose of 0.5 mg/kg of 6–8 h (orally or intravenously) during the first 72 h (3, 4, 10, 24) with later tapering until its complete stop in about 2 weeks (evidence D) (3, 7, 10, 23).

Antibiotics

As discussed above, the use of antibiotics in the management of AECOPD is a highly controversial topic. It is generally thought that infections of the tracheobronchial tree (both of viral and bacterial origin) are the main cause (but clearly not the only one) of AECOPD (25). This idea is supported by some evidence. First, using invasive techniques bacteria can be isolated from the tracheobronchial tree in about 65% of patients with AECOPD (12). However, under stable conditions, about 35% of patients are chronically colonized by bacteria (8, 12). If this is considered, then only in about 30% of the episodes of AECOPD could new bacterial pathogens be identified. Clearly, viruses can also play a mechanistic role and, in fact, using the polymerase chain reaction, viruses can be identified in about 30% of episodes of AECOPD (26). However, for the purposes of discussing the adequacy of antibiotic usage in AECOPD, viruses are irrelevant. In summary, available evidence suggests that bacteria probably play a mechanistic role in some (but certainly not all) AECOPD. Accordingly, in theory, antibiotics should be indicated only in these cases. The problem, obviously, is how to identify reliably the episodes of AECOPD due to bacterial infection. This is an area that clearly needs research. In the meantime, antibiotic treatment is normally recommended in those episodes of AECOPD that fulfill at least two of the following criteria: increased breathlessness, fever, increased volume of expectoration or increased sputum purulence (evidence B) (3, 4, 7, 10, 17). Antibiotics can also be indicated in those AECOPD episodes that are accompanied by acute (or acute on chronic) respiratory failure (evidence B) (3, 6, 7, 27).

The most common bacteria isolated in AECOPD are *S. pneumoniae*, *H. influenzae*, and *M. catarrhalis* (12). In patients with severe COPD (i.e., with an FEV_1 of less than 35% of the reference value) Gram-negative bacilli, particularly enterobacteria and *Pseudomonas*, can also play a role (28). Due to these considerations, the empirical antibiotic regime recommended for the hospital management of AECOPD normally includes the use of cephalosporins, wide-spectrum penicillin and quinolones with antipseudomonas activity (2, 8, 15, 28). In any case, the prescription of a given antibiotic in AECOPD should consider both the level of antibiotic resistance in the local community as well as the usage of other antibiotics by the individual patient prior to hospitalization.

Other Pharmacological Measures

Low-weight molecular heparin is generally recommended in patients with restricted mobility, in those with significant polycythemia and/or significant dehydration, as well as in those with previous pulmonary emboli.

Diuretics are indicated in case of overt right-heart failure, as indicated by the presence of peripheral edema and raised jugular venous pressure.

Because magnesium, calcium, phosphate, and potassium deficits are not rare in COPD and can worsen during AECOPD, close monitoring of fluid and electrolyte balance, and proper correction if needed, is generally advised (2, 10).

Patients with COPD are often undernourished (29). This can be significantly worsened during AECOPD requiring hospitalization (29). Yet, parenteral nutrition is recommended only in severely malnourished patients in whom adequate enteral support cannot be achieved (10).

Despite its wide use in some countries, there is no evidence that ventilatory stimulants such as doxapram, almitrine, protriptyine, medroxyprogesterone, or acetazolamide offer significant benefit in AECOPD (21, 30, 31) and, in general, their use is not recommended (2–5).

B. Nonpharmacological Measures

Oxygen Therapy

Respiratory failure is almost invariably present in patients hospitalized because of AECOPD. Thus, restoration of an adequate arterial oxygenation is one of the therapeutic cornerstones in these patients. In this context, the goal of oxygen therapy is to achieve an arterial partial pressure of oxygen (PaO_2) greater than 60 mmHg (8.0 kPa), which results in an arterial oxyhemoglobin saturation (SaO_2) greater than 90%, avoiding, if possible, significant CO_2 retention that may result in acidosis (evidence A) (2–5, 10). To this end, the use of an inspiratory fraction of oxygen (FiO_2) of 0.24 or 0.28 is normally enough (3, 4, 15).

In hospitalized patients with AECOPD, oxygen therapy can be administered either by nasal prongs (less cumbersome and more comfortable for the patient) or venturi masks (which allow a more precise control of FiO_2) (3, 10, 32). If an $FiO_2 > 0.40$ is required to achieve adequate arterial oxygenation, nonrebreathing masks equipped with a reservoir and a 1-way valve are recommended (2).

Given that FiO_2 is chosen empirically and that its effects upon arterial oxygenation, CO_2 retention and pH cannot be predicted accurately in any given individual patient, arterial blood gases should be measured 30 min after every FiO_2 change. This will allow the correct assessment of the FiO_2 chosen and its further adjustment (up or down) if needed. Likewise, and for the same reasons, whenever the clinical condition of the patient changes significantly or FiO_2 is again changed (up or down), another arterial blood gas measurement should be performed (21). The use of pulse oxymetry to monitor noninvasively the level of arterial oxygen saturation is acceptable only when there is certainty that arterial pH and $PaCO_2$ values are correct (3).

Physiotherapy

There is no evidence that physiotherapy is useful in the routine management of hospitalized patients with COPD (actually, it may be deleterious because it can cause a transient decrease in FEV_1) (3, 6, 7, 33). However, in selected patients with significant (>25 mL/day) mucus production, techniques such as huff coughing and postural drainage (with or without the aid of vibration or percussion methods) may be useful (evidence D) (2, 10). The use of mucolytic drugs as well as overhydration have not been proved to be useful in these patients (6, 7).

Noninvasive Ventilatory Support

The use of noninvasive ventilatory support (NIVS) outside of the intensive care unit is also a controversial issue. In principle, the authors believe that NIVS in the ward should be restricted to selected patients. Its pros and cons, as well as the inclusion/exclusion criteria, are analyzed below, in conjunction with other ventilatory support modalities.

V. Management in the Intensive Care Unit

A. General Measures and Pharmacology

All the general and pharmacological measures discussed above for the management of the AECOPD patient hospitalized in a general ward (bronchodilators, steroids, antibiotics, oxygen therapy, etc.), are equally applicable to those patients requiring intensive care (Table 5), and will not be discussed further here.

B. Mechanical Ventilation

Patients with severe AECOPD may require ventilatory support. This can be provided invasively (that is, by means of an endotracheal tube connected to a ventilator) or noninvasively (by means of a nasal or facial mask that avoids the need of the endotracheal tube). In both instances, however, the therapeutic goals are the same: to reduce the morbidity–mortality of AECOPD; and to improve the symptoms of the patient.

Noninvasive Ventilatory Support

A recent consensus conference on the topic concluded that NIVS is useful for the treatment of patients with AECOPD and ventilatory failure (34). In these patients, NIVS (1) reduces $PaCO_2$ and increases arterial pH; (2) improves the symptoms arising from respiratory muscle fatigue (such as dyspnea); (3) shortens the length of

Table 5 Indications for Admission in ICU

Severe dyspnea despite maximum treatment
Impaired mental status or respiratory muscle fatigue
Life-threatening hypoxemia despite maximum treatment
Life-threatening acidosis (pH <7.30) despite maximum treatment
Need for mechanical ventilation

Table 6 Inclusion and Exclusion Criteria for NIPPV

Inclusion criteria	Exclusion criteria (any may be present)
pH <7.35 and PaCO$_2$ >45 mmHg	Respiratory arrest
	Nonrespiratory system failure
	Impaired mental status (Glasgow scale value <10)
	Severe upper gastrointestinal bleeding
	Cardiovascular Instability (hypotension, arrhythmias, myocardial infarction)
	Surgery, craniofacial trauma or facial deformity
	Upper airway obstruction
	Uncooperative patient
	High aspiration risk/viscous or copious secretions
	Extreme obesity

Source: Modified from Ref. 10.

stay in hospital (evidence A); and (4) reduces the need for orotracheal intubation as well as hospital mortality (35–37). Table 6 shows the inclusion/exclusion criteria for NIVS in AECOPD.

This same international consensus conference indicates that NIVS should be used only in the ICU or in units that can guarantee an adequate (high) level of monitoring (evidence D) (34). The use of NIVS in a general hospitalization ward is controversial (38, 39). In principle, NIVS in the ward should be restricted to those patients with AECOPD who have not responded adequately to the initial therapeutic measures, as shown by the presence of (1) PaCO$_2$ values that result in pH $\geq$ 7.30 (evidence D) (34); and (2) cannot be treated in an ICU due to clinical reasons (age, comorbidity) or operational conditions (lack of availability of ICU beds). NIVS can be initiated in the emergency room only if there are experienced personnel and adequate monitoring capabilities (34).

The correct use of NIVS requires (evidence D) (1) proper monitorization of SaO$_2$, arterial blood gases and vital signs; (2) adequate adaptation of the patient to the device, avoidance of gross air leaks and a preserved capacity to clear bronchopulmonary secretions; and (3) human (and technological) resources with adequate experience as to face and solve potential complications.

In patients with AECOPD four different modalities of NIVS have been used: (1) volume-cycled NIVS (35); (2) positive-pressure support ventilation (36); (3) pressure-cycled ventilation (37); and, (4) bilevel pressure ventilation (BiPAP) (i.e., different inspiratory and expiratory pressure levels) (38, 40). The selection of a particular ventilatory mode basically depends on the availability of equipment and the experience of the involved personnel.

NIVS must be adjusted individually keeping in mind the following therapeutic goals: (1) improved symptoms; (2) improved pulmonary gas exchange; and (3) avoidance of undesired side effects (34). NIVS requires the use of a mask to interface the ventilator and the patient. Two different types of masks can be used in this setting: (1) facial masks (covering both the nose and the mouth); and (2) nasal masks (covering only the former). There is no evidence to support that one type of mask is better (or worse) than the other. Yet facial masks normally allow higher pressure levels with less air leaks, require less patient collaboration and permit mouth breathing. By contrast, they are less comfortable than nasal masks and interfere with other physiological functions, such as speaking and eating. On the other hand, nasal masks require a higher degree of patient collaboration, who have to maintain their mouth closed to avoid air leaks. The selection of a particular type of mask in a particular patient depends on availability, previous experience of the caring team, and, importantly, on the goodness of the adaptation of the individual patient to a particular type of mask. In any case, NIVS is normally used intermittently, only during a limited period of time per day (6–12 h).

Invasive Mechanical Ventilation

Despite the fact that NIVS offer some advantages with respect to invasive mechanical ventilation (MV) (36), the latter has some clear indications in AECOPD, which are listed in Table 7. The therapeutic goals of MV include: (1) normalization of their pulmonary gas exchange and respiratory acidosis (41); (2) provision of adequate vital support while treatment for a specific cause of AECOPD (pneumonia, pulmonary emboli, severe bronchospasm) is given ("buy time"); and (3) resting (and recovering) the fatigued respiratory muscles (42). However, MV is not free of complications. These include: (1) barotrauma (43); (2) ultrastructural lesion of the pulmonary parenchyma, with increased pulmonary permeability and edema (44); and (3) ventilator-associated pneumonia (45). Mortality in patients with AECOPD who need MV is not higher than that of other patients who also require MV due to causes other than AECOPD (10).

Tracheal Intubation

In an emergency situation, the oral route is preferred for tracheal intubation (TI) (46). TI through the nose increases the risk of sinusitis (47), increases airway

Table 7 Indications for Invasive Mechanical Ventilation

Absolute indications	Potential indications
Respiratory arrest	Severe dyspnea with use of accessory muscles and paradoxical abdominal motion
NIPPV failure or exclusion criteria present	Respiratory rate >35 breaths/min
Life-threatening hypoxemia (PaO_2 <40 mmHg) despite maximum treatment	Cardiovascular complications (hypotension shock, heart failure)
Life-threatening acidosis (pH <7.25) despite maximum treatment	Other complications (pneumonia, pulmonary embolism, etc.)

Source: Modified from Ref. 10.

resistance (due to the smaller diameter of the tubes used) (48), and limits the efficacy of aerosolized therapy (49). Fiberoptic bronchoscopy can be used to guide TI in difficult situations (such as facial anatomic abnormalities).

Ventilatory Strategies

In patients with AECOPD, two different ventilatory strategies can be used: (1) assisted-controlled MV (CMV), either volume-cycled or pressure-cycled; and (2) pressure-support ventilation (PSV). No previous study has compared the efficacy and side effects of these different ventilatory modes in AECOPD.

Assisted-Controlled MV (ACMV). An important goal of MV in patients with AECOPD is to reduce the degree of intrinsic end-expiratory pressure (PEEPi) and dynamic hyperinflation (DH). To achieve this goal, the ventilatory strategy used during ACMV in these patients normally combines low tidal volume (VT) values (8–10 mL/kg) with increased expiratory time (TE)/inspiratory time (TI) ratios. This requires the use of low breathing frequencies and high inspiratory flows (50) and/or the use of an external end-expiratory pressure (PEEPe) to balance PEEPi (51). The latter allows (1) a reduction of the work of breathing; and (2) a reduction of air trapping (thus, PEEPi) due to the recruitment of collapsed alveolar units. To avoid an accentuation of the degree of DH, however, the level of PEEPe used should be lower than those of PEEPi (52, 53). Another ventilatory strategy that can be used in patients with AECOPD is the so-called controlled hypoventilation with permissive hypercapnia (CHPH). This is widely used in patients with adult respiratory distress syndrome (ARDS) to avoid the undesired side effects of CMV (54). In patients with AECOPD and severe airflow limitation, CHPH can improve the increased levels of PEEPi and DH (evidence D) (46). In any case, whenever CMV is used, it is imperative to monitor PEEPi levels and the peak and plateau pressure levels. The former informs on changes of respiratory mechanics and airway resistance, while the latter reflects the degree of pulmonary hyperinflation and distensibility. Plateau pressures greater than 30–35 cmH$_2$O should be avoided because they carry a high risk of barotrauma (41).

Pressure-Support Ventilation (PSV). PSV is a more comfortable mode of MV than ACMV because the patient (not the ventilator) controls VT. PSV also allows a reduction of DH and PEEPi. PSV should be individually tailored taking into account VT and the breathing frequency (f), which has to be lower than 30 breaths per minute (55). PSV can be used only in patients with AECOPD who can maintain adequate values of VT and f. In those requiring absolute rest of the respiratory muscles and in those who cannot adapt to PSV, CMV should be used preferably.

Sedation, Analgesia, and Paralysis

During MV some degree of sedation and analgesia is always necessary. In patients with AECOPD, this is normally required for the proper adaptation of the patient to the ventilator which, in turn, contributes to reduce DH as well as oxygen uptake and CO$_2$ production (46). Unless otherwise contraindicated, propofol is normally used for this purpose. This drug has some bronchodilator effect (56) and avoids the need of paralytic agents (57). Benzodiazepines and opioids, either alone or in combination, are valid alternatives. Haloperidol is normally used during weaning because it does not affect the respiratory centers. These drugs are normally administered on demand (not regularly) (58, 59). Continuous sedation prolongs the time during which MV is needed as well as the associated health-care costs. Paralytic agents should be administered in patients with severe DH or in those unable to adapt to the ventilator properly.

Bronchodilator Treatment During MV

Bronchodilator treatment is effective (and should be used) in patients with AECOPD requiring MV (60–62). It can be delivered using MDI devices or nebulizers with similar results (63). Systemic bronchodilators (and steroids) should be used following the same indications and dosages as in patients managed outside the ICU.

Weaning

Weaning is be considered when the cause of AECOPD has been corrected (or improved significantly) and the patient is clinically stable. Premature weaning attempts can (1) increase mortality (due to cardiac arrest, pneumonia and/or aspiration) (64); (2) prolong hospitalization in the ICU; and (3) increase the rehabilitation requirements (65). Weaning can be facilitated by using either a T tube (66) or NIVS (67). In patients with AECOPD, the latter strategy (1) reduces the duration of the weaning procedure; (2) reduces the hospitalization time in the ICU; (3) reduces the risk of nosocomial pneumonia; and (4) improves survival during the first 60 days after discharge from the ICU (evidence B) (67).

VI. Criteria for Discharge

A. From the ICU

There are no clearly defined criteria to discharge a patient with AECOPD requiring MV from the ICU. Clinical experience shows that, in order to consider discharge from ICU, these patients should comply with the following criteria: (1) correction (or significant improvement) of the cause of AECOPD; (2) absence of relevant medical complications that can potentially interfere with the clinical stability of the patient; (3) no need of ventilatory support; and (4) no need of intensive monitoring.

B. From the Ward

The optimal length of stay in a ward of a patient hospitalized because of AECOPD is unclear. This is mostly due to the absence of a defined set of objective criteria for discharge, which are normally based upon expert opinion (2, 10). Table 8 shows those proposed recently by the GOLD initiative (10).

C. Home-Support and Early-Discharge Programs

The scenario outlined in Table 8 may change with the recent introduction of home-support and early-discharge programs. There are now several published studies that show the feasibility, security, acceptance and health-economic consequences of these

Table 8   Discharge Criteria

Patient has been clinically stable for 24 h
Arterial blood gases has been stable for 24 h
Patient (or home caregiver) fully understands correct use of medications
Follow-up and home-care arrangements have been completed
Patient, family, and physician are confident patient can manage successfully

Source: Modified from Ref. 10.

alternative programs (68, 69–72). These studies have shown that about 20 to 30% of patients with AECOPD attended at the emergency room, who would otherwise qualify for hospitalization, can be sent home directly and managed there safely and efficiently if adequate nurse support is provided (68–70). Likewise, these studies have clearly highlighted the possibility of combining a short hospital stay during the first few hours of AECOPD and early discharge with home support (71, 72). This latter alternative can be offered to a wider group of patients with equally good results (71, 72).

D.   Ambulatory Follow-Up

It is normally advised that patients discharged from hospital because of an AECOPD should be visited in the ambulatory clinic between 4 and 6 weeks after discharge (evidence D) (10). Table 9 lists the main variables to check in that control visit. If the patient presented respiratory failure during AECOPD, arterial blood gases must be investigated at this point to decide whether or not the patient needs domiciliary oxygen therapy. This decision cannot be taken on the basis of the arterial blood gas measurements obtained at discharge (10). After this initial post-hospitalization visit, ambulatory follow up should be that of any patient with stable COPD.

VII.   Summary and Future Prospects

Despite that many aspects of COPD management have changed significantly over the past few years (73) including, perhaps, the natural history of the disease (74), episodes of hospitalization due to AECOPD still constitute a big burden for health

Table 9   Follow-Up Assessment 4 to 6 Weeks After Discharge from Hospital for AECOPD

Measurement of FEV_1
Reassessment of inhaler technique
Understanding of recommended treatment regimen
Need for long-term oxygen therapy or home nebulizer (for patients with severe COPD)

Source: Modified from Ref. 10.

care all over the world. In this chapter, we have reviewed the basic principles of their hospital management trying to provide the level of evidence for each of the statements made whenever available. By doing so, this review has also highlighted several management gaps which lack the necessary level of evidence and, therefore, need more research. The following are examples of what the authors believe are items that require further investigation.

A. Better Understanding of the Basic Mechanisms of AECOPD

The pathophysiology of many AECOPD episodes is unclear and, until we have a better understanding of the mechanisms underlying many of these episodes, treatment will continue to be mostly symptomatic. Traditionally, the hypothesis that AECOPD basically equates "airway infection" has prevailed. However, even with the aid of invasive and sophisticated techniques, in a substantial percentage of AECOPD episodes (perhaps in as much as 50% of them) bacterial pathogens cannot be clearly identified (12). This observation is often overlooked but, in the opinion of the authors, it clearly indicates the need of a more open-minded approach in this area. For instance, the "infective approach" discussed above is based upon the idea of an "external" trigger for AECOPD (in this case, a virus and/or a bacteria). In theory, however, it is also possible that AECOPD (at least, a given percentage of them) are not really due to any "external" trigger but to an "internal" one. In fact, many nonpulmonary chronic inflammatory diseases (e.g., rheumatoid arthritis) also present "episodes of exacerbation" which, at variance to COPD, are normally thought to be an integral part of the disease process. Whether this may occur in COPD (also a chronic inflammatory disease) is not known, but a better understanding of these aspects of the pathophysiology of AECOPD may very likely provide new insights in the future that may eventually lead to new and more rational therapeutic alternatives.

B. Clarification of the Role of Existing Therapeutic Options

Several therapeutic options currently available for AECOPD still lack the necessary scientific evidence for their proper positioning in the global strategy of their hospital management. For instance, the role of long acting β_2-agonist for the treatment of AECOPD has not been analyzed. Likewise, despite that NIV has clear beneficial effects when used in the ICU (34), it is still unclear when and how to use it outside the ICU (38, 39). Finally, the use of antibiotics for the hospital management of AECOPD is a long-standing, unresolved issue. Probably, this will continue to be so until we have some surrogate marker of *bacterial* airway infection that can identify reliably those patients who can benefit most from this treatment.

C. Evidence-Based Criteria for Hospitalization and Discharge

The criteria for hospitalization and discharge discussed above are based on clinical experience and "expert opinion" (2–5). Over the past few years, new forms of hospital management of AECOPD have been published, including full home support and short hospitalization followed by early discharge and home support (68, 69–72). These new forms of care require a better definition (based on evidence, if possible) of the criteria for hospitalization and discharge. This will result in a better and more comfortable care of the patient as well as in a more rational use of health-care resources.

References

1. Rodriguez-Roisin R. Toward a consensus definition for COPD exacerbations. Chest 2000; 117(5 suppl 2):398S–401S.
2. Standards for the diagnosis and care of patients with chronic obstructive pulmonary disease. American Thoracic Society. Am J Respir Crit Care Med 1995; 152(5 Pt 2):S77–S121.
3. BTS guidelines for the management of chronic obstructive pulmonary disease. The COPD Guidelines Group of the Standards of Care Committee of the BTS. Thorax 1997; 52(suppl 5):S1–S28.
4. Barbera J, Peces-Barba G, Agustí A, Izquierdo J, Monso E, Montemayor T, Viejo J. Clinical guidelines for diagnosing and treating chronic obstructive pulmonary disease. Arch Bronconeumol 2001; 37(6):297–316.
5. Siafakas NM, Vermeire P, Pride NB, Paoletti P, Gibson J, Howard P, Yernault JC, Decramer M, Higenbottam TW, Postma DS, Rees J. Optimal assessment and management of chronic obstructive pulmonary disease (COPD). European Respiratory Society consensus statement. Eur Respir J 1995; 8:1398–1420.
6. Snow V, Lascher S, Mottur-Pilson C. Evidence base for management of acute exacerbations of chronic obstructive pulmonary disease. Ann Intern Med 2001; 134:595–599.
7. Bach PB, Brown C, Gelfand SE, McCrory DC. Management of acute exacerbations of chronic obstructive pulmonary disease: a summary and appraisal of published evidence. Ann Intern Med 2001; 134(7):600–620.
8. Madison JM, Irwin RS. Chronic obstructive pulmonary disease. Lancet 1998; 352(9126):467–473.
9. Voelkel NF, Tuder R. COPD: exacerbation. Chest 2000; 117(5 suppl 2):376S–379S.
10. Pauwels RA, Buist AS, Calverley PM, Jenkins CR, Hurd SS. Global strategy for the diagnosis, management, and prevention of chronic obstructive pulmonary disease. NHLBI/WHO Global Initiative for Chronic Obstructive Lung Disease (GOLD) Workshop summary. Am J Respir Crit Care Med 2001; 163(5):1256–1276.
11. Niewoehner DE, Erbland ML, Deupree RH, Collins D, Gross NJ, Light RW, Anderson P, Morgan NA. Effect of systemic glucocorticoids on exacerbations of chronic obstructive pulmonary disease. Department of Veterans Affairs Cooperative Study Group. N Engl J Med 1999; 340(25):1941–1947.
12. Monso E, Ruiz J, Rosell A, Manterola J, Fiz J, Morera J, Ausina V. Bacterial infection in chronic obstructive pulmonary disease. A study of stable and exacerbated outpatients using the protected specimen brush. Am J Respir Crit Care Med 1995; 152(4 Pt 1):1316–1320.
13. Fagon JY, Chastre J, Trouillet JL, Domart Y, Dombret MC, Bornet M, Gibert C. Characterization of distal bronchial microflora during acute exacerbation of chronic bronchitis. Use of the protected specimen brush technique in 54 mechanically ventilated patients. Am Rev Respir Dis 1990; 142(5):1004–1008.

14. Gump DW, Phillips CA, Forsyth BR, McIntosh K, Lamborn KR, Stouch WH. Role of infection in chronic bronchitis. Am Rev Respir Dis 1976; 113(4):465–474.
15. Sherk PA, Grossman RF. The chronic obstructive pulmonary disease exacerbation. Clin Chest Med 2000; 21(4):705–721.
16. Soler N, Torres A, Ewig S, Gonzalez J, Celis R, El Ebiary M, Hernandez C, Rodriguez-Roisin R. Bronchial microbial patterns in severe exacerbations of chronic obstructive pulmonary disease (COPD) requiring mechanical ventilation. Am J Respir Crit Care Med 1998; 157(5 Pt 1):1498–1505.
17. Anthonisen NR, Manfreda J, Warren CP, Hershfield ES, Harding GK, Nelson NA. Antibiotic therapy in exacerbations of chronic obstructive pulmonary disease. Ann Intern Med 1987; 106(2):196–204.
18. McCrory DC, Brown CD. Inhaled short-acting β_2-agonists versus ipratropium for acute exacerbations of chronic obstructive pulmonary disease (Cochrane Review). Cochrane Database Syst Rev 2001; 2:CD002984.
19. Barbera JA, Reyes A, Roca J, Montserrat JM, Wagner PD, Rodriguez-Roisin R. Effect of intravenously administered aminophylline on ventilation/perfusion inequality during recovery from exacerbations of chronic obstructive pulmonary disease. Am Rev Respir Dis 1992; 145(6):1328–1333.
20. Murciano D, Aubier M, Lecocguic Y, Pariente R. Effects of theophylline on diaphragmatic strength and fatigue in patients with chronic obstructive pulmonary disease. N Engl J Med 1984; 311(6):349–353.
21. Ferguson GT. Update on pharmacologic therapy for chronic obstructive pulmonary disease. Clin Chest Med 2000; 21(4):723–738.
22. McEvoy CE, Niewoehner DE. Corticosteroids in chronic obstructive pulmonary disease. Clinical benefits and risks. Clin Chest Med 2000; 21(4):739–752.
23. Davies L, Angus RM, Calverley PMA. Oral corticosteroids in patients admitted to hospital with exacerbations of chronic obstructive pulmonary disease: a prospective randomised trial. Lancet 1999; 354:456–460.
24. Jantz MA, Sahn SA. Corticosteroids in acute respiratory failure. State of the art. Am J Respir Crit Care Med 1999; 160:1079–1100.
25. Sethi S. Infectious etiology of acute exacerbations of chronic bronchitis. Chest 2000; 117(5 suppl 2):380S–385S.
26. Banner AS. Emerging role of corticosteroids in chronic obstructive pulmonary disease. Lancet 1999; 354:440–441.
27. Saint S, Bent S, Vittinghoff E, Grady D. Antibiotics in chronic obstructive pulmonary disease exacerbations. A meta-analysis. JAMA 1995; 273:957–960.
28. Eller J, Ede A, Schaberg T, Niederman MS, Mauch H, Lode H. Infective exacerbations of chronic bronchitis: relation between bacteriologic etiology and lung function. Chest 1998; 113(6):1542–1548.
29. Schols AM, Wouters EF. Nutritional abnormalities and supplementation in chronic obstructive pulmonary disease. Clin Chest Med 2000; 21(4):753–762.
30. Greenstone M. Doxapram for ventilatory failure due to exacerbations of chronic obstructive pulmonary disease. Cochrane Database Syst Rev 2000; (2):CD000223.
31. Jones PW, Greenstone M. Carbonic anhydrase inhibitors for hypercapnic ventilatory failure in chronic obstructive pulmonary disease (Cochrane Review). Cochrane Database Syst Rev 2001; 1:CD002881.
32. Agusti AG, Carrera M, Barbe F, Munoz A, Togores B. Oxygen therapy during exacerbations of chronic obstructive pulmonary disease. Eur Respir J 1999; 14(4):934–939.

33. Jones AP, Rowe BH. Bronchopulmonary hygiene physical therapy for chronic obstructive pulmonary disease and bronchiectasis. Cochrane Database Syst Rev 2000; (2):CD000045.

34. International Consensus Conferences in Intensive Care Medicine: noninvasive positive pressure ventilation in acute respiratory failure. Am J Respir Crit Care Med 2001; 163(1):283–291.

35. Bott J, Carroll MP, Conway JH, Keilty SE, Ward EM, Brown AM, Paul EA, Elliott MW, Godfrey RC, Wedzicha JA. Randomised controlled trial of nasal ventilation in acute ventilatory failure due to chronic obstructive airways disease. Lancet 1993; 341(8860):1555–1557.

36. Brochard L, Mancebo J, Wysocki M, Lofaso F, Conti G, Rauss A, Simonneau G, Benito S, Gasparetto A, Lemaire F. Noninvasive ventilation for acute exacerbations of chronic obstructive pulmonary disease. N Engl J Med 1995; 333(13):817–822.

37. Plant PK, Owen JL, Elliott MW. Non-invasive ventilation in acute exacerbations of chronic obstructive pulmonary disease: long term survival and predictors of in-hospital outcome. Thorax 2001; 56(9):708–712.

38. Barbe F, Togores B, Rubi M, Pons S, Maimo A, Agusti AG. Noninvasive ventilatory support does not facilitate recovery from acute respiratory failure in chronic obstructive pulmonary disease. Eur Respir J 1996; 9(6):1240–1245.

39. Plant PK, Owen JL, Elliott MW. Early use of non-invasive ventilation for acute exacerbations of chronic obstructive pulmonary disease on general respiratory wards: a multicentre randomised controlled trial. Lancet 2000; 355(9219):1931–1935.

40. Kramer N, Meyer TJ, Meharg J, Cece RD, Hill NS. Randomized, prospective trial of noninvasive positive pressure ventilation in acute respiratory failure. Am J Respir Crit Care Med 1995; 151(6):1799–1806.

41. Slutsky AS. Mechanical ventilation. American College of Chest Physicians' Consensus Conference. Chest 1993; 104(6):1833–1859.

42. Aldrich TK. Respiratory muscle fatigue. Clin Chest Med 1988; 9(2):225–236.

43. Jantz MA, Pierson DJ. Pneumothorax and barotrauma. Clin Chest Med 1994; 15(1):75–91.

44. Webb HH, Tierney DF. Experimental pulmonary edema due to intermittent positive pressure ventilation with high inflation pressures. Protection by positive end-expiratory pressure. Am Rev Respir Dis 1974; 110(5):556–565.

45. Cook DJ, Walter SD, Cook RJ, Griffith LE, Guyatt GH, Leasa D, Jaeschke RZ, Brun-Buisson C. Incidence of and risk factors for ventilator-associated pneumonia in critically ill patients. Ann Intern Med 1998; 129(6):433–440.

46. Sethi JM, Siegel MD. Mechanical ventilation in chronic obstructive lung disease. Clin Chest Med 2000; 21(4):799–818.

47. Michelson A, Schuster B, Kamp HD. Paranasal sinusitis associated with nasotracheal and orotracheal long-term intubation. Arch Otolaryngol Head Neck Surg 1992; 118(9):937–939.

48. Wright PE, Marini JJ, Bernard GR. In vitro versus in vivo comparison of endotracheal tube airflow resistance. Am Rev Respir Dis 1989; 140(1):10–16.

49. Crogan SJ, Bishop MJ. Delivery efficiency of metered dose aerosols given via endotracheal tubes. Anesthesiology 1989; 70(6):1008–1010.

50. Connors AF, Jr., McCaffree DR, Gray BA. Effect of inspiratory flow rate on gas exchange during mechanical ventilation. Am Rev Respir Dis 1981; 124(5):537–543.

51. Smith TC, Marini JJ. Impact of PEEP on lung mechanics and work of breathing in severe airflow obstruction. J Appl Physiol 1988; 65(4):1488–1499.

52. Ranieri VM, Giuliani R, Cinnella G, Pesce C, Brienza N, Ippolito EL, Pomo V, Fiore T, Gottfried SB, Brienza A. Physiologic effects of positive end-expiratory pressure in patients with chronic obstructive pulmonary disease during acute ventilatory failure and controlled mechanical ventilation. Am Rev Respir Dis 1993; 147(1):5–13.
53. Georgopoulos D, Giannouli E, Patakas D. Effects of extrinsic positive end-expiratory pressure on mechanically ventilated patients with chronic obstructive pulmonary disease and dynamic hyperinflation. Intens Care Med 1993; 19(4):197–203.
54. Tobin MJ. Advances in mechanical ventilation. N Engl J Med 2001; 344(26):1986–1996.
55. MacIntyre NR. Respiratory function during pressure support ventilation. Chest 1986; 89(5):677–683.
56. Conti G, Dell'Utri D, Vilardi V, De Blasi RA, Pelaia P, Antonelli M, Bufi M, Rosa G, Gasparetto A. Propofol induces bronchodilation in mechanically ventilated chronic obstructive pulmonary disease (COPD) patients. Acta Anaesthesiol Scand 1993; 37(1):105–109.
57. Santamaria LB, Fodale V, Mandolfino T, Lucanto T, de LV, I, Ballistreri I, Spavara M. [Transdermal scopolamine reduces nausea, vomiting and sialorrhea in the postoperative period in teeth and mouth surgery]. Minerva Anestesiol 1991; 57(9):686–687.
58. Kress JP, Pohlman AS, O'Connor MF, Hall JB. Daily interruption of sedative infusions in critically ill patients undergoing mechanical ventilation. N Engl J Med 2000; 342(20):1471–1477.
59. Kollef MH, Levy NT, Ahrens TS, Schaiff R, Prentice D, Sherman G. The use of continuous i.v. sedation is associated with prolongation of mechanical ventilation. Chest 1998; 114(2):541–548.
60. Manthous CA, Chatila W, Schmidt GA, Hall JB. Treatment of bronchospasm by metered-dose inhaler albuterol in mechanically ventilated patients. Chest 1995; 107(1):210–213.
61. O'Riordan TG, Greco MJ, Perry RJ, Smaldone GC. Nebulizer function during mechanical ventilation. Am Rev Respir Dis 1992; 145(5):1117–1122.
62. Dhand R, Duarte AG, Jubran A, Jenne JW, Fink JB, Fahey PJ, Tobin MJ. Dose-response to bronchodilator delivered by metered-dose inhaler in ventilator-supported patients. Am J Respir Crit Care Med 1996; 154(2 Pt 1):388–393.
63. Rabatin JT, Gay PC. Noninvasive ventilation. Mayo Clin Proc 1999; 74(8):817–820.
64. Esteban A, Alia I, Gordo F, Fernandez R, Solsona JF, Vallverdu I, Macias S, Allegue JM, Blanco J, Carriedo D, Leon M, De La Cal MA, Taboada F, Gonzalez D, Palazon E, Carrizosa F, Tomas R, Suarez J, Goldwasser RS. Extubation outcome after spontaneous breathing trials with T-tube or pressure support ventilation. The Spanish Lung Failure Collaborative Group. Am J Respir Crit Care Med 1997; 156(2 Pt 1):459–465.
65. Epstein SK, Ciubotaru RL, Wong JB. Effect of failed extubation on the outcome of mechanical ventilation. Chest 1997; 112(1):186–192.
66. Esteban A, Frutos F, Tobin MJ, Alia I, Solsona JF, Valverdu I, Fernandez R, De La Cal MA, Benito S, Tomas R. A comparison of four methods of weaning patients from mechanical ventilation. Spanish Lung Failure Collaborative Group. N Engl J Med 1995; 332(6):345–350.
67. Nava S, Ambrosino N, Clini E, Prato M, Orlando G, Vitacca M, Brigada P, Fracchia C, Rubini F. Noninvasive mechanical ventilation in the weaning of patients with respiratory failure due to chronic obstructive pulmonary disease. A randomized, controlled trial. Ann Intern Med 1998; 128(9):721–728.
68. Gravil JH, Al Rawas OA, Cotton MM, Flanigan U, Irwin A, Stevenson RD. Home treatment of exacerbations of chronic obstructive pulmonary disease by an acute respiratory assessment service. Lancet 1998; 351(9119):1853–1855.

69. Skwarska E, Cohen G, Skwarski KM, Lamb C, Bushell D, Parker S, MacNee W. Randomised controlled trial of supported discharge in patients with exacerbations of chronic obstructive pulmonary disease. Thorax 2000; 55:907–912.
70. Davies L, Wilkinson M, Bonner S, Calverley PMA, Angus RM. "Hospital at home" versus hospital care in patients with exacerbations of chronic obstructive pulmonary disease: prospective randomised controlled trial. Br Med J 2000; 321:1265–1268.
71. Cotton MM, Bucknall, CE, Dagg KD, Johnson MK, MacGregor G, Stewart C, Stevenson RD. Early discharge for patients with exacerbations of chronic obstructive pulmonary disease: a randomised controlled trial. Thorax 2000; 55:902–906.
72. Sala E, Alegre L, Carrera M, Ibars M, Orriols X, Carceles F, Beltran S, Mata F, Font I, August AGN. Supported discharge shortens hospital stay in patients hospitalised because of an exacerbation of chronic obstructive pulmonary disease (COPD). Eur Respir J 2001; 17:1138–1142.
73. Agustí AGN. What's new in the COPD management? Monaldi Arch Chest Dis 2000; 55(6):506–508.
74. Carrera M, Sauleda J, Bauzá F, Bosch M, Togores B, Barbé F, Agustí AGN. Resultados de la actuación de una unidad de control de la oxigenoterapia domiciliaria. Arch Bronco-neumol 1999; 35:33–38.

31

Acute Exacerbation of Chronic Obstructive Pulmonary Disease as Outcome of Therapeutic Interventions

NIKOS M. SIAFAKAS and MARIOS E. FROUDARAKIS

University Hospital of Heraklion
Heraklion, Crete, Greece

JOHN KOTTAKIS

University General Hospital and Thrace Medical School
Alexandroupolis, Crete, Greece

I. Introduction

COPD is the fourth leading cause of death in the world and mortality rates for this disease are increasing (1–3). In addition, acute exacerbations of COPD (AECOPD) are common and associated with an increase in hospitalization rates and health-care utilization and cost (1–3). Furthermore, whereas the severity of stable COPD is associated with longer term mortality, acute exacerbations are associated with significant short-term mortality. In hospitalized AECOPD patients, short-term or hospital mortality has been reported to range between 4 to 26% (1–3). Primarily in COPD, the effects of therapeutic interventions have been assessed spirometrically. However, since pulmonary function tests do not always correlate with the patient's health status, there has been a switch of focus from FEV_1 measurements to the assessment of symptoms, quality of life, exertion tolerance, pharmacoeconomics, and survival (4–7). Despite the high prevalence of the disease and the significance of AECOPD, little is known about the ability of currently available treatments to prevent AECOPD. This may be due to lack of a consistent and universally accepted definition of what exactly constitutes an AECOPD and the consequent lack of a consistent design in the clinical trials evaluating the results of therapeutic interventions (3).

Until now, evaluating the rate and frequency of AECOPD to assess the effectiveness of therapeutic interventions has been infrequent, although a beneficial effect on AECOPD may have an effect on the natural history, quality of life, mortality, and cost of the disease (8). This chapter reviews studies investigating the effect of various modes of treatment on the frequency and/or severity of AECOPD. The importance of AECOPD as a primary or secondary outcome in the assessment of various interventions on COPD is stated.

II. Bronchodilators

Current state-of-the art management of acute exacerbation of COPD includes the use of bronchodilating agents (9, 10). When maximal bronchodilation is achieved with one bronchodilating agent, some patients showed additional benefit from the addition of a second bronchodilator (11). In a clinical trial by Lloberes and coworkers, it was shown that significantly higher doses of salbutamol and ipratropium (than usually used for stable disease) were required to achieve maximal bronchodilation in at least half of the patients in a group of 13 AECOPD patients (12).

Three randomized controlled trials investigated the use of intravenous aminophylline on AECOPD. Aminophylline failed to confer additional benefit in lung function across all three studies (13–15). However, in one of the three studies, i.v. aminophylline was able to significantly decrease hospital admissions (15).

Friedman and coworkers performed a post hoc evaluation of two double-blind, randomized, parallel group studies of 12 weeks duration each in patients with stable COPD. In both studies, the therapeutic intervention tested was a single inhaler containing albuterol and ipratropium bromide versus the monotherapies. They found that comparable rates of exacerbation were observed with four times daily treatment with conventional doses of albuterol and ipratropium given together, or ipratropium monotherapy, whereas an increased number of exacerbations was observed under albuterol monotherapy (16).

An assessment of the effect of salmeterol on the acute exacerbation of COPD has been investigated as a secondary objective in a number of recently published clinical trials. Boyd et al. (17) randomized 674 patients with COPD to treament with salmeterol 50 μg b.i.d., salmeterol 100 μg b.i.d., or placebo for a period of 16 weeks in a parallel group fashion. The definition of what constitutes an acute COPO exacerbation used in their investigation was the need for additional therapy and/or a hospitalization for COPD treatment. No differences were reported over placebo with 21%, 25%, and 26% of patients experiencing at least one COPD exacerbation in the salmeterol 50 μg, salmeterol 100 μg, and placebo treatment groups, respectively (17).

Mahler et al. (18) compared 361 COPD patients randomized over a period of 12 weeks to salmeterol 50 μg b.i.d., ipratropium bromide 40 μg q.i.d., or placebo. Analysis of the time to first exacerbation demonstrated that the salmeterol-treated patients had a delayed onset of an AECOPD, compared to placebo ($p = 0.0052$) and ipratropium bromide ($p = 0.0411$). The authors speculated that this finding may be attributed to the prolonged bronchodilation with salmeterol. In the same investigation, 20.7%, 30.8%, and 32.9% of the salmeterol, ipratropium, and placebo-treated patients experienced at least one COPD exacerbation during the 12 weeks of the study (18).

Van Noord et al. (19) and Zu Wallack et al. (20) performed two 12-week-long clinical trials comparing salmeterol monotherapy with the combination of salmeterol plus ipratropium bromide (19) and the combination of theophylline and salmeterol with salmeterol monotherapy and theophylline monotherapy in the second investigation. In both investigations, AECOPD was identified by the requirement for additional treatment for a AECOPD and/or hospitalization due to AECOPD. Both studies showed a significant effect of the combination treatment on the frequency of AECOPD versus placebo ($p = 0.01$) in the first study and versus theophylline monotherapy ($p = 0.023$) in the second study: the percentage of patients with at least one AECOPD was 12.8% with the salmeterol plus theophylline combination as compared to 20% and 17.8% with the theophylline and salmeterol monotherapy, respectively, in the study by ZuWallack (20) and 13% with the salmeterol plus ipratropium combination as compared to 23% in the salmeterol only and 36% in the placebo-treated group in the van Noord investigation (19).

Three recently published clinical trials have included 974 patients and studied the assessment of the effects of formoterol fumarate on the acute exacerbation of COPD as secondary outcome (21–23). In the first two trials, formoterol given in doses of 12 µg and 24 µg twice daily was compared with ipratropium bromide 40 µg four times daily over a period of 3 months (21) and titrated to therapeutic levels oral slow-release theophylline over a period of 12 months (22). In the third clinical trial with a crossover design, a regimen of formoterol 12 µg twice daily plus ipratropium bromide 40 µg four times daily was compared with a regimen of salbutamol 200 µg four times daily plus ipratropium bromide 40 µg four times daily over a period of 3 weeks (23). In these clinical trials, the definitions used to identify and assess AECOPD were similar. Dahl et al. (21) and Rossi et al. (22) evaluated AECOPD by defining three levels of exacerbation. The first level, corresponding to mild exacerbations, identified days during which patients experienced relatively mild symptoms and/or a decrease in PEF from personal best of at least 20% ("bad days"). Second-level exacerbations were those requiring a course of additional therapy (e.g., antibiotics, corticosteroids, oxygen) and corresponded to a moderate AECOPD. Third-level exacerbations comprised hospitalizations due to an AECOPD (severe exacerbation). D'Urzo et al. (23), in their assessment of AECOPD in the third drug trial, identified only mild and severe exacerbations using the same criteria as above.

In the first study, Dahl et al. (21) reported a decrease in the number of "bad days" (first-level AECOPD) in the formoterol-treated patients compared to patients treated with ipratropium bromide or placebo. There was no statistical significant difference among the treatment groups in the numbers of days with additional COPD-related therapy (second-level exacerbation). Finally, third-level AECOPD comprising onc hospitalization for AECOPD was similar in the three groups.

In the second study, Rossi et al. (22) reported that patients who received regular therapy with formoterol, or oral slow-release theophylline, showed marked differences in the total number of severe third-level AECOPD as compared to the group of patients treated with placebo. In fact, this difference was particularly pronounced in the formoterol 24 µg twice-daily-treated group of patients, as compared to the placebo-treated patients; the difference in the mean frequency was five severe AECOPD in the formoterol-treated patients versus 20 severe AECOPD in the placebo group over the 12 months of treatment. Also, the mean percentage of days requiring additional therapy for COPD (second-level moderate AECOPD) was lower in the group of patients who received formoterol 24 µg twice daily, or oral slow-release theophylline compared to the placebo. As far as mild exacerbations were concerned, the authors reported a superior effect of formoterol to theophylline or placebo with statistical significant differences in the percentage of days with symptoms and/or a 20% or more drop in PEF over the 12-month treatment period.

However, D'Urzo et al. (23) did not find any difference between treatment regimens as to the number of mild or severe AECOPD experienced by patients participating in the third clinical trial. Their investigation was not placebo controlled, and thus did not allow for the identification of an effect on exacerbations of one, or both, drugs over placebo.

Recently, a new long-acting anticholinergic, tiotropium bromide, was aproved for COPD treatment and beneficial effects on exacerbations have been reported in placebo and active-treatment controlled studies (24–27). Compared with ipratropium, tiotropium significantly reduced the incidence of COPD exacerbations (35 vs. 46%), the number of exacerbations (0.73 vs. 0.96 events·patients/year) and the number of exacerbation days (10.8 vs. 17.7 days·patients/year). Tiotropium treatment also lengthened the time to first exacerbation and time to first hospitalization for exacerbation, compared to ipratropium. The proportion of patients hospitalized and the number of hospitalizations were not statistically different between tiotropium and ipratropium (24, 25). Compared to salmeterol (26), there was a tendency for fewer tiotropium-treated patients to have COPD exacerbations (36.8% vs. 38.5%), but failed to achieve statistical significance. In the placebo-controlled trials, fewer tiotropium than placebo patients has at least one COPD exacerbation (36% vs. 42%; $p < 0.05$) and statistically significant differences in favor of tiotropium treatment were also reported for the total number of exacerbations and the time-to-first exacerbation (27).

III. Corticosteroids

The effects of corticosteroids in AECOPD has been discussed in detail in Chapter 22. In summary, the beneficial effect of short-term treatment with systemic corticosteroids has been well demonstrated in AECOPD (28).

Recent clinical trials have investigated the effects of treatment of stable COPD with inhaled corticosteroids on AECOPD; however, only one encompassed AECOPD as primary assessment outcome (29). Indeed, Paggiaro and coworkers (29) performed a 6-month investigation administrating 500 µg of fluticasone twice daily in patients with moderate-to-severe COPD. Primary efficacy outcome was the number of patients with at least one AECOPD. No significant difference over placebo was noted; however, the number of moderate-to-severe exacerbations was less in the fluticasone-treated group.

Two recent, 3-year-long, clinical trials have included the assessment of the AECOPD as a secondary outcome: the Copenhagen City Lung Study and the ISOLDE (30, 31). Only in the ISOLDE study, in which moderate-to-severe patients with a mean FEV_1 of 50% of predicted were enrolled, an effect of treatment with high-dose fluticasone (1000 µg/day) on exacerbations was noted; the median yearly exacerbation rate in the fluticasone group was 0.99 compared with 1.32 of the placebo ($p = 0.026$) (30). A meta-analysis (32) of three studies of 2-year treatment duration with high-dose inhaled budesonide in the one (33), high-dose beclomethasone dipropionate in the second (34), and medium-dose beclomethasone in the third (35) demonstrated a "no effect" on exacerbations in moderate-to-severe COPD patients (32).

Don D. Sin and Jack V. Tu (36) looked retrospectively—by means of a large population-based cohort study ($n = 22, 260$)—at the relationship between inhaled corticosteroids and the subsequent risk of rehospitalization and death in patients admitted to the hospital for AECOPD. They found that patients who received inhaled corticosteroid therapy post discharge from the hospital experienced fewer repeat hospitalizations and were less likely to die. However, because of the design of their study, they could not rule out the inclusion of asthmatics from the database used.

In conclusion, an effect of high-dose inhaled corticosteroids on COPD exacerbations and on the risk for hospitalization in patients with severe COPD has been observed in two prospective randomized studies (30, 31), although a meta-analysis of three other studies has failed to replicate it (32). In the face of conflicting results, future investigations are warranted, designed and powered to look at the effect of inhaled steroids on AECOPD as the primary investigational outcome.

IV. Antibiotics

Respiratory tract infections are considered as the common cause of AECOPD. In the 1960s several large-scale studies had shown that the prophylactic, continuous use of antibiotics had no effect on the frequency of AECOPD (37–39).

In addition, Johnston et al. investigated the efficacy of winter chemoprophylaxis and noticed that there was no beneficial effect (40). Based on the above studies, the prophylactic use of antibiotics is not recommended (1, 41, 42).

The efficacy of antibiotic therapy during an AECOPD has been the subject of controversial reports (43–46), since the specific role of bacterial infections in these patients is under debate (47). A meta-analysis published by Saint et al. showed a small but statistically significant improvement due to antibiotic therapy in patients with exacerbations of COPD. This antibiotic-associated improvement may be clinically significant, especially in patients with low baseline lung function (46).

Recently, Adams and coworkers (48) have reviewed the admissions for patients with AECOPD due to respiratory infections. Their primary interest was the relapse rate: an admission and/or consultation to the emergency department for AECOPD within 14 days following the initial presentation for an interval of 2 years. They included 173 patients with 362 visits. In 270 patient-visits, antibiotics were prescribed, and 19% of those visits have relapsed. From the 192 patient-visits that have not received antibiotics, 32% have relapsed ($p < 0.001$). Amoxycillin had the higher (54%) relapse risk than ciprofloxacine (22%). Amoxicillin-clavulanate and cephalosporins showed the lowest rate of exacerbations, respectively—8 and 4% (48). Although the study has the limitation of a retrospective one, the authors concluded that COPD patients should receive antibiotics during AECOPD.

Controversy exists whether the new-generation antibiotics have a better impact on exacerbation relapse. In a recent study using ciprofloxacine versus first-line antibiotics, Grossman and coworkers (44) found that there was a trend, although not significant, of lower incidence of symptoms, duration of exacerbation, and rate of hospitalizations for exacerbations, and better quality of life for the group of patients treated with ciprofloxacine. The symptom-free interval was not affected by either treatment, but was affected by the severity of the disease and the number of the exacerbations during previous year. However, Destache et al. found that the use of amoxicillin/clavulanate, ciprofloxacine, or azithromycin was associated with lower rate of hospitalization for AECOPD and a longer exacerbation-free interval than the use of amoxicillin, erithromycin, or tetracycline (49). Again, this study was a retrospective evaluation (48). During AECOPD in mechanically ventilated patients, a recent study showed the significant benefit of ofloxacin versus placebo on the survival ($p = 0.01$) and on the need for additional antibiotic therapy ($p = 0.006$). The duration of mechanical ventilation and hospital stay was also significantly shorter in the ofloxacin group than in the placebo group (absolute difference 4.2 days, 95% Cl 2.5–5.9; and 9.6 days, 3.4–12.8, respectively) (50).

V. Others

A. Mucolytics, Mucoregulators, and Antioxidants

The role of the above medications in AECOPD has not yet been clearly established because of the lack of well-designed clinical trials and because the mechanism of action of most of these drugs is unknown (10, 51–53).

Recently, Poole and Black published a meta-analysis (54). The aim was to assess the effects of oral mucolytics in adults with stable chronic bronchitis and chronic obstructive pulmonary disease. They reviewed all randomized controlled trials that compared at least 2 months of regular oral mucolytic drugs with placebo. The outcome measured was exacerbations, days of illness, lung function, and adverse events. Compared to placebo, the number of AECOPD was significantly reduced (29%) in subjects taking oral mucolytics ($p < 0.0001$). Days of illness also fell significantly ($p < 0.0001$). The number of subjects who had no AECOPD in the study period was significantly larger in the mucolytic group ($p < 0.0001$). There was no difference in lung function or in adverse events reported between treatments.

Cost-effective treatment would be in patients with poor lung function who have frequent or prolonged exacerbations or are repeatedly admitted to the hospital (53).

A European group initiated a phase III double-blind, placebo-controlled, parallel group, multicenter randomized trial, to assess the effect of N-acetylcysteine (NAC) in altering the decline in FEV_1, exacerbation rate and quality of life in patients with moderate-to-severe COPD (55). In addition, cost-utility of the treatment will be estimated. Patients will be followed for 3 years. The final results of the trial will be available in about 2 years. This study will provide objective data on the effects of N-acetylcysteine on outcome variables in COPD including exacerbations. Finally, the widespread use of the above agents is not recommended on the basis of the present evidence of their effect on AECOPD (1).

B. Immunostimulating Agents

Immunostimulating agents are a class of medication that contains antigens derived from several bacterial strains. Their potential beneficial results may come from stimulation of the nonspecific components of the immune system, such as activation of macrophages resulting in an increased specific response of either T or B lymphocytes and macrophage phagocytosis, thus putting the immune system in a "state of alert" against any microbial invader (56). In the last 10 years, randomized clinical trials with immunostimulating agents showed an improvement in the symptoms and a reduction in acute exacerbations by 20 to 30% compared to placebo (57, 58). Moreover, the mean number of infections was significantly reduced, associated with a significantly lower use of antibiotics (57).

Recently, a Canadian group reported the results of a controlled trial (59). The risk of AECOPD between the Broncho-Vaxom treated patients and the control subjects was found to be equal (44.5% vs. 43.7%; $p = 0.87$), and no difference in the mortality rates was observed between the two groups (59). However, the total hospital stay was significantly reduced in the treated group (287 days vs. 642 days), with a significant difference in the mean hospital stay in favor of the treated group (1.5 days vs. 3.4; $p = 0.037$). Although they have not studied the impact of other therapies in their analysis, they suggested that this agent might be beneficial for patients with COPD by reducing the likelihood of severe respiratory events leading to hospitalization. The same team suggests that immunostimulants may become a key element in the improved control of COPD, as these agents may decrease the disease-related cost (60). These results have not been duplicated thus far; more studies are needed before a worldwide recommendation of those drugs can be issued (1).

C. Vaccinations

Infections are important triggers for COPD exacerbations, especially those of the upper respiratory tract. About 30 to 40% of AECOPD are attributed to viral infections, while half of them are attributed to *Haemophilus influenza*, *Moraxella catarrhalis*, or *Streptococcus pneumoniae*. These infections occur commonly in the winter months (61, 62).

Which common viruses cause AECOPD is still controversial. However, recent studies using modern molecular techniques isolated rhinoviruses and respiratory sincytial virus (RSV) (63, 64), while it was believed that influenzae is the most common virus met in exacerbated COPD patients (61, 65). Nichol and associates have clearly demonstrated the reduction in the rate of hospitalization and the risk of death in elderly patients with chronic lung disease due to influenza vaccination (66, 67). Although few randomized controlled trials are available specifically in COPD patients, a recent meta-analysis confirmed that AECOPD is significantly reduced (68). Thus, influenza vaccination is highly recommended (1, 69).

The value of pneumococcal vaccination in patients with COPD is under debate: two randomized controlled trials evaluating the efficacy of this vaccine failed to show any significant benefit in relation to the number of exacerbations (70, 71). A possible explanation is that pneumonoccocal vaccine provides partial protection against bacteremic pneumonococcal pneumonia but not against other manifestations such as simple bronchitis (61, 70, 72). In addition, this effect was seen in low-risk, but not in high-risk adults, such as with COPD (72). Due to these results, the use of pneumococcal vaccination in COPD patients is not yet justified (1).

D. Long-Term Oxygen Therapy

Since the early 1980s, long-term oxygen therapy (LTOT) has proved its efficacy in increasing the survival of patients with COPD and chronic respiratory failure (73, 74). However, the MRC study (69) did not show any significant difference in number of days spent in the hospital due to exacerbations between the oxygen-treated and control groups. Recent studies confirmed these findings (75, 76). Furthermore, LTOT was found to be a risk factor for exacerbation in the retrospective analysis of Dewan and coworkers' study (77) and confirmed in the prospective study of Kessler and coworkers, although no association remained when adjusting for physiological parameters, suggesting that LTOT was probably a marker of severity in those patients (76). In contrast, a recent prospective study investigating the potential risk factors of hospitalization in patients with COPD reported that underprescription of LTOT was an independent risk factor (78).

It is well established that quality of life in COPD patients is closely related to the rate of hospital admissions due to acute exacerbations (79, 80). However, it is unclear whether LTOT significantly affects quality of life since the overall hospital stay for AECOPD may not be improved (75, 81). Further studies are needed to clarify the role of LTOT on AECOPD.

VI. Nondrug Interventions

A. Noninvasive Ventilation

Hypercapnea is an indicator of poor prognosis in COPD patients and most of these patients worsen their $PaCO_2$ during AECOPD (82). Recently, significant benefits have been reported by the use of noninvasive ventilation (NIV) during AECOPD. Studies reported that NIV may unload the diaphragm and reduce hyperinflation in COPD patients (83, 84), improving daytime blood gases (85). However, minimal data are available to assess the usefulness of NIV in COPD patients on a long-term basis (86). Few randomized prospective studies are being completed in Europe and the first results showed that NIV was associated with a reduction in hospitalization for chronic respiratory failure decompensation (87).

Clini and coworkers (87) showed that home-care programs with NIV and LTOT may significantly reduce hospital admissions in patients with hypercapnic COPD for a period of 18 months. They also reported a decrease in the days of hospitalization, although no significant difference in mortality was observed (87). Later, in 1998, the same team conducted a randomized trial with the aim of evaluating the long-term survival, clinical effectiveness, and side effects of NIV (88). Forty-nine stable hypercapnic COPD patients on LTOT were assigned to two groups: in Group 1, 28 patients performed NIV by pressure support modality in addition to LTOT; in Group 2, 21 patients continued their usual LTOT regimen. Mortality rate, hospital stay, and ICU admissions were recorded in the two groups. PFTs and respiratory muscle function, dyspnea, and exercise capacity (by 6-min walk test) were evaluated baseline and every 3 to 6 months up to 3 years. Mortality rate was no different between the two groups. PFTs and respiratory muscle function did not significantly change over time. Hospitalizations significantly decreased in both groups (from 37 ± 29 to 15 ± 12 and from 32 ± 18 to 17 ± 11 days/pt/yr in groups 1 and 2, respectively; $p < 0.001$), whereas ICU admissions significantly decreased only in patients using NIV (from 1.0 ± 0.7 to 0.2 ± 0.3/pt/yr; $p < 0.0001$). They concluded that the addition of NIV by pressure support modality to LTOT does not improve long-term survival but significantly reduces ICU admissions and improves exercise capacity in severe COPD with hypercapnia (87).

Bardi et al. compared 30 patients with an early administration of NIV (group A), to medical therapy only (group B) (89). In-hospital mortality, need for endotracheal intubation, and mean length of hospitalization were lower in group A, although the difference was not statistically significant. In addition, FEV_1 and tidal volume (VT) improved significantly in group A patients only; survival rates were significantly higher in group A than in group B ($p < 0.02$). New hospital admissions for AECOPD relapse over 1 year were more frequent in group B than in group A (84).

Confalioneri et al. published a study (90) assessing short- and 1-year outcome of early administration of NIV in 24 patients with respiratory failure due to exacerbated COPD (group A) in comparison with 24 matched historical control patients treated conventionally (group B). In-hospital survival rate was not significantly different in group A versus group B, but patients treated with NIV showed an earlier improvement in blood gases and a better pH and respiratory rate at discharge. Only two patients from group A needed endotracheal intubation as compared with 9 from group B. Hospital stay was significantly reduced in survivors of group A versus group B. The number and length of further hospitalizations for AECOPD were significantly higher in group B compared with group A. The survival rate at 12 months was significantly lower in group B than in group A (50% vs. 71%). They concluded that NIV administration in patients with respiratory failure due to AECOPD improves not only immediate but also long-term outcomes.

In contrast, Casanova et al. (86) in a prospective randomized study in patients with severe stable COPD, recently showed no benefit from the addition of NIV to LTOT during a 1-year period. They enrolled 52 patients with severe COPD ($FEV_1 = 45\%$) to either NIV plus "standard care" (96% patients with LTOT) or to standard care alone (93% patients with LTOT). One-year survival was similar in both groups (78%). The number of AECOPD was similar at all time points in patients receiving NIV compared with control subjects. The number of hospital admissions was decreased at 3 months in the NIV group (5% vs. 15% of patients; $p = 0.05$), but this difference was not seen at 6 months (18% vs. 19%, respectively). The only beneficial differences were observed in the Borg dyspnea scale, which dropped from 6 to 5 ($p = 0.039$), and in one of the neuropsychological tests (psychomotor coordination) for the NIV group at 6 months. They concluded that over 1 year, NIV does not affect the natural course of the disease and is of marginal benefit in outpatients with stable severe COPD (91).

The longest follow-up (7 years) of the effect of NIV on AECOPD was reported recently by Janssen et al. (92) and showed that there was a significant reduction in the number of days spent in the hospital up to 2 years. Thereafter, the difference was no longer significant. However, the number of COPD patients that were followed was extremely small (only 24) (92).

Even if such studies are difficult to perform, there is clearly a need for prospective studies comparing LTOT and NIV in a large number of patients and for several years (86). Despite adequate NIV and/or LTOT, the high rate of exacerbation relapse is more likely to occur in these patients with more severe clinical and functional status (93).

B. Pulmonary Rehabilitation Studies

The effect of rehabilition on AECOPD patients has been studied initially in uncontrolled trials already from the early 1970s showing a reduced rate of hospitalization per year and per patient (94, 95). This effect also seemed to be long lasting (94, 95). Thus, Burton et al. studied 80 COPD patients on rehabilitation program and found that the mean days of hospitalization were reduced from 19 to 6 days (94). More impressive was the result obtained by Hudson et al., who studied 44 COPD patients in a self-care program without exercise (95). They showed an important reduction in days of overall hospitalization from 529 days in the year prior to the program to 145 days in the year following rehabilitation. This result of pulmonary rehabilitation on hospitalization days could indicate an indirect beneficial effect on AECOPD. However, more important is the effect of rehabilitation on the overall cost of treatment, which may lead to a wide application of rehabilitation (94–96).

Despite the optimistic results of these studies, methodological problems must be addressed as difficulties arise in designing randomized controlled studies of rehabilitation (96), such as the mode of pulmonary rehabilitation and the selection of patients (6, 97). Thus, more studies are needed to clarify those issues, although some studies showed that there is a benefit in days of hospitalization and in overall cost from rehabilitation (98, 99).

VII. Conclusion

AECOPD is an important clinical event in the natural history of the disease. AECOPD is related to the quality of life, mortality, and overall cost of the disease. Thus, the number and severity of AECOPD should be included in the outcomes of every study investigating modes of interventions. This chapter reviews the available literature on the effects of drug and nondrug interventions on AECOPD. Evidence of effectiveness was reported for bronchodilators, steroids, noninvasive mechanical ventilation, and rehabilitation. Antibiotics should be used during an exacerbation if needed, but not prophylactically. On the basis of limited data, the use of mucolytics, antioxidants, and immunoregulators cannot be recommended for worldwide use.

References

1. Global Initiative for Chronic Obstructive Lung Disease. Global strategy for the diagnosis, management and prevention of Chronic Obstructive Pulmonary Disease. NHLBI/WHO workshop report. Bethesda, MD: National Heart, Lung and Blood Institute, 2001:1–100.
2. World Health Organization, eds. World Health Report 2000. Geneva: WHO, 2000.
3. Rodriguez-Roisin R. Towards a consensus definition for COPD exacerbations. Chest 2000; 117:398S–401S.
4. Connors AF, Jr, Dawson NV, Thomas C, Harrell FE, Jr, Desbiens N, Fulkerson WJ, Kussin P, Bellamy P, Goldman L, Knaus WA. Outcomes following acute exacerbation of severe chronic obstructive lung disease. The SUPPORT investigators (Study to Understand Prognoses and Preferences for Outcomes and Risks of Treatments). Am J Respir Cut Care Med 1996; 154:959–967.
5. Friedman M, Hilleman DE. Economic burden of chronic obstructive pulmonary disease. Impact of new treatment options. Pharmacoeconomics 2001; 19:245–254.
6. Gosselink R, Troosters T, Decramer M. Exercise training in COPD patients: the basic questions. Eur Respir J 1997; 10:2884–2891.
7. Jones PW. Issues concerning health-related quality of life in COPD. Chest 1995; 107:187S–193S.
8. Johnson M, Rennard S. Alternative mechanisms for long-acting beta(2)-adrenergic agonists in COPD. Chest 2001; 120:258–270.
9. Siafakas NM, Bouros D. Management of acute exacerbations of chronic obstructive pulmonary disease. Eur Respir Mon 1998; 7:264–277.
10. Barnes PJ. Chronic obstructive pulmonary disease. Med Progr 2000; 343:269–280.
11. McCrory DC, Brown C, Gelfand SE, Bach PB. Management of acute exacerbations of COPD: a summary and appraisal of published evidence. Chest 2001; 119:1190–1209.
12. Lloberes P, Ramis L, Montserrat JM, Serra J, Campistol J, Picado C, Agusti-Vidal A. Effect of three different bronchodilators during an exacerbation of chronic obstructive pulmonary disease. Eur Respir J 1988; 1:536–539.

13. Seidenfeld JJ, Jones WN, Moss RE, Tremper J. Intravenous aminophylline in the treatment of acute bronchospastic exacerbations of chronic obstructive pulmonary disease. Ann Emerg Med 1984; 13:248–252.

14. Rice KL, Leatherman JW, Duane PG, Snyder LS, Harmon KR, Abel J, Niewoehner DE. Aminophylline for acute exacerbations of chronic obstructive pulmonary disease. A controlled trial. Ann Intern Med 1987; 107:305–309.

15. Wrenn K, Slovis CM, Murphy F, Greenberg RS. Aminophylline therapy for acute bronchospastic disease in the emergency room. Ann Intern Med 1991; 115:241–247.

16. Friedman M, Serby CW, Menjoge SS, Wilson JD, Hilleman DE, Witek TJ, Jr. Pharmacoeconomic evaluation of a combination of ipratropium plus albuterol compared with ipratropium alone and albuterol alone in COPD. Chest 1999; 115:635–641.

17. Boyd G, Morice AH, Pounsford JC, Siebert M, Peslis N, Crawford C. An evaluation of salmeterol in the treatment of chronic obstructive pulmonary disease (COPD). Eur Respir J 1997; 10:815–821.

18. Mahler DA, Donohue JF, Barbee RA, Goldman MD, Gross NJ, Wisniewski ME, Yancey SW, Zakes BA, Rickard KA, Anderson WH. Efficacy of salmeterol xinafoate in the treatment of COPD. Chest 1999; 115:957–965.

19. van Noord JA, de Munck DR, Bantje TA, Hop WC, Akveld ML, Bommer AM. Long-term treatment of chronic obstructive pulmonary disease with salmeterol and the additive effect of ipratropium. Eur Respir J 2000; 15:878–885.

20. ZuWallack RL, Mahler DA, Reilly D, Church N, Emmett A, Rickard K, Knobil K. Salmeterol plus theophylline combination therapy in the treatment of COPD. Chest 2001; 119:1661–1670.

21. Dahl R, Greefhorst LA, Nowak D, Nonikov V, Byrne AM, Thomson MH, Till D, Della Cioppa G. Inhaled formoterol dry powder versus ipratropium bromide in chronic obstructive pulmonary disease. Am J Respir Crit Care Med 2001; 164:778–784.

22. Rossi A, Kristufek P, Levine BE, Thomson MH, Till D, Kottakis J, Della Cioppa G. Comparison of the efficacy, tolerability and safety of formoterol dry powder and oral slow-release theophylline in COPD. Chest 2002; 121:1058–1069.

23. D'Urzo AD, De Salvo MC, Ramirez-Rivera A, Almeida J, Sichletidis L, Rapatz G, Kottakis J. In patients with COPD, treatment with a combination of formoterol and ipratropium is more effective than a combination of salbutamol and ipratropium: a 3-week, randomized, double-blind, within-patient, multicenter study. Chest 2001; 119:1347–1356.

24. Hvizdos KM, Goa KL. Tiotropium bromide. Drugs 2002; 62:1195–1203.

25. van Noord JA, Bantje TA, Eland ME, Korducki L, Cornelissen PJ. A randomised controlled comparison of tiotropium and ipratropium in the treatment of chronic obstructive pulmonary disease. The Dutch Tiotropium Study Group. Thorax 2000; 55:289–294.

26. Donohue JF, van Noord JA, Bateman ED, Langley SJ, Lee A, Witek TJ, Jr, Kesten S, Towse L. A 6-month, placebo-controlled study comparing lung function and health status changes in COPD patients treated with tiotropium or salmeterol. Chest 2002; 122:47–55.

27. Vincken W, van Noord JA, Greefhorst AP, Bantje TA, Kesten S, Korducki L, Cornelissen PJ. Improved health outcomes in patients with COPD during 1 year's treatment with tiotropium. Eur Respir J 2002; 19:209–216.

28. Stanbrook MB, Goldstein RS. Steroids for acute exacerbations of COPD: How long is enough? Chest 2001; 119:675–676.

29. Paggiaro PL, Dahle R, Bakran I, Frith L, Hollingworth K, Efthimiou J. Multicentre randomised placebo-controlled trial of inhaled fluticasone propionate in patients with

chronic obstructive pulmonary disease. International COPD Study Group. Lancet 1998; 351:773–780.

30. Burge PS, Calverley PM, Jones PW, Spencer S, Anderson JA, Maslen TK. Randomised, double blind, placebo controlled study of fluticasone propionate in patients with moderate to severe chronic obstructive pulmonary disease: the ISOLDE trial. Br Med J 2000; 320:1297–1303.

31. Pauwels RA, Lofdahl CG, Laitinen L, Schouten JP, Postma DS, Pride NB, Ohlsson SV. Long-term treatment with inhaled budesonide in persons with mild chronic obstructive pulmonary disease who continue smoking. European Respiratory Society Study on Chronic Obstructive Pulmonary Disease. N Engl J Med 1999; 340:1948–1953.

32. van Grunsven PM, van Schayck CP, Derenne JP, Kerstjens HA, Renkema TE, Postma DS, Similowski T, Akkermans RP, Pasker-de Jong PC, Dekhuijzen PN, van Herwaarden CL, van Weel C. Long term effects of inhaled corticosteroids in chronic obstructive pulmonary disease: a meta-analysis. Thorax 1999; 54:7–14.

33. Renkema TE, Schouten JP, Koeter GH, Postma DS. Effects of long-term treatment with corticosteroids in COPD. Chest 1996; 109:1156–1162.

34. Derenne JP. Effects of high dose inhaled beclomethasone in the rate of decline FEV_1 in patients with chronic obstructive pulmonary disease: results of a 2 years prospective multicentre study. Am J Respir Crit Care Med 1995; 151:A463.

35. Kerstjens HA, Overbeek SE, Schouten JP, Brand PL, Postma DS. Airways hyperresponsiveness, bronchodilator response, allergy and smoking predict improvement in FEV1 during long-term inhaled corticosteroid treatment. Eur Respir J 1993; 6: 868–876.

36. Sin DD, Tu JV. Inhaled corticosteroids and the risk of mortality and re-admission in elderly patients with chronic obstructive pulmonary disease. Am J Respir Crit Care Med 2001; 164:580–584.

37. Francis RS, May JR, Spicer CC. Chemotherapy of bronchitis: influence of penicillin and tetracycline administered daily, or intermittently for exacerbations. Br Med J 1961; 2:979–985.

38. Francis RS, Spicer CC. Chemotherapy in chronic bronchitis: Influence of daily penicillin and tetracycline on exacerbations and their cost. A report to the research committee of the British Tuberculosis Association by their Chronic Bronchitis Subcommittee. Br Med J 1960; 1:297–303.

39. Fletcher CM, Ball JD, Carstairs LW, Couch AHC, Crofton JM, Edge JR et al. Value of chemoprophylaxis and chemotherapy in early chronic bronchitis. A report to the Medical Research Council by their Working Party on trials of chemotherapy in early chronic bronchitis. Br Med J 1966; 1:1317–1322.

40. Johnson RN, McNeill RS, Spith DH, Dempster MB, Nairn JR, Purvi MS et al. Five year winter chemoprophylaxis for chronic bronchitis. Br Med J 1969; 4:265–269.

41. Isada CM, Stoller JK. Chronic bronchitis: the role of antibiotics. In: Nederman MS, Sarosi GA, Glassroth J, eds. Respiratory Infections: A Scientific Basis for Management. London: WB Saunders; 1994:621–633.

42. Siafakas NM, Bouros D. Management of acute exacerbation of chronic obstructive pulmonary disease. In: Postma DS, Siafakas NM, eds. Management of Chronic Obstructive Pulmonary Disease. Sheffield: ERS Monograph, 1998:264–277.

43. Chodosh S. Treatment of acute exacerbations of chronic bronchitis: state of the art. Am J Med 1991; 91:87S–92S.

44. Grossman RF. The value of antibiotics and the outcomes of antibiotic therapy in exacerbations of COPD. Chest 1998; 113:249S–255S.

45. Nicotra MB, Rivera M. Chronic bronchitis: when and how to treat. Semin Respir Infect 1988; 3:61–71.
46. Saint S, Bent S, Vittinghoff E, Grady D. Antibiotics in chronic obstructive pulmonary disease exacerbations. A meta-analysis. JAMA 1995; 273:957–960.
47. Fagon JY, Chastre J. Severe exacerbations of COPD patients: the role of pulmonary infections. Semin Respir Infect 1996; 11:109–118.
48. Adams SG, Melo J, Luther M, Anzueto A. Antibiotics are associated with lower relapse rates in outpatients with acute exacerbations of COPD. Chest 2000; 117:1345–1352.
49. Destache CJ, Dewan N, O'Donohue WJ, Campbell JC, Angelillo VA. Clinical and economic considerations in the treatment of acute exacerbations of chronic bronchitis. J Antimicrob Chemother 1999; 43(suppl 3):107–113.
50. Nouira S, Marghli S, Belghith M, Besbes L, Elatrous S, Abroug F. Once daily oral ofloxacin in chronic obstructive pulmonary disease exacerbation requiring mechanical ventilation: a randomised placebo-controlled trial. Lancet 2001; 358:2020–2025.
51. Barnes PJ. Nonantimicrobial aspects of therapy. Semin Respir Infect 2000; 15:52–58.
52. Celli BR. Standards for the optimal management of COPD: a summary. Chest 1998; 113:283S–287S.
53. Rogers DF. Mucoactive drugs for asthma and COPD: any place in therapy? Expert Opin Investig Drugs 2002; 11:15–35.
54. Poole PJ, Black PN. Oral mucolytic drugs for exacerbations of chronic obstructive pulmonary disease: systematic review. Br Med J 2001; 322:1271–1274.
55. Decramer M, Dekhuijzen PN, Troosters T, van Herwaarden C, Rutten-van Molken M, van Schayck CP, Olivieri D, Lankhorst I, Ardia A. The Bronchitis Randomized On NAC Cost-Utility Study (BRONCUS): hypothesis and design. BRONCUS-trial Committee. Eur Respir J 2001; 17:329–336.
56. Mauël J, Van Pham T, Kreis B, Bauer J. Stimulation by a bacterial extract (Broncho-Vaxom) of the metabolic and functional activities of murine macrophages. Int J Immunopharmacol 1989; 11:637–645.
57. Derenne JP, Delclaux B. Clinical experience with OM-85 BV in upper and lower respiratory tract infections. Respiration 1992; 59(suppl 3):29–31.
58. Xynogalos S, Duratsos D, Varonos D. Clinical effectiveness of Broncho-Vaxom in patients with chronic obstructive pulmonary disease. Int J Immunother 1993; 9:135–142.
59. Collet JP, Shapiro P, Ernst P, Renzi T, Ducruet T, Robinson A. Effects of an immuno-stimulating agent on acute exacerbations and hospitalizations in patients with chronic obstructive pulmonary disease. The PARI-IS Study Steering Committee and Research Group. Prevention of Acute Respiratory Infection by an Immunostimulant. Am J Respir Crit Care Med 1997; 156:1719–1724.
60. Collet JP, Ducruet T, Haider S, Shapiro S, Robinson A, Renzi PM, Contandriopoulos AP, Ernst P. Economic impact of using an immunostimulating agent to prevent severe acute exacerbations in patients with chronic obstructive pulmonary disease. Can Respir J 2001; 8:27–33.
61. Sherk PA, Grossman RE. The chronic obstructive pulmonary disease exacerbation. Clin Chest Med 2000; 21:705–721.
62. Wedzicha JA. Exacerbations: etiology and pathophysiologic mechanisms. Chest 2002; 121(Suppl):136S–141S.
63. Seemungal TA, Harper-Owen R, Bhowmik A, Jeffries DJ, Wedzicha JA. Detection of rhinovirus in induced sputum at exacerbations of chronic obstructive pulmonary disease. Eur Respir J 2000; 16:677–683.

64. Seemungal TAR, Bhowmik A, McCallum P, Johnston SL, Wedzicha JA. Evidence for prolonged infection with RSV in COPD patients. Am J Respir Crit Care Med 2001; 163:A51.
65. Sethi S. Infectious etiology of acute exacerbations of chronic bronchitis. Chest 2000; 117(Suppl 2):380S–385S.
66. Nichol KL, Margolis KL, Wuorenma J, Von Sternberg. The efficacy and cost effectiveness of vaccination against influenza among elderly persons living in the community. N Engl J Med 1994; 331:778–784.
67. Nichol KL, Baken L, Nelson A. Relation between influenza vaccination and outpatient visits, hospitalization, and mortality in elderly persons with chronic lung disease. Ann Intern Med 1999; 130:397–403.
68. Poole PJ, Chacko E, Wood-Baker RW, Cates CJ. Influenza vaccine for patients with chronic obstructive pulmonary disease. Cochrane Database Syst Rev 2000:4.
69. Nathan RA, Geddes D, Woodhead M. Management of influenza in patients with asthma or chronic obstructive pulmonary disease. Ann Allergy Asthma Immunol 2001; 87:447–454, 487.
70. Davis AL, Aranda CP, Schiffman G, Christianson LC. Pneumococcal infection and immunologic response to pneumococcal vaccine in chronic obstructive pulmonary disease. A pilot study. Chest 1987; 92:204–212.
71. Leech JA, Gervais A, Ruben FL. Efficacy of pneumococcal vaccine in severe chronic obstructive pulmonary disease. Can Med Assoc J 1987; 136:361–365.
72. Fine MJ, Smith MA, Carson CA, Meffe F, Sankey SS, Weissfeld LA, Detsky AS, Kapoor WN. Efficacy of pneumococcal vaccination in adults. A meta-analysis of randomized controlled trials. Arch Intern Med 1994; 154:2666–2677.
73. Nocturnal Oxygen Therapy Group. Continuous or nocturnal oxygen therapy in hypoxaemic chronic obstructive lung disease: a clinical trial. Ann Intern Med 1980; 93:391–398.
74. Medical Research Council. Long term domiciliary oxygen therapy in chronic hypoxic cor pulmonale complicating chronic bronchitis and emphysema. Lancet 1981; 1:681–686.
75. Janssens JP, Rochat T, Frey JG, Dousse N, Pichard C, Tschopp JM. Health-related quality of life in patients under long-term oxygen therapy: a home-based descriptive study. Respir Med 1997; 91:592–602.
76. Kessler R, Faller M, Fourgault G, Mennecier B, Weitzenblum E. Predictive factors of hospitalization for acute exacerbation in a series of 64 patients with chronic obstructive pulmonary disease. Am J Respir Crit Care Med 1999; 159:158–164.
77. Dewan NA, Rafique S, Kanwar B, Satpathy H, Ryschon K, Tillotson GS, Niederman MS. Acute exacerbation of COPD: factors associated with poor treatment outcome. Chest 2000; 117:662–671.
78. Garcia-Aymerich J, Monso E, Marrades RM, Escarrabill J, Felez MA, Sunyer J, Anto JM. Risk factors for hospitalization for a chronic obstructive pulmonary disease exacerbation. EFRAM study. Am J Respir Crit Care Med 2001; 164:1002–1007.
79. Osman IM, Godden DJ, Friend JA, Legge JS, Douglas JG. Quality of life and hospital re-admission in patients with chronic obstructive pulmonary disease. Thorax 1997; 52:67–71.
80. Seemungal TA, Donaldson GC, Paul EA, Bestall JC, Jeffries DJ, Wedzicha JA. Effect of exacerbation on quality of life in patients with chronic obstructive pulmonary disease. Am J Respir Crit Care Med 1998; 157:1418–1422.
81. Zielinski J. Indications for long-term oxygen therapy: a reappraisal. Monaldi Arch Chest Dis 1999; 54:178–182.

82. Burrows B, Earle RH. Prediction of survival in patients with chronic airway obstruction. Am Rev Respir Dis 1969; 99:865–871.

83. Carrey Z, Gottfried SB, Levy RD. Ventilatory muscle support in respiratory failure with nasal positive pressure ventilation. Chest 1990; 97:150–158.

84. Ambrosino N, Nava S, Bertone P, Fracchia C, Rampulla C. Physiologic evaluation of pressure support ventilation by nasal mask in patients with stable COPD. Chest 1992; 101:385–391.

85. Leger P, Bedicam JM, Cornette A, Reybet-Degat O, Langevin B, Polu JM, Jeannin L, Robert D. Nasal intermittent positive pressure ventilation. Long-term follow-up in patients with severe chronic respiratory insufficiency. Chest 1994; 105:100–105.

86. Cuvelier A, Muir JF. Noninvasive ventilation and obstructive lung diseases. Eur Respir J 2001; 17:1271–1281.

87. Clini E, Vitacca M, Foglio K, Simoni P, Ambrosino N. Long-term home care programmes may reduce hospital admissions in COPD with chronic hypercapnia. Eur Respir J 1996; 9:1605–1610.

88. Clini E, Sturani C, Porta R, Scarduelli C, Galavotti V, Vitacca M, Ambrosino N. Outcome of COPD patients performing nocturnal non-invasive mechanical ventilation. Respir Med 1998; 92:1215–1222.

89. Bardi G, Pierotello R, Desideri M, Valdisserri L, Bottai M, Palla A. Nasal ventilation in COPD exacerbations: early and late results of a prospective, controlled study. Eur Respir J 2000; 15:98–104.

90. Confalonieri M, Parigi P, Scartabellati A, Aiolfi S, Scorsetti S, Nava S, Gandola L. Noninvasive mechanical ventilation improves the immediate and long-term outcome of COPD patients with acute respiratory failure. Eur Respir J 1996; 9:422–430.

91. Casanova C, Celli BR, Tost L, Soriano E, Abreu J, Velasco V, Santolaria F. Long-term controlled trial of nocturnal nasal positive pressure ventilation in patients with severe COPD. Chest 2000; 118:1582–1590.

92. Janssens JP, Derivaz S, Breitenstin E, de Muralt B, Fitting JW, Chevrolet JC, Rochat T. Changing patterns in long-term nonivasive ventilation. A 7-year prospective study in the Geneva Lake Area. Chest 2003; 123:67–79.

93. Moretti M, Cilione C, Tampieri A, Fracchia C, Marchioni A, Nava S. Incidence and causes of non-invasive mechanical ventilation failure after initial success. Thorax 2000; 55:819–825.

94. Burton GG, Gee GN, Hodgkin JE, Dunham JK. Cost effectiveness studies in respiratory care: an oveview and some possible solutions. Hospitals 1975; 49:61–71.

95. Hudson LD, Tyler ML, Petty TL. Hospitalization needs during an outpatient rehabilitation program for a severe chronic airway obstruction. Chest 1976; 70:606–610.

96. Vestbo J, Decramer M. Pulmonary rehabilitation and medical consumption. Eur Respir Mon 2000; 13:26–40.

97. Donner CF, Lusuardi M. Selection of candidates and programmes. Eur Respir Mon 2000; 13:132–142.

98. Jensen PS. Risk, protective factors, and supportive interventions in chronic airway obstruction. Arch Gen Psychiatry 1983; 40:1203–1207.

99. Toevs CD, Kaplan RM, Atkins CJ. The costs and effects of behavioral programs in chronic obstructive pulmonary disease. Med Care 1984; 22:1088–1100.

32

Future Research on Acute Exacerbations of Chronic Obstructive Pulmonary Disease

PETER J. BARNES

National Heart and Lung Institute
Imperial College London
London, England

I. Introduction

Acute exacerbations account for a high proportion of the medical costs for COPD, as well as accounting for considerable morbidity. Prevention of exacerbations therefore remains a major aim of therapy and novel drugs will be assessed for their ability to prevent exacerbations. However, despite their frequency, there is relatively little information about the cellular and molecular mechanisms involved in an exacerbation and an important focus for research in the future is to define the basic mechanisms and the sequence of cellular and molecular events responsible for the different types of exacerbation. This should lead to the more logical development of therapy to prevent and treat exacerbations. An exacerbation may be an amplification of existing pathology, or may represent an additional novel pathological mechanism that is added to the existing pathology.

This chapter considers some of the future research approaches that may be useful in better understanding of exacerbations.

II. The Inflammatory Process

A. Inflammatory Cells

In chronic stable COPD there is chronic inflammation in the airways and lung parenchyma which involves multiple cells and inflammatory mediators, including cytokines (1). This inflammation is dominated by increased numbers of activated macrophages, neutrophils, and CD8$^+$ (cytotoxic) T-lymphocytes (2–4). This is markedly different from the inflammation found in asthma, which is characterized by eosinophils, activated mast cells and CD4$^+$ (helper) T-lymphocytes (5). During an exacerbation of COPD, the cellular pattern may change with a 30-fold increase in eosinophils in bronchial biopsies (6), so that it becomes more like asthma (7). Similarly, eosinophil numbers as well as neutrophils are increased in bronchoalveolar lavage fluid during exacerbations (8). However, this does not appear to apply to the sputum where there is no obvious increase in eosinophils, as seen in exacerbations of asthma. The mechanisms for increased eosinophil recruitment in the airways of patients with COPD during an exacerbation needs to be further investigated. It is unlikely to be due to expression of interleukin (IL-5), but may be due to upregulation of eosinophil chemotactic factors. Future research should identify which chemokines are increased during an exacerbation and which chemokine receptors are activated. Several chemokine receptor antagonists are now in clinical development and may therefore be of potential value in treating and preventing exacerbations (9).

It is likely that during an acute exacerbation there is also an increase in the underlying inflammatory process, with increased numbers of neutrophils, T-cells and macrophages. Indeed, the increase in neutrophils, with release of myeloperoxidase, accounts for the purulence of sputum during an exacerbation. This suggests that there is an increase in neutrophil chemotactic factors during an exacerbation. In stable COPD there are increased concentrations of IL-8 and leukotriene (LT) B$_4$ in the airways, both of which are potent neutrophil chemoattractants (2, 10, 11). In addition, there is an increase in the proinflammatory cytokines tumor necrosis factor-α (TNF-α) and IL-6 (2, 12). In acute exacerbations there are increases in all of these mediators (11–14). The cytokine granulocyte-macrophage colony-simulating factor (GM-CSF), which is important for prolonging survival of neutrophils and eosinophils, is also elevated in bronchoalveolar lavage fluid during exacerbations (8). Using exhaled breath condensate, a noninvasive method to assess pulmonary inflammation (15), we have also demonstrated a marked increase in the concentrations of LTB$_4$ during an exacerbation (16). This suggests that an acute exacerbation of COPD shows an amplification of the inflammatory pattern seen in stable disease. It is likely that macrophages and epithelial cells play a critical role and these my be activated by infective agents and by air pollutants to release cytokines that amplify the inflammatory process (Fig. 1).

Endothelin-1, a potent bronchoconstrictor and vasoconstrictor peptide is also increased in sputum of patients with COPD during exacerbations (17), but its role in the pathophysiology of exacerbations is not yet certain. Several ET-1 antagonists are now in clinical development, so it may be possible to study their effects in exacerbation in the future.

B. Transcription Factors

Transcription factors play a critical role in the activation of inflammatory genes that orchestrate the chronic inflammatory process (18). Several transcription factors may

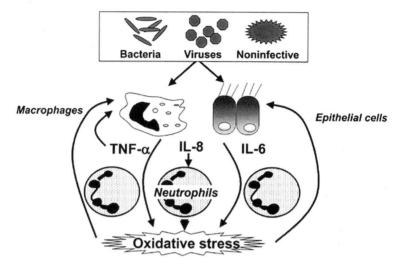

Figure 1 Macrophages and epithelial cells may be activated by bacteria, viruses and atmospheric pollution to release cytokines, such as interleukin(IL)-8 and tumor necrosis factor-α (TNF-α) that recruit neutrophils. Oxidative stress may further amplify the inflammatory process.

be involved in COPD, but so far there is little research in this area. Many of the inflammatory cytokines involved in COPD are regulated by the transcription factor nuclear factor-κB (NF-κB) and there is evidence that this is activated to a greater extent in acute exacerbations (19). NF-κB may be activated by bacterial and viral infections and by oxidative stress (20, 21) (Fig. 2). This provides a molecular basis for exacerbations and is a logical target for the development of novel therapies that may inhibit NF-κB activation (22). There are several possible approaches to inhibition of NF-κB, including gene transfer of the inhibitor of NF-κB (IκB), a search for inhibitors of IκB kinases (IKK), NF-κB-inducing kinase (NIK) and IκB ubiquitin ligase, which regulate the activity of NF-κB, and the development of drugs that inhibit the degradation of IκB (22). One concern about this approach is that effective inhibitors of NF-κB may result in immune suppression and impair host defenses, since knock-out mice which lack NF-κB proteins succumb to septicemia. However, there are alternative pathways of NF-κB activation that might be more important in inflammatory disease (23).

III. Oxidative Stress

Oxidative stress is increased in patients with COPD and may play an important role in amplifying the inflammatory and destructive process (24). Oxidative stress may now be monitored by several noninvasive techniques (15), so that it may be measured during exacerbations of the disease. The concentrations of hydrogen

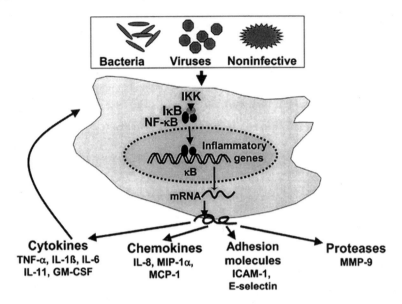

Figure 2   Causal agents activate nuclear factor-kappa B (NF-κB), via activation of IκB kinase (IKK) which switches on multiple inflammatory genes, including cytokines, chemokines, adhesion molecules and proteases. TNF-α = tumor necrosis factor-α; IL = interleukin; GM-CSF = granulocyte-macrophage colony-stimulating factor; ICAM = intercellular adhesion molecule; MMP = matrix metalloprotease.

peroxide (H_2O_2) are increased in exhaled breath condensate of patients with COPD and there is a further increase in exacerbations (25). H_2O_2 in exhaled breath is relatively unstable, giving variable results, but the novel prostanoid 8-isoprostane (8-epi prostaglandin $F_{2\alpha}$) formed by the effect of oxidative stress on arachidonic acid is more stable and a more reliable marker of oxidative stress (26). The concentrations of 8-isoprostane are increased in exhaled breath condensate of patients with COPD, even in patients who have quit smoking (27). The levels of 8-isoprostane are further increased during an exacerbation and remain elevated for several weeks (28). Another marker of oxidative stress is the volatile hydrocarbon ethane formed by lipid peroxidation. Increase concentrations of ethane are detected in the exhaled breath of patients with COPD and are related to disease severity (29), but no measurements have yet been made during exacerbations. The availability of these noninvasive markers of oxidative stress now makes it possible to monitor the increase in oxidative stress during exacerbations of COPD and during the recovery period. The prolonged increase in oxidative stress associated with an exacerbation is consistent with the prolonged effect of an exacerbation on health status of patients with COPD (30). The increase in oxidative stress during an exacerbation may play an important role in its pathophysiology since H_2O_2 is able to activate NF-κB and thus further increased the expression of inflammatory mediators such as TNF-α and IL-8, which increase neutrophilic inflammation.

This suggests that antioxidants may be of use in the therapy of acute exacerbations of COPD. *N*-acetyl cysteine (NAC) provides cysteine for enhanced production of glutathione (GSH) and has antioxidant effects in vitro and in vivo. Recent reviews of studies with oral NAC in COPD suggest small but significant reductions in exacerbations (31, 32). More effective antioxidants, including stable glutathione compounds and selenium-based drugs, are now in development for clinical use (33). Spin-trap antioxidants, such as α-phenyl-*N*-tert-butyl nitrone, are much more potent and inhibit the formation of intracellular reactive oxygen species by forming stable compounds, but these drugs have toxicity that may preclude clinical development. Further studies are now indicated on the use of antioxidants to treat and prevent acute exacerbations, using more potent antioxidants or giving existing antioxidants via the inhaled route.

IV. Causal Mechanisms

Although it was always assumed that bacterial infections accounted for most acute exacerbations of COPD, there is increasing evidence for an important role for virus infections and for noninfective causes (34, 35). Bacterial products, such as endotoxin and polyglycans, and virus infections, such as rhinovirus, activate NF-κB and thereby switch on an increase in the existing neutrophilic inflammatory response (36, 37). However, other transcription factors in addition to NF-κB are also involved in rhinovirus-induced increased transcription of inflammatory genes (38). What is not clear is whether there is any difference in the exacerbation activated by bacteria and virus infections, in terms of the nature of the inflammatory response. Antibiotics are commonly used to treat exacerbations, but are presumably only of benefit when exacerbations are due to bacterial infections. At the moment there is no easy way to distinguish between these infective causes, but future research may identify noninvasive markers that might differentiate between bacterial and viral infections, so that antibiotics may be used selectively in bacterial infections. Noninvasive markers may include the profile of inflammatory mediators, or protein products of specific bacteria detected by proteomics.

Some patients appear to suffer frequent exacerbations. While this is predicted to some extent by disease severity, there are clearly differences between patients of matching severity. The reasons for these differences are not yet understood, but may be genetically determined or may be related to colonization of the respiratory tract during the stable state. There is a relationship between the number of bacterial colonies and the intensity of the neutrophilic inflammatory response and concentrations of IL-8 and LTB$_4$ (39). Those patients with higher bacterial counts may be more susceptible to exacerbations as less increase is required to initiate an exacerbation.

The infecting bacteria may also determine the nature of the exacerbation. There is some evidence that *Pseudomonas* and *Enterococci* are more common in exacerbations of patients with severe disease (FEV$_1$ < 35% predicted) (40, 41). The pathogen may influence the nature of the inflammatory response. For example, acute exacerbations associated with *Haemophilus influenzae* was associated with higher concentrations of IL-8, TNF-α and neutrophil elastase in sputum compared to infection with *H. parainfluenzae* (42). Further studies are needed relating different infections agents and bacterial load to the inflammatory response in acute exacerbations.

V. Extrapulmonary Effects

Extrapulmonary manifestations are an important feature of severe COPD and become prominent during exacerbations (43). These systemic features appear to reflect the inflammatory process and are mediated by cytokines, such as TNF-α. During exacerbations of COPD there are increases in plasma ET-1, IL-6, and fibrinogen (17, 35, 44). Recently increases in plasma leptin concentrations have been linked to the increased systemic inflammatory response during acute exacerbations (45). This may contribute to the energy imbalance and weight loss associated with exacerbations. More research is needed to understand the role of inflammatory mediators in producing systemic features such as muscle wasting, weight loss, fatigue, and depression that result in severe impairment in the quality of life. Exacerbations in COPD have a profound and long-lasting influence on health status (30), but more research is needed to identify the molecular mechanisms of these effects and to understand their prolonged course. The prolonged course over several weeks outlasts any infective process and suggests that the infection initiates a sequence of inflammatory events that are self-perpetuating. The mechanisms for these prolonged effects need to be dissected so that effective treatments can be instituted. TNF-α is a very good target for inhibition and it is likely that TNF inhibitors may have a beneficial effect on the extrapulmonary effects of an exacerbation.

Humanized monoclonal TNF antibodies (such as infliximab) and soluble TNF receptors (etanercept) that are effective in other chronic inflammatory diseases, such as rheumatoid arthritis and inflammatory bowel disease (46, 47). There may be problems with long-term administration because of the development of blocking antibodies and repeated injections are inconvenient. TNF-α converting enzyme (TACE), which is required for the release of soluble TNF-α, may be a more attractive target as it is possible to discover small molecule TACE inhibitors, some of which are also matrix metalloproteinase inhibitors (48, 49). General anti-inflammatory drugs such as phosphodiesterase-4 inhibitors and p38 MAP kinase inhibitors also potently inhibit TNF-α expression.

VI. Corticosteroids

Because there is chronic inflammation in COPD airways it was argued that inhaled corticosteroids might be useful in treatment and in particular may prevent the progression of the disease. However, four large 3-year controlled trials of inhaled corticosteroids have demonstrated no reduction in disease progression (50–53). This might be predicted by the demonstration that neither inhaled nor oral corticosteroids have any significant effect on neutrophil counts, granule proteins, inflammatory or proteases in induced sputum (54–56). Inhaled corticosteroids do not inhibit neutrophilic inflammation induced by ozone in humans (57) and this may reflect that corticosteroids prolong neutrophil survival (58). There may also be an active resistance to corticosteroids due to an inhibitory effect of cigarette smoke on histone deacetylation, which is required for corticosteroids to switch off inflammatory genes (59). Although inhaled corticosteroids do not prevent progression of COPD or reduce the inflammatory response, they may reduce the number of exacerbations in patients with severe disease (52, 60). However, this is a very small effect that is less than seen with bronchodilators alone.

In contrast to the trivial effect of inhaled corticosteroids in preventing exacerbations, systemic corticosteroids appear to have some beneficial role in the treatment of acute exacerbations of COPD (61, 62). The reasons for the greater efficacy of corticosteroids during an acute exacerbation compared to the chronic stable state suggests that they may be acting on some component of the disease that is different in acute exacerbations. This might be airway edema or an eosinophilic infiltration that has been described during acute exacerbations (6, 63). More research is needed to identify which components of the acute exacerbation respond to corticosteroids, using noninvasive techniques, such as induced sputum or exhaled breath markers.

VII. Novel Therapies

There is a pressing need to develop new therapies for COPD and particularly drugs that may reduce the chronic inflammatory process. It is likely that suppression of the inflammatory process would not only reduce the relentless progression of the disease, but would also prevent exacerbations and be useful in the management of acute exacerbations. The inflammation of COPD is largely corticosteroid-resistant and therefore there is a need to develop novel anti-inflammatory treatments or to find drugs that can unlock the resistance to steroids. Several novel types of anti-inflammatory drug are now in development for COPD and these drugs are predicted to reduce the frequency, severity or duration of acute exacerbations (9, 64). These drugs include antagonists of LTB_4 and the CXCR2 receptor for chemokines, such as IL-8, which should inhibit neutrophilic inflammation, and inhibitors of TNF-α. As discussed above, antioxidants have already been shown to reduce acute exacerbation of COPD and in the future more effective antioxidants may be introduced. Anti-inflammatory drugs with a broader spectrum of action include inhibitors of phosphodiesterase-4 (PDE4), p38 MAP kinase inhibitors and NF-κB inhibitors. So far, only PDE-4 inhibitors have been tested in clinical trial in COPD. PDE4 is the predominant PDE expressed in neutrophils, $CD8^+$ cells and macrophages (65), suggesting that PDE4 inhibitors would be effective in controlling inflammation in COPD. Selective PDE4 inhibitors, such as cilomilast and roflumilast, are active in animal models of neutrophil inflammation (66, 67). Cilomilast has some beneficial clinical effect in improving lung function and symptoms in COPD patients (68). Larger studies over 6 months also show a beneficial effect of cilomilast, including a reduction in exacerbations (69). Thus, over 6 months there was an almost 50% reduction in hospitalizations. PDE4 inhibitors are limited by side effects, particularly nausea and other gastrointestinal effects, but it might be possible to develop isoenzyme subtype selective inhibitors in the future which are less likely to be dose-limited by adverse effects in the future.

VIII. Future Research

Although acute exacerbations have a major impact on patients with COPD and account for a large proportion of associated health care costs, there is relatively little research into underlying mechanisms. This is partly because of the difficulties in studying patients who are acutely ill. It is likely that the enormous developments in noninvasive exhaled markers of inflammation and oxidative stress will provide important new insights into the inflammatory mechanisms involved in different types of acute exacerbation (15). Because these measurements are entirely non-invasive and may be performed repeatedly even in patients who are severely ill, it is possible to study the kinetics of the acute exacerbations and also the effects of various therapeutic interventions. This should provide information about the involvement of specific mediators in exacerbations and may enable a distinction to be made between causal mechanisms. Future research should also identify factors that are predictive for patients who have frequent exacerbations. Current studies suggest that higher concentrations of IL-6 and IL-8 and lower concentrations of secretory leukoprotease inhibitor (SLPI) in sputum are found in patients with more frequent exacerbations (> 3/year), suggesting that these features may be predictive (12, 70). Genetic factors may play a role in predisposing toward COPD in cigarette smokers, but they may also determine susceptibility to exacerbations (71, 72). Powerful techniques, including high-density DNA arrays (gene chips), are able to identify multiple polymorphisms, differential display may identify the expression of novel genes and proteomics of novel proteins expressed.

References

1. Barnes PJ. Chronic obstructive pulmonary disease. New Engl J Med 2000; 343:269–280.
2. Keatings VM, Collins PD, Scott DM, Barnes PJ. Differences in interleukin-8 and tumor necrosis factor-α in induced sputum from patients with chronic obstructive pulmonary disease or asthma. Am J Respir Crit Care Med 1996; 153:530–534.
3. Jeffery PK. Structural and inflammatory changes in COPD: a comparison with asthma. Thorax 1998; 53:129–136.
4. Saetta M, Turato G, Maestrelli P, Mapp CE, Fabbri LM. Cellular and structural bases of chronic obstructive pulmonary disease. Am J Respir Crit Care Med 2001; 163:1304–1309.
5. Barnes PJ. Mechanisms in COPD: differences from asthma. Chest 2000; 117:10S–14S.

6. Saetta M, Di Stefano A, Maestrelli P, Turato G, Mapp CE, Pieno M, Zanguochi G, Del Prete G, Fabbri LM. Airway eosinophilia and expression of interleukin-5 protein in asthma and in exacerbations of chronic bronchitis [see comments]. Clin Exp Allergy 1996; 26:766–774.

7. Fabbri L, Beghe B, Caramori G, Papi A, Saetta M. Similarities and discrepancies between exacerbations of asthma and chronic obstructive pulmonary disease. Thorax 1998; 53:803–808.

8. Balbi B, Bason C, Balleari E, Fiasella F, Pesci A, Ghio R, Fabiano F. Increased bronchoalveolar granulocytes and granulocyte/macrophage colony-stimulating factor during exacerbations of chronic bronchitis. Eur Respir J 1997; 10:846–850.

9. Barnes PJ. New treatments for chronic obstructive pulmonary disease. Curr Opin Pharmacol 2001; 1:217–222.

10. Yamamoto C, Yoneda T, Yoshikawa M, Fu A, Tokuyama T, Tsukaguchi K, Narita N. Airway inflammation in COPD assessed by sputum levels of interleukin-8. Chest 1997; 112:505–510.

11. Hill AT, Bayley D, Stockle RA. The interrelationship of sputum inflammatory markers in patients with chronic bronchitis. Am J Respir Crit Care Med 1999; 160:893–898.

12. Bhowmik A, Seemungal TA, Sapsford RJ, Wedzicha JA. Relation of sputum inflammatory markers to symptoms and lung function changes in COPD exacerbations. Thorax 2000; 55:114–120.

13. Aaron SD, Angel JB, Lunau M, Wright K, Fex C, Le Saux N, Dales RE. Granulocyte inflammatory markers and airway infection during acute exacerbation of chronic obstructive pulmonary disease. Am J Respir Crit Care Med 2001; 163:349–355.

14. Crooks SW, Bayley DL, Hill SL, Stockley RA. Bronchial inflammation in acute bacterial exacerbations of chronic bronchitis: the role of leukotriene B_4. Eur Respir J 2000; 15:274–280.

15. Kharitonov SA, Barnes PJ. Exhaled markers of pulmonary disease. Am J Respir Crit Care Med 2001; 163:1693–1772.

16. Biernacki W, Kharitonov SA, Barnes PJ. Leukotriene B_4 in exhaled breath condensate of patients with exacerbations of COPD. Am J Respir Crit Care Med 2002:165.

17. Roland M, Bhowmik A, Saps ford RJ, Seemungal TA, Jeffries DJ, Warner TD, Wedzicha JA. Sputum and plasma endothelin-1 levels in exacerbations of chronic obstructive pulmonary disease. Thorax 2001; 56:30–35.

18. Barnes PJ, Adcock IM. Transcription factors and asthma. Eur Respir J 1998; 12: 221–234.

19. Caramori G, Romagnoli M, Casolari P, Bellettato C, Casoni G, Boschetto P, Fan Chung K, Barnes PK, Adcock IM, Ciaccia A, Fabbri LM, Papi A. Nuclear localisation of p65 in sputum macrophages but not in sputum neutrophils during COPD exacerbations. Thorax 2003; 58:348–351.

20. Barnes PJ, Karin M. Nuclear factor-κB: a pivotal transcription factor in chronic inflammatory diseases. New Engl J Med 1997; 336:1066–1071.

21. Karin M, Ben-Neriah Y. Phosphorylation meets ubiquitination: the control of NF-κB activity. Annu Rev Immunol 2000; 18:621–663.

22. Delhase M, Li N, Karin M. Kinase regulation in inflammatory response. Nature 2000; 406:367–368.

23. Nasuhara Y, Adcock IM, Catley M, Barnes PJ, Newton R. Differential IKK activation and IκBα degradation by interleukin-1β and tumor necrosis factor-α in human U937 monocytic cells: evidence for additional regulatory steps in κB-dependent transcription. J Biol Chem 1999; 274:19965–19972.

24. Macnee W. Oxidants/Antioxidants and COPD. Chest 2000; 117:303S–317S.
25. Dekhuijzen PNR, Aben KHH, Dekker I, Aarts LPHJ, Wielders PLM, van Herwarden CLA, Bast A. Increased exhalation of hydrogen peroxide in patients with stable and unstable chronic obstructive pulmonary disease. Am J Respir Crit Care Med 1996; 154:813–816.
26. Morrow JD, Roberts LJ. The isoprostanes. Current knowledge and directions for future research. Biochem Pharmacol 1996; 51:1–9.
27. Montuschi P, Collins JV, Ciabattoni G, Lazzeri N, Corradi M, Kharitonov SA, Barnes PJ. Exhaled 8-isoprostane as an *in vivo* biomarker of lung oxidative stress in patients with COPD and healthy smokers. Am J Respir Crit Care Med 2000; 162:1175–1177.
28. Biernacki W, Kharitonov SA, Barnes PJ. 8-Isoprostane in exhaled condensate in patients with exacerbations of COPD. Am J Respir Crit Care Med 2002:165.
29. Paredi P, Kharitonov SA, Leak D, Ward S, Cramer D, Barnes PJ. Exhaled ethane, a marker of lipid peroxidation, is elevated in chronic obstructive pulmonary disease. Am J Respir Crit Care Med 2000; 162:369–373.
30. Seemungal TA, Donaldson GC, Paul EA, Bestall JC, Jeffries DJ, Wedzicha JA. Effect of exacerbation on quality of life in patients with chronic obstructive pulmonary disease. Am Respir Crit Care Med 1998; 157:1418–1422.
31. Grandjean EM, Berthet P, Ruffmann R, Leuenberger P. Efficacy of oral long-term N-acetylcysteine in chronic bronchopulmonary disease: a meta-analysis of published double-blind, placebo-controlled clinical trials. Clin Ther 2000; 22:209–221.
32. Poole PJ, Black PN. Oral mucolytic drugs for exacerbations of chronic obstructive pulmonary disease: systematic review. Br Med J 2001; 322:1271–1274.
33. Cuzzocrea S, Riley DP, Caputi AP, Salvemini D. Antioxidant therapy: a new Pharmacological approach in shock, inflammation, and ischemia/reperfusion injury. Pharmacol Rev 2001; 53:135–159.
34. Seemungal T, Harper-Owen R, Bhowmik A, Jeffries DJ, Wedzicha JA. Detection of rhinoviruses in induced sputum at exacerbations of chronic obstructive pulmonary disease. Eur Respir J 2000; 16:677–683.
35. Seemungal T, Harper-Owen R, Bhowmik A, Moric I, Sanderson G, Message S, Maccallum P, Meade TW, Jeffries DJ, Johnston SL, Wedzicha JA. Respiratory viruses, symptoms, and inflammatory markers in acute exacerbations and stable chronic obstructive pulmonary disease. Am J Respir Crit Care Med 2001; 164:1618–1623.
36. Zhu Z, Tang W, Ray A, Wu Y, Einarsson O, Landry ML, Gwaltney J, Elias JA. Rhinovirus stimulation of interleukin-6 in vivo and in vitro. Evidence for nuclear factor κB-dependent transcription activation. J Clin Invest 1996; 97:421–430.
37. Xu Z, Dziarski R, Wang Q, Swartz K, Sakamoto KM, Gupta D. Bacterial peptidoglycan-induced TNF-α transcription is mediated through the transcription factors Egr-1, Elk-1, and NF-κB. J Immunol 2001; 167:6975–6982.
38. Kim J, Sanders SP, Siekierski ES, Casolaro V, Proud D. Role of NF-κB in cytokine production induced from human airway epithelial cells by rhinovirus infection. J Immunol 2000; 165:3384–3392.
39. Hill AT, Campbell EJ, Hill SL, Bayley DL, Stockley RA. Association between airway bacterial load and markers of airway inflammation in patients with stable chronic bronchitis. Am J Med 2000; 109:288–295.
40. Eller J, Ede A, Schaberg T, Niederman MS, Mauch H, Lode H. Infective exacerbations of chronic bronchitis: relation between bacteriologic etiology and lung function. Chest 1998; 113:1542–1548.

41. Miravitlles M, Espinosa C, Fernandez-Laso E, Martos JA, Maldonado D, Gallego M. Relationship between bacterial flora in sputum and functional impairment in patients with acute exacerbations of COPD. Chest 1999; 116:40–46.
42. Sethi S, Muscarella K, Evans N, Klingman KL, Grant BJ, Murphy TF. Airway inflammation and etiology of acute exacerbations of chronic bronchitis. Chest 2000; 118:1557–1565.
43. Schols AM, Buurman WA, Staal van den Brekel AJ, Dentener MA, Wouters EF. Evidence for a relation between metabolic derangements and increased levels of inflammatory mediators in a subgroup of patients with chronic obstructive pulmonary disease. Thorax 1996; 51:819–824.
44. Wedzicha JA, Seemungal TA, MacCallum PK, Paul EA, Donaldson GC, Bhowmik A, Jeffries DJ, Meade TW. Acute exacerbations of chronic obstructive pulmonary disease are accompanied by elevations of plasma fibrinogen and serum IL-6 levels. Thromb Haemost 2000; 84:210–215.
45. Creutzberg EC, Wouters EF, Vanderhoven-Augustin IM, Dentener MA, Schols AM. Disturbances in leptin metabolism are related to energy imbalance during acute exacerbations of chronic obstructive pulmonary disease. Am J Respir Crit Care Med 2000; 162:1239–1245.
46. Markham A, Lamb HM. Infliximab: a review of its use in the management of rheumatoid arthritis. Drugs 2000; 59:1341–1359.
47. Jarvis B, Faulds D. Etanercept: a review of its use in rheumatoid arthritis. Drugs 1999; 57:945–966.
48. Barlaam B, Bird TG, Lambert-Van DB, Campbell D, Foster SJ, Maciewicz R. New alpha-substituted succinate-based hydroxamic acids as TNF-α convertase inhibitors. J Med Chem 1999; 42:4890–4908.
49. Rabinowitz MH, Andrews RC, Becherer JD, Bickett DM, Bubacz DG, Conway JG, Cowan DJ, Gaul M, Glennon K, Lambert MH, Leesnitzer MA, McDougald DL, Moss ML, Musso DL, Rizzolio MC. Design of selective and soluble inhibitors of tumor necrosis factor-alpha converting enzyme (TACE). J Med Chem 2001; 44:4252–4267.
50. Vestbo J, Sorensen T, Lange P, Brix A, Torre P, Viskum K. Long-term effect of inhaled budesonide in mild and moderate chronic obstructive pulmonary disease: a randomised controlled trial. Lancet 1999; 353:1819–1823.
51. Pauwels RA, Lofdahl CG, Laitinen LA, Schouten JP, Postma DS, Pride NB, Ohlsson SV. Long-term treatment with inhaled budesonide in persons with mild chronic obstructive pulmonary disease who continue smoking. N Engl J Med 1999; 340:1948–1953.
52. Burge PS, Calverley PMA, Jones PW, Spencer S, Anderson JA, Maslen T. Randomised, double-blind, placebo-controlled study of fluticasone propionate in patients with moderate to severe chronic obstructive pulmonary disease; the ISOLDE trial. Br Med J 2000; 320:1297–1303.
53. Lung Health Study Research Group. Effect of inhaled triamcinolone on the decline in pulmonary function in chronic obstructive pulmonary disease. N Engl J Med 2000; 343:1902–1909.
54. Barnes PJ. Inhaled corticosteroids are not helpful in chronic obstructive pulmonary disease. Am J Respir Crit Care Med 2000; 161:342–344.
55. Keatings VM, Jatakanon A, Worsdell YM, Barnes PJ. Effects of inhaled and oral glucocorticoids on inflammatory indices in asthma and COPD. Am J Respir Crit Care Med 1997; 155:542–548.
56. Culpitt SV, Nightingale JA, Barnes PJ. Effect of high dose inhaled steroid on cells, cytokines and proteases in induced sputum in chronic obstructive pulmonary disease. Am J Respir Crit Care Med 1999; 160:1635–1639.

57. Nightingale JA, Rogers DF, Chung KF, Barnes PJ. No effect of inhaled budesonide on the response to inhaled ozone in normal subjects. Am J Respir Crit Care Med 2000; 161:479–486.

58. Meagher LC, Cousin JM, Secki JR, Haslett C. Opposing effects of glucocorticoids on the rate of apoptosis in neutrophilic and eosinophilic granulocytes. J Immunol 1996; 156:4422–4428.

59. Ito K, Lim S, Caramori G, Chung KF, Barnes PJ, Adcock IM. Cigarette smoking reduces histone deacetylase 2 expression, enhances cytokine expression and inhibits glucocorticoid actions in alveolar macrophages. FASEB J 2001; 15:1100–1102.

60. Paggiaro PL, Dahle R, Bakran I, Frith L, Hollingworth K, Efthimou J. Multicentre randomised placebo-controlled trial of inhaled fluticasone propionate in patients with chronic obstructive pulmonary disease. Lancet 1998; 351:773–780.

61. Davies L, Angus RM, Calverley PM. Oral corticosteroids in patients admitted to hospital with exacerbations of chronic obstructive pulmonary disease: a prospective randomised controlled trial. Lancet 1999; 354:456–460.

62. Niewoehner PE, Erbland ML, Deupree RH, Collins D, Gross NJ, Light RW, Anderson P, Morgan NA. Effect of systemic glucocorticoids on exacerbations of chronic obstructive pulmonary disease. N Engl J Med 1999; 340:1941–1947.

63. Saetta M, Distefano A, Maestrelli P, Graziella T, Rugieri MP, Roggeri A, Calcagni P, Mapp CE, Ciaccia A, Fabbri LM. Airway eosinophilia in chronic bronchitis during exacerbations. Am J Resp Crit Care Med 1994; 150:1646–1652.

64. Barnes PJ. Future Advances in COPD Therapy. Respiration 2001; 68:441–448.

65. Souness JE, Aldous D, Sargent C. Immunosuppressive and anti-inflammatory effects of cyclic AMP phosphodiesterase (PDE) type 4 inhibitors. Immunopharmacology 2000; 47:127–162.

66. Spond J, Chapman R, Fine J, Jones H, Kreutner W, Kung TT, Minnicozzi M. Comparison of PDE4 inhibitors, rolipram and SB 207499 (Ariflo), in a rat model of pulmonary neutrophilia. Pulm Pharmacol Ther 2001; 14:157–164.

67. Bundschuh DS, Eltze M, Barsig J, Wollin L, Hatzelmann A, Beume R. In vivo efficacy in airway disease models of roflumilast, a novel orally active PDE4 inhibitor. J Pharmacol Exp Ther 2001; 297:280–290.

68. Compton CH, Gubb J, Nieman R, Edelson J, Amit O, Bakst A, Ayres JG, Creemers JP, Schultze-Werninghaus G, Brambilla C, Barnes NC. Cilomilast, a selective phosphodiesterase-4 inhibitor for treatment of patients with chronic obstructive pulmonary disease: a randomised, dose-ranging study. Lancet 2001; 358:265–270.

69. Edelson J, Compton CH, Nieman R, Robinson CB, Amit O, Bagchi I. Cilomilast (Ariflo) a potent, selective phosphodiesterase 4 inhibitor, reduces exacerbations in COPD patients: results of a 6-month trial. Am J Respir Crit Care Med 2001; 163:A771.

70. Gompertz S, Bayley DL, Hill SL, Stockley RA. Relationship between airway inflammation and the frequency of exacerbations in patients with smoking related COPD. Thorax 2001; 56:36–41.

71. Barnes PJ. Molecular genetics of chronic obstructive pulmonary disease. Thorax 1999; 54:245–252.

72. Sandiford AJ, Weir TD, Pare PD. Genetic risk factors for chronic obstructive pulmonary disease. Eur Respir J 1997; 10:1380–1391.

Index